AAOS
AMERICAN ACADEMY OF ORTHOPAEDIC SURGEONS

ECSI
EMERGENCY CARE
& SAFETY INSTITUTE

# First Aid, CPR, and AED Advanced

**Seventh Edition**

## Alton L. Thygerson, EdD, FAWM
Medical Writer

## Steven M. Thygerson, PhD, MSPH
Medical Writer

## Benjamin Gulli, MD, FAAOS
Medical Editor

## Howard K. Mell, MD, MPH, FACEP
Medical Editor

## Bob Elling, MPA, EMT-P
Series Editor

American College of
Emergency Physicians®
ADVANCING EMERGENCY CARE

JONES & BARTLETT
LEARNING

**World Headquarters**
Jones & Bartlett Learning
5 Wall Street
Burlington, MA 01803
978-443-5000
info@jblearning.com
www.jblearning.com

Substantial discounts on bulk quantities of Jones & Bartlett Learning publications are available to corporations, professional associations, and other qualified organizations. For details and specific discount information, contact the special sales department at Jones & Bartlett Learning via the above contact information or send an email to specialsales@jblearning.com.

Jones & Bartlett Learning books and products are available through most bookstores and online booksellers. To contact Jones & Bartlett Learning directly, call 800-832-0034, fax 978-443-8000, or visit our website, www.jblearning.com.

**Production Credits**
General Manager, Executive Publisher: Kimberly Brophy
VP, Product Development and Executive Editor: Christine Emerton
Acquisitions Editor: Tiffany Sliter
Development Editor: Carly Mahoney
Senior Production Editor: Jessica deMartin
VP, Sales, Public Safety Group: Matt Maniscalco
Director of Sales, Public Safety Group: Patricia Einstein
Marketing Manager: Jessica Carmichael

VP, Manufacturing and Inventory Control: Therese Connell
Composition: diacriTech
Cover Design: Kristin E. Parker
Rights & Media Specialist: Robert Boder
Media Development Editor: Shannon Sheehan
Cover Image: © SeanShot/iStock/Getty; Science Photo Library/Getty; pixelaway/Shutterstock
Printing and Binding: LSC Communications
Cover Printing: LSC Communications

**Library of Congress Cataloging-in-Publication Data**
Names: Thygerson, Alton L., author. | Thygerson, Steven M., author.
Title: First aid, CPR, and AED. Advanced / Alton L. Thygerson, Steven M. Thygerson.
Description: Seventh edition. | Burlington, MA : Jones & Bartlett Learning, [2017] | Includes index.
Identifiers: LCCN 2016004372 | ISBN 9781284105315
Subjects: | MESH: First Aid | Emergencies | Cardiopulmonary Resuscitation | Electric Countershock
Classification: LCC RC86.7 | NLM WA 292 | DDC 616.02/52—dc23
LC record available at http://lccn.loc.gov/2016004372

6048

Printed in the United States of America
20 19 18 17 16   10 9 8 7 6 5 4 3 2

# Content

# Flowcharts

# Skill Sheets

# Welcome

## Welcome to the Emergency Care & Safety Institute

Welcome to the Emergency Care & Safety Institute (ECSI), brought to you by the American Academy of Orthopaedic Surgeons (AAOS) and the American College of Emergency Physicians (ACEP).

ECSI is an internationally renowned organization that provides training and certifications that meet job-related requirements as defined by regulatory authorities such as Occupational Safety & Health Administration (OSHA), The Joint Commission, and state offices of Emergency Medical Services (EMS), Education, Transportation, and Health. Our courses are delivered throughout a range of industries and markets worldwide, including colleges and universities, business and industry, government, public safety agencies, hospitals, private training companies, and secondary school systems.

ECSI programs are offered in association with the AAOS and ACEP. AAOS, the world's largest medical association of musculoskeletal specialists, is known as the original name in EMS publishing with the very first EMS textbook in 1971, and ACEP is widely recognized as the leading name in all of emergency medicine.

## ECSI Course Catalog

Individuals seeking training from ECSI can choose from among various traditional classroom-based courses or alternative online courses such as:

- Advanced Cardiac Life Support (ACLS)
- Bloodborne and Airborne Pathogens
- Babysitter Safety
- CPR (layperson and health care provider levels)
- Emergency Medical Responder
- First Aid (multiple courses available), and more!

ECSI offers a wide range of textbooks, instructor and student support materials, and interactive technology, including eBooks and online courses. ECSI student manuals are the center of an integrated teaching and learning system that offers resources to better support instructors and train students. The instructor supplements provide practical hands-on, time-saving tools like PowerPoint presentations, skill demonstration videos, and web-based distance learning resources. Technology resources provide interactive exercises and simulations to help students become prepared for any emergency.

The ECSI website fully supports instructors by providing a course roster system for easy upload and management of student information. Digital course completion certificates and cards attesting to ECSI's recognitions of satisfactory course completion will be issued to those who successfully meet the course requirements. Instructors can distribute the completion certificates and cards to students via email or can print them out and issue on-site.

Visit www.ECSInstitute.org today!

# Background Information

## ▶ Why Is First Aid Important?

A large truck swings around a corner and crashes into an automobile, and pushes it over an embankment. Bystanders rush to the rescue. They extricate the injured driver of the car, lift him to his feet, stop a passing car, and send the injured man to a nearby hospital in a sitting position. Because of the lack of knowledge and unskilled handling, the man's spinal cord is injured by the sharp edge of a broken vertebra, and he will remain paralyzed for the rest of his life. This tragic outcome could have been avoided if someone had known what to do in an emergency.

A backcountry hiker is bitten by a rattlesnake. Her frantic companion cuts and sucks the bitten area, not realizing that this is an outdated and harmful procedure. By the time the woman seeks appropriate medical care, she has suffered extensive tissue damage. A trained first aid provider would have known the proper procedures to care for this person.

A group of beachgoers removes an unresponsive swimmer from the water. No one helps because no one knows cardiopulmonary resuscitation (CPR). The emergency medical services (EMS) ambulance arrives too late to revive the swimmer. CPR would have served as an interim action and preserved life for the few minutes needed until the ambulance arrived.

Late at night, a man who had earlier smashed a finger in a car door can no longer stand the excruciating pain caused by the pressure of blood accumulating underneath the fingernail. He drives himself to a hospital emergency department where a physician relieves a blood clot. The man later receives an expensive hospital bill. If he had known the proper first

## Chapter
### at a glance

▶ **Why Is First Aid Important?**

▶ **Who Needs First Aid?**

▶ **What Is First Aid?**

▶ **First Aid and the Law**

▶ **Injury Prevention**

aid procedure, he could have relieved the pain sooner and saved money.

These cases clearly point out the need for first aid training. *It is better to know it and not need it than to need it and not know it.* Everyone should be able to perform first aid, because most people will eventually find themselves in a situation requiring it for another person or for themselves. First aid providers do not diagnose (this is what physicians do), but they can suspect what the problem is and then give first aid.

## ▶ Who Needs First Aid?

Just as heart disease and cancer demand public attention because of the critical health risks they pose in the United States, injuries—both unintentional and intentional—must be recognized as a major threat to public health. This threat has been called the neglected epidemic. Table 1-1 shows the role of injury as a cause of death by age group and ranking compared with other causes of death.

Death statistics do not always reflect the extent or severity of the injury issue. Most injuries and sudden illnesses do not result in death, but rather result in hospitalization, treatment in an emergency department or from a general practitioner, or treatment from a first aid provider. According to the World Health Organization, in the world's high-income countries, for every person killed by injury, 30 people are hospitalized and 300 people are treated in emergency departments; even more are treated in other health care facilities and by first aid providers.

## Table 1-1 Ten Leading Causes of Death by Age Group, United States, 2014

| Rank | <1 | 1-4 | 5-9 | 10-14 | 15-24 | 25-34 | 35-44 | 45-54 | 55-64 | 65+ | Total |
|---|---|---|---|---|---|---|---|---|---|---|---|
| 1 | Congenital anomalies 4,746 | Unintentional injury 1,216 | Unintentional injury 730 | Unintentional injury 750 | Unintentional injury 11,836 | Unintentional injury 17,357 | Unintentional injury 16,048 | Malignant neoplasms 44,834 | Malignant neoplasms 115,282 | Heart disease 489,722 | Heart disease 614,348 |
| 2 | Short gestation 4,173 | Congenital anomalies 399 | Malignant neoplasms 436 | Suicide 425 | Suicide 5,079 | Suicide 6,569 | Malignant neoplasms 11,267 | Heart disease 34,791 | Heart disease 74,473 | Malignant neoplasms 413,885 | Malignant neoplasms 591,699 |
| 3 | Maternal pregnancy complications 1,574 | Homicide 364 | Congenital anomalies 192 | Malignant neoplasms 416 | Homicide 4,144 | Homicide 4,159 | Heart disease 10,368 | Unintentional injury 20,610 | Unintentional injury 18,030 | Chronic lower respiratory disease 124,693 | Chronic lower respiratory disease 147,101 |
| 4 | SIDS 1,545 | Malignant neoplasms 321 | Homicide 123 | Congenital anomalies 156 | Malignant neoplasms 1,569 | Malignant neoplasms 3,624 | Suicide 6,706 | Suicide 8,767 | Chronic lower respiratory disease 16,492 | Cerebro-vascular causes 113,308 | Unintentional injury 136,053 |
| 5 | Unintentional injury 1,161 | Heart disease 149 | Heart disease 69 | Homicide 156 | Heart disease 953 | Heart disease 3,341 | Homicide 2,588 | Liver disease 8,627 | Diabetes mellitus 13,342 | Alzheimer disease 92,604 | Cerebro-vascular causes 133,103 |
| 6 | Placenta cord membranes 965 | Influenza & pneumonia 109 | Chronic lower respiratory disease 68 | Heart disease 122 | Congenital anomalies 377 | Liver disease 725 | Liver disease 2,582 | Diabetes mellitus 6,062 | Liver disease 12,792 | Diabetes mellitus 54,161 | Alzheimer disease 93,541 |
| 7 | Bacterial sepsis 544 | Chronic lower respiratory disease 53 | Influenza & pneumonia 57 | Chronic lower respiratory disease 71 | Influenza & pneumonia 199 | Diabetes mellitus 709 | Diabetes mellitus 1,999 | Cerebro-vascular causes 5,349 | Cerebro-vascular causes 11,727 | Unintentional injury 48,295 | Diabetes mellitus 76,488 |
| 8 | Respiratory distress 460 | Septicemia 53 | Cerebro-vascular causes 45 | Cerebro-vascular causes 43 | Diabetes mellitus 181 | HIV 583 | Cerebro-vascular causes 1,745 | Chronic lower respiratory disease 4,402 | Suicide 7,527 | Influenza & pneumonia 44,836 | Influenza & pneumonia 55,227 |
| 9 | Circulatory system disease 444 | Benign neoplasms 38 | Benign neoplasms 36 | Influenza & pneumonia 41 | Chronic lower respiratory disease 178 | Cerebro-vascular causes 579 | HIV 1,174 | Influenza & pneumonia 2,731 | Septicemia 5,709 | Nephritis 39,957 | Nephritis 48,146 |
| 10 | Neonatal hemorrhage 441 | Perinatal period 38 | Septicemia 33 | Benign neoplasms 38 | Cerebro-vascular causes 177 | Influenza & pneumonia 549 | Influenza & pneumonia 1,125 | Septicemia 2,514 | Influenza & pneumonia 5,390 | Septicemia 29,124 | Suicide 42,773 |

*Data Source:* National Vital Statistics System, National Center for Health Statistics, CDC.

Produced by: National Center for injury Prevention and Control, CDC using WISQARS™.

**OSHA Regulations**

(Standards-29 CFR 1910.151) Medical Services and First Aid—General Industry:

"In the absence of an infirmary, clinic, or hospital in near proximity to workplace which is used for the treatment of all injured employees, a person or persons shall be adequately trained to render first aid. Adequate first aid supplies shall be readily available."

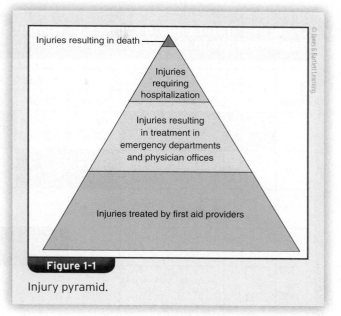

Injuries resulting in death

Injuries requiring hospitalization

Injuries resulting in treatment in emergency departments and physician offices

Injuries treated by first aid providers

**Figure 1-1**

Injury pyramid.

The injury pyramid, as shown in **Figure 1-1**, helps illustrate the distribution of injury severity. The top of the pyramid is composed of deaths caused by injury. Although deaths from injury are fewer in number than other types of injuries, they are more visible because they are considered newsworthy and often appear on television and in newspapers. The second category is composed of severe injuries that result in hospitalization and disability. Severe injuries are followed on the pyramid by less-severe injuries, those that require emergency department care, and those that are treated in basic health care facilities. Finally, at the bottom of the pyramid are injuries that do not require medical care and that are instead treated by a first aid provider.

**Table 1-2** shows the leading causes of nonfatal injuries treated at hospital emergency departments by age group in the United States. Each year, one in four people experiences a nonfatal injury serious enough to need medical care or to restrict activity for at least 1 day. More sports-related nonfatal injuries are treated in hospital emergency departments than any other type of unintentional injury.

Death occurs when a person's heart stops. Therefore, what a bystander does can mean the difference between life and death. Fortunately, most injuries and sudden illnesses do not require lifesaving efforts. During their entire lifetimes, most people will rarely, if ever, see a life-threatening condition outside of a medical facility. Saving lives is important, but first aid providers are more frequently called upon to provide initial care for less-severe conditions. If not properly treated, these less-severe injuries can evolve into something more serious. As such, these skills demand attention during first aid training.

Each year, the injuries of millions of Americans go unreported. For many of these people, the injury causes temporary pain and inconvenience; for others, however, the injury leads to disability, chronic pain, and a profound change in lifestyle. Given the size of the injury and sudden illness issue, everyone should be prepared to deal with an emergency.

## Value of First Aid to Self

Although many people learn first aid to help others, the training primarily helps oneself. It enables a person to give proper immediate care to one's own injuries and sudden illnesses. If people are too seriously injured to help themselves, they could be able to direct others in proper care. First aid training also helps develop safety awareness. Discussing injuries teaches people how injuries occur and thus promotes injury prevention.

## Value of First Aid to Others

People with first aid training are more likely to give proper assistance to injured family members. Although the main beneficiaries are the trained person and his or her family, the benefits of knowing appropriate first aid techniques extend further, usually to coworkers, acquaintances, and strangers.

## Value of First Aid in Remote Areas

Should an injury or sudden illness require medical care, time, distance, and availability are major considerations. EMS can reach most people who are severely injured or suddenly ill within 10 to 20 minutes. However, some

**Table 1-2  Ten Leading Causes of Nonfatal Injuries Treated in Hospital Emergency Departments in the United States, 2013**

| Rank | <1 | 1-4 | 5-9 | 10-14 | 15-24 | 25-34 | 35-44 | 45-54 | 55-64 | 65+ | Total |
|---|---|---|---|---|---|---|---|---|---|---|---|
| 1 | Fall 134,229 | Fall 852,884 | Fall 624,890 | Struck by/against 561,690 | Struck by/against 905,659 | Fall 742,177 | Fall 704,264 | Fall 913,871 | Fall 930,521 | Fall 2,495,397 | Fall 8,771,656 |
| 2 | Struck by/against 28,786 | Struck by/against 336,917 | Struck by/against 403,522 | Fall 558,177 | Fall 814,829 | Overexertion 638,745 | Overexertion 530,422 | Overexertion 461,114 | Struck by/against 266,126 | Struck by/against 281,279 | Struck by/against 4,214,125 |
| 3 | Other bite/sting 12,186 | Other bite/sting 158,587 | Cut/pierce 112,633 | Overexertion 294,669 | Overexertion 672,946 | Struck by/against 599,340 | Struck by/against 444,089 | Struck by/against 390,931 | Struck by/against 261,840 | Overexertion 212,293 | Overexertion 3,256,567 |
| 4 | Foreign body 10,650 | Foreign body 139,597 | Other bite/sting 107,975 | Cut/pierce 114,285 | MV-occupant 627,565 | MV-occupant 526,303 | MV-occupant 374,231 | Other specified 385,221 | MV-occupant 227,620 | MV-occupant 197,646 | MV-occupant 2,462,684 |
| 5 | Other specified 10,511 | Cut/pierce 83,575 | Overexertion 93,612 | Pedal cyclist 84,732 | Cut/pierce 431,691 | Cut/pierce 402,197 | Other specified 300,154 | MV-occupant 343,470 | Other specified 212,168 | Cut/pierce 156,693 | Cut/pierce 2,077,775 |
| 6 | Fire/burn 9,816 | Overexertion 81,588 | Pedal cyclist 74,831 | Unknown/unspecified 84,668 | Other assault, struck by/against 381,522 | Other assault, struck by/against 342,514 | Cut/pierce 297,769 | Cut/pierce 282,353 | Cut/pierce 189,440 | Poisoning 100,988 | Other specified 1,767,630 |
| 7 | Inhalation/suffocation 8,294 | Other specified 65,120 | Foreign body 63,450 | MV-occupant 73,692 | Other specified 321,914 | Other specified 336,990 | Other assault, struck by/against 207,287 | Poisoning 237,328 | Poisoning 153,767 | Other bite/sting 90,850 | Other assault, struck by/against 1,291,100 |
| 8 | Cut/pierce 7,139 | Fire/burn 52,884 | MV-occupant 58,114 | Other bite/sting 64,848 | Other bite/sting 177,665 | Other bite/sting 180,448 | Poisoning 175,870 | Other assault, struck by/against 169,688 | Other bite/sting 97,474 | Other specified 86,729 | Other bite/sting 1,174,267 |
| 9 | Unknown/unspecified 5,735 | Unknown/unspecified 41,297 | Dog bite 43,499 | Other assault, struck by/against 62,829 | Unknown/unspecified 163,923 | Poisoning 180,448 | Other bite/sting 138,410 | Other bite/sting 145,349 | Other assault, struck by/against 73,674 | Unknown/unspecified 74,864 | Poisoning 1,055,960 |
| 10 | Overexertion 4,985 | Poisoning 32,443 | Unknown/unspecified 35,303 | Other transport 35,609 | Poisoning 152,962 | Unknown/unspecified 129,308 | Unknown/unspecified 106,498 | Unknown/unspecified 110,102 | Unknown/unspecified 67,974 | Other transport 68,022 | Unknown/unspecified 819,878 |

\* With the exception of the "Other assault" category, all causes of injury in this table are unintentional.

MV = motor vehicle.

*Source:* Office of Statistics and Programming, National Center for Injury Prevention and Control, CDC.

people are long distances from medical care. Although most people associate long distances and lack of medical care with wilderness settings involving outdoor recreational activities (eg, hiking, camping, hunting, and snowmobiling), other settings also demand that people be prepared to give first aid for an extended time. The following are some examples:

- Urban areas after a disaster that destroys or overwhelms EMS
- Remote areas relating to one's occupation (eg, farming, ranching, commercial fishing, and forestry)
- Remote communities
- Developing countries

First aid needed in remote locations is similar to that needed in urban settings, but extra skills are sometimes required. See Chapter 24, *Wilderness First Aid*, for information on delivering first aid in remote locations.

## ▶ What Is First Aid?

In the latest International Liaison Committee on Resuscitation (ILCOR) guidelines, the First Aid Task Force defines **first aid** as the helping behaviors and initial care provided for an acute illness or injury. According to the guidelines, the goals of the first aid provider include "preserving life, alleviating suffering, preventing further illness or injury, and promoting recovery." First aid, which includes self-care, can be initiated by anyone in any situation but should be based on medical and scientific evidence or expert consensus. First aid competencies include:

- Recognizing, assessing, and prioritizing the need for first aid
- Providing care by using appropriate knowledge, skills, and behaviors
- Recognizing limitations and seeking additional care when needed

First aid does not take the place of proper medical care. However, in many cases, medical care is unnecessary and the ill or injured person will safely recover.

## Q&A

**What level of care am I expected to give?**

The level of care required of a provider is referred to as the **standard of care**. A first aid provider cannot provide the same level of care as a physician or an emergency medical technician. When you are providing first aid, you must do the following to meet the standard of care: (1) do what is expected of someone with first aid training and experience working under similar conditions and (2) treat the person to the best of your ability. If the first aid you provide is not up to the expected standard, you may be held liable for your actions.

## ▶ First Aid and the Law

Legal and ethical issues concern all first aid providers. For example, are you required to stop and give care at an automobile crash? Are you allowed to treat a child with a broken arm even when the parents cannot be contacted for their consent? These and many other legal and ethical questions confront first aid providers.

A first aid provider can be sued. However, do not become overly concerned about being sued; it rarely happens. Ways to minimize the risk of a lawsuit include the following:

- Obtain the person's consent before touching him or her.
- Follow this text's guidelines and do not exceed your training level.
- Explain any first aid you are about to give.
- Once you have started to care for a person, stay with that person. You are legally bound

to remain with the person until care is turned over to an equally or better trained person.

## Consent

A first aid provider must have the person's **consent** (permission) before giving first aid. Touching another person without his or her consent (which is known as **battery**) is unlawful and could be grounds for a lawsuit. Likewise, giving first aid without the person's consent is unlawful.

### Informed (Expressed) Consent

Consent must be obtained from every alert, mentally competent (able to make a rational decision) person of legal age. Tell the person that you have first aid training and explain what you will be doing. The person may give permission verbally or with a nod of the head, which would indicate **expressed consent**.

### Implied Consent

**Implied consent** involves an unresponsive person with a life-threatening condition. It is assumed or implied that an unresponsive person would consent to lifesaving interventions. An alert person who does not resist the administrations of a first aid provider is also assumed to have given implied consent.

### Children and Incompetent Adults

Consent must be obtained from the parent or guardian of a child, as legally defined by the state. In some states, a minor can give consent to receive medical care, depending on the minor's age and maturity. In many states, minors who are married, are members of the armed services, or are parents are legally considered adults. Consent must also be obtained from the parent or guardian of an adult who is mentally incompetent (unable to make a rational decision).

When life-threatening situations exist and a parent or legal guardian is not available for consent, first aid should be given based on implied consent. Do not withhold first aid just to obtain consent from a parent or guardian.

Psychiatric emergencies present difficult issues of consent. Under most conditions, a police officer is the only person with the authority to restrain and transport a person against that person's will. A first aid provider should not intervene unless directed to do so by a police officer or unless it is obvious that the person is about to do life-threatening harm to himself or herself or to others.

## Refusing Help

Although it seldom happens, a person might refuse assistance for countless reasons, such as religious grounds, avoidance of possible pain, or the desire to be examined by a physician rather than by a first aid provider. Whatever the reason for refusing medical care, or even if no reason is given, the alert and mentally competent adult can reject help.

Generally, the wisest approach is for you to inform the person of his or her medical condition, what you propose to do, and why the help is necessary. If the person understands the consequences and still refuses treatment, there is little else you can do. Call 9-1-1 and, while awaiting arrival, do the following:

- Try again to persuade the person to accept care, and encourage others at the scene to persuade the person. A person could change his or her mind after a short time.
- Make certain you have witnesses. A person could refuse consent and then deny having done so.
- Consider calling for law enforcement assistance. In most locations, the police can place a person in protective custody and require him or her to go to a hospital.

## Abandonment

**Abandonment** means leaving a person after starting to give help without first ensuring that the person will receive continued care at the same level or higher. Once you have responded to an emergency, you must not leave a person who needs continuing first aid until another competent and trained person takes responsibility for the person. This might seem obvious, but

cases exist in which critically ill or injured people were left unattended and then died. Thus, a first aid provider must stay with the person until another equally or better trained person takes over.

## Negligence

**Negligence** means not following the accepted standards of care, resulting in further injury to the person. Negligence involves the following:

1. Having a duty to act (ie, an obligation to give first aid)
2. Breaching that duty (either by not giving care or by giving substandard care)
3. Causing injury and damages
4. Exceeding your level of training

### Duty to Act

No one is required to give first aid unless a legal **duty to act** exists. Usually, the decision to help in an emergency is an ethical (moral) one. However, a legal duty to act could apply in the following situations:

- *When employment requires it.* If your employer designates you as the person responsible for providing first aid to meet Occupational Safety and Health Administration (OSHA) requirements and you are called to an injury scene, you have a duty to act. Examples of occupations that involve a legal obligation to give first aid include law enforcement officers, park rangers, athletic trainers, lifeguards, flight attendants, and firefighters.

  A person's employment-related duty to act may extend to off-duty hours. Some states require certain people who are licensed by the state to give emergency care regardless of their on- or off-duty status. In other words, these people are considered to be always on duty. Other states require such people to act when on duty but not generally when they are off duty, unless they are in uniform or have other visible insignia and appear to be on duty—in which case these people must respond.
- *When a preexisting responsibility exists.* You might have a preexisting relationship with other people that makes you responsible for them, which means you must give first aid should they need it. For example, a parent has a preexisting responsibility for a child, and a driver for a passenger.

- *When you were involved in the events that led to the person's injuries.* Regardless of who was at fault, if you possess first aid training, you are legally obligated to offer care to any person who has been injured or becomes ill as a result of actions in which you are involved.

Duty to act means following guidelines for standards of care. Standards of care ensure quality care and protection for injured or suddenly ill people. The elements that make up standards of care include the following:

- *The type of rescuer.* A first aid provider should provide the level and type of care expected of a reasonable person with the same amount of training and in similar circumstances. Different standards of care apply to physicians, nurses, emergency medical technicians (EMTs), and first aid providers.
- *Published guidelines.* Organizations and societies devoted to emergency care publish recommended first aid procedures. For example, the American Heart Association publishes guidelines for giving CPR, and the Wilderness Medical Society publishes guidelines for assisting people who are in remote locations.

### Breach of Duty

A **breach of duty** happens when a first aid provider fails to provide the type of care that would be given by a person having the same or similar training. A breach of duty can occur in two ways: through omission and through commission. An **act of omission** is the failure to do what a reasonably prudent person with the same or similar training would do in the same or similar circumstances. An **act of commission** is doing something that a reasonably prudent person would not do under the same or similar circumstances. Forgetting to apply a dressing is an act of omission; cutting the site of a snakebite is an act of commission.

### Injury and Damages Inflicted

The unfortunate outcome of a breach of duty is harm to the person in need of care. The most obvious harm is the physical damage produced at the point of contact. However, injury and damage can include subsequent physical pain and suffering, mental anguish, medical expenses, and sometimes loss of earnings and earning capacity. First aid providers can help prevent such adverse outcomes, and can avoid any liability should they occur, by conforming to the appropriate standard of care.

### Level of Training Restrictions

As mentioned in the discussion of duty to act, the standard of care expected of a provider depends on the provider's training level and on organizational recommendations. It may seem that meeting the prescribed standard of care is the bare minimum to which a provider should aspire and that going beyond this standard would be commendable. However, in meeting the standard of care, doing the minimum is enough. Providers should not exceed their skill level. Doing more than what is defined by the standard of care may be dangerous to the injured or ill person, and possibly even to the provider. If a provider chooses to exceed the standard of care, he or she can be held liable for any damage done in the process.

## Confidentiality

First aid providers might learn confidential information. It is important that you be extremely cautious about revealing information you learn while caring for someone. The law recognizes that people have the right to privacy. Do not discuss what you know with anyone other than those who have a medical need to know. The exception to this rule is when state laws require the reporting of certain incidents, such as rape, abuse, and gunshot wounds.

## Good Samaritan Laws

Starting in the late 1950s, a number of states (beginning with California in 1959) enacted laws designed to protect physicians and other medical personnel from legal actions that might arise from emergency treatment they provided while not in the line of duty. These laws, known as **Good Samaritan laws**, encourage people to assist others in distress by granting them protection from lawsuits. Although the laws vary from state to state, Good Samaritan protection generally applies only when the rescuer (1) is acting during an emergency; (2) is acting in good faith, which means he or she has good intentions; (3) is acting without compensation; and (4) is not guilty of malicious misconduct or gross negligence toward the person (deviating from rational first aid guidelines).

Although Good Samaritan laws primarily cover health care providers, many states have expanded them to include laypeople serving as first aid providers. In fact, some states have several Good Samaritan laws that cover different types of people in various situations. These laws will not protect first aid providers who have caused further injury to a person. Good Samaritan laws are not a protection for poorly given first aid; nor do they license providers to exceed their scope of training. Fear of lawsuits has made some people hesitant of becoming involved in emergency situations. First aid providers, however, are rarely sued.

## Q&A

**What is the rescue doctrine?**

The rescue doctrine is an unfamiliar concept to most first aid providers and emergency personnel. The rescue doctrine says that a person who is injured while performing a rescue may, unless he or she has acted rashly or recklessly, recover damages from the person whose negligence created the peril that necessitated the rescue in the first place. In other words, in some cases, an injured first aid provider has the right to recover for injuries sustained while attempting to assist others who caused the dangerous rescue. The following are examples of situations covered by the rescue doctrine:

- A person intervenes to rescue another person who is being attacked by a dog and the rescuer is injured. The owner of the dog will be held responsible for the injury.
- A distracted driver fails to see a stop sign. A person who is standing on a nearby street curb realizes that the driver is about to hit a pedestrian and runs into the street to push the pedestrian out of the way. The vehicle hits the rescuer instead. The driver will be liable for Mr. Smith's injury as well for any injuries to the other pedestrian.

## ▶ Injury Prevention

"An ounce of prevention is worth a pound of cure" refers to the fact that it is easier to prevent an injury or illness than it is to treat one. Effective prevention requires a combination of interventions known as the **3Es**: education, enforcement, and engineering.

Educational interventions are the most well known because they are the easiest to implement. Education attempts to change behavior by informing a target group about potential hazards, explaining risks, and persuading people to adopt safer behavior.

Enforcement tries to reduce dangerous behaviors through enforcing laws and regulations. For most laws to be effective, they should incorporate the following elements:

- A perceived high likelihood of apprehension
- Swift penalty delivery
- Penalties that do not always have to be extreme or severe

Engineering makes changes to the environment or product design to protect everyone automatically. This is called a passive or automatic intervention because it requires no work on the part of the person.

Examples of interventions are listed in **Table 1-3**.

## Haddon Matrix

The **Haddon Matrix** is a strategy for identifying interventions that can be applied to any type of illness or injury. As seen in **Table 1-4**, the three major phases go horizontally left to right and can be viewed as time phases:

- *Pre-event.* In this phase, interventions attempt to stop or hinder an event (eg, drowning) from happening. This phase involves prevention efforts.
- *Event.* This phase attempts to modify the consequences of such events either to prevent or to reduce the severity of an injury (eg, airbag inflating on impact).
- *Post-event.* This phase focuses on returning the person to optimal functioning in society after an injury or illness. This phase involves rescue, first aid, medical treatment, and rehabilitation.

Table 1-4 shows examples of interventions related to crashes, poisoning, and drowning.

## Table 1-3  Examples of Interventions

| Education/Persuasion | Enforcement/Laws | Engineering/Technology |
|---|---|---|
| • Swimming lessons<br>• Gun safety course<br>• DVD showing a safety procedure or message<br>• Weather and road condition alerts for drivers | • Laws requiring seat belt and helmet use<br>• Prohibition of fireworks<br>• Laws requiring that personal flotation devices be worn when boating<br>• Building codes and inspections | • Airbags in cars<br>• Helmets<br>• Child-resistant packaging on medications and chemicals<br>• Smoke and carbon monoxide detectors |

## Table 1-4  Sample Haddon Matrix

| Injury Type | Pre-event | Event | Post-event |
|---|---|---|---|
| Motor vehicle crash | Passing drinking and driving laws | Wearing seat belts | Initiating rapid EMS response |
| Poisoning | Labeling toxic products | Packaging poisons in small, nonlethal amounts | Calling the National Poison Control telephone number |
| Drowning | Constructing fences around backyard swimming pools | Wearing personal flotation devices | Performing CPR |

# prep kit

## ▶ Ready for Review

- Everyone should be able to perform first aid because most people will eventually find themselves in a situation requiring it for another person or for themselves.
- First aid is the immediate care given to an injured or suddenly ill person. First aid does not take the place of proper medical care.
- Legal and ethical issues concern all first aid providers.
- A first aid provider must have the person's consent (permission) before giving first aid.
- First aid providers might learn confidential information. It is important that you be extremely cautious about revealing information you learn while caring for someone.
- Varying from state to state, Good Samaritan laws encourage people to assist others in distress by granting them protection from lawsuits.

## ▶ Vital Vocabulary

**abandonment** Failure to continue first aid until relieved by someone with an equal or higher level of training.

**act of commission** A breach of duty in which the provider does something that a reasonably prudent person would not do under the same or similar circumstances.

**act of omission** A breach of duty in which the provider fails to do what a reasonably prudent person with the same or similar training would do in the same or similar circumstances.

**battery** Touching a person or providing first aid without consent.

**breach of duty** Failure of a first aid provider to deliver the type of care that would be given by a person having the same or similar training.

**consent** An agreement by a person in need of care to accept treatment offered as explained by medical personnel or first aid providers.

**duty to act** A person's responsibility to provide care.

**expressed consent** Permission for care that a person gives verbally or with a head nod.

**first aid** Immediate care given to an injured or suddenly ill person.

**Good Samaritan laws** Laws that encourage people to voluntarily help an injured or suddenly ill person by minimizing the liability for errors made while rendering emergency care in good faith.

**Haddon Matrix** A strategy for identifying interventions that can be applied to any type of illness or injury. Interventions proceed through three stages: pre-event, event, and post-event.

**implied consent** The legally permissible assumption that an unconscious person in need of emergency lifesaving treatment would accept treatment, were he or she alert and able.

**negligence** Deviation from the accepted standard of care that results in further injury to the person.

**standard of care** The level of care legally and ethically required of a provider. To meet the standard of care when providing first aid, a provider must (1) do what is expected of someone with first aid training and experience working under similar conditions and (2) treat the person to the best of his or her ability.

**3Es** A strategy to produce effective prevention by combining three types of intervention: education, enforcement, and engineering.

## ▶ Assessment in Action

Toward the end of the ski season, you hear that a ski resort in a neighboring state is almost vacant of skiers and the resort is offering reduced fees during weekdays. You decide to take advantage of reduced ski fees and take a few days off to go skiing. As you ski down the mountain on a run with trees bordering on both sides, you come across a man lying motionless in the snow near a tree that he may have crashed into. No other skiers are in sight and you are alone. As you approach the person, you see no obvious injuries. You have no first aid supplies. Your first aid certification is current.

*Directions:* Circle Yes if you agree with the statement; circle No if you disagree.

Yes No **1.** You have to stop to help the man.

Yes No **2.** You have implied consent to help this man.

Yes   No   **3.** After tapping on the man's shoulder to see if he is okay, he remains unresponsive but is breathing. You can leave and assume that the ski patrol will be coming shortly.

Yes   No   **4.** You are an off-duty paramedic and you decide to help. Can you expect to be paid for helping?

## ▶ Check Your Knowledge

*Directions:* Circle Yes if you agree with the statement; circle No if you disagree.

Yes   No   **1.** Because an ambulance can arrive within minutes in most locations, most people do not need to learn first aid.

Yes   No   **2.** Correct first aid can mean the difference between life and death.

Yes   No   **3.** During your lifetime, you are likely to encounter many life-threatening emergencies.

Yes   No   **4.** All injured people require medical care.

Yes   No   **5.** Before giving first aid to an alert, competent adult, you must get consent (permission) from the person.

Yes   No   **6.** If you ask an injured adult if you can help, and he or she says, "No," you can ignore him or her and proceed to provide care.

Yes   No   **7.** People who are designated as first aid providers by their employers must give first aid to injured employees while on the job.

Yes   No   **8.** First aid providers who help injured people are rarely sued.

Yes   No   **9.** Good Samaritan laws provide a degree of protection for first aid providers who act in good faith and without compensation.

Yes   No   **10.** You are required to provide first aid to any injured or suddenly ill person you encounter.

# Action at an Emergency

## 2

## Emergencies

Emergencies have the following distinctive characteristics:

- *Dangerous.* People's lives, well-being, or property are threatened.
- *Unusual and rare.* The average person will probably encounter fewer than a half dozen serious emergencies in a lifetime.
- *Different from one another.* Each emergency presents a unique set of issues.
- *Unforeseen.* Emergencies happen suddenly and without warning.
- *Urgent.* If the emergency is not dealt with immediately, the situation will escalate.

## ► Bystander Actions

The bystander is a vital link between <u>emergency medical services (EMS)</u> and the injured or suddenly ill person. Typically it is a bystander who recognizes a situation as an emergency and acts to help the person. If a bystander is to intervene in an emergency, he or she must make not just one but a series of decisions and actions quickly and reliably. These include the following:

1. Recognizing the emergency
2. Deciding to help
3. Calling 9-1-1 if EMS is needed

**4.** Checking the injured or ill person
**5.** Giving first aid

Compared with health care providers, ordinary bystanders are significantly less likely to offer help in emergencies that occur in public places. Some reasons for this include the following:

- Lack of knowledge
- Confusion about what constitutes an emergency
- Characteristics of the emergency (eg, unpleasant physical appearance of the person, the presence of other bystanders)

### Lack of Knowledge

The average layperson is unaware of many aspects of emergency care and has difficulty recognizing common medical emergencies and deciding to call 9-1-1 for help. Also, a person who does not feel competent to deal with an emergency is not likely to offer even minimal help. The person who does not feel competent can escape this uncomfortable feeling by failing to acknowledge the situation as an emergency. The implication is that bystanders who are uncertain of their ability to deal with a seriously injured person are more likely to assume that the person is not seriously injured.

### Confusion About What Is an Emergency

Sometimes, laypeople have difficulty deciding when an emergency exists **Figure 2-1**. For example, motor vehicle crashes can be easier to recognize as emergencies than heart attacks. Underestimating the severity of an emergency can lead to delays in calling 9-1-1 and to inappropriate decisions, such as transporting people with life-threatening conditions by private vehicles rather than calling 9-1-1.

### Other Factors That Influence Whether a Bystander Helps

In addition to lack of knowledge and confusion, bystanders encounter other barriers that can slow or prevent action in an emergency. Many people are put off by unpleasant physical characteristics such as blood, vomitus, or alcohol on the breath. An unwillingness to approach or touch a person who is bleeding is a common impediment to providing care. Concerns about contracting such diseases as human immunodeficiency virus (HIV) and acquired immunodeficiency syndrome (AIDS) can worsen this issue.

**Figure 2-1**

It is not always clear at first glance whether an emergency exists.

Another factor involved in helping behavior is the bystander's time of arrival. A bystander who sees the emergency happen is more likely to help than a bystander who arrives after the event.

### Quality of Help Provided by Bystanders

First aid and other assistance given by bystanders can be inadequate or potentially dangerous. Failure to keep an open airway and the decision to transport the person in a private vehicle rather than by EMS are two examples. Many people, trained decades ago or remembering a home remedy, might use outdated and unproven first aid procedures for various injuries or sudden illnesses. A few examples include the following:

- Putting butter on a burn
- Treating a nosebleed by tilting the head back
- Using hydrogen peroxide to clean a wound
- Sticking an object between the teeth of a person experiencing a seizure to prevent the person from biting his or her tongue
- Giving syrup of ipecac for a swallowed poison

## ▶ What Should Be Done?

As stated at the beginning of this chapter, injured or suddenly ill people would benefit if bystanders could quickly and reliably do the following **Flowchart 2-1** :

**1.** Recognize the emergency.
**2.** Decide to help.
**3.** Call 9-1-1 if EMS is needed.
**4.** Check the person.
**5.** Give first aid.

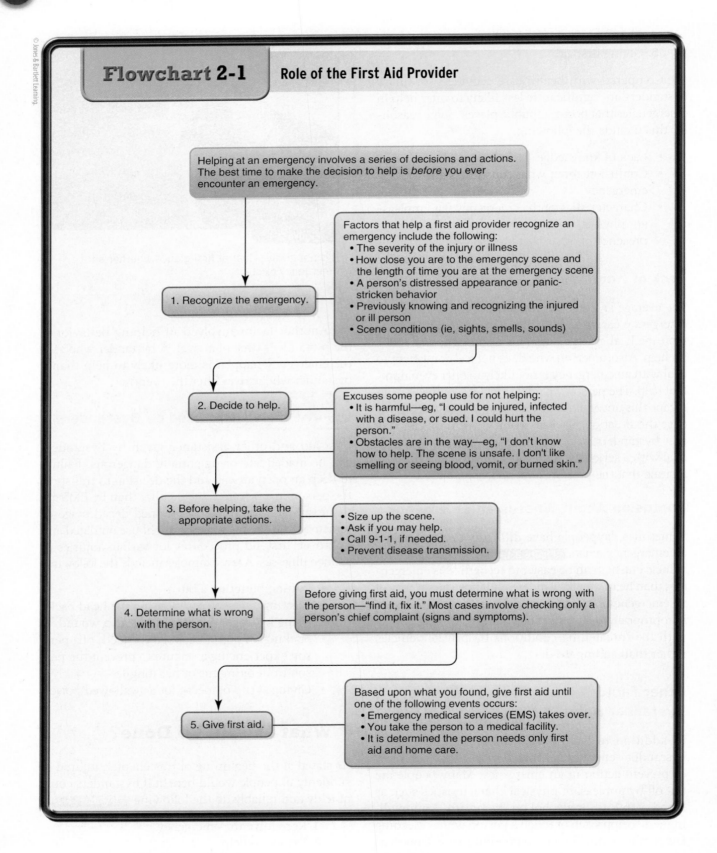

# Flowchart 2-1    Role of the First Aid Provider

Helping at an emergency involves a series of decisions and actions. The best time to make the decision to help is *before* you ever encounter an emergency.

**1. Recognize the emergency.**

Factors that help a first aid provider recognize an emergency include the following:
- The severity of the injury or illness
- How close you are to the emergency scene and the length of time you are at the emergency scene
- A person's distressed appearance or panic-stricken behavior
- Previously knowing and recognizing the injured or ill person
- Scene conditions (ie, sights, smells, sounds)

**2. Decide to help.**

Excuses some people use for not helping:
- It is harmful—eg, "I could be injured, infected with a disease, or sued. I could hurt the person."
- Obstacles are in the way—eg, "I don't know how to help. The scene is unsafe. I don't like smelling or seeing blood, vomit, or burned skin."

**3. Before helping, take the appropriate actions.**

- Size up the scene.
- Ask if you may help.
- Call 9-1-1, if needed.
- Prevent disease transmission.

**4. Determine what is wrong with the person.**

Before giving first aid, you must determine what is wrong with the person—"find it, fix it." Most cases involve checking only a person's chief complaint (signs and symptoms).

**5. Give first aid.**

Based upon what you found, give first aid until one of the following events occurs:
- Emergency medical services (EMS) takes over.
- You take the person to a medical facility.
- It is determined the person needs only first aid and home care.

## Recognize the Emergency

To help in an emergency, the bystander first has to notice that something is wrong. Factors that help a first aid provider recognize that something is wrong include the following:

- *Severity*. Severe, catastrophic emergencies such as a motor vehicle crash involving an overturned vehicle or several vehicles attract attention.
- *Physical distance*. The closer a bystander is to an emergency situation, the more likely he or she is to notice it.
- *Relationship*. Knowing the person increases the likelihood of noticing an emergency. For example, you would notice your child's injuries before you might notice the same injuries on a stranger.
- *Time exposed*. Evidence indicates that the longer a bystander is aware of the situation, the more likely he or she is to recognize it as an emergency.
- *Scene conditions*. Gory sights, terrible smells, and gruesome sounds repel many people.
- *Person's appearance*. A bystander is likely to notice a person who has a distressed appearance or is exhibiting panic-stricken behavior.

## Decide to Help

At some time, everyone will have to decide whether to help another person. Unless the decision to act in an emergency is considered well in advance of an actual emergency, the many obstacles that make it difficult or unpleasant for a bystander to help a stranger are almost certain to impede action. One important strategy that people use to avoid action is to refuse (consciously or unconsciously) to acknowledge the emergency. Many emergencies do not look like the ones portrayed on television, and the uncertainty of the real event can make it easier for the bystander to avoid acknowledging the emergency.

Bystanders are more likely to promptly get involved at the time of an emergency if they have previously considered the possibility of helping others. Thus, the most important time to make the decision to help is before ever encountering an emergency. Deciding to help is an attitude about emergencies and about one's ability to deal with emergencies. It is an attitude that takes time to develop and is affected by a number of factors. To develop such a helping attitude, people must do the following:

- Appreciate the importance of bystander help to an injured or suddenly ill person.
- Feel confident about helping someone who is seriously injured or suddenly ill, even if someone else is present.
- Be willing to take the time to help.
- Be able to put the potential risks of helping in perspective.
- Feel comfortable about taking charge at an emergency scene.
- Feel comfortable about seeing or touching a person who is bleeding or vomiting or who appears dead.

## Deciding Not to Help

A bystander could always find excuses for not helping in emergency situations. The following are reasons, some of them more legitimate than others, that people often give for not aiding others:

- *Helping could be harmful*. Bystanders have lost their lives or been severely injured while attempting to rescue others. The fear of being sued or contracting a disease such as HIV or tuberculosis can also act as a deterrent. And some would-be first aid providers have been attacked by dogs protecting their disabled owners. The sight of blood, vomit, and other unpleasant conditions sometimes found at emergency scenes may be all that some would-be first aid providers need to justify not getting involved.
- *Helping is not worth the effort*. Some bystanders might feel that the person is getting what he or she deserves. Rewards, if any, are not significant for first aid providers, possibly consisting of a newspaper write-up or a small cash prize. Often the first aid provider gets nothing more than a hurried "Thanks," and in some cases, first aid providers are never known.
- *Helping requires advanced training and skills*. Many bystanders do not know how to help. They cannot swim, do not know how to

control bleeding or perform cardiopulmonary resuscitation (CPR), or do not have other necessary rescue and first aid skills.

- *No other bystanders are helping.* The likelihood that a person will help in an emergency decreases as the number of bystanders increases. When bystanders see that others are not taking action, they may conclude that the situation is not serious. Further, the presence of other bystanders may encourage a person to leave the situation to someone else.

### Call 9-1-1 if EMS Is Needed

People sometimes make the wrong decision about calling 9-1-1. They may delay calling 9-1-1 until absolutely sure that an emergency exists, or decide to bypass EMS and transport the person to medical care in a private vehicle. Such actions can endanger a person. Fortunately, most injuries and sudden illnesses do not require medical care—only first aid.

### Check the Person

You must decide whether life-threatening conditions exist and what kind of help a person needs. See Chapter 4, *Finding Out What is Wrong,* for details.

**FYI**

**Actual Versus Perceived EMS Response Time**

People's perceptions of ambulance response times are inaccurate. They tend to overestimate response time while underestimating scene time and time to medical care.
*Source:* Harvey AH, Gerard WC, Rice GF, Finch H. Actual vs. perceived EMS response time. *Prehosp Emerg Care* 1999;3(1):11-14.

### Give First Aid

Often the most critical life support measures are effective only if started immediately by the nearest available person. That person usually will be a layperson—a bystander.

**Q&A**

**Should the family be present during resuscitation?**

Controversy exists regarding this question. Studies indicate that most family members want to be present. Offering select family members the opportunity to be present is reasonable. If family members are present during resuscitation, be sensitive to them by answering their questions, clarifying information, and providing them comfort.
*Source:* Morrison LJ, et al. 2010 American Heart Association guidelines for cardiopulmonary resuscitation and emergency cardiovascular care science. *Circulation* 2010;122: S670.

## ▶ Seeking Medical Care

Knowing when to call 9-1-1 for help from EMS is important. To know when to call, you must be able to tell the difference between a minor injury or illness and a life-threatening one. For example, upper abdominal pain may be attributed to something as simple as indigestion or ulcers, but it may also be an early sign of a heart attack. Wheezing could be related to a person's asthma, for which the person can use his or her prescribed inhaler for quick relief, or it can be as serious as a severe allergic reaction from a bee sting.

Not every cut requires stitches, nor does every burn require medical care. It is, however, always best to err on the side of caution. According to the American College of Emergency Physicians (ACEP), if the answer to any of the following questions is "yes," or if you are unsure, call 9-1-1 for help:

- Is the condition life-threatening?
- Could the condition get worse on the way to the hospital?
- If you move the person, will it cause further injury?
- Does the person need the skills or equipment of EMS?
- Would distance or traffic cause a delay in getting the person to the hospital?

ACEP also recommends immediate transport to the hospital emergency department, by EMS or by private vehicle, for the following conditions that are warning signs of more serious conditions:

- Difficulty breathing, especially if it does not improve with rest
- Chest or upper abdominal pain or pressure lasting 2 minutes or more

- A fast heartbeat (more than 120 to 150 beats per minute) at rest, especially if associated with shortness of breath or feeling faint
- Fainting (passing out) or unresponsiveness
- Difficulty speaking, or numbness or weakness of any part of the body
- Sudden dizziness
- Confusion or changes in mental status, unusual behavior, or difficulty walking
- Sudden blindness or vision changes
- Bleeding from any wound that will not stop with direct pressure
- Broken bones visible through an open wound, or a broken leg
- Drowning (submersion)
- Choking
- Severe burn
- Allergic reaction, especially if there is any difficulty breathing
- Extremely hot or cold body temperature
- Poisoning or drug overdose
- Sudden, severe headache
- Any sudden or severe pain
- Severe or persistent vomiting or diarrhea
- Coughing or vomiting of blood
- Behavioral emergencies (threatening to hurt or kill themselves or someone else)

Wounds requiring immediate medical care include the following (see Chapter 9, *Wounds*, for additional information on wounds requiring medical care):

- Bleeding from a cut that does not slow during the first 15 minutes of steady direct pressure
- Signs of shock
- Breathing difficultly resulting from a cut to the neck or chest
- A deep cut to the abdomen that causes moderate to severe pain
- A cut to the eyeball
- A cut that amputates or partially amputates an extremity

When a serious situation occurs, call 9-1-1 *first*. **DO NOT** call your physician, the hospital, a friend, relatives, or neighbors for help before you call 9-1-1. Calling anyone else first only wastes time. Calling 9-1-1 has several advantages over driving to the hospital emergency department by private vehicle:

- Many injured or suddenly ill people should not be moved except by trained personnel.

- The EMS personnel who arrive with the ambulance know what to do. In addition, they are in radio contact with hospital physicians.
- Care provided by EMS personnel at the scene and on the way to the hospital can increase a person's chances of survival and rate of recovery. The condition could get worse and become life threatening on the way to the hospital, in which case, the presence of trained professionals is vital.
- An EMS ambulance usually can get a person to the hospital more quickly.

If the situation is not an emergency, call your physician. However, if you have *any* doubt about whether the situation is an emergency, call 9-1-1. Later chapters identify when to call 9-1-1 for specific conditions.

## ▶ How to Call EMS

In most communities, to receive emergency assistance of any kind, call 9-1-1 **Figure 2-2**. Check to confirm that this is the method used in your community. Emergency telephone numbers are usually listed on the inside front cover of telephone directories. Keep these numbers near or on every telephone. In the case of cell phones, store the numbers under emergency contacts. Dial 0 (the operator) if you do not know the emergency number. A community 9-1-1 number has some benefits:

- There is only one number to remember.
- Calls are received by specially trained personnel.
- Response time is reduced.

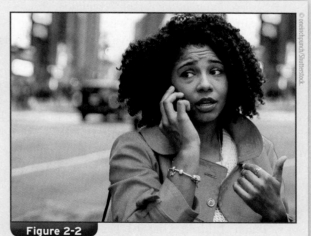

**Figure 2-2**

For help, call 9-1-1 or the local emergency number.

According to the National Emergency Number Association, over 98% of the people in the United States and Canada are covered by some type of 9-1-1 service. Many areas also have Enhanced 9-1-1, which allows the dispatcher to see the caller's phone number and address if the call is placed on a landline. When you call 9-1-1 from a cell phone, however, Enhanced 9-1-1 cannot identify your exact address, because cell phone signals only provide a general location. Because of this key difference, make sure you know your exact address or location to give the 9-1-1 dispatcher.

When you call 9-1-1, speak slowly and clearly. Be ready to give the dispatcher the following information:

1. *The person's location.* Give the address, names of intersecting roads, and other landmarks, if possible. Location details are the most important information you can provide. Also, tell the specific location of the person. (For example, "in the basement" or "in the backyard.")
2. *The phone number you are calling from and your name.* This information allows dispatchers to detect false reports, thus minimizing their frequency, and it allows a dispatch center without Enhanced 9-1-1 to call back if disconnected or if additional information is needed.
3. *A description of what happened.* State the nature of the emergency. (For example, "My husband fell off a ladder and is not moving.")
4. *The number of people needing help and any special conditions.* (For example, "There was a car crash involving two cars. Three people are trapped.")
5. *A description of the person's condition.* (For example, "My husband's head is bleeding.") List any first aid you have attempted, such as pressing on the site of the bleeding.

**DO NOT** hang up the phone unless the dispatcher instructs you to do so **Figure 2-3**. Enhanced 9-1-1 systems can track a call, but some communities lack this technology. Also, the EMS dispatcher could tell you how best to care for the person. If you send someone else to call, have the person report back to you so you can be sure the call was made. Other tips include the following:

- Teach children what 9-1-1 is for and how and when to call. Refer to "nine-one-one," not "nine-eleven," because children might expect

**Figure 2-3**

9-1-1 dispatch center.

to find an eleven on the dial or on the push buttons.
- Do not hang up without explanation if you call 9-1-1 by mistake; if you hang up, the dispatcher will have to call back to see if you need help.
- If your area does not have a 9-1-1 system, add the numbers for EMS, fire, and police services to a list by your phones, or in the emergency contacts of your cell phone. During an emergency, you might not have the time or presence of mind to find a directory listing.

## ▶ Rescuer Reactions

The sight of blood and the cries of people can be upsetting to people attempting to rescue and help an injured person. Seeing a grotesque amputation, being splattered with vomit or blood, or smelling disagreeable odors from urine and feces can be unnerving. More than one first aid provider has felt nauseated and weak, vomited, or fainted when helping injured people. Even the toughest of physicians and emergency medical technicians have difficult moments when exposed to certain situations.

It is essential that first aid providers stay alert and keep working at an injury scene. A first aid provider who collapses while aiding an injured person diverts attention from the original person, whose condition is usually more serious. All the knowledge and skills a first aid provider has are useless if he or she collapses or has to leave the scene because of weakness or fainting.

## Desensitization

Some emergency care providers seem to have ice in their veins. They always appear calm and unaffected by even the worst injuries. These people might seem callous, but the proper psychological term is *desensitized*. A specialty within psychology deals with **desensitization** and suggests ways of overcoming anxieties caused by unpleasant sights and sounds. Desensitization is a deconditioning or a counterconditioning process that can reduce fears and anxieties. The idea is to weaken an undesirable response such as fainting by strengthening an incompatible response. When responses are incompatible (calmness versus anxiety), the occurrence of either one prevents the occurrence of the other. By desensitizing, you learn to associate relaxation with situations that elicit anxiety so that eventually you do not experience anxiety. But you first need to learn how to invoke relaxation before gradually exposing yourself to anxiety-producing situations such as the sight of blood.

A simple way to desensitize (calm) yourself while helping another person is to change your thought patterns from the unpleasant to the pleasant by singing a favorite song to yourself (not out loud, of course, for the obvious reason of how you might appear to the person or observers). You can begin a process of gradual exposure to unpleasant scenes by viewing television programs, movies, or pictures of injuries in medical journals. You might eventually consider volunteering at a hospital emergency department where you can see injuries.

## Physical-Emotional Intersect

A provider's ability to withstand emotional strains can be directly affected by his or her physical condition. In a number of cases, a first aid provider who fainted had failed to eat breakfast. It is strongly recommended that everyone maintain an adequate blood glucose level through proper eating habits. Eating breakfast is especially important.

## Postcare Reactions

After giving first aid for severe injuries, a person might feel an emotional letdown, which is frequently overlooked. A stressful event can be psychologically overwhelming and can result in a condition known as **posttraumatic stress disorder (PTSD)**. Its symptoms include depression and flashbacks of the event.

Discussing your feelings, fears, and reactions within 24 to 72 hours of helping at an emergency helps prevent later emotional conditions. You could discuss your feelings with a trusted friend, a mental health professional, or a member of the clergy. Bringing out your feelings quickly can relieve personal anxieties and stress.

## ▶ Scene Size-up

If you are at the scene of an emergency situation, do a 10-second **scene size-up** `Flowchart 2-2`, trying to answer the following questions:

1. Are hazards present that could be dangerous to you, the injured or suddenly ill person or people, or bystanders?
2. How many people are involved?
3. What is wrong?
4. What happened?
5. Are bystanders available to help?

As you approach an emergency scene, scan the area for immediate dangers to yourself or to the person `Figure 2-4`. For example, if a car crash is obstructing traffic, you have to consider whether you can safely approach the vehicle of the person requiring help. Or you might notice that gasoline is dripping from the gas tank and that the battery has shorted out and is sparking. Other conditions include hazardous conditions such as chemical spills, toxic fumes, explosives, gas leaks, or live electric wires. In some locations, dangers such as an avalanche, landslides, fires, flash floods, or attack dogs might exist. If the scene is dangerous, stay away and call 9-1-1. You are not being cowardly, merely realistic. Never attempt a rescue that you have not been specifically trained to do. You cannot help another person if you also become injured or ill. For details about hazards at an emergency scene, refer to Chapter 26, *Disaster Preparedness*.

The second step is to try to determine the cause of the injury. For example, if the emergency department physician knows that a person was thrown against a steering wheel, he or she will check for liver, spleen, and cardiac injuries. Be sure to tell EMS personnel about your findings so they can identify the extent of any injuries.

Finally, determine how many people are involved. There could be more than one person in need of help, so look around and ask about others involved.

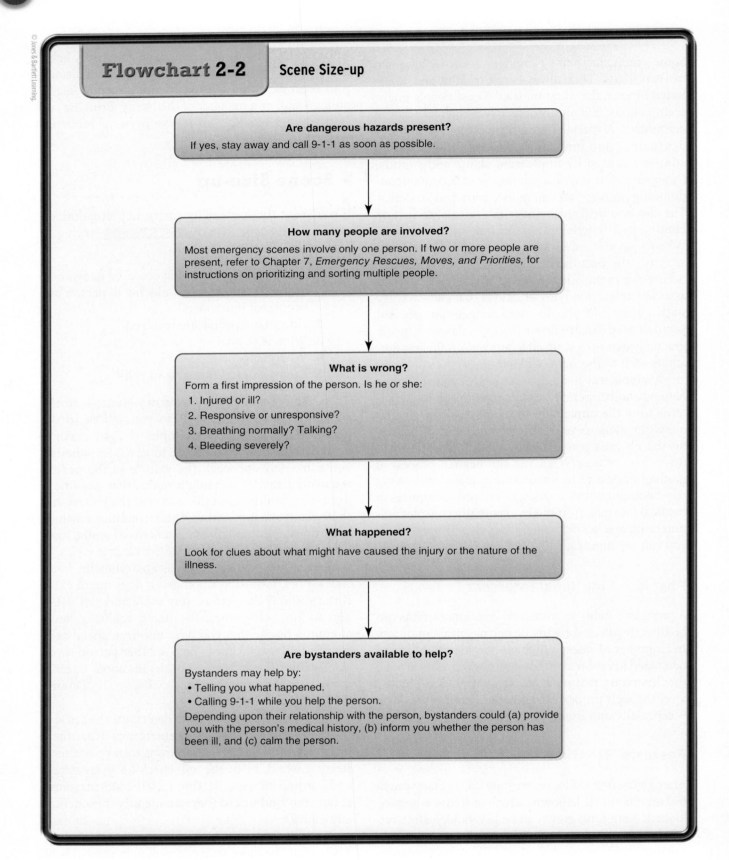

**Flowchart 2-2**    Scene Size-up

**Are dangerous hazards present?**

If yes, stay away and call 9-1-1 as soon as possible.

**How many people are involved?**

Most emergency scenes involve only one person. If two or more people are present, refer to Chapter 7, *Emergency Rescues, Moves, and Priorities*, for instructions on prioritizing and sorting multiple people.

**What is wrong?**

Form a first impression of the person. Is he or she:

1. Injured or ill?
2. Responsive or unresponsive?
3. Breathing normally? Talking?
4. Bleeding severely?

**What happened?**

Look for clues about what might have caused the injury or the nature of the illness.

**Are bystanders available to help?**

Bystanders may help by:

- Telling you what happened.
- Calling 9-1-1 while you help the person.

Depending upon their relationship with the person, bystanders could (a) provide you with the person's medical history, (b) inform you whether the person has been ill, and (c) calm the person.

**Figure 2-4**

The scene size-up includes evaluating the scene for hazardous conditions.

**Q&A**

**Should I leave my headlights on at a scene?**

Always turn your hazard lights on at a scene. Unless your headlights are needed to light up the scene, turn off your headlights when parked. Your headlights can blind approaching vehicles, making it difficult for the drivers to see rescue personnel walking around the scene.

## ▶ Disease Precautions

First aid providers must understand the risks from infectious diseases, which can range in severity from mild to life threatening. First aid providers should know how to reduce the risk of contamination to themselves and to others.

An **infectious disease** is a medical condition caused by the growth and spread of small, harmful organisms within the body. A **communicable disease** is a disease that can spread from one person to another. Immunizations, protective techniques, and handwashing can minimize the risk of infection. Because there are so many different infectious diseases to be concerned about, the Centers for Disease Control and Prevention (CDC) developed a set of **standard precautions**, which advise you to assume that all people are infected and can spread an organism that poses a risk for transmission of

infectious diseases. These protective measures are designed to prevent first aid providers from coming into direct contact with infectious agents Flowchart 2-3 .

### Handwashing

Handwashing is one of the simplest, yet most effective ways to control disease transmission Figure 2-5 . Even if you are wearing gloves, you should wash your hands before, if possible, and definitely after every contact with an ill or injured person. The longer the germs remain with you, the greater their chance of infecting you.

The proper procedure for washing your hands is as follows:

1. Use soap and warm water, if possible. All types of soap are acceptable when washing with water.
2. Rub your hands together for 15 to 20 seconds to work up a lather. Wash all surfaces well, including wrists, palms, backs of hands, and fingers. Clean the dirt from under your fingernails.
3. Rinse the soap from your hands.
4. Dry your hands completely with a clean towel if possible (this helps remove the germs). If towels are not available, however, it is okay to allow your hands to air dry.

If soap and water are not available, use an alcohol-based hand sanitizer to clean your hands Figure 2-6 . Apply the gel to one hand and rub your hands together, covering all surfaces of your hands and fingers, until the hands are dry. If your mucous membranes (eg, your eyes, nose, or mouth) are splashed by blood or body fluid, immediately flush the area with clean water.

### Personal Protective Equipment

**Personal protective equipment (PPE)** includes exam gloves, mouth-to-barrier devices, eye protection, and gowns. PPE provides a barrier between the first aid provider and infectious diseases.

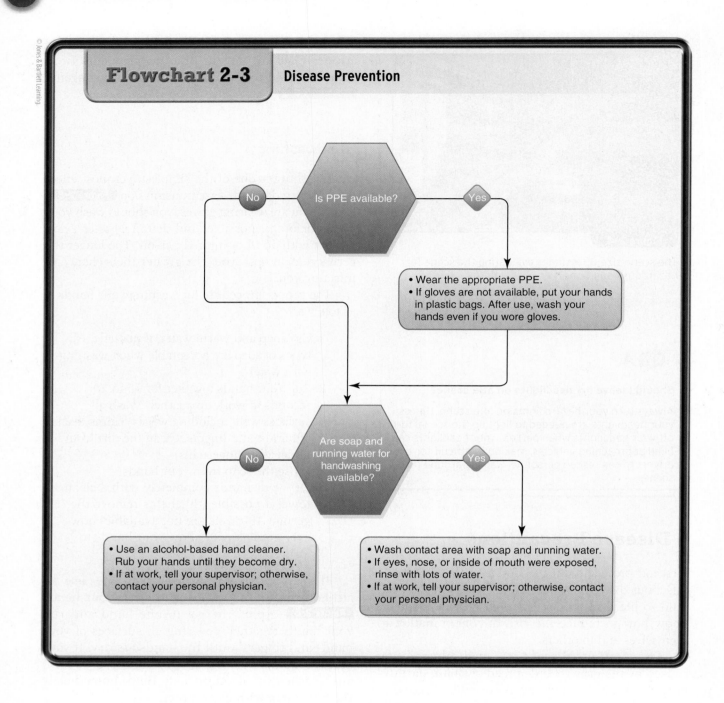

**Flowchart 2-3** | **Disease Prevention**

Is PPE available?

No

Yes
- Wear the appropriate PPE.
- If gloves are not available, put your hands in plastic bags. After use, wash your hands even if you wore gloves.

Are soap and running water for handwashing available?

No
- Use an alcohol-based hand cleaner. Rub your hands until they become dry.
- If at work, tell your supervisor; otherwise, contact your personal physician.

Yes
- Wash contact area with soap and running water.
- If eyes, nose, or inside of mouth were exposed, rinse with lots of water.
- If at work, tell your supervisor; otherwise, contact your personal physician.

## Exam Gloves

Exam gloves are the most common type of PPE and should always be worn when there is any possibility of exposure to blood or body fluids. The Food and Drug Administration (FDA), the CDC, and the Occupational Safety and Health Administration (OSHA) have stated that both vinyl and latex gloves provide adequate protection. Research indicates that latex has fewer micropores (very small holes) and,

thus, offers the most protection. However, latex tends to break down faster (within several years) while the gloves are in a first aid kit waiting to be used. Another option is nitrile gloves. All first aid kits should contain several pairs of gloves **Figure 2-7** . Because some rescuers have allergic reactions to latex, latex-free gloves should also be available.

It is important to use the proper technique when removing used gloves so you do not contaminate

**Figure 2-5**

Handwashing.

**Figure 2-7**

Disposable gloves.

**Figure 2-6**

Use a waterless handwashing solution if there is no running water available.

yourself. When removing used gloves, do not touch their outer surface . The proper method of removing gloves is as follows:

1. Pinch one glove on the outside near the wrist (**Step 1**).
2. Gently pull the glove off, keeping the inside out (**Step 2**).
3. Hold the removed glove in your gloved hand (**Step 3**).
4. Slide two fingers of your bare hand inside the remaining glove at the wrist (**Step 4**).
5. Gently stretch the glove away from the hand and gently pull the glove off, keeping the inside out. The first glove remains inside the glove just removed (**Step 5**).

6. Dispose of the gloves in a biohazard container or a sealed plastic bag. Wash your hands with soap and running water. If they are not available, use an alcohol-based hand sanitizer (**Step 6**).

You might consider putting on a second pair of gloves over the first if there is major, significant external bleeding or body fluid. If the gloves are cut or torn, replace them.

## Q&A

**Why is the use of latex gloves a concern?**

Natural latex, which is used in latex gloves, contains natural proteins that have been shown to sensitize and cause allergic reactions in some people over time with repeated use. During the processing and manufacturing of latex gloves, many impurities are left in the gloves and eventually attach to the cornstarch that is placed in the gloves for ease of donning. When the gloves are removed, the natural proteins, which are attached to the cornstarch, are aerosolized into the air and inhaled by everyone nearby. The person who removed the gloves may further sensitize himself or herself by touching the nose, eyes, or mucous membranes while the powder is still on the hands.

People who are sensitive or allergic to latex may experience a wide variety of symptoms, including rash, asthma, severe food allergies, anaphylaxis, and death. A large amount of literature is available regarding concerns over the use of latex gloves. Alternative materials used in making gloves are nitrile, neoprene, and vinyl.

## Skill Sheet

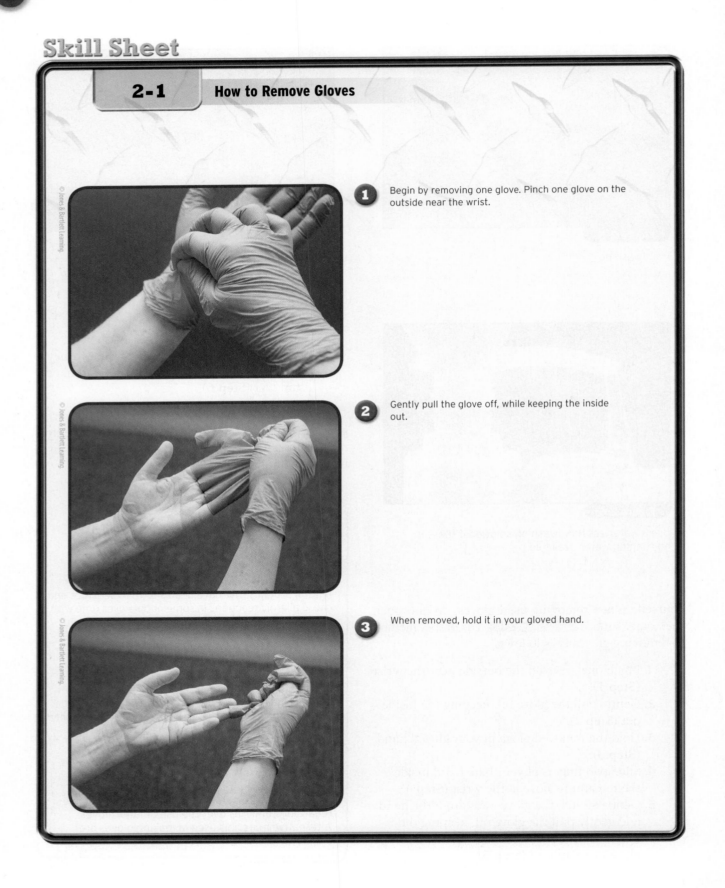

| 2-1 | How to Remove Gloves |

**1** Begin by removing one glove. Pinch one glove on the outside near the wrist.

**2** Gently pull the glove off, while keeping the inside out.

**3** When removed, hold it in your gloved hand.

© Jones & Bartlett Learning.

# Skill Sheet Continued

| 2-1 | How to Remove Gloves |

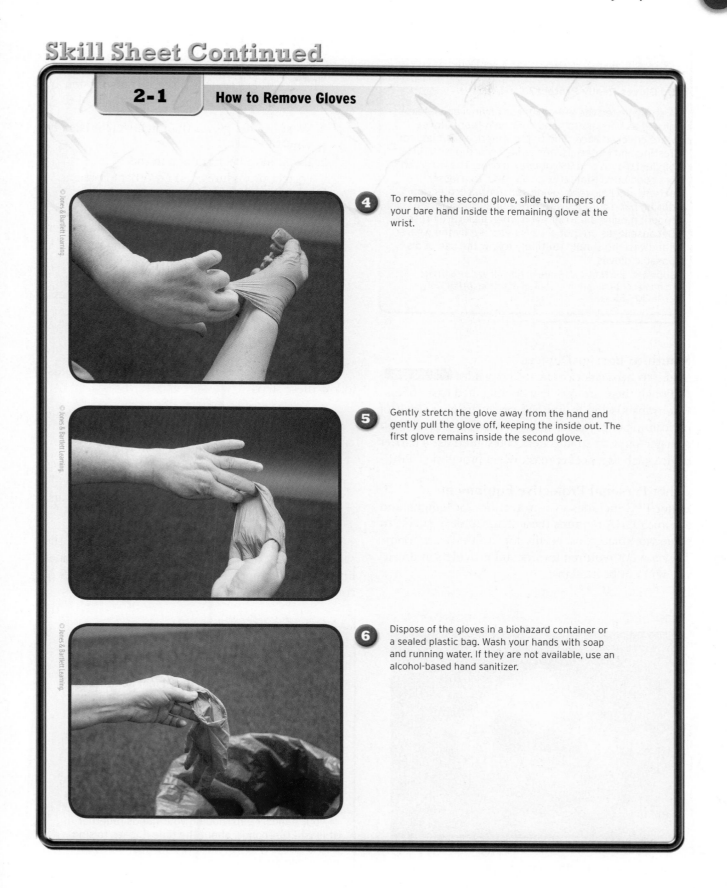

**4** To remove the second glove, slide two fingers of your bare hand inside the remaining glove at the wrist.

**5** Gently stretch the glove away from the hand and gently pull the glove off, keeping the inside out. The first glove remains inside the second glove.

**6** Dispose of the gloves in a biohazard container or a sealed plastic bag. Wash your hands with soap and running water. If they are not available, use an alcohol-based hand sanitizer.

## Mouth-to-Barrier Devices

Mouth-to-barrier devices are recommended **Figure 2-8**. Although there are very few documented cases of disease transmission to first aid providers as a result of performing unprotected mouth-to-mouth resuscitation on a person with an infection, you should use a barrier device such as a pocket mask when providing CPR.

## Other Personal Protective Equipment

Other PPE includes eye protection and gowns and aprons. OSHA requires these items to be available in some workplaces, especially for health care workers. They are not required for first aid providers and usually will not be available.

## Cleaning Up After an Emergency

When cleaning up blood or other body fluids, protect yourself and others against disease transmission by following these steps:

1. Wear heavier gloves than lightweight latex or vinyl.
2. If you have been trained in the correct procedures, use absorbent barriers to soak up blood or other infectious materials.
3. Clean the spill area using soap and water. After cleaning, disinfect with a bleach and water solution at a 1:10 dilution. Isopropyl alcohol can also be used to disinfect. These solutions can corrode or discolor certain fabrics, leathers, vinyl, or other synthetic materials.
4. Discard contaminated materials in an appropriate waste disposal container.

If you have been exposed to blood or body fluids, follow these steps:

1. Use soap and water to wash the parts of your body that have been contaminated.
2. If the exposure happened at work, report the incident to your supervisor. Otherwise, contact your personal physician. If the exposure was significant, seek medical care. Early action can prevent the development of certain infections.

The best protection against disease is using the safeguards described here. By following these guidelines, first aid providers can decrease their chances of contracting bloodborne illnesses.

**Figure 2-8**

Pocket face mask with a one-way valve.

## Some Diseases of Special Concern

### Bloodborne Diseases

Some diseases are carried in the blood of a person with an infection (**bloodborne diseases**). **Human immunodeficiency virus (HIV)** is the virus that can cause AIDS. The virus is transmitted by direct contact with infected blood, semen, or vaginal secretions; there is no scientific documentation that the virus is transmitted by contact with sweat, saliva, tears, sputum, urine, feces, vomitus, or nasal secretions, unless these fluids contain visible signs of blood. No vaccine is currently available to prevent HIV infection.

**Hepatitis B virus (HBV)** is also spread by direct contact with infected blood. The term *hepatitis* refers to an inflammation (and often infection) of the liver. A vaccine is available for HBV and is recommended

---

**FYI**

**On-the-Job Protection**

People infected with HBV or HIV might not show symptoms and might not even know they are infected. For that reason, consider all human blood and body fluids potentially infectious, and take precautions to avoid contact. Standard precautions recommend that you assume that *all* body fluids are a possible risk. EMS personnel routinely follow standard precautions, even if blood or body fluids are not visible.

OSHA requires any company with employees who are expected to give first aid in an emergency to follow standard precautions. OSHA applies the "Good Samaritan" definition to an employee who assists another with a nosebleed or a cut. Such acts, however, are not considered occupational exposure unless the employee who provides the assistance is a member of a first aid team or is designated or expected to provide first aid as part of his or her job. In essence, OSHA's requirement excludes unassigned employees who perform unanticipated first aid.

Whenever there is a chance that you could be exposed to bloodborne pathogens, your employer must provide appropriate PPE, which might include eye protection, gloves, gowns, and masks. The PPE must be accessible, and your employer must provide training to help you choose the right PPE for your work.

EMS personnel follow standard precautions, and OSHA requires designated work-site first aid providers to follow standard precautions. But what procedures should a typical first aid provider follow? It makes sense for first aid providers to follow standard precautions and assume that *all* blood and body fluids are infectious.

---

**FYI**

**Emergency Medical Services**

If you or someone you know is ever sick or injured and needs emergency help, remember, there are a lot of people who are specially trained to help you!

- *Emergency medical technicians.* Emergency medical technicians (EMTs) have different amounts of training, depending on their jobs. Sometimes EMTs are dispatchers who answer calls for help and send ambulances and rescue vehicles to the scene of the emergency. Other EMTs drive the ambulance, assist with rescues, and perform basic emergency medical care. An EMT course requires about 150 hours of training.
- *Paramedics.* Paramedics are EMTs with the highest level of training. They are able to perform many medical procedures at the scene of the emergency or in the ambulance on the way to the hospital. Using a radio to communicate, paramedics often get instructions from a physician at the emergency room or at the base station (the paramedic's headquarters).
- *Emergency nurses.* If you were a patient in the emergency department, an emergency nurse would probably be the first person you would see. One of the nurse's jobs is to ask you questions about your medical condition and help decide when you can see the physician. Emergency nurses are specially trained to help treat emergency patients.
- *Emergency physicians.* Emergency physicians are specially trained to take care of a certain type of patient: emergency patients. Physicians who are specially trained are often called specialists. Emergency physicians specialize in helping people who are injured or who become sick very suddenly, such as someone who is having a heart attack or has a very high fever.
- *Emergency medical responders.* Police officers and firefighters are some of the other people who might help you, especially if you have to be rescued.

*Source:* American College of Emergency Physicians.

---

for all infants and for adults who might have contact with carriers of the disease or with blood. **Hepatitis C virus (HCV)** can cause liver disease or cancer. It cannot be cured, and no vaccine exists.

### Airborne Diseases

**Airborne diseases** are transmitted through the air by coughing or sneezing. **Tuberculosis (TB)**, a chronic bacterial disease that usually affects the lungs, is becoming a common condition and is hard to distinguish from other diseases. People who present the highest risk often have a cough. TB is more common in people who have lived in a homeless shelter or in a developing country. New and re-emerging diseases can be potentially life threatening. If a surgical mask is available, wear it or wrap a handkerchief over your nose and mouth.

## ▶ Death and Dying

Few incidents are as emotionally stressful as a life-and-death situation. Witnessing death and dying is an unfortunate possibility accepted by those who provide emergency care.

### The Dying Person

Assisting a person who is dying presents a difficult situation. The following guidelines can help you provide compassionate, effective care:

- Avoid negative statements about the person's condition. Even an unresponsive person can hear what is being said.
- Assure the person that you will locate and inform his or her family of what has happened. Attempt to have family members present; they can provide great comfort to the person.
- Allow some hope. Do not tell the person that he or she is dying. Instead, say something like, "I will not give up on you, so do not give up on yourself."
- Do not volunteer information about the person or others who might also be injured. However, if the person asks a question about a family member, tell the truth. Provide simple, honest, clear information if it is requested, and repeat it as often as necessary.
- Use a gentle tone of voice.
- Use a reassuring touch, if appropriate.
- Let the person know that everything that can be done to help will be done.

### The Stages of Grieving

People who lose a loved one go through a **grieving process**. This process generally involves five stages,

but not all people move through the process in the same way or at the same pace.

1. *Denial* ("Not me."). The person cannot believe what is happening. This stage serves as a buffer for the person experiencing the situation. This reaction is normal.
2. *Anger* ("Why me?"). First aid providers and bystanders could be the target of the anger. Do not take the anger or insults personally. Be tolerant, use good listening skills, and be empathetic.
3. *Bargaining* ("OK, but first let me . . ."). In the person's mind, an agreement will postpone an unpleasant event, such as death.
4. *Depression* ("But I have not . . ."). This stage is characterized by sadness and despair. The person is usually silent and retreats into his or her own world.
5. *Acceptance* ("OK, I am not afraid."). Acceptance does not mean a person is happy about the situation. The family often requires more support during this stage than the person does.

With an understanding of these five stages, you can better understand the reactions of those who are grieving and also your reactions to stressful situations.

### Interacting With Survivors

Interact with the family members of a dead or dying person as follows:

- Do not pronounce death; leave the confirmation of death to a physician.
- Allow survivors to grieve in whatever way seems right to them (eg, anger, rage, crying).
- Provide simple, honest, clear information as it is requested, and repeat it as often as necessary.
- Offer as much support and comfort as possible by your presence and by your words. Do not leave an individual survivor alone, but respect that person's right to privacy.
- Use a gentle tone of voice.
- Use a reassuring touch, if appropriate.

## ▶ Ready for Review

- Emergencies are dangerous, unusual, rare, and unforeseen, and they must be dealt with before the situation becomes worse.
- A bystander is a vital link between the EMS system and the person in need of care.
- Injured or suddenly ill people would benefit if bystanders could quickly and reliably do the following:
  - Recognize the emergency.
  - Decide to help.
  - Call 9-1-1 if EMS is needed.
  - Check the person.
  - Give first aid.
- Knowing when to call 9-1-1 is important. To do so, you must be able to tell the difference between a minor injury or illness and a life-threatening one.
- In most communities, call 9-1-1 to receive emergency assistance.
- The sight of blood and the cries of people at an emergency scene can be upsetting, but it is essential that first aid providers remain alert and keep working at an injury scene.
- If you are at the scene of an emergency situation, do a 10-second scene size-up looking for hazards, the cause of the injury or illness, and the number of people involved.
- First aid providers should take precautions to protect against infectious diseases.
- Few incidents are as emotionally stressful as the life-and-death situations that you might face when providing emergency care.

## ▶ Vital Vocabulary

**airborne disease** An infection transmitted through the air, such as tuberculosis (TB).

**bloodborne disease** An infection transmitted through the blood, such as human immunodeficiency virus (HIV) or hepatitis B virus (HBV).

**communicable disease** A disease that can spread from person to person, or from animal to person.

**desensitization** A process of deconditioning or counterconditioning designed reduce a person's fears and anxieties. The idea is to weaken an undesirable response such as fainting by strengthening an incompatible response.

**emergency medical services (EMS)** A system that represents the combined efforts of several professionals and agencies to provide emergency medical care.

**grieving process** The emotional process that a person works through after a stressful situation that causes personal pain. People go through several stages of grieving.

**hepatitis B virus (HBV)** A viral infection of the liver for which a vaccine is available.

**hepatitis C virus (HCV)** A viral infection of the liver for which no vaccine is available.

**human immunodeficiency virus (HIV)** The virus that can cause acquired immunodeficiency syndrome (AIDS).

**infectious disease** A medical condition caused by the growth of small, harmful organisms within the body.

**personal protective equipment (PPE)** Equipment, such as exam gloves, used to block the entry of an organism into the body.

**posttraumatic stress disorder (PTSD)** A delayed stress reaction to a prior emergency event.

**SARS (severe acute respiratory syndrome)** A potentially life-threatening viral infection that usually starts with flulike symptoms.

**scene size-up** A quick assessment of the scene and the surroundings for safety issues, the cause of injury or nature of illness, and the number of people; it is completed before starting first aid.

**standard precautions** Protective measures that have traditionally been developed by the Centers for Disease Control and Prevention (CDC) for use in dealing with objects, blood, body fluids, or other potential exposure risks of communicable disease.

**tuberculosis (TB)** A bacterial disease usually affecting the lungs.

# prep kit

## ▶ Assessment in Action

You are walking from house to house in an unfamiliar neighborhood collecting donated clothing for a local charitable organization. You find no one home at a particular house but hear a loud explosion in the garage. You decide to see what happened. Upon entering the garage, you find a teenage boy lying on the ground. There is a strong gasoline odor. You have a cell phone with you.

*Directions:* Circle Yes if you agree with the statement; circle No if you disagree.

Yes    No    **1.** This scene could be dangerous.

Yes    No    **2.** You should not be concerned about other people.

Yes    No    **3.** In most communities, 9-1-1 can be used to contact EMS.

Yes    No    **4.** If you do not know the exact address of the emergency, be prepared to give a description of the location as best as you can.

## ▶ Check Your Knowledge

*Directions:* Circle Yes if you agree with the statement; circle No if you disagree.

Yes    No    **1.** A scene survey should be done before giving first aid to an injured person.

Yes    No    **2.** For a severely injured person, call the person's physician before calling for an ambulance.

Yes    No    **3.** Dial 0 (for the telephone operator) if you do not know the emergency telephone number.

Yes    No    **4.** First aid providers should assume that blood and all body fluids are infectious.

Yes    No    **5.** If you are exposed to blood while on the job, report it to your supervisor, and if off the job, to your personal physician.

Yes    No    **6.** First aid kits should contain exam gloves.

Yes    No    **7.** Wash your hands with soap and water after giving first aid.

Yes    No    **8.** Vaccinations are available for both HBV and HCV.

Yes    No    **9.** Exam gloves can be made of almost any material as long as they fit the hand well.

Yes    No    **10.** TB is a bloodborne disease.

# The Human Body

**3**

## The Human Body

To assess a person's condition adequately and to give effective first aid, a first aid provider must be familiar with the basic structure and functions of the human body. This knowledge provides a solid cornerstone for building the essentials of quality assessment and emergency first aid. By using the proper medical terms, you will be able to communicate more effectively with the person you are assessing and with medical care providers.

## ▶ Directional Terms

When you are discussing where an injury is located or how a pain moves throughout the body, you need to know the correct directional terms **Figure 3-1**. The terms *right* and *left* refer to the person's right and left sides, not to your right and left sides. **Anterior** refers to the front of the body and **posterior** refers to the back of the body. **Superior** parts of the body are closer to the head; the parts closer to the feet are called **inferior**. **Lateral** (outer) parts of the body are farther from the middle of the body; the parts closer to the middle of the body are called **medial** (inner).

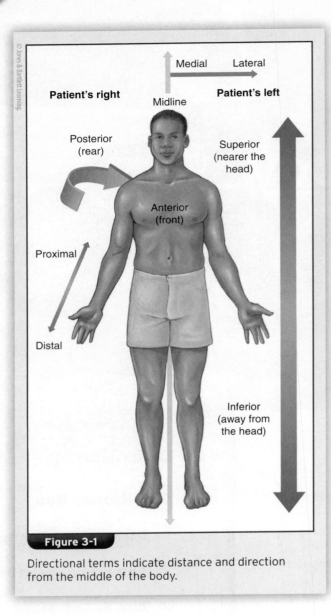

**Figure 3-1**

Directional terms indicate distance and direction from the middle of the body.

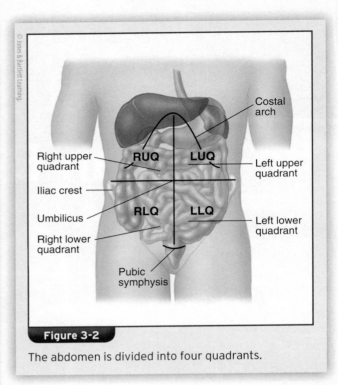

**Figure 3-2**

The abdomen is divided into four quadrants.

vertical line intersecting at the umbilicus (navel), dividing the **abdomen** into four equal areas. These areas are referred to as the right upper quadrant, left upper quadrant, right lower quadrant, and left lower quadrant **Figure 3-2** .

The terms *proximal* and *distal* are used when discussing an arm or leg. **Proximal** (close) refers to areas that are close to the point where the arm or leg is attached to the body. **Distal** (distant) refers to areas that are distant from the point of attachment.

**Superficial** means closer to or on the skin. **Deep** means farther inside the body and away from the skin.

The term **quadrant** indicates a section of the abdominal cavity. Imagine a horizontal line and a

## ▶ The Body Systems

In injuries and illnesses, most life-threatening conditions affect the respiratory, circulatory, and nervous systems. These three body systems include the most important and sensitive organs: the lungs, the heart, the brain, and the spinal cord. The other body systems are also important, and thorough assessment of the person can locate injury and/or sudden illnesses affecting them as well. The major body systems described in this chapter are the respiratory, circulatory, nervous, skeletal, and muscular systems. The skin is also described. The other body systems—including the endocrine, gastrointestinal, and genitourinary systems—are summarized in **Table 3-1** .

## Table 3-1  The Human Body Systems

| System | Function | Major Components | Interactions With Other Systems |
|---|---|---|---|
| Digestive | • Takes in food (ingestion)<br>• Digests food into smaller molecules and absorbs nutrients<br>• Removes indigestible food from body (feces) | • Mouth<br>• Esophagus<br>• Stomach<br>• Small intestine<br>• Large intestine<br>• Rectum<br>• Anus<br>• Salivary glands<br>• Pancreas<br>• Liver<br>• Gallbladder | • Circulatory system: Absorbs and delivers the digested nutrients to the cells<br>• Muscular system: Controls the contractions of many of the digestive organs to pass food along<br>• Nervous system: Hypothalamus maintains homeostasis by triggering appetite (stomach growling) |
| Circulatory | Transports materials to and from cells | • Heart<br>• Veins<br>• Arteries<br>• Capillaries<br>• Blood | • Respiratory system: Delivers $O_2$ from lungs to cells and drops off $CO_2$ from cells to lungs<br>• Digestive system: Absorbs and delivers digested nutrients to cells<br>• Excretory system: Kidneys filter cellular waste out of blood for removal<br>• Lymphatic system: Transports tissue fluid back to the circulatory system<br>• Immune system: Transports WBCs throughout the body to fight disease<br>• Nervous system: Brain controls heartbeat<br>• Endocrine system: Transports hormones |
| Nervous | • Gathers and interprets information<br>• Responds to information<br>• Helps maintain homeostasis | • Brain<br>• Spinal cord<br>• Nerves<br>• Neurons | • Controls all other systems<br>• Maintains homeostasis by working with all systems |
| Excretory | • Removes waste products from cellular metabolism<br>• Filters blood | • Kidneys<br>• Ureters<br>• Bladder<br>• Urethra<br>• Lungs<br>• Skin<br>• Liver | • Circulatory system: Filters waste out of blood<br>• Lungs: Removes excretory waste<br>• Integumentary system: Removes excretory waste |
| Respiratory | Takes in $O_2$ and removes $CO_2$ and water | • Nose<br>• Trachea<br>• Bronchi<br>• Bronchioles<br>• Alveoli<br>• Lungs | • Circulatory system: Takes in $O_2$ for delivery to cells and removes $CO_2$ brought from cells<br>• Excretory system: Removes excretory waste<br>• Nervous system: Controls breathing<br>• Muscular system: Diaphragm controls breathing |
| Skeletal | • Protects organs<br>• Provides shape and support<br>• Stores materials (fats, minerals)<br>• Produces blood cells<br>• Allows movement | • Bones<br>• Cartilage<br>• Ligaments | • Muscular system: Allows movement<br>• Circulatory system: Produces blood cells<br>• Immune system: Produces WBCs<br>• Circulatory and respiratory systems: Protects its organs |

*(Continues)*

## Table 3-1 The Human Body Systems, Continued

| System | Function | Major Components | Interactions With Other Systems |
|---|---|---|---|
| Muscular | Allows for movement by contracting | • Skeletal muscle<br>• Tendons | • Skeletal system: Allows movement<br>• Digestive system: Allows organs to contract to push food through<br>• Respiratory system: Diaphragm controls breathing<br>• Circulatory system: Controls pumping of blood<br>• Nervous system: Controls all muscle contractions |
| Endocrine | Regulates body activities using hormones (slow response, long lasting) | • Glands<br>  • Hypothalamus<br>  • Pituitary<br>  • Thyroid<br>  • Thymus<br>  • Adrenal<br>  • Pancreas<br>  • Ovaries<br>  • Testes | • Circulatory system: Transports hormones to target organs<br>• Nervous system: Maintains homeostasis, hormone release<br>• Reproductive system: Controlled by hormones<br>• Skeletal system: Controls growth of bones |
| Immune | Fights off foreign invaders in the body | • WBCs<br>  • T cells<br>  • B cells<br>  • Macrophages<br>• Skin | • Circulatory system: Transports WBCs to fight invaders<br>• Lymphatic system: Has lots of WBCs to fight invaders; spleen filters bacteria/viruses out of blood<br>• Skeletal system: WBCs made in bone marrow<br>• Integumentary system: Prevents invaders from getting in |
| Integumentary | • Acts as barrier against infection<br>• Helps regulate body temperature<br>• Removes excretory waste<br>• Protects against sun's ultraviolet rays<br>• Produces vitamin D | • Skin<br>  • Epidermis<br>  • Dermis | • Excretory system: Removes cellular waste<br>• Nervous system: Controls body temperature<br>• Immune system: Prevents pathogens from entering |
| Lymphatic | • Stores and carries WBCs that fight disease<br>• Collects excess fluid and returns it to blood (acts as a second circulatory system; reaches places other circulatory system cannot) | • Lymph (liquid part of blood)<br>• Lymph vessels<br>• Lymph nodes<br>• WBCs | • Immune system: Holds lots of WBCs to fight pathogens<br>• Circulatory system: Transports materials from cells |
| Reproductive | Allows organisms to reproduce, which prevents their species from becoming extinct | • Ovaries<br>• Testes | • Endocrine system: Controls production of sex cells<br>• Muscular system: Uterus contracts to give birth; controlled by hormones |

$CO_2$ = carbon dioxide; $O_2$ = oxygen; WBCs = white blood cells.

# ▶ The Respiratory System

The body can store food to last several weeks and water to last several days, but it can store enough oxygen for only a few minutes. Ordinarily, this limited oxygen reserve is not a concern because we only have to inhale air to get the oxygen we need. However, if the body's oxygen supply is cut off, as in drowning, choking, or smothering, death will result in about 4 to 6 minutes unless the oxygen intake is restored. Oxygen from air is made available to the blood through the **respiratory system** Figure 3-3 and then to the body cells by the circulatory system.

## Nose

Air normally enters the body during inhalation through the nostrils. It is warmed, moistened, and filtered as it flows over the damp, mucous membrane (sticky lining) of the nose. When a person breathes through the mouth instead of the nose, there is less filtration and warming. After passing through the nasal passages, air enters the nasal portion of the **pharynx** (throat).

## Pharynx and Trachea

From the back of the nose or the mouth, the air enters the pharynx. The pharynx is a common passageway for food and air. At its lower end, the pharynx divides into two passageways: one for food and the other for air. Muscular control in the back of the throat routes food to the **esophagus** (food tube), which leads to the stomach; air is routed from the pharynx to the **trachea** (windpipe), which leads to the lungs. The trachea and the esophagus are separated by a small flap of tissue,

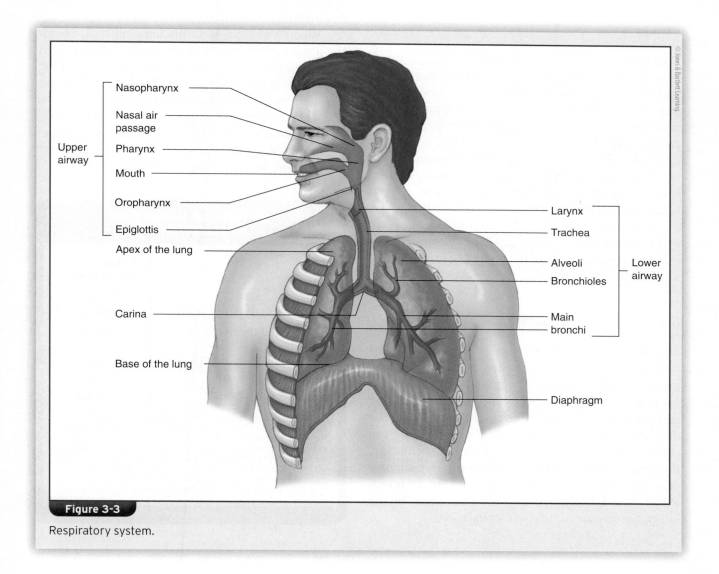

**Figure 3-3**

Respiratory system.

the **epiglottis**, which diverts food away from the trachea. Usually this diversion works automatically to keep food out of the trachea and to prevent air from entering the esophagus. If the muscles of the pharynx and larynx are not coordinated, food or other liquid can enter the trachea instead of the esophagus.

Normal swallowing controls do not operate if a person is unresponsive. That is why a first aid provider should never pour liquid into the mouth of an unresponsive person in an attempt to revive him or her. The liquid could flow into the windpipe and suffocate the person. Foreign objects, such as false teeth or a piece of food, might also lodge in the throat or windpipe and cut off the passage of air. In the upper 2 inches (5 cm) of the trachea, just below the epiglottis, is the **larynx** (voice box), which contains the vocal cords. The larynx can be felt in the front of the throat (**Adam's apple**).

## Lungs

The trachea branches into two tubes (**bronchial tubes** or bronchi), one for each lung. Each bronchus divides and subdivides somewhat like the branches of a tree. The smallest bronchioles end in thousands of tiny pouches (**alveoli**, or air sacs), just as the twigs of a tree end in leaves. Each air sac is enclosed in a network of capillaries. The walls that separate the air sacs and the capillaries are very thin. Through those walls, oxygen combines with the hemoglobin in red blood cells to form oxyhemoglobin, which is carried to all parts of the body. Carbon dioxide and certain other waste gases in the blood move across the capillary walls into the air sacs and are exhaled from the body. The lungs occupy most of the chest cavity.

## Mechanics of Breathing

The passage of air into and out of the lungs is called respiration. Breathing in is called inhalation; breathing out is called exhalation. Ventilation is a mechanical process brought about by alternately increasing and decreasing the size of the chest cavity. When the **diaphragm** (the dome-shaped muscle dividing the chest from the abdomen) contracts, the chest expands, drawing air into the lungs (inhalation). An exchange of oxygen and carbon dioxide takes place in the lungs. When the diaphragm relaxes, it exerts pressure on the lungs, causing air to flow out (exhalation).

Infants and children differ from adults. Their respiratory structures are smaller and more easily obstructed than those of adults. Infants' and children's tongues take up proportionally more space in the mouth than do the tongues of adults. The trachea is more flexible in infants and children. The primary cause of cardiac arrest in infants and children is an uncorrected respiratory condition.

The average rate of breathing in an adult at rest is 12 to 20 complete respirations per minute Table 3-2 . Normal rates for children are 18 to 40 respirations per minute; infant rates are 30 to 60 respirations per minute. Normally the rate slows when a person is lying down and speeds up during vigorous exercise. The rate of breathing is controlled by a nerve center in the brain. Signs of inadequate breathing include a rate of breathing outside the normal range, cool or clammy skin that is pale or cyanotic (blue-purple), and nasal flaring, especially in children.

When a person performs hard muscular work, the lungs cannot get rid of carbon dioxide or take in oxygen fast enough at the normal rate of breathing. As carbon dioxide increases in the blood and tissues, the brain sends impulses along its nerves to cause deeper and more rapid respirations. At the same time, the heart rate increases. This faster heart rate increases the supply of oxygen available to the body as the heart pumps more blood through the lungs.

### Table 3-2 Normal Ranges for Respirations

| Age | Range (breaths/min) |
| --- | --- |
| Adults | 12 to 20 |
| Adolescents (13 to 18 years) | 12 to 16 |
| School-aged children (6 to 12 years) | 18 to 30 |
| Preschoolers (4 to 5 years) | 22 to 34 |
| Toddlers (1 to 3 years) | 24 to 40 |
| Infants | 30 to 60 |

*Note:* Adult respiratory ranges are per the NHTSA 2009 EMT National EMS Education Standards. Pediatric ranges are modified from Pediatric Advanced Life Support, 2012, the American Heart Association. Ranges presented in other sources may vary. To obtain the respiratory rate in a person, count the number of breaths in a 30-second period and multiply by 2. A person's awareness that respirations are being counted can influence the respiratory rate, so avoid letting the person know you are counting respirations.

© Jones & Bartlett Learning

# ▶ The Circulatory System

The <u>circulatory system</u> Figure 3-4 is made up of the blood, the heart, and the blood vessels. Blood is the delivery system for cells throughout the body. It carries nutrients and other products from the digestive tract in its plasma, and it carries oxygen from the lungs in its hemoglobin. It also transports wastes produced by the cells to the lungs, kidneys, and other excretory organs for removal from the body.

## Heart

The human circulatory system is a completely closed circuit of tubelike vessels through which blood flows. The <u>heart</u> Figure 3-5 , by contracting and relaxing, pumps blood through the vessels. It is a powerful, hollow, muscular organ about as big as a man's clenched fist, shaped like a pear, and located in the left center of the chest, behind the sternum (breast bone). The heart is divided by a wall in the middle. Right and left compartments are divided into two chambers, the atrium above and the ventricle below. Check valves are located between each atrium and its corresponding ventricle and at the exit of the major arteries leading out of each ventricle. The opening and shutting of these valves at just the right time in the heartbeat keeps the blood from backing up.

**Figure 3-4**

Circulatory system.

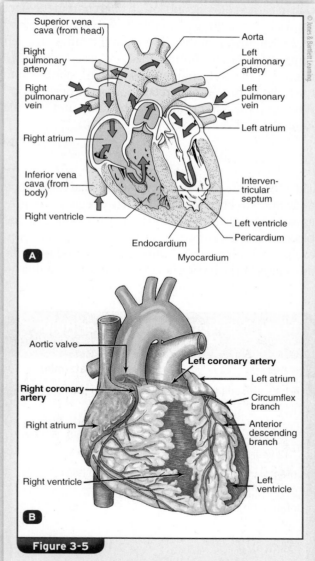

**Figure 3-5**

The heart. **A.** Circulation (internal view). **B.** The two main coronary arteries supply the heart with blood.

**Did You Know?**

The carotid arteries along the neck convey the blood to the head, and if pressure is applied to them, the individual becomes unconscious, seeming to drop off into a stupor or slumber. Hence, the Greeks called these arteries the *karotides* from the Greek word *karoun*, meaning "to stupefy."

*Source:* Skinner HA. *The Origin of Medical Terms*. 2nd ed. Baltimore, MD: Williams & Wilkins; 1961.

At each beat, or contraction, the heart pumps blood rich in carbon dioxide and low in oxygen from the right ventricle to the lungs and returns oxygen-rich blood to the left atrium of the heart from the lungs. The left ventricle pushes freshly obtained, oxygen-rich blood to the rest of the body and returns oxygen-poor blood to the right atrium. At each relaxation of the heart, blood flows into the left atrium from the lungs and into the right atrium from the rest of the body .

## Blood Vessels

The **arteries** are elastic, muscular tubes that carry blood away from the heart **Figure 3-6**. They begin at the heart as two large tubes: the pulmonary artery, which carries blood to the lungs for the carbon dioxide and oxygen exchange, and the **aorta**, which carries blood to all the other parts of the body. The aorta divides and subdivides

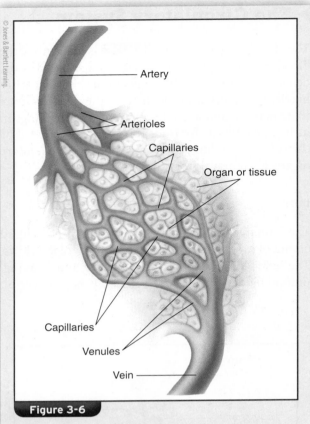

**Figure 3-6**

Blood enters an organ or tissue through the arteries and leaves through the veins. This process provides adequate blood flow to the tissue to meet the cells' needs.

until it ends in networks of extremely fine vessels (**capillaries**) smaller than hairs. Through the thin walls of the capillaries, oxygen and nourishment pass out of the bloodstream into the stationary cells of the body, while the body cells discharge their waste products into the bloodstream. In the capillaries of the lungs, carbon dioxide is released and oxygen is absorbed. Capillaries, having reached their limit of subdivision, begin to join together again into veins. The **veins** become larger and

| Table 3-3 Normal Ranges for Pulse Rate | |
|---|---|
| **Age** | **Range (beats/min)** |
| Adults and children (older than 10 years) | 60 to 100 |
| Preschoolers and school-aged children (2 years to 10 years) | 60 to 140 |
| Infants and toddlers (3 months to 2 years) | 100 to 190 |
| Infants (up to 3 months of age) | 85 to 205 |

*Data From Pediatric Advanced Life Support, 2012, the American Heart Association.*

*Note:* An adult's pulse rate can be affected by his or her physical condition (adults in good cardiovascular condition may have heart rates near 40 beats/min), age, medications, and gender (females 12 years and older tend to have faster pulse rates than males).

**Word Origins**

Arteries received their name from the Greek term for windpipe because the Greek physician Praxagoras thought they carried air. In corpses, they are usually empty and that was probably where his observations were made.

*Source:* Skinner HA. *The Origin of Medical Terms*. 2nd ed. Baltimore, MD: Williams & Wilkins; 1961.

larger and finally form major trunks that empty blood returning from the body into the right atrium and blood from the lungs into the left atrium.

It is impossible to prick normal skin anywhere without puncturing capillaries. Because the flow of blood through the capillaries is relatively slow and under little pressure, blood merely oozes from a punctured capillary and usually has time to clot, promptly plugging the leak.

Each time the heart contracts, the surge of blood can be felt as a **pulse** at any point where an artery lies close to the surface of the body, near the skin surface and over a bone. When an artery is cut, blood spurts out. There is no pulse in a vein because the pulse is lost by the time the blood has passed through the capillaries. Hence, blood from a cut vein flows out in a steady stream. It has much less pressure behind it than blood from a cut artery.

Major locations for feeling pulses include the following **Figure 3-7** :

- **Carotid artery**: The major artery of the neck, which supplies the head with blood. Pulsations can be palpated (felt) on either side of

the neck (do not try to feel both at the same time). Health care providers use the carotid artery to check an unresponsive person's pulse.
- **Femoral artery**: The major artery of the thigh, which supplies the lower extremities with blood. Pulsations can be palpated in the groin area (the crease between the abdomen and the thigh).
- **Radial artery**: The major artery of the lower arm. Pulsations can be palpated at the palm side of the wristwrist on the thumb side. Use the radial location to check an alert person's pulse.
- **Brachial artery**: An artery of the upper arm. Pulsations can be palpated on the inside of the arm between the elbow and the armpit. Health care providers use the brachial location to determine a pulse in an infant.
- **Posterior tibial artery**: Located behind the inside ankle knob (medial malleolus). Pulsations can be palpated behind the posterior surface of the medial malleolus.
- **Dorsalis pedis artery**: Pulsations can be palpated on the top surface of the foot (many people have no pulsations here).

## Blood Pressure

Blood pressure is a measure of the pressure exerted by the blood on the walls of the flexible arteries. Blood pressure might be high or low according to the resistance offered by the walls to the passage of blood. This difference in resistance could have several causes. For example, if blood does not fill the system, as occurs following a hemorrhage, the pressure will be low (hypotension). High blood pressure (hypertension) might be present when the arterial walls have become hard and cannot expand readily.

## Blood

**Blood** has liquid and solid portions. The liquid portion is called plasma. The solid portion, which is transported by the plasma, includes disklike red blood cells; slightly larger, irregularly shaped white blood cells; and smaller bodies called **platelets**.

**Plasma**, the liquid part of the blood, is about 90% water, in which minerals, sugar, and other materials are dissolved. Plasma carries food materials picked up from the digestive tract and transports them to the body cells. It also carries waste materials produced by cells to the kidneys, digestive tract, sweat glands, and lungs for elimination (excretion) in urine, feces, sweat, and expired breath.

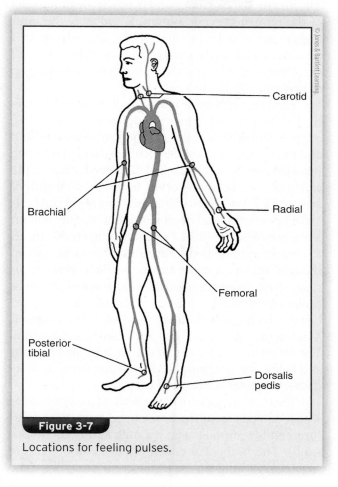

© Jones & Bartlett Learning.

Carotid

Brachial

Radial

Femoral

Posterior tibial

Dorsalis pedis

**Figure 3-7**

Locations for feeling pulses.

The <u>red blood cells</u>, which give blood its color, carry oxygen to the organs. The <u>white blood cells</u> are part of the body's defense against infection. These cells can go wherever they are needed in the body to fight infection, such as to a wound in the skin or to other tissue that is diseased or injured. Pus, a sign of wound infection, gets its yellow-white color from the innumerable white blood cells that are fighting the invading bacteria.

Platelets are essential for the formation of blood clots. If blood plasma did not clot at the site of a wound, the slightest cut or abrasion would produce death from bleeding. Clots plug the openings through which blood escapes from punctured blood vessels. Bleeding from a large blood vessel could be too rapid to permit the formation of a clot. *Hemorrhage* is the term for profuse bleeding.

<u>Perfusion</u> refers to the circulation of blood through an organ or a structure. Hypoperfusion is the inadequate circulation of blood through an organ or a structure. The average-size man has about 6 quarts (12 pints [roughly 6 L]) of blood.

Inadequate circulation is known as shock (hypoperfusion). Shock is a state of profound depression of the vital processes of the body and may be characterized by the following signs and symptoms: pale or cyanotic (blue) skin; cool, clammy skin; rapid pulse; rapid breathing; restlessness, anxiety, or mental dullness; nausea and vomiting; reduction in total blood volume; low or decreasing blood pressure; and subnormal body temperature.

## ▶ The Nervous System

The <u>nervous system</u> is a complex collection of nerve cells (neurons) that coordinate the work of all parts of the human body and keep the individual in touch with the outside world. Neurons receive stimuli from the environment and transmit impulses to nerve centers in the brain and spinal cord. Then, through a complicated process that includes signals from the conscious thoughts of the person, in addition to reflex and automatic reactions, they produce nerve impulses that regulate and coordinate all bodily movements and functions and govern behavior and consciousness.

Once neurons have been destroyed, the body cannot regenerate them. Some limited nerve repair is possible, however, as long as the vital cell body is intact. If a nerve fiber is cut or injured, the section attached to the cell body remains alive, but the part beyond the injury withers away.

The nervous system can be classified in different ways. From a structural standpoint, it can be divided into the <u>central nervous system (CNS)</u> and the <u>peripheral nervous system</u>. The CNS includes the brain and the spinal cord. The peripheral nervous system is a network of nerve cells that originates in the brain and spinal cord and extends to all parts of the body, including the muscles, the surface of the skin, and the special sense organs, such as the eyes and the ears. The peripheral nervous system is further subdivided into the voluntary and the autonomic (involuntary) nervous systems.

## Central Nervous System

The CNS consists of the brain, which is enclosed within the skull, and the spinal cord, which is housed in a semiflexible bony column of vertebrae. The CNS serves as the controlling organ of the body. The brain enables us to think, judge, and act. The spinal cord is a major communication pathway between the brain and the rest of the body.

### Brain

The <u>brain</u> **Figure 3-8** , which is the headquarters of the human nervous system, is probably the most highly specialized organ in the body. It weighs about 3 pounds (1.4 kg) in the average adult, is richly supplied with blood vessels, and requires considerable oxygen to perform effectively.

The brain has three main subdivisions: the <u>cerebrum</u> (large brain), which occupies nearly all (75%) of the cranial cavity; the <u>cerebellum</u> (small brain); and the <u>brainstem</u>. The cerebrum is divided into two hemispheres by a deep cleft. The outer surface of the cerebrum, the cerebral cortex, is about one-eighth of an inch (3.2 mm) thick, composed mainly of cell bodies of nerve cells, and often referred to as gray matter.

Certain sections of the cerebrum are localized to control specific body functions such as sensation, thought, and associative memory, which allows us to store, recall, and make use of past experiences. The sight center of the brain is located at the back of the cerebrum, which is called the occipital lobe. The temporal lobes, at the sides of the head, direct smell and hearing. The cerebellum is located at the back of the <u>cranium</u> and below the cerebrum. Its main function is to coordinate muscular activity and balance.

The third major area of the brain is the brainstem, which extends from the base of the cerebrum to the <u>foramen magnum</u> (a large opening at the base of the skull). The brainstem controls automatic functions such as breathing and heart rate.

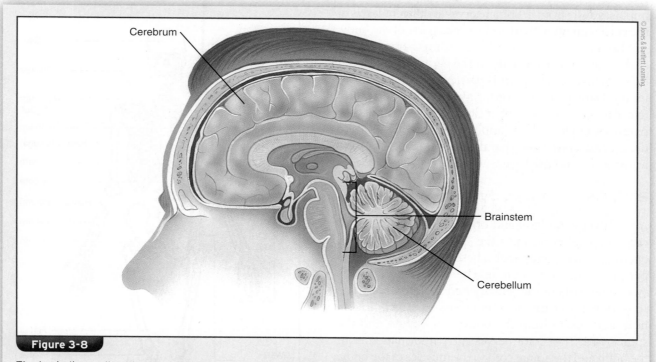

**Figure 3-8**

The brain lies well protected within the skull. Its principal subdivisions are the cerebrum, the cerebellum, and the brainstem.

Small cavities in the brain contain the **cerebrospinal fluid (CSF)**, a clear, watery solution similar to blood plasma. Circulating around the brain and the spinal cord, CSF serves as a protective cushion and exchanges food and waste materials. The total quantity of CSF in the brain–spinal cord system is 100 to 150 mL, although up to several liters can be produced daily. It is constantly being produced and reabsorbed.

Knowledge of nerve structure and function enables physicians to locate diseased brain sections. Because nerves from one side of the body eventually connect with the opposite side of the brain, a person whose left arm is paralyzed after a stroke will have suffered damage to the right side of the brain.

### Spinal Cord

The **spinal cord** is a soft column of nerve tissue continuous with the lower part of the brain that is enclosed in the bony vertebral column **Figure 3-9**. The spinal cord exits the brain through the foramen magnum, which is a hole in the base of the skull. Thirty-one pairs of spinal nerves branch from the spinal cord. These nerves are large trunks that are similar to telephone cables because they house many nerve fibers. Some fibers carry impulses into the spinal cord; others carry

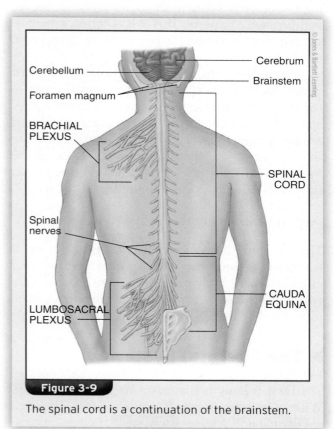

**Figure 3-9**

The spinal cord is a continuation of the brainstem.

impulses away from it. Spinal nerves at different levels of the cord regulate activities of various parts of the body.

Because the spinal cord lies within the bony walls of the vertebrae, especially in the cervical (neck) and thoracic (chest) regions, it is particularly vulnerable to injury. Damage to the cord is almost always irreversible. An injury to the lumbar (lower back) spine causes paralysis and loss of sensation in the legs; an injury to the cervical cord causes paralysis and loss of sensation in the arms and the legs.

## Peripheral Nervous System

At each vertebral level and on each side of the spinal cord, a spinal nerve exits the spinal cord through an opening in the bony canal. These nerves make up the peripheral nervous system. The peripheral nervous system consists of the sensory and motor nerves. The sensory nerves carry sensations such as smell, touch, heat, and sound from the body to the brain and the spinal cord. The motor nerves carry information from the brain and the spinal cord to the muscles of the body.

If a nerve is cut or seriously damaged, disrupting the connection between the brain and the body, the body part will not be able to work. For example, if the motor nerve going to the right leg is cut, the leg will be unable to move. This loss of function may be permanent. Injuries to the nerves in the spinal cord can be very serious.

Fortunately, the CNS is well protected against injury. The brain is enclosed in the cranial cavity of the skull. The spinal cord is contained in the hollow space of the vertebrae. The brain and the spinal cord are also protected by three layers of tissue known as the meninges. The space between the layers of the meninges is filled with CSF, which also helps protect the brain and spinal cord from injury.

## Autonomic Nervous System

The autonomic nervous system consists of a group of nerves that control heart rate, digestion, sweating, and other automatic body processes. These processes are not controlled by the conscious mind, but they can be influenced by the CNS to a limited extent.

## ▶ The Skeletal System

The human body is shaped by its bony framework. Without its bones, the body would collapse. The adult **skeleton** has 206 bones **Figure 3-10** . **Bones** are composed of living cells surrounded by hard deposits of

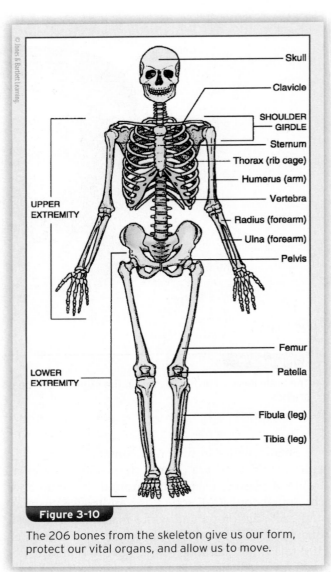

**Figure 3-10**

The 206 bones from the skeleton give us our form, protect our vital organs, and allow us to move.

calcium. The bone cells are well supplied by blood vessels and nerves. The calcium deposits give bones their strength and rigidity. Broken bones are repaired by bone-building cells within the bone and its covering sheath, the periosteum. New bone is formed at the site of the break, much as two pieces of steel are welded together.

## Skull

The skull rests at the top of the spinal column. It contains the brain, certain special-purpose glands (such as the pituitary and the pineal), and the centers of special senses—sight, hearing, taste, and smell. The skull has two parts, the brain case (cranium) and the face **Figure 3-11** . Blood vessels and nerve trunks pass to and from the brain through openings in the skull, mostly at the base. The largest opening is the foramen

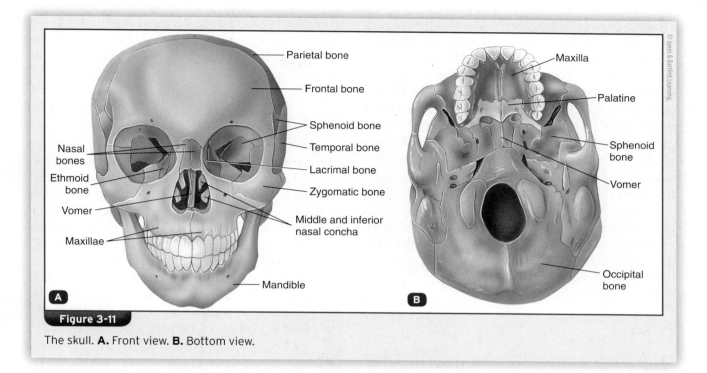

**Figure 3-11**

The skull. **A.** Front view. **B.** Bottom view.

magnum, where the spinal cord exits the skull and joins the brain. The brain, which fits snugly in the cranium, is covered by the meninges. The very narrow spaces between the meninges are filled with CSF.

Although the skull is very tough, a blow can fracture it. Even if there is no fracture, a sudden impact can tear or bruise the brain and cause it to swell, just as any soft tissue swells following an injury or a bruise. Because the skull does not "give," injury to the brain is magnified by the contained pressure within the skull. Unresponsiveness or even death could result from swelling (edema), a tearing wound (laceration), bleeding, or other damage to the brain. The face extends from the eyebrows to the chin and contains the eyes, nose, cheeks, mouth, and lower jaw (mandible).

## Spinal Column

The spinal column **Figure 3-12** is made up of irregularly shaped bones called **vertebrae** (singular is vertebra). Lying one on top of the other to form a strong, flexible column, the vertebrae are bound firmly together by strong **ligaments**. Between every two vertebrae is an intervertebral disk, a pad of tough elastic cartilage that acts as a shock absorber.

The spinal column can be damaged by disease or by injury. A crushed or displaced vertebra can squeeze, stretch, tear, or sever the spinal cord. Careless handling of an injured person by well-meaning but uninformed people or movement of the disabled part

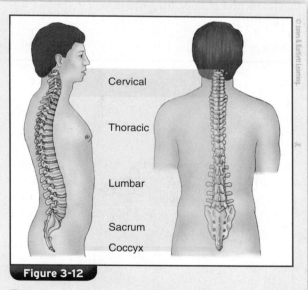

**Figure 3-12**

The spinal column (spine) is composed of 33 bones.

by the injured person can result in additional injury to the cord and possibly permanent paralysis. For that reason, a person with a back or neck injury must be handled with extreme care.

## Thorax

The **thorax** (rib cage) is made up of ribs and the sternum (breast bone). The **sternum** is a flat, narrow bone in the middle of the front wall of the chest.

The lowest portion of the sternum is the <u>**xiphoid process**</u>. The collar bones and certain ribs are attached to the sternum. The 24 ribs are semiflexible arches of bone. There are 12 on each side of the chest. The back ends of the 12 pairs of ribs are attached to the 12 thoracic vertebrae. Strong ligaments bind the back ends of the ribs to the backbone but allow slight gliding or tilting movements. The front ends of the top 10 pairs of ribs are attached to the sternum by cartilage. The front ends of the last two pairs (pairs 11 and 12) hang free, giving them the name <u>**floating ribs**</u>.

Fractures of the sternum or the ribs usually result from crushing or squeezing the chest. A fall, blow, or penetration of the chest wall by an object can have the same effect. The chief danger from such injuries is that the lungs might be punctured by the sharp ends of the broken bones.

## Pelvis

The two hipbones and the sacrum form the pelvic girdle (pelvis). Muscles help connect the pelvic bones, the trunk, the thighs, and the legs. The pelvis forms the floor of the abdominal cavity. The lower part of the cavity, sometimes called the pelvic cavity, holds the bladder, rectum, and internal parts of the reproductive organs. The floor of the pelvic cavity helps to support the intestines.

## Leg Bones

### Upper Leg (Thigh)

At the outer side of each hipbone is a deep socket into which the round head of the thigh bone (<u>**femur**</u>) fits, forming a ball-and-socket joint. The lower end of the femur is flat and has two knobs. These knobs articulate with the shin bone (tibia) at the knee joint. Although the femur is the longest and strongest bone in the skeleton, it is a common fracture site. A fractured femur is always serious because it is difficult to align the broken or splintered ends. Because of the force required to break the femur, laceration of the surrounding tissues, pain, and blood loss could be extensive.

### Knee

The knee joint is the largest joint in the body and is a strong hinge joint **Figure 3-13**. The joint is protected and stabilized in the front by the knee cap (patella).

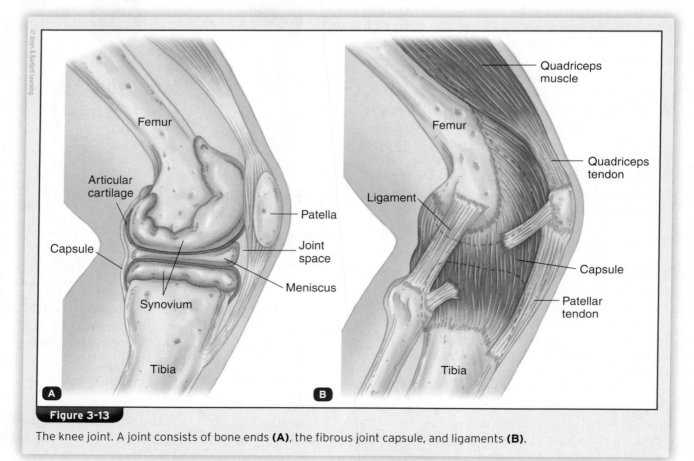

**Figure 3-13**

The knee joint. A joint consists of bone ends **(A)**, the fibrous joint capsule, and ligaments **(B)**.

The <u>patella</u> is a small, triangular-shaped bone in front of and between the femur and the tibia and within the tendon of the large muscle (the quadraceps) of the front of the thigh. Because the patella usually receives the force of falls or blows to the knee, it is frequently bruised or dislocated and sometimes fractured.

## Lower Leg

The lower leg refers to the portion of the lower extremity between the knee and the ankle. Its two bones are the tibia and the fibula **Figure 3-14**. The <u>tibia</u> (shin bone) is at the front and inner side of the leg. It is palpable throughout its length. Its broad upper surface receives the end of the femur to form the knee joint. The lower end, much smaller than the upper end, forms the inner rounded knob of the ankle (medial malleolus). The <u>fibula</u>, which is not a part of the true knee joint, is attached at the top to the tibia. Its lower end forms the outside ankle knob (lateral malleolus). The fibula is more often fractured alone than is the tibia.

## Ankles, Feet, and Toes

The ends of the tibia and fibula form the socket of the ankle joint. Both ankle knobs are easily palpated. The seven ankle bones (tarsals) are bound firmly together by tough ligaments. The heel bone (calcaneus) transmits the weight of the body to the ground and forms a base for the muscles of the calf of the leg when walking **Figure 3-15**. The sole and the instep of the foot are formed by the five long metatarsals. These bones articulate with the tarsals and with the front row of toe bones (phalanges).

## Shoulder

The collar bone (clavicle) and the shoulder blade (scapula) form the shoulder girdle. Each <u>clavicle</u>—a long, slightly double-curved bone—is attached to the sternum at its inner end and to the scapula at its outer end. Each clavicle can be palpated throughout its length. Fractures are common because the clavicle lies close to the surface and must absorb blows. Each

**Figure 3-14**

The principal parts of the lower extremity include the thigh, leg, and foot. The principal parts of the lower leg include the tibia and fibula.

**Figure 3-15**

**A.** The surface landmarks of the foot and ankle include the medial malleolus, the calcaneus, and the phalanges. **B.** Soft tissue of the ankle.

scapula—a large, flat, triangular bone—is located over the upper ribs at the back of the thorax.

## Arm Bones

### Upper Arm

The bone of the upper arm, the **humerus**, is the arm's largest bone. Its upper end (the head) is round; its lower end is flat. The round head fits into a shallow cup in the shoulder blade, forming a ball-and-socket joint. This is the most freely movable joint in the body and is easily dislocated. Dislocations can tear the capsule of the joint (synovial membrane) and cause damage. Improper manipulation during attempts to reduce or set the dislocation could add to the damage. Therefore, it is important to treat dislocations of the shoulder with gentle care.

### Forearm

The two bones of the forearm (radius and ulna) lie side by side. The larger of the two, the **ulna**, is on the little finger side, and part of it forms the elbow. The flat, curved lower end of the humerus fits into a big notch at the upper end of the ulna to form the elbow joint. This hinge joint permits movement in one direction only. The **radius**, shorter and smaller than the ulna, is on the thumb side of the forearm Figure 3-16 .

## Wrist, Hand, and Fingers

The wrist is composed of eight small, irregularly shaped bones (carpals) united by ligaments. Tendons extending from the muscles of the forearm to the bones of the hand and fingers pass down the front and the back of the wrist close to the surface. Wrist lacerations could sever these tendons, resulting in total or partial immobility of the fingers.

The palm of the hand has five long bones (metacarpals). The 14 bones of the fingers (phalanges) give the hand its great flexibility. The thumb is the most important digit. A functioning thumb and one or two fingers make a far more useful hand than four fingers minus the thumb Figure 3-17 .

## Joints

A **joint** is where two or more bones meet or join. Some joints, such as those in the cranium, allow little, if any, movement of the bones. Other joints, such as the hip and the shoulder, allow a wide range of motion. In a typical joint, a layer of cartilage (gristle), which is softer than bone, acts as a pad or buffer. The bones of such a joint are held in place by firmly attached ligaments, which are bands of very dense, tough, but

**Figure 3-16**

The principal bones in the arm and forearm include the humerus, the radius, and the ulna.

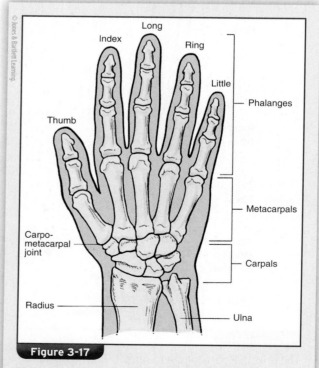

**Figure 3-17**

The principal bones in the wrist and hand include the carpals, the metacarpals, and the phalanges.

flexible connective tissue. Joints are enclosed in a capsule, a layer of thin, tough material, strengthened by the ligaments. The inner side of the capsule (synovial membrane) secretes a thick fluid (synovial fluid) that lubricates and protects the joint.

## ▶ The Muscular System

Body movement is due to work performed by muscles. Examples are walking, breathing, the beating of the heart, and the movements of the stomach and the intestines. What enables muscle tissue to perform work is its ability to contract—that is, to become shorter and thicker—when stimulated by a nerve impulse. The cells of a muscle, usually long and threadlike, are called fibers. Each muscle has countless bundles of closely packed, overlapping fibers bound together by connective tissue. The three kinds of muscles are skeletal muscle (voluntary), smooth muscle (involuntary), and cardiac muscle (heart). They differ in appearance and in the specific jobs they do **Figure 3-18**.

© Jones & Bartlett Learning

Cardiac muscle

Skeletal muscle

Smooth muscle

**Figure 3-18**

The three types of muscles are skeletal, smooth, and cardiac.

The **voluntary muscles**, which are under the control of a person's will, make possible all deliberate acts, including walking, chewing, swallowing, smiling, frowning, talking, and moving the eyeballs. Also called **skeletal muscles**, most voluntary muscles are attached by one or both ends to the skeleton by tendons. However, some muscles are attached to skin, cartilage, and special organs (such as the eyeball) or to other muscles, such as the tongue.

Muscles help to shape the body and to form its walls. Most skeletal muscles end in tough, whitish cords (**tendons**) that attach them to the bones they move. Tendons continue into the fascia, which covers the skeletal muscles. The fascia is much like the skin of a sausage in that it surrounds the muscle tissue. At either end of the muscle, the fascia extends beyond the muscle to attach to a bone. Tendons are covered with a synovial membrane, which secretes a lubricating substance, the synovial fluid. This lubrication makes it easier for the tendon to move when the muscle contracts or relaxes. Muscular contraction pulls the bone in the direction permitted by a joint.

When they are not working, muscles become comparatively slack. Normally, muscles never completely relax; some fibers are contracting all the time. They always have some tension (muscle tone). Loss of muscle tone can be a sign of nerve injury. Muscles can be injured in many ways. Overexerting a muscle can break fibers. Muscles can be bruised, crushed, cut, torn, or otherwise injured, with or without breaking the skin. Muscles injured in any of those ways are likely to become swollen, tender, painful, or weak.

A person has little or no control over the **smooth muscles** and usually is not conscious of them. Smooth muscles line the walls of tubelike structures such as the gastrointestinal tract, the urinary system, the blood vessels, and the bronchi of the lungs. **Cardiac muscle** is a specialized form of muscle found only in the heart. A continuous supply of oxygen and glucose is needed for cardiac muscle to work properly.

## ▶ The Skin

The skin covers the entire body, protecting the deep tissues from being injured, drying out, or being invaded by bacteria and other foreign bodies. The skin helps to regulate body temperature by aiding in the elimination of water and various salts. The skin senses heat, cold, touch, pressure, and pain and transmits that information to the brain and the spinal cord.

The skin consists of two layers: the outer layer (**epidermis**) and the inner layer (**dermis**) **Figure 3-19**. The epidermis varies in thickness in different parts of the body (the palms and the soles of the feet are thickest), and its dead cells are constantly worn off. The dermis has a rich supply of blood vessels and nerve endings. Hair grows from the dermis through openings called hair follicles. Sweat glands and oil glands in the dermis empty onto the surface of the epidermis through pores in the skin. Beneath the dermis is the subcutaneous (meaning "under the skin") layer, which is well supplied with fat cells and blood vessels.

Sweat glands, which create perspiration, occur in nearly all parts of the skin. Sweat contains essentially the same minerals as blood plasma and urine, but it is more diluted. Normally, only traces of the waste products excreted in urine are in sweat. But when sweating is profuse or when the kidneys are diseased, the amounts of such wastes excreted in the sweat could be considerable. Several mineral salts are removed from the body in sweat. Chief among those in quantity is sodium chloride (the same mineral as common table salt).

**Figure 3-19**

The skin has two main layers: the epidermis and the dermis. Below the skin is a layer of subcutaneous tissue.

## prep kit

## ▶ Ready for Review

- A first aid provider must be familiar with the basic structure and functions of the human body.
- The circulatory system is made up of the blood, heart, and blood vessels.
- The nervous system is a complex collection of nerve cells that coordinate the work of all parts of the human body.
- The skeletal system is the bony framework that shapes the body.
- The muscular system lets the body move.
- Skin covers the entire body and protects the deep tissues.

## ▶ Vital Vocabulary

**abdomen** The body cavity that contains the major organs of digestion and excretion. It is located below the diaphragm and above the pelvis.

**Adam's apple** The projection on the anterior surface of the neck, formed by the thyroid cartilage over the larynx.

**alveoli** The air sacs of the lungs in which the exchange of oxygen and carbon dioxide takes place.

**anterior** The front surface of the body.

**aorta** The principal artery leaving the left side of the heart and carrying freshly oxygenated blood to the body.

**artery** A blood vessel, consisting of three layers of tissue and smooth muscle, that carries blood away from the heart.

**blood** The fluid that circulates through the heart, arteries, capillaries, and veins, carrying nutrients and oxygen to the body cells and removing waste products such as carbon dioxide and various metabolic products for excretion.

**bones** The hard form of connective tissue that constitutes most of the skeleton in humans.

**brachial artery** The artery of the arm that branches at the elbow into the radial and ulnar arteries; used to determine an infant's pulse.

**brain** The soft, large mass of nerve tissue that is contained in the cranium.

**brainstem** The area of the brain between the spinal cord and cerebrum, surrounded by the cerebellum; controls automatic functions that are necessary for life, such as respirations.

**bronchial tubes** The passageways from the trachea to the lungs.

**capillaries** The small blood vessels through whose walls various substances pass into and out of the tissues and on to the cells.

**cardiac muscle** The heart muscle.

**carotid artery** The major arteries that supply blood to the head and brain.

**central nervous system (CNS)** The brain and spinal cord.

**cerebellum** One of the three major subdivisions of the brain; coordinates voluntary body movements.

**cerebrospinal fluid (CSF)** A clear, watery solution similar to blood plasma.

**cerebrum** The largest part of the three subdivisions of the brain, made up of several lobes that control movement, hearing, balance, speech, visual perception, emotions, and personality.

**circulatory system** The arrangement of connected tubes, including the arteries, arterioles, capillaries, venules, and veins, that moves blood, oxygen, nutrients, carbon dioxide, and cellular waste throughout the body.

**clavicle** The collar bone.

**cranium** The area of the head above the ears and eyes; the part of the skull that contains the brain.

**deep** Located further inside the body and away from the skin.

**dermis** The inner layer of the skin, containing hair follicles, sweat glands, nerve endings, and blood vessels.

**diaphragm** A muscular dome that forms the undersurface of the thorax, separating the chest from the abdominal cavity. Contraction of the diaphragm brings air into the lungs. Relaxation allows air to be expelled from the lungs.

**distal** Located farther away from the point where the arm or leg attaches to the body.

**dorsalis pedis artery** The artery on the anterior (top) surface of the foot between the first and second metatarsals.

**epidermis** The outer layer of the skin, which is made up of cells that are sealed together to form a watertight protective covering for the body.

# prep kit

**epiglottis** A small flap of tissue that allows air to pass into the trachea but prevents food and liquid from entering.

**esophagus** A collapsible tube that extends from the pharynx to the stomach. Contractions of the muscle in the wall of the esophagus propel food and liquids through it to the stomach.

**femoral artery** The principal artery of the thigh. It supplies blood to the lower abdominal wall, external genitalia, and legs. It can be palpated in the groin area.

**femur** The thigh bone; the longest and one of the strongest bones in the body.

**fibula** The outer and smaller bone of the two bones of the lower leg.

**floating ribs** The 11th and 12th ribs, which do not attach to the sternum.

**foramen magnum** A large opening at the base of the skull through which the brain connects to the spinal cord.

**heart** A hollow, muscular organ that receives blood from the veins and propels it into the arteries.

**humerus** The supporting bone of the upper arm.

**inferior** Located closer to the feet.

**joint** The place where two bones come into contact.

**larynx** The voice box.

**lateral** Located farther from the middle of the body.

**ligament** A band of the fibrous tissue that connects bones to bones. It supports and strengthens a joint.

**medial** Located closer to the middle of the body.

**nervous system** The system that controls virtually all activities of the body, both voluntary and involuntary.

**patella** The knee cap; a specialized bone that lies within the tendon of the quadriceps muscle.

**perfusion** The circulation of oxygenated blood within an organ or tissue in adequate amounts to meet the cells' current needs.

**peripheral nervous system** A network of nerve cells that originates in the brain and spinal cord and extends to all parts of the body, including the muscles, the surface of the skin, and the special sense organs, such as the eyes and the ears.

**pharynx** The throat.

**plasma** A sticky, yellow fluid that carries the blood cells and nutrients and transports cellular waste material to the organs of excretion.

**platelets** Tiny, disk-shaped elements that are much smaller than cells. They are essential in the initial formation of a blood clot, the mechanism that stops bleeding.

**posterior** The back surface of the body.

**posterior tibial artery** The artery just posterior to the medial malleolus; supplies blood to the foot.

**proximal** Located closer to the point where the arm or leg attaches to the body.

**pulse** The wave of pressure created as the heart contracts and forces blood out of the left ventricle and into the major arteries.

**quadrant** A section of the abdominal cavity. Imagine a horizontal and a vertical line intersecting at the umbilicus, dividing the abdomen into four equal areas.

**radial artery** The major artery in the forearm. It is palpable at the wrist on the thumb side.

**radius** The bone on the thumb side of the forearm.

**red blood cells** Cells that carry oxygen to the body tissues; also called erythrocytes.

**respiratory system** All the structures of the body that contribute to the process of breathing, consisting of the upper and lower airways and their component parts.

**skeletal muscle** Muscle that is attached to bones and usually crosses at least one joint. It is striated, or voluntary, muscle.

**skeleton** The framework that gives us our recognizable form; also designed to allow motion of the body and protection of vital organs.

**smooth muscle** Muscle that constitutes the bulk of the gastrointestinal tract and is present in nearly every organ to regulate automatic activity. It is nonstriated, or involuntary, muscle.

**spinal cord** An extension of the brain, composed of virtually all the nerves carrying messages between the brain and the rest of the body. It lies inside of and is protected by the spinal canal.

sternum The breast bone.

superficial Located closer to or on the skin.

superior Located closer to the head.

tendons The fibrous connective tissue that attaches muscle to bone.

thorax The chest cavity that contains the heart, lungs, esophagus, and great vessels.

tibia The shin bone; the larger of the two bones of the lower leg.

trachea The windpipe; the main trunk for air passing to and from the lungs.

ulna The inner bone of the forearm, on the side opposite the thumb.

vein Any blood vessel that carries blood from the tissues to the heart.

vertebrae The 33 bones that make up the spinal column.

voluntary muscle Muscle that is under direct voluntary control of the brain and can be contracted or relaxed at will; skeletal or striated muscle.

white blood cells Blood cells involved in the body's immune defense mechanisms against infection.

xiphoid process The lowest part of the sternum.

## ▶ Assessment in Action

You are helping a friend with her human anatomy and physiology homework during your lunch break. Having taken the same class, you feel confident that you can help explain how the human body works. Your friend seems impressed when you explain the different types of muscles. After taking a bite of her lunch, your friend clutches her throat and appears to be choking. You ask her if she is choking and she nods her head "yes." You ask her to say something but she cannot and continues clutching her throat. You notice that she had been eating a hot dog.

*Directions:* Circle Yes if you agree with the statement; circle No if you disagree.

Yes   No   **1.** You should not panic. Your friend is young and with a little more time the hot dog will pass into the esophagus.

Yes   No   **2.** Because your friend is alert and responsive, she can survive without breathing for over 10 minutes.

Yes   No   **3.** Her face begins to turn blue and she collapses to the floor. Her chest is not moving, which is a sign that she is not breathing.

Yes   No   **4.** If your friend is not breathing, her tissues and organs are not getting enough carbon dioxide.

## ▶ Check Your Knowledge

*Directions:* Circle Yes if you agree with the statement; circle No if you disagree.

Yes   No   **1.** A first aid provider does not have to understand how the human body works in order to effectively provide care.

Yes   No   **2.** The human body can store oxygen for hours.

Yes   No   **3.** Blood is the delivery system for cells throughout the body.

Yes   No   **4.** The heart is a pear-shaped, muscular organ.

Yes   No   **5.** Once neurons have been destroyed, the body can replace them.

Yes   No   **6.** The autonomic nervous system consists of a group of nerves that control heart rate, digestion, sweating, and other automatic body processes.

Yes   No   **7.** The adult skeleton has 228 bones.

Yes   No   **8.** A joint is where two or more bones meet or join.

Yes   No   **9.** There are three kinds of muscle: skeletal, smooth, and cardiac.

Yes   No   **10.** Skin transmits information to the brain and helps regulate body temperature.

# Finding Out What is Wrong

**4**

## Assessment Overview

During emergency situations when panic exists, knowing what to do and what not to do is crucial. An assessment is a sequence of actions that helps determine what is wrong and thus helps provide safe and appropriate first aid. Becoming familiar with the process of assessment will enable you to act quickly and decisively in hectic emergency situations. Assessment is an important first aid skill. It requires an understanding of each assessment step as well as decision-making skills.

Finding out what is wrong with a person will be influenced by whether the person is suffering from an illness or an injury, whether the person is responsive or unresponsive, and whether life-threatening conditions exist. Conduct a **primary check** first and care for any conditions you uncover before going on with the assessment.

Different conditions require different approaches for determining what is wrong. Not all parts of an assessment apply to every person, and the sequencing can vary depending on the person's medical condition. Most people do not require a complete assessment. For example, a person who cut a finger while whittling a stick will not require a complete assessment; however, a person who cut a finger while sliding down a mountainside will require a full assessment because this person might have sustained other injuries. **Table 4-1** gives a preview of the assessment sequence for the different presentations of injuries and illnesses that you may encounter as a first aid provider.

## Table 4-1 Sequence of Assessment

| | Injured Person | | | Suddenly Ill Person | |
|---|---|---|---|---|---|
| | | Responsive | | | |
| Unresponsive | With Significant COI | Without Significant COI | Unresponsive | Responsive | |
| • Primary check<br>• Physical exam using the DOS parts of DOTS<br>• SAMPLE history from others | • Primary check<br>• Physical exam using DOTS<br>• SAMPLE history | • Primary check<br>• Examination of chief complaint using DOTS<br>• SAMPLE history | • Primary check<br>• Physical exam using the DOS parts of DOTS<br>• SAMPLE history from others | • Primary check<br>• SAMPLE history<br>• Examination of chief complaint | |

COI = cause of injury (also known as mechanism of injury); DOTS = deformity, open wounds, tenderness, swelling; SAMPLE = signs and symptoms, allergies, medications, pertinent past medical history, last oral intake, and events leading up to the illness or injury.

An assessment can provide important information about a condition and help you determine how to treat it and whether medical care is needed Flowchart 4-1. If the person requires medical care, pass what you found during the assessment to the emergency medical services (EMS) personnel or health care providers. Call 9-1-1 for any person with a significant **cause (mechanism) of injury** or **nature of illness**, and for any unresponsive person.

You should check the person systematically Skill Sheet 4-1. You can do this by performing three steps:

1. Perform a primary check **(Step 1)**.
2. Perform a physical exam, also known as a head-to-toe exam **(Step 2)**.
3. Obtain the person's SAMPLE history **(Step 3)**.

A primary check (also known as a primary survey or initial assessment) consists of identifying and treating immediate, life-threatening conditions involving breathing impairments and severe bleeding. People with immediate, life-threatening conditions can die within minutes unless the cause is quickly recognized and treated.

A physical exam follows the primary check. (For a critically injured person, you may not go beyond the primary check.) These procedures can reveal information that will help you identify the injury or illness, judge its severity, and determine what first aid is needed. You will gain detailed information about the person's injury (eg, a painful ankle or bleeding nose) or **chief complaint** (eg, chest pain or itchy skin).

Performing the physical exam right after the primary check and before doing the **SAMPLE history** allows an injury to be found and cared for sooner than if the SAMPLE history comes before the physical exam. In some cases, especially when caring for a stranger, performing the SAMPLE history before the physical exam involves a conversation with the stranger, which may ease the person's anxiety about having you conduct a physical exam. Also, in cases of illness, performing the SAMPLE history before the physical exam can indicate which part of the physical exam should be performed first.

### Q&A

**Can I make a diagnosis as to what is wrong?**

No. Diagnosing a medical condition is best left to a physician. A layperson diagnosing a medical condition could be accused of practicing medicine without a license, which has legal consequences. However, a first aid provider can suspect what may be wrong based on the signs and symptoms found.

## ▶ Scene Size-up

Every time you encounter a person with an injury or illness, first check out the scene. The **scene size-up** determines the safety of the scene, the cause of injury or nature of illness, and the number of people involved.

Without a scene size-up, a potentially hazardous situation could result in further injury to the person or injury to you and bystanders. Hazards come in

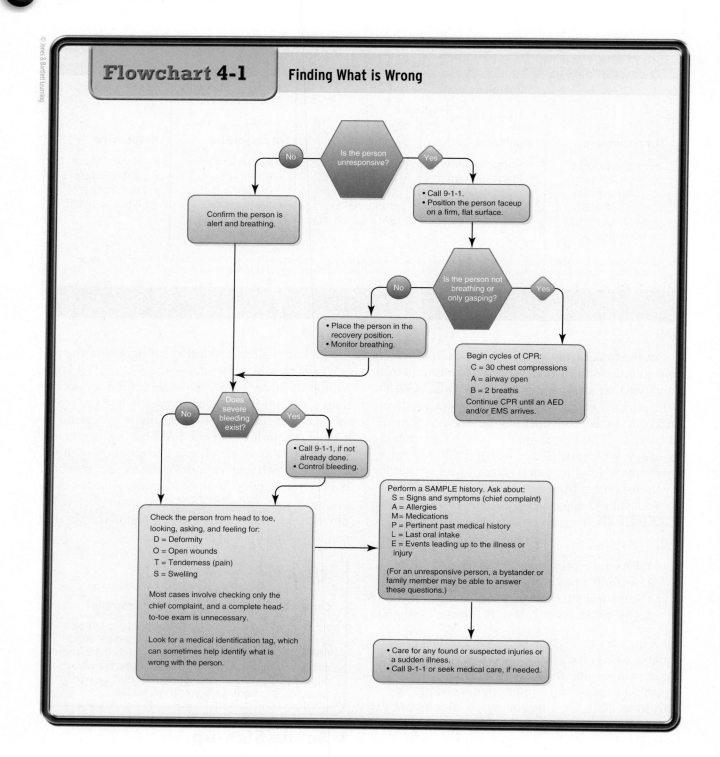

## Flowchart 4-1    Finding What is Wrong

**Is the person unresponsive?**

No → Confirm the person is alert and breathing.

Yes →
- Call 9-1-1.
- Position the person faceup on a firm, flat surface.

**Is the person not breathing or only gasping?**

No →
- Place the person in the recovery position.
- Monitor breathing.

Yes →
Begin cycles of CPR:
- C = 30 chest compressions
- A = airway open
- B = 2 breaths
Continue CPR until an AED and/or EMS arrives.

**Does severe bleeding exist?**

No ↓

Yes →
- Call 9-1-1, if not already done.
- Control bleeding.

Check the person from head to toe, looking, asking, and feeling for:
- D = Deformity
- O = Open wounds
- T = Tenderness (pain)
- S = Swelling

Most cases involve checking only the chief complaint, and a complete head-to-toe exam is unnecessary.

Look for a medical identification tag, which can sometimes help identify what is wrong with the person.

Perform a SAMPLE history. Ask about:
- S = Signs and symptoms (chief complaint)
- A = Allergies
- M = Medications
- P = Pertinent past medical history
- L = Last oral intake
- E = Events leading up to the illness or injury

(For an unresponsive person, a bystander or family member may be able to answer these questions.)

- Care for any found or suspected injuries or a sudden illness.
- Call 9-1-1 or seek medical care, if needed.

## Skill Sheet

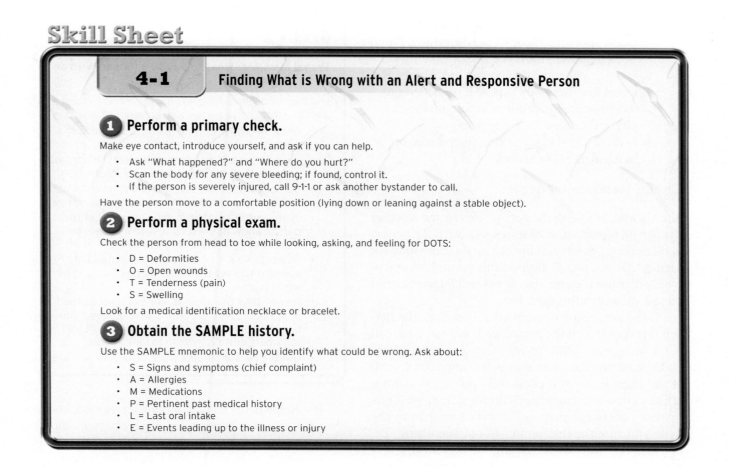

**4-1          Finding What is Wrong with an Alert and Responsive Person**

**1  Perform a primary check.**

Make eye contact, introduce yourself, and ask if you can help.

- Ask "What happened?" and "Where do you hurt?"
- Scan the body for any severe bleeding; if found, control it.
- If the person is severely injured, call 9-1-1 or ask another bystander to call.

Have the person move to a comfortable position (lying down or leaning against a stable object).

**2  Perform a physical exam.**

Check the person from head to toe while looking, asking, and feeling for DOTS:

- D = Deformities
- O = Open wounds
- T = Tenderness (pain)
- S = Swelling

Look for a medical identification necklace or bracelet.

**3  Obtain the SAMPLE history.**

Use the SAMPLE mnemonic to help you identify what could be wrong. Ask about:

- S = Signs and symptoms (chief complaint)
- A = Allergies
- M = Medications
- P = Pertinent past medical history
- L = Last oral intake
- E = Events leading up to the illness or injury

---

many different forms (eg, chemicals, electricity, water, fires, explosions, carbon monoxide). They exist at most motor vehicle crash scenes. Some scenes have the potential for violence—violent people, distraught family members, angry bystanders, gangs, and unruly crowds. Be observant for weapons. If the scene appears hazardous, do not enter the area. You cannot help a person if you become injured or ill yourself.

Reduce exposure to potentially dangerous body substances that can carry disease. Disease transmission is very rare; however, you should wear exam gloves and assume that all people are infected.

Determining whether an injury or an illness exists is also an important step. Making this distinction gives you a starting point and determines the order of the assessment. If the scene size-up or primary check suggests serious illness or injury, call 9-1-1.

## ▶ Primary Check

The purpose of the primary check is to identify life-threatening conditions so you can immediately take action to treat the conditions. The primary check

includes checking the person's responsiveness, checking circulation, checking for breathing, and checking for severe bleeding.

## Form a First Impression of the Person

While approaching the person, form an immediate **first impression**. The first impression has also been referred to as a general impression, look test, or gut reaction. Using the scene size-up and your first impression of the person, determine the following:

1. Does the person appear to have an injury or an illness? If you are unable to determine whether the person is ill or injured, proceed as though he or she is injured. Impressions can come from such things as the person's position and the person's breathing sounds.
2. Is the person obviously responsive or unresponsive?
3. Is the person obviously breathing adequately or normally? If the person is able to talk, there is a good chance he or she is breathing adequately.

4. Are signs of obvious bleeding present—blood spurting, blood-soaked clothing, blood pooled on the ground or floor?
5. Is there a chance of exposure to the person's blood or other body fluids? If so, be sure to use standard precautions before making physical contact with the person.
6. Is there any danger to you, the person, or bystanders at the scene?

## Check Responsiveness

Shortly after reaching the person, determine whether the person is responsive or unresponsive. If the person is motionless, gently tap his or her shoulder and ask loudly, "Are you okay?" Beyond this point, how and in what order you conduct the checks will largely depend on the answer to this question.

If the person answers, moans, or moves, the person is responsive. If the person does not respond, call 9-1-1 to activate EMS. In the unresponsive person, observe for regular breathing by taking a quick look at the chest to see if it rises and falls. If you cannot see any chest movement and cannot hear any sounds (except occasional gasping) of air coming from the nose and mouth, the person is not breathing. Do not mistake occasional gasping for breathing—it is not! Take immediate steps to begin cardiopulmonary resuscitation (CPR), starting with 30 chest compressions followed by 2 breaths (1 second each). See Chapter 5, *CPR*, for directions on how to perform CPR.

A person's level of responsiveness can range from fully responsive (conscious) to unresponsive (unconscious). Not all responsive people are fully alert, and they may respond to different levels of stimulation.

For an alert person, begin by introducing yourself. Tell the person that you are trained in first aid and ask permission to help. For an alert, responsive person, you can evaluate the person's ability to remember by asking about the following:

- Person—What is your name?
- Place—Do you know where you are?
- Time—What is the month and year?
- Event—What happened?

For a motionless person, tap his or her shoulder and ask, "Are you okay?" If there is no response, check for breathing.

For an unresponsive person, the steps resemble the steps used when beginning to perform CPR—which are remembered with the mnemonic RAB-CAB—although most unresponsive people do not need CPR (see Chapter 5, *CPR*):

---

### FYI

**Verbal First Aid: What to Say to a Person With an Injury or Illness**

Use these guidelines for gaining rapport and calming an alert and responsive person with an injury or illness:

- Avoid negative statements that could add to a person's distress and anxiety.
- Your first words to a person are very important because they set the tone of your interaction.
- Do not ask unnecessary questions unless it aids treatment or satisfies the person's need to talk.
- Tears and/or laughter can be normal. Let the person know this if such responses seem to make him or her feel embarrassed.
- Stress the positive. For example, instead of saying, "You will not have any pain," say, "The worst is over."
- Do not deny the obvious. For example, instead of saying, "There is nothing wrong," say, "You have had quite a fall and probably do not feel too well, but we are going to look at you."
- Use the person's name while providing first aid.

---

**R** = *Responsive?* For any motionless person, check responsiveness by gently tapping the person's shoulder and shouting, "Are you okay?" Speak loudly enough to wake the person if he or she is sleeping.

**A** = *Activate EMS.* If there is no response, activate EMS by calling 9-1-1.

**B** = *Breathing?* After activating EMS, position the person on his or her back on a flat, firm surface. Check for no breathing or only gasping. If the person is breathing, place him or her in the recovery position and check for severe bleeding. If the person is not breathing, give CPR.

An unresponsive, breathing person can receive other first aid, especially to control severe bleeding. Providing care would be covered by implied consent. (Refer to Chapter 1, *Background Information*.)

You are more likely to see an alert, responsive person. Responsive people rarely need the type of primary check used for unresponsive people. However, a responsive person may be developing an airway obstruction, may have severe bleeding, may be having a heart attack, or may be in the early stages of shock or some other serious condition. Each of these conditions is considered a medical emergency, and immediate care must be provided if you suspect any of them. Follow these steps to care for an alert, responsive person:

1. While approaching a responsive person, make eye contact, introduce yourself as a

trained first aid provider, and give your name. Next, ask if you can help; in doing so, you are asking for the person's expressed consent to help. With permission from the person, perform an assessment.

2. If the person appears to be severely injured or ill, activate EMS.
3. Position the person in a comfortable position (eg, lying down, tripod position, leaning against a stable object).
4. Check for severe bleeding.
5. Monitor breathing; check for abnormal breathing sounds (eg, wheezing, gurgling) or fast breathing.

## Q&A

**When should I interrupt a primary check?**

When a life-threatening condition is identified during the primary check, immediately begin first aid. For example, if a person has an obstructed airway, treat the obstruction before going through the other assessment steps. Once the life-threatening condition (eg, choking) has been cared for and/or corrected, continue the primary check of the person until completed.

## Check Breathing

Check for adequate breathing by looking for chest rise and fall and listening for normal or abnormal breath sounds. Distinguish between effective and ineffective breathing efforts. Cyanosis (blue discoloration around lips and mouth) and ashen (gray) skin are signs of inadequate oxygenation. See Table 4-2 for breathing sounds that may indicate inadequate breathing.

## Check for Severe Bleeding

Check for severe bleeding by quickly looking over the person's entire body for blood (eg, blood-soaked clothing or blood pooling on the floor or the ground). This is not a head-to-toe exam, but a search for large amounts of blood around the person or in the person's clothing. In most cases, placing a sterile dressing over the wound and applying direct pressure with a hand or a pressure bandage controls the bleeding. Life-threatening external bleeding is rare, but when found, it must be controlled immediately or the person can bleed to death. Avoid contact with the person's blood whenever possible by using exam gloves or extra layers of dressings or cloth.

## Position the Person

Most people should not be moved, especially if a spinal injury is suspected. However, you may need to safely reposition the person if the position in which you find the person is impeding the primary check or if repositioning can otherwise improve the person's outcome. Such circumstances include the following:

- When the person and first aid provider(s) are in an unsafe location, you may need to first call 9-1-1 to enlist assistance. Depending on the situation, you may need to delay your primary check until law enforcement or rescue services have ensured a safe scene. If you can safely do so, you may move the person only as needed to reach a safe location.
- When an unresponsive person is facedown (prone position) and needs CPR, turn the person faceup (supine position) on a firm, flat surface to be in a position to receive CPR.
- When an unresponsive person is breathing, place the person in the recovery position to help maintain a clear airway Skill Sheet 4-2 .

## Table 4-2  Abnormal Breathing Sounds

| Breathing Sound | Possible Cause |
|---|---|
| Snoring | Airway partially blocked (usually by tongue) |
| Gurgling (breaths passing through liquid) | Fluids in throat |
| Crowing (noisy creak or squeak) | Spasm of the larynx; foreign body |
| Wheezing | Spasm or partial obstruction in bronchi (asthma, emphysema) |
| Occasional gasping breaths (known as agonal respirations) | Breathing after the heart has stopped |

## Skill Sheet

| 4-2 | Placing an Unresponsive Breathing Person in the Recovery Position |

*Note:* **DO NOT** move a person with a suspected spinal injury. Leave the person in the position in which he or she was found. If the person's airway is blocked or the area is unsafe, move the person only as needed to open the airway or to reach a safe location.

If a person is unresponsive and breathing, place him or her in a side-lying recovery position.

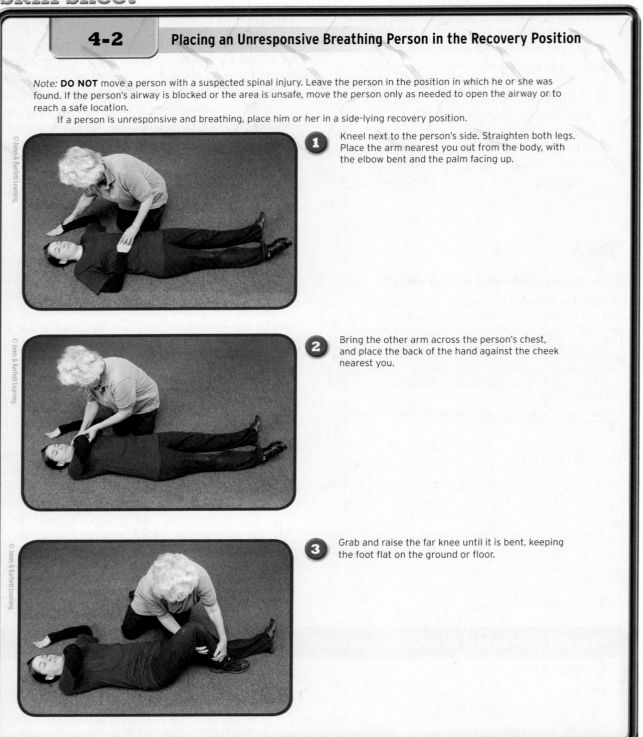

**1** Kneel next to the person's side. Straighten both legs. Place the arm nearest you out from the body, with the elbow bent and the palm facing up.

**2** Bring the other arm across the person's chest, and place the back of the hand against the cheek nearest you.

**3** Grab and raise the far knee until it is bent, keeping the foot flat on the ground or floor.

© Jones & Bartlett Learning.

# Skill Sheet Continued

**4-2**   **Placing an Unresponsive Breathing Person in the Recovery Position**

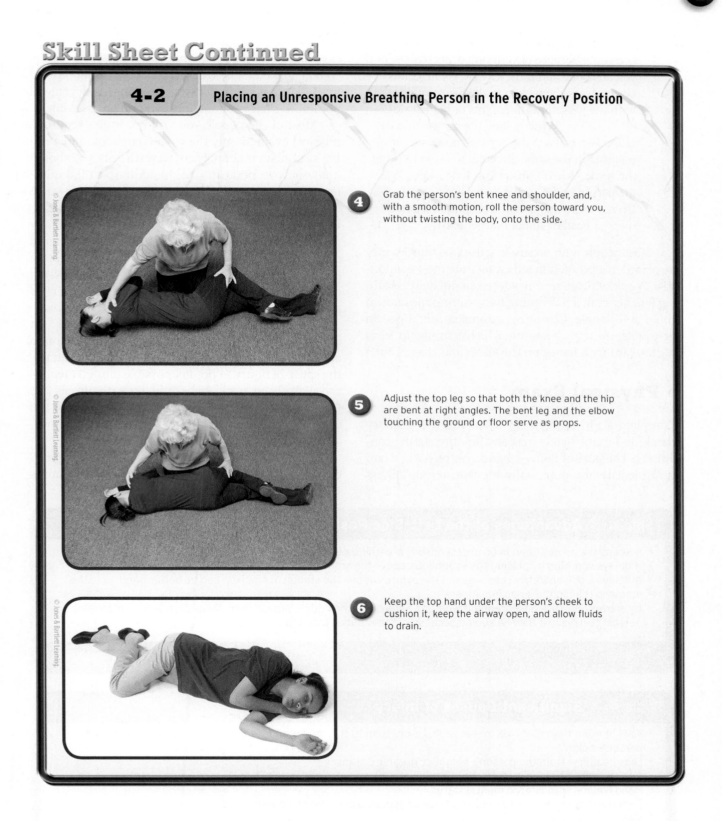

**4** Grab the person's bent knee and shoulder, and, with a smooth motion, roll the person toward you, without twisting the body, onto the side.

**5** Adjust the top leg so that both the knee and the hip are bent at right angles. The bent leg and the elbow touching the ground or floor serve as props.

**6** Keep the top hand under the person's cheek to cushion it, keep the airway open, and allow fluids to drain.

© Jones & Bartlett Learning.

- In some cases when the person has difficulty breathing because of vomiting or secretions, or if you are alone and must leave to get help, it is best to place the person in the recovery position, with the person resting on his or her left side **Table 4-3**. While rolling the person into the side position, keep the person's nose and navel pointing in the same direction to avoid twisting the spine. When signs of shock develop, place the person on his or her back (supine position). Do not move the person if suspected leg fractures or head or spinal injuries exist.

Most people with no suspected spinal injuries may be placed in a position in which they are most comfortable. People with chest pain, nausea, or difficulty breathing fare better in a half-sitting (semi-sitting) position at about a 45° angle. During an asthma attack, a person may prefer the tripod position, which is sitting up, leaning forward with hands on the knees and elbows out.

## ▶ Physical Exam

Complete a **physical exam** following the primary check, and immediately treat any life-threatening conditions. The goal of doing a hands-on physical exam is to identify any potentially life-threatening illness or injury requiring first aid. A good physical exam is essential in discovering what is wrong. The adage of "Find it, fix it" stresses the fact that you cannot provide first aid unless you know what is wrong. And, you will not know what is wrong until you do an assessment.

Most of the people you will encounter require a physical exam of only the chief complaint, and a full physical exam is not needed. Nevertheless, you should know how to perform one. In addition to the question, "What is wrong?" or "What happened to you?" another important question to ask of the person who has been injured is "Do you hurt anywhere?" Many people view a physical exam with apprehension and anxiety. They feel vulnerable and exposed. Maintain dignity throughout the assessment. Show compassion toward the person and his or her family members. If possible, the person should be sitting or lying down.

Start by reconsidering the cause of injury that you identified during the scene size-up. Ask the person to describe what happened in detail, so that you can use the cause of injury to predict possible injured areas—especially head, neck, spine, and internal injuries (see Chapter 2, *Action at an Emergency*). Establishing the cause of injury helps to determine which first aid procedures to use.

Determine whether the cause of injury was significant **Table 4-4**. In addition to the significant causes

### Table 4-3 Advantages of the Left-Side Position

- It keeps the airway open in an unresponsive, breathing person.
- It delays vomiting by placing the esophagus above the stomach.
- It delays a poison's effects by keeping the pylorus above the stomach. A poison can be better handled in the stomach than in the small intestines.
- It relieves pressure on a pregnant woman's vena cava (the body's largest vein). Many pregnant women faint or at least feel dizzy if they lie supine because of the reduced blood flow.

### Table 4-4 Significant Causes of Injury

- Falls of more than 15 ft (4.6 m) for adults, more than 10 ft (3 m) for children, or more than three times the person's height
- Falls headfirst from the person's height or greater distance
- Vehicle collisions involving ejection, a rollover, high speed, a pedestrian, a motorcycle, or a bicycle
- Head trauma with altered mental status
- Penetrations of the head, chest, or abdomen (eg, stab or gunshot wounds)
- Major burn injury
- Vehicle collisions involving death of an occupant in the same vehicle
- Pedestrian hit by a vehicle

of injury, assume that a person with a head injury also has a spinal injury until proven otherwise.

For a responsive person, check for a spinal injury by asking the person the following questions (refer to Chapter 12, *Head and Spinal Injuries*):

- Can you feel me squeezing your fingers and toes? (Before doing this, have the person look away or close his or her eyes. While you are squeezing, ask the person which finger or toe you are squeezing.)
- Can you wiggle your fingers and toes?
- Can you squeeze my hand, and can you push your foot against my hand?

Stabilize the person against any movement, and tell him or her not to move.

For an unresponsive person whom you suspect has a spinal injury, do not move the person's head or neck.

**Q&A**

**Do I have to perform a complete assessment for every person with an injury or sudden illness?**

No. Perform a primary check for every person and acquire as much of each person's SAMPLE history as you can. Performing a complete head-to-toe physical exam is crucial for the unresponsive person with an illness or significant injury. However, for the responsive person with an illness or nonsignificant injury, the physical exam focuses primarily on the person's chief complaint.

A physical exam assesses the person's entire body from head to toe; you will note the person's signs and symptoms:

- <u>Signs</u> refer to your observations of the person's conditions—what you can see, feel, hear, or smell.
- <u>Symptoms</u> refer to things the person feels and is able to describe. The primary symptom is known as the chief complaint.

To check a part of the body, look and feel (mnemonic is LAF) for the following signs and symptoms of injury: deformities, open wounds, tenderness, and swelling. The mnemonic <u>DOTS</u> is helpful for

remembering the signs and symptoms of an injury
**Figure 4-1**:

**D** = *Deformity*. The shape of the body part is abnormal. Compare the body part to the opposite uninjured part, if applicable. Deformities occur when bones are broken or joints are dislocated.

**O** = *Open wounds*. The skin is broken and bleeding is present.

**T** = *Tenderness*. The person reports sensitivity, discomfort, or pain when touched.

**S** = *Swelling*. The area looks larger than usual. Swelling is caused by excess fluid in the tissue. When possible, compare one side of the body with the other side (eg, if an ankle appears swollen, look at the other one).

**Q&A**

**When might an assessment be unreliable?**

Use caution when assessing any person who has an altered mental status or a painful injury that could distract from other injuries or illness (eg, femur fracture), or who has ingested alcohol or drugs.

## Person With a Significant Cause of Injury

For a person with a significant cause of injury, perform a hands-on, full-body, head-to-toe assessment, taking no more than 2 minutes to complete. The person may be responsive or unresponsive. Assume that an unresponsive person has a spinal injury and stabilize the head and neck against movement. When a man examines a woman, it is wise, if possible, to have another woman present. Follow the steps in **Skill Sheet 4-3** to perform a physical exam:

1. *Check the head.* Use both hands to check the scalp for DOTS. A deformity may be a bump or a depression. Do not move the person's head during this procedure. Check the skin condition for temperature, color, and moisture.
2. *Check the eyes.* Compare the pupils, the black center of the eye. Pupils should be the same

**Figure 4-1**

Examine an area by looking and feeling for DOTS: D = deformity **(A)**, O = open wounds **(B)**, T = tenderness **(C)**, and S = swelling **(D)**.

# Skill Sheet

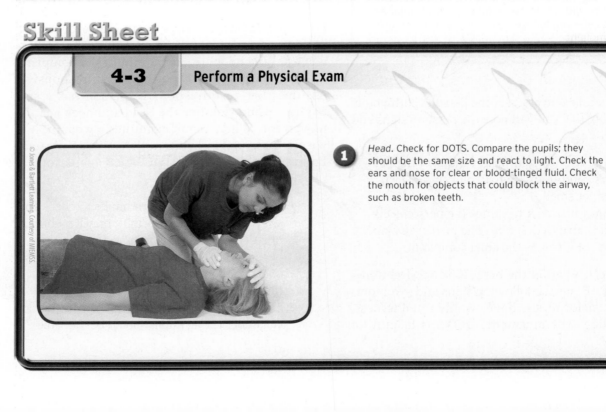

| 4-3 | Perform a Physical Exam |
|-----|--------------------------|

**1** *Head.* Check for DOTS. Compare the pupils; they should be the same size and react to light. Check the ears and nose for clear or blood-tinged fluid. Check the mouth for objects that could block the airway, such as broken teeth.

# Skill Sheet Continued

**4-3** **Perform a Physical Exam**

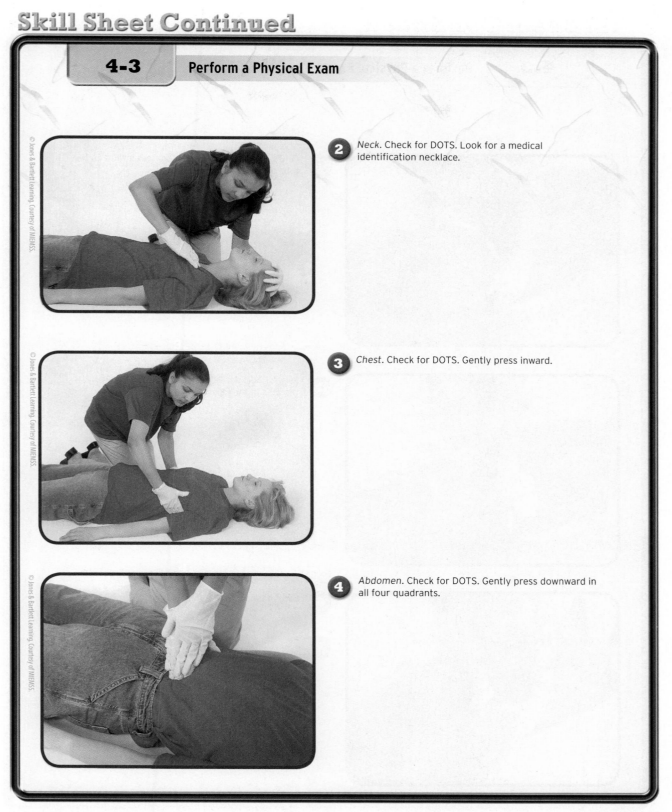

**2** *Neck.* Check for DOTS. Look for a medical identification necklace.

**3** *Chest.* Check for DOTS. Gently press inward.

**4** *Abdomen.* Check for DOTS. Gently press downward in all four quadrants.

© Jones & Bartlett Learning. Courtesy of MIEMSS.

*(Continues)*

# Skill Sheet Continued

**4-3**    **Perform a Physical Exam**

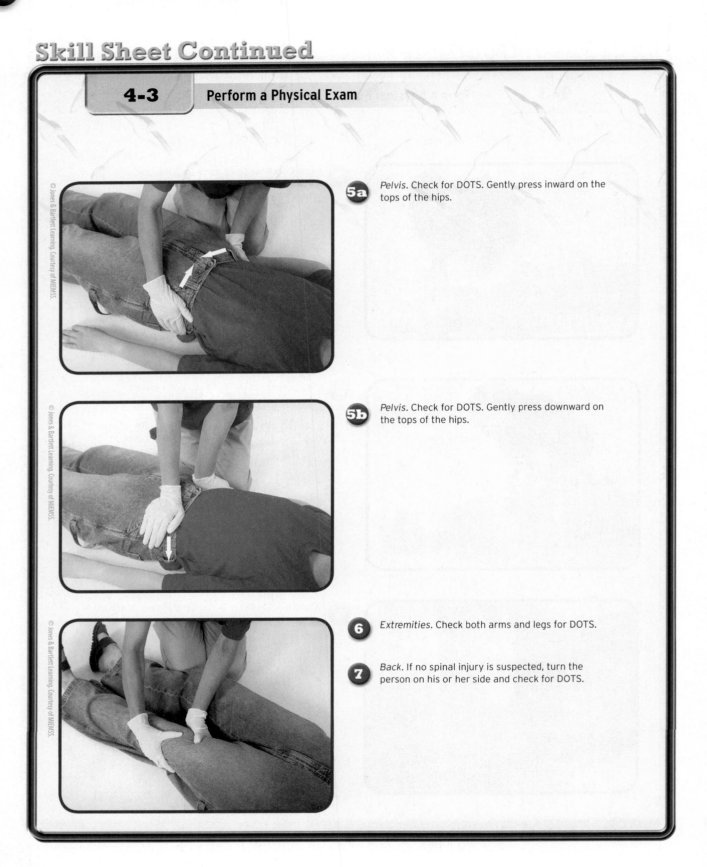

© Jones & Bartlett Learning. Courtesy of MIEMSS.

**5a**   *Pelvis.* Check for DOTS. Gently press inward on the tops of the hips.

© Jones & Bartlett Learning. Courtesy of MIEMSS.

**5b**   *Pelvis.* Check for DOTS. Gently press downward on the tops of the hips.

© Jones & Bartlett Learning. Courtesy of MIEMSS.

**6**   *Extremities.* Check both arms and legs for DOTS.

**7**   *Back.* If no spinal injury is suspected, turn the person on his or her side and check for DOTS.

size and react to light **Figure 4-2**. Use a flashlight to determine whether the pupils are reactive. If a flashlight is not present, cover one of the person's eyes with your hand and observe the pupil's reaction when the eye is uncovered. Normally, the pupil constricts (gets smaller) within 1 second. No pupil reaction to light could mean death, coma, cataracts (in older people), or an artificial eye. Pupil dilation happens within 30 to 60 seconds of cardiac arrest.

Look for unequal pupils. A difference in the size of the two pupils is almost always a sign of a medical emergency, such as a stroke or a brain injury. However, the unequal condition occurs normally in 2% to 4% of the population. Also, an artificial eye may give the appearance of unequal pupils.

Lastly, observe the inner eyelid surface. Pink is normal in all healthy people regardless of skin pigmentation. A pale color may indicate poor blood circulation.

3. *Check the ears and nose* for clear or blood-tinged fluid. Check the nose for DOTS.

4. *Check the mouth* for swelling or objects (eg, broken teeth, dentures, chewing gum, vomit, food, and foreign objects), which could block the airway (**Step 1**).

5. *Check the neck* for DOTS. Look for a medical identification necklace chain and tag (**Step 2**).

6. *Check the chest* for DOTS. Warn the person that you are going to apply pressure to the sides of the chest. Gently squeeze the chest inward and ask if doing so is painful. Pain from squeezing or compressing the sides may indicate a rib fracture (**Step 3**).

7. *Check the abdomen* for DOTS. Feel the abdomen for tenderness by pushing gently downward in all four of the abdominal quadrants (divide the abdomen into four parts by two imaginary lines intersecting at right angles at the navel). If a chief complaint is abdominal pain, ask the person to point to where it hurts. Do not push on the area that hurts. Begin on the opposite side from the spot, and press gently on each abdominal quadrant. As you press on an area, ask the person if it hurts. Feel for abnormal lumps and hardened areas. Do not push too deeply. The person may "guard" an area if it is tender by tightening abdominal muscles or

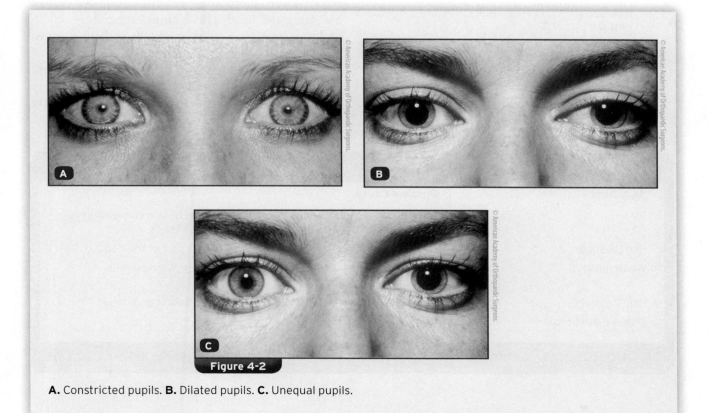

**Figure 4-2**

**A.** Constricted pupils. **B.** Dilated pupils. **C.** Unequal pupils.

protecting that area with his or her hands. Anything protruding from the abdomen will be obvious, but be sure to check for penetrating objects (**Step 4**).

8. *Check the pelvis* for DOTS. If the person does not report pain, gently press inward on the tops of the hip bones and then, if the person still does not report pain, press downward on the same bones. Before pressing, warn the person about possible tenderness (**Step 5**).

9. *Check all four extremities* for DOTS. Use both hands to encircle an extremity. Gently but firmly squeeze each part of the extremity for any sign of tenderness. Compare the two sides of the body. Look for a medical identification bracelet on a wrist (**Step 6**).

10. *Check all four extremities* for circulation, sensation, and movement (CSM):

    **C** = *Circulation.* For arms, feel for radial (on the wrist's thumb side) pulse, and for legs, feel the posterior tibial pulse behind the ankle bone (malleolus) on the inner (medial) side of the ankle.

    **S** = *Sensation.* Pinch the end of the person's fingers and toes (have the person close his or her eyes and tell you which finger or toe is being squeezed).

    **M** = *Movement.* Have the person wiggle his or her fingers and toes.

11. *Check the back.* If no spinal injury is suspected, turn the person onto his or her side and check for DOTS. You may have to turn the person toward one side to check half of the back and then turn the person the other direction to check the other half of the back (**Step 7**).

   If you suspect a neck or spinal injury and the person's position is stable, tell the person not to move while you are performing the check. If the person is uncooperative or in an unstable position, you may have to stop at that point and stabilize the person's head and neck manually until more help arrives.

## Person With No Significant Cause of Injury

When a person has no significant cause of injury, a full-body physical exam from head to toe is not needed. Instead, focus the assessment on the chief complaints (the areas that the person complains about). For most first aid providers, this will be the more frequently performed type of assessment.

## Special Considerations

### Skin Condition

A quick check of the person's skin can also provide information about the person's condition. When assessing the head, check skin temperature, color, and moisture. Skin color, especially in light-skinned people, reflects the circulation under the skin as well as oxygen status (Table 4-5). For those with dark complexions, changes might not be readily apparent but can be assessed by the appearance of the nail beds, the inside of the mouth, and the inner eyelids.

### Table 4-5 Skin Color

| Skin Color | Possible Cause |
| --- | --- |
| Pink | Normal color in nonpigmented areas regardless of skin complexion—lining of the eyelids, inside of mouth, fingernail beds |
| Red (flushed) | Dilated blood vessels; excess circulation to that part of the body |
| White (pale) | Constricted blood vessels from blood loss, shock, hypothermia, emotional distress |
| Blue (cyanotic) | Lack of oxygen in the blood from breathing or heart conditions |
| Yellow (jaundiced) | Liver disease or failure |

You can get a rough idea of skin temperature by putting the back of your hand or wrist on the person's forehead to determine whether the temperature is elevated or decreased. Dry skin is normal. Skin that is wet, moist, or excessively dry and hot suggests a medical condition Table 4-6 .

## Capillary Refill Test

Some first aid providers use the capillary refill technique to check adequacy of blood circulation in an extremity. To perform the technique, gently press a fingernail or toenail for a few seconds and then release the pressure Figure 4-3 . When released, the blanched skin should return to its normal color within 2 seconds. (Saying "capillary refill" takes 2 seconds.) A refill time of greater than 2 seconds indicates poor circulation, which requires medical care. Some medical experts question the capillary refill test's reliability in adults because of various factors (eg, exposure to cold, heavy tobacco use, medications, and preexisting medical conditions). It appears to be more accurate in children and infants.

## Exposing the Injury

You might have to remove items of clothing from the person to check for an injury and to give proper first aid. If you need to remove clothing, explain what you intend to do (and why) to the person and any family members or bystanders. Remove as much clothing as necessary, try to maintain privacy, and prevent exposure to cold. Damage clothing only if necessary, and do so by cutting along the seams Figure 4-4 .

### Table 4-6 Skin Temperature

| Skin Temperature/Moisture | Possible Cause |
| --- | --- |
| Warm and dry | Normal |
| Hot and dry or moist | Excessive body heat (heat stroke, high fever) |
| Cool and moist (clammy) | Poor circulation, heat exhaustion, shock, acute stress reaction |
| Cold and moist | Body is losing heat |
| Cold and dry | Exposed to cold and has lost considerable heat (hypothermia) |

© Jones & Bartlett Learning.

© American Academy of Orthopaedic Surgeons.

Figure 4-3

**A.** To test capillary refill, gently compress the fingertip until it blanches. **B.** Release the fingertip and count until it returns to its normal pink color.

**Figure 4-4**

Expose the injury. Remove as much clothing from the person as necessary, while trying to maintain privacy.

**A**

**B**

**Figure 4-5**

Medical identification tag. **A.** Front of tag. **B.** Back of tag.

## Checking for Medical Identification Tags

Look for a medical identification tag or for a medical information card in the person's wallet or purse. (Note that this search might be illegal in some states.) Such information can be beneficial in identifying allergies, medications, or medical history **Figure 4-5**. A medical identification tag, worn as a necklace or as a bracelet, contains the wearer's medical condition(s) and a 24-hour telephone number that offers, in case of an emergency, access to the person's medical history plus names of physicians and close relatives.

These sources of information can be especially useful when the wearer is unresponsive or not old enough to answer questions. Necklaces and bracelets are durable, instantly recognizable, and less likely than cards to be separated from the person in an emergency. If looking through a person's wallet or purse, always do so in the presence of another person at the scene to protect yourself against later accusations, should money or credit cards be missing.

## ▶ SAMPLE History

The information in a SAMPLE history can help you identify what is wrong with the person and what first aid is needed **Table 4-7**.

In the best of circumstances, the person will be able to answer all questions about his or her chief complaint and medical history. In other cases, you may obtain this information from family, friends, bystanders, medical identification jewelry, or other medical information sources.

### Check for Clues

In addition to a medical identification tag, you may find other clues in determining the cause of the person's injury or illness. A medicine bottle label gives the name of the medication, but you may not know why the medication was prescribed. Suspect a diabetic emergency if you find glucose tablets or gel or insulin with a person. An inhaler indicates that a person has asthma. An auto-injector could point to a person's susceptibility to severe, life-threatening allergic reactions.

The direct cause (mechanism) of injury (such as a sharp object, broken glass, or bent steering wheel) can provide crucial details about an injury. Additionally, objects at the scene that are not the cause of an injury can offer a clue as to what may be wrong with a person. Examples include a fallen ladder or an open medicine bottle.

## Table 4-7 SAMPLE History

| Description | Questions |
|---|---|
| S = Signs and symptoms | What is wrong? Where do you hurt? |
| A = Allergies | Are you allergic to anything? |
| M = Medications | Are you taking any prescription or nonprescription medications? What are they for? |
| P = Pertinent past medical history | Have you had this condition before? Have you had recent medical conditions? |
| L = Last oral intake | When did you last eat or drink anything? What was it? How much? |
| E = Events leading up to the illness or injury | Injury: How did you get hurt?<br>Illness: What led to this condition? |

## ▶ What to Do Until Medical Care Is Available

The primary check, physical exam, and SAMPLE history are done quickly so that injuries and illnesses can be identified and given first aid. After the most serious conditions have been cared for, regularly recheck the person who has a serious injury or illness such as having breathing difficulties, has major blood loss, or has experienced a significant cause of injury. When in doubt, keep checking the person as frequently as possible. Remaining calm and reassuring the person that help is on the way may be the best treatment you can provide for the person.

# prep kit

## ▶ Ready for Review

- Assessment is a sequence of actions that helps determine what is wrong and thus ensures safe and appropriate first aid.
- Every time you encounter a person, first perform a scene size-up.
- Assessment will be influenced by whether the person is suffering from an illness or an injury, whether the person is responsive or unresponsive, and whether life-threatening conditions are present.
- The primary check determines whether there are life-threatening conditions requiring quick care.
- The goal of a hands-on physical exam is to identify any potentially life-threatening illness or injury.
- Look for medical identification tags on the person.
- The information in a SAMPLE history can help you identify what is wrong with the person and can indicate the needed first aid.

## ▶ Vital Vocabulary

cause (mechanism) of injury The force that causes an injury.

chief complaint The primary symptom a person complains about; also, the person's response to questions such as "What is wrong?" or "What happened?"

DOTS A mnemonic for assessment in which each area of the body is evaluated for deformities, open wounds, tenderness, and swelling.

first impression The part of the assessment that helps identify any immediately or potentially life-threatening conditions.

nature of illness The general type of illness a person is experiencing.

physical exam A part of the assessment process in which a detailed, area-by-area exam is performed on people whose conditions cannot be readily identified or when more specific information is needed about a condition.

primary check A step of the assessment process in which a first aid provider checks for life-threatening injuries and gives care for any that are found.

SAMPLE history A brief history of a person's condition to determine signs and symptoms, allergies, medications, pertinent past medical history, last oral intake, and events leading to the illness/injury.

scene size-up A quick assessment of the scene and the surroundings for safety issues, the cause of injury or nature of illness, and the number of people; completed before starting first aid.

sign Evidence of an injury or disease that can be seen, heard, or felt.

symptom What a person tells a first aid provider about what he or she feels.

## ▶ Assessment in Action

You are in a crowded mall doing some last-minute holiday shopping. You hear someone yell for help at a nearby store. You are the first to arrive on the scene. Bystanders begin to approach and ask what is going on. The person who called for help witnessed a man collapse.

*Directions:* Circle Yes if you agree with the statement; circle No if you disagree.

Yes No **1.** The first thing you should do is conduct a physical exam.

Yes No **2.** Your primary check of the man includes identifying and treating immediate life-threatening conditions such as issues with his breathing and severe bleeding.

Yes No **3.** The man is responsive and alert. Ask permission from him before beginning first aid.

Yes No **4.** The man asks you to stay until medical help arrives. You should continue to do regular checks of him until medical help arrives.

## ▶ Check Your Knowledge

*Directions:* Circle Yes if you agree with the statement; circle No if you disagree.

Yes    No    **1.** The purpose of a primary check is to find life-threatening conditions.

Yes    No    **2.** Most injured people require a complete physical exam.

Yes    No    **3.** For a physical exam, you usually begin at the head and work down the body.

Yes    No    **4.** The mnemonic DOTS helps in remembering what information to obtain about the person's history that could be useful.

Yes    No    **5.** For all injured and suddenly ill people, look for a medical identification tag during a physical exam.

Yes    No    **6.** The mnemonic SAMPLE can remind you how to examine an area for signs of an injury.

Yes    No    **7.** A gurgling sound heard while checking for breathing indicates possible fluid in the throat.

# CPR

**5**

## Chapter
### at a glance

## Heart Attack and Cardiac Arrest

A **heart attack** occurs when heart muscle tissue dies because its blood supply is severely reduced or stopped. The cause of this impaired blood supply is often a clot in one or more coronary arteries. The signs of a heart attack and the steps for caring for a heart attack are discussed in detail in Chapter 17, *Sudden Illnesses*.

If damage to the heart muscle is too severe, the person's heart can stop beating—a condition known as **cardiac arrest**. Sudden cardiac arrest is a leading cause of death in the United States.

## ▶ Caring for Cardiac Arrest

Few people experiencing sudden cardiac arrest outside of a hospital survive unless a rapid sequence of events takes place. One way of describing the ideal sequence of care that should take place when a cardiac arrest occurs is to think about the links in a chain. Each link is dependent on the others for strength and success. In this way, the links form a **chain of survival**.

The five events (links) that must occur rapidly and in an integrated manner during cardiac arrest outside of a hospital are as follows Figure 5-1 :

1. *Recognition and action.* Responders must recognize the early warning signs of cardiac arrest and immediately call 9-1-1 to activate emergency medical services (EMS).

**Figure 5-1**

Out-of-hospital chain of survival.

2. *CPR.* The chest compressions delivered during **cardiopulmonary resuscitation (CPR)** circulate blood to the heart and brain. Effective chest compressions are critical to buying time until a defibrillator and EMS personnel are available.

3. *Defibrillation.* Administering a shock to the heart can restore the heartbeat in some people. Time is a critical factor. The earlier the shock, the better the chance of success.

4. *Advanced care.* Paramedics provide advanced cardiac life support to people experiencing sudden cardiac arrest. This support includes providing IV fluids, medications, advanced airway devices, and rapid transport to the hospital.

5. *Post-arrest care.* The hospital can provide life-saving medications, surgical procedures, and advanced medical care to enable the person of sudden cardiac arrest to survive and recover.

## ▶ Performing CPR

When a person's heart stops beating, he or she quickly needs CPR, defibrillation, and the help of EMS professionals. CPR consists of moving blood to the heart and brain by giving **chest compressions** and providing periodic breaths to place oxygen into the person's lungs. CPR techniques are similar for infants (birth to 1 year), children (1 year to puberty), and adults (puberty and older), with just slight variations.

### Q&A

**For CPR purposes, what defines a person as an adult, child, or infant?**

- Infants are those less than 1 year of age.
- A child ranges from 1 year to puberty. (Puberty can be recognized by hair in the armpits of boys and breast development in girls.)
- Adults include those at puberty and older.

## Check for Responsiveness

In a motionless person, check for responsiveness by tapping the person's shoulder and asking if he or she is okay. If the person does not respond (ie, does not answer, move, or moan), he or she is said to be unresponsive.

## Activate the EMS System

After you check for responsiveness, shout for nearby help. Activate the EMS system by calling or asking a bystander to call 9-1-1. Using a mobile phone, you can call EMS without leaving the person's side. If a mobile phone is used, it should be kept by the person's side, if possible. If a mobile phone is not available, leave the person to call 9-1-1 and get an AED. If you are alone with a child or infant, give CPR for five sets of 30 compressions and 2 breaths (2 minutes); then call 9-1-1.

**Figure 5-2**

The hand position for chest compressions is in the center of the chest.

---

## FYI

### Risk Factors of Cardiovascular Disease

Several factors contribute to an increased risk of developing heart disease. Risk factors you cannot change are as follows:

- *Heredity.* Tendencies appear in family lines.
- *Gender.* Men have a greater risk. After menopause, the death rate from heart disease in women increases. Coronary heart disease is the leading cause of death in American men and women.
- *Age.* Over 80% of those who die of heart disease are 65 years or older.

Risk factors you can change are as follows:

- *Tobacco smoking.* People who smoke have a two to four times greater chance of developing heart disease than do people who do not smoke.
- *High blood pressure.* This condition increases the heart's workload.
- *High cholesterol.* Too much cholesterol can cause a buildup in the walls of the arteries.
- *Diabetes.* This condition affects blood cholesterol and triglyceride levels.
- *Overweight and obesity.* Excess body fat, especially around the waist, increases the likelihood of developing heart disease. Being overweight affects blood pressure and cholesterol and places an added strain on the heart.

## Check for Breathing

Check breathing for 5 to 10 seconds by looking for the rise and fall of the person's chest. No breathing and occasional gasps (may sound like a groan or snore) indicate that a person needs CPR.

## Give Chest Compressions

Place the person faceup on a firm, flat surface. Perform chest compressions with two hands for an adult, one or two hands for a child, and two fingers for an infant. Effective compressions require first aid providers to push hard and push fast. The chest of an adult should be compressed at least 2 inches (5 cm) but no more than 2.4 inches (6 cm), the chest of a child about 2 inches (5 cm), and the chest of an infant about 1.5 inches (4 cm). The desired hand position for chest compressions is in the center of the chest (lower half of the sternum [breast bone]) **Figure 5-2**.

Give compressions at a rate of 100 to 120 compressions per minute for adults, children, and infants. The beat of the Bee Gees song "Stayin' Alive" is helpful for maintaining the speed of compressions. The 100- to 120-compression rate is not the actual number of compressions given in a minute; it is the speed of compressions.

## Open the Airway

Before giving breaths during CPR, open the airway using the head tilt–chin lift maneuver.

To perform the **head tilt–chin lift maneuver**, follow these steps:

1. Place one hand on the person's forehead and the fingertips of the other hand on the bony part of the chin nearest you.
2. While applying firm backward pressure with your hand, lift the chin upward to help tilt the person's head back.

First aid providers should use this maneuver even when a cervical spine injury is suspected, whereas health care providers would use a jaw-thrust maneuver.

## FYI

### Oxygen Use in First Aid

Supplemental oxygen is useful for various medical conditions (eg, carbon monoxide poisoning); however, its use is not considered a first aid skill and requires special training. If using supplemental oxygen, be sure to keep any possible source of fire (eg, glowing cigarette, spark) away from the area.

## Give Rescue Breaths

Breathing for a person who is not breathing is known as rescue breathing. Keep the person's airway open using the head tilt–chin lift maneuver **Figure 5-3** . Pinch the person's nose shut with your thumb and index finger, take a normal breath, and blow gently into the person's mouth for 1 second. Remove your mouth and take a breath for yourself, then give a second breath. Watch for chest rise to determine if the breaths go in. You only need to make the person's chest gently rise. Rescue breaths can cause stomach distention; minimize this condition by limiting the force of your breath.

A barrier device (ie, mask or face shield) is a protective device used during rescue breathing; it features a plastic barrier placed on a person's face to prevent contact with secretions, vomitus, and gases. This device is a safety precaution to prevent possible disease transmission. Provide mouth-to-mouth breathing without a barrier device only when a barrier device is unavailable.

Continue CPR until an automated external defibrillator (AED) becomes available, the person shows signs of life, EMS personnel take over, or you are too tired to continue. Keep interruptions in compressions to a minimum. If other first aid providers are available, they can rotate performing chest compressions after every five sets of 30 compressions and 2 breaths (2 minutes) or after an AED delivers a shock.

### Mouth-to-Mouth Breathing

To perform mouth-to-mouth breathing, follow these steps:

1. Position yourself beside the person's head.
2. Pinch the person's nostrils together with a thumb and index finger.
3. Open the airway with the head tilt–chin lift maneuver. Press on the forehead to maintain a backward tilt of the head.
4. Place your mouth over the person's mouth and gently breathe into the person's mouth for 1 second. The person's chest should rise.
5. Remove your mouth and take a breath for yourself before giving the next breath.

### Mouth-to-Mask Breathing

To perform mouth-to-mask breathing, follow these steps:

1. Position yourself beside the person's head.
2. Place the mask over the person's mouth and nose. The mask's nose notch should be on the nose and not on the chin.
3. Open the airway with the head tilt–chin lift maneuver. Press on the forehead to maintain a backward tilt of the head.
4. Place your mouth on the mouthpiece and gently breathe into the mouthpiece for 1 second. The person's chest should rise.
5. Remove your mouth and take a breath for yourself before giving the next breath.

### Mouth-to-Face Shield Breathing

To perform mouth-to-face shield breathing, follow these steps:

1. Position yourself beside the person's head.
2. Place the shield over the person's mouth.

Tongue blocking air passage
Air passage

© Jones & Bartlett Learning

© Jones & Bartlett Learning

**A**

**B**

**Figure 5-3**

**A.** Relaxation of the tongue back into the throat causes airway obstruction. **B.** To perform the head tilt-chin lift maneuver, place one hand on the person's forehead and apply firm backward pressure with your palm to tilt the head back. Next, place the tips of the index and middle fingers of your other hand under the lower jaw near the bony part of the chin. Lift the chin upward, bringing the entire lower jaw with it, helping to tilt the head back.

3. Pinch the person's nostrils together with a thumb and index finger.
4. Open the airway with the head tilt–chin lift maneuver. Press on the forehead to maintain a backward tilt of the head.

5. Place your mouth over the shield and gently breathe into the person's mouth for 1 second. The person's chest should rise.
6. Remove your mouth and take a breath for yourself before giving the next breath.

---

## FYI

### Rescue Breaths

Other methods of rescue breathing are as follows:
- Mouth-to-breathing device
- Mouth-to-nose method
- Mouth-to-stoma method

### Mouth-to-Breathing Device

A breathing device is placed in the person's mouth or over the person's mouth and nose as a precaution against disease transmission. There are several different types of barrier devices **Figure 5-4**.

### Mouth-to-Nose Method

If you cannot open the person's mouth, the person's mouth is severely injured, or you cannot make a good seal with the person's mouth (eg, because there are no teeth), use the mouth-to-nose method. With the head tilted back, push up on the person's chin to close the mouth. Make a seal with your mouth over the person's nose and provide rescue breaths.

### Mouth-to-Stoma Method

Some diseases of the vocal cords may result in surgical removal of the larynx. People who have this surgery breathe through a small permanent opening in the neck called a stoma. To perform mouth-to-stoma breathing, close the person's mouth and nose and breathe through the opening in the neck.

---

## Adult and Child CPR

To perform CPR on an adult or child, follow the steps in **Skill Sheet 5-1** and **Flowchart 5-1**.

## Infant CPR

To perform CPR on an infant, follow the steps in **Skill Sheet 5-2** and **Flowchart 5-2**.

**Figure 5-4**

Barrier devices. **A.** Face shield. **B.** Mask.

# Skill Sheet

## 5-1   Adult and Child CPR

*Note:* Whenever possible, use a mouth-to-barrier device to prevent disease transmission. Use the **RAB-CAB** mnemonic to remember what to do.

**1** **R = Responsive?** Tap the person on the shoulder and shout, "Are you okay?" If the person does not respond, continue to Step 2. If the person responds:

- Ask the person about chief complaints.
- Use the SAMPLE (signs and symptoms, allergies, medications, pertinent past medical history, last oral intake, events leading up to the illness or injury) history questions.
- Check the person for DOTS (deformities, open wounds, tenderness, and swelling) if an injury is suspected.

**2** **A = Activate** EMS. If you are alone:

- Shout for help.
- Activate EMS by calling 9-1-1 or the local emergency number. If a cell phone is used, it should be kept by the person's side, if possible.
- If a cell phone is not available, leave the person to activate EMS and get an AED before starting CPR.

If another person arrives or is nearby, have him or her activate EMS and get an AED.

**3** **B = Breathing?**

- Place the person faceup on a flat, firm surface.
- Observe the person's chest for movement (rise and fall); take 5 sec but no more than 10 sec.
- If the person is not breathing or is only gasping, continue to Step 4.
- If the person is breathing normally, continue to monitor his or her breathing until EMS arrives.

*(Continues)*

# Skill Sheet Continued

**5-1**    **Adult and Child CPR**

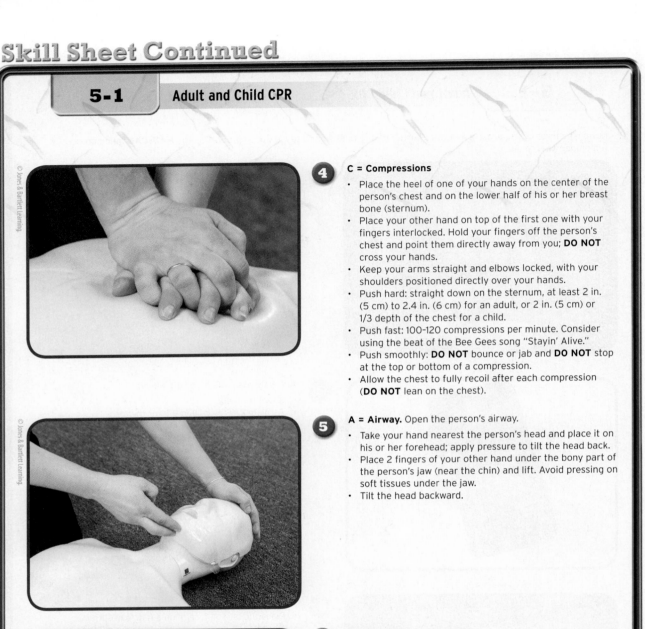

**4** **C = Compressions**
- Place the heel of one of your hands on the center of the person's chest and on the lower half of his or her breast bone (sternum).
- Place your other hand on top of the first one with your fingers interlocked. Hold your fingers off the person's chest and point them directly away from you; **DO NOT** cross your hands.
- Keep your arms straight and elbows locked, with your shoulders positioned directly over your hands.
- Push hard: straight down on the sternum, at least 2 in. (5 cm) to 2.4 in. (6 cm) for an adult, or 2 in. (5 cm) or 1/3 depth of the chest for a child.
- Push fast: 100-120 compressions per minute. Consider using the beat of the Bee Gees song "Stayin' Alive."
- Push smoothly: **DO NOT** bounce or jab and **DO NOT** stop at the top or bottom of a compression.
- Allow the chest to fully recoil after each compression (**DO NOT** lean on the chest).

**5** **A = Airway.** Open the person's airway.
- Take your hand nearest the person's head and place it on his or her forehead; apply pressure to tilt the head back.
- Place 2 fingers of your other hand under the bony part of the person's jaw (near the chin) and lift. Avoid pressing on soft tissues under the jaw.
- Tilt the head backward.

**6** **B = Breaths.** Give 2 breaths.
- Pinch the person's nose shut.
- Give 2 breaths, each lasting 1 sec. (Take a normal breath for yourself after each breath.)
- Watch for chest rise to determine if your breaths go in.
- Allow for chest deflation after each breath.
- If you see chest rise after the 2 breaths, give 30 chest compressions.
- If the first breath does not make the chest rise, retilt the person's head and give a second breath. If the second breath does not make the chest rise, begin CPR (30 compressions and 2 breaths). Each time before giving the first of the 2 breaths, open the mouth and look for an object; if seen, remove it.
- If you cannot use the person's mouth (ie, seriously injured mouth, ineffective seal, mouth cannot be opened, person is in water), use the head tilt-chin lift maneuver. Seal your mouth around the person's nose and breathe.

# Skill Sheet Continued

**5-1**   Adult and Child CPR

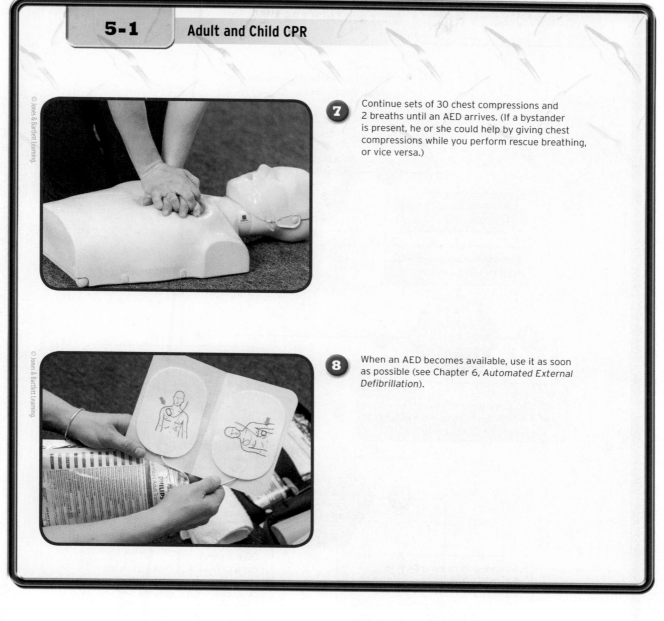

**7** Continue sets of 30 chest compressions and 2 breaths until an AED arrives. (If a bystander is present, he or she could help by giving chest compressions while you perform rescue breathing, or vice versa.)

**8** When an AED becomes available, use it as soon as possible (see Chapter 6, *Automated External Defibrillation*).

© Jones & Bartlett Learning.

## Flowchart 5-1 — Adult and Child CPR

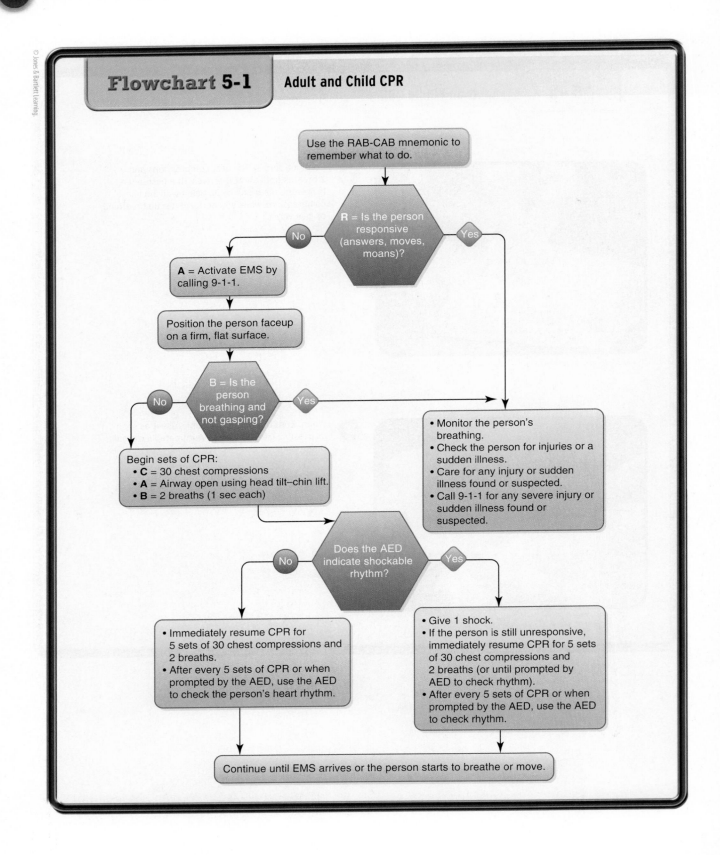

Use the RAB-CAB mnemonic to remember what to do.

**R** = Is the person responsive (answers, moves, moans)?

**No** → **A** = Activate EMS by calling 9-1-1.

Position the person faceup on a firm, flat surface.

**B** = Is the person breathing and not gasping?

**Yes** →

- Monitor the person's breathing.
- Check the person for injuries or a sudden illness.
- Care for any injury or sudden illness found or suspected.
- Call 9-1-1 for any severe injury or sudden illness found or suspected.

**No** → Begin sets of CPR:
- **C** = 30 chest compressions
- **A** = Airway open using head tilt–chin lift.
- **B** = 2 breaths (1 sec each)

Does the AED indicate shockable rhythm?

**No** →
- Immediately resume CPR for 5 sets of 30 chest compressions and 2 breaths.
- After every 5 sets of CPR or when prompted by the AED, use the AED to check the person's heart rhythm.

**Yes** →
- Give 1 shock.
- If the person is still unresponsive, immediately resume CPR for 5 sets of 30 chest compressions and 2 breaths (or until prompted by AED to check rhythm).
- After every 5 sets of CPR or when prompted by the AED, use the AED to check rhythm.

Continue until EMS arrives or the person starts to breathe or move.

# Skill Sheet

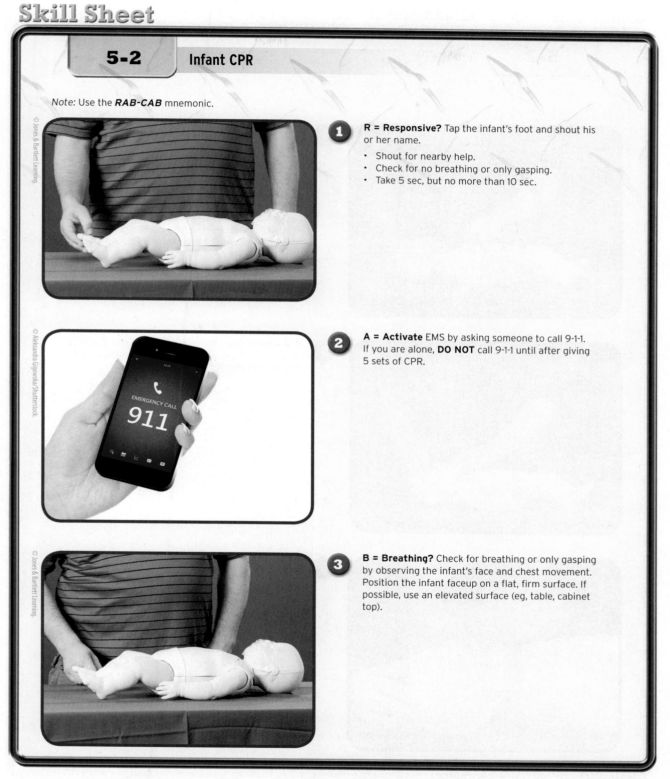

**5-2**    Infant CPR

*Note:* Use the **RAB-CAB** mnemonic.

**1**  **R = Responsive?** Tap the infant's foot and shout his or her name.

- Shout for nearby help.
- Check for no breathing or only gasping.
- Take 5 sec, but no more than 10 sec.

**2**  **A = Activate** EMS by asking someone to call 9-1-1. If you are alone, **DO NOT** call 9-1-1 until after giving 5 sets of CPR.

**3**  **B = Breathing?** Check for breathing or only gasping by observing the infant's face and chest movement. Position the infant faceup on a flat, firm surface. If possible, use an elevated surface (eg, table, cabinet top).

*(Continues)*

© Jones & Bartlett Learning

© Aleksandra Gigowska/Shutterstock.

© Jones & Bartlett Learning.

## Skill Sheet Continued

**5-2**    Infant CPR

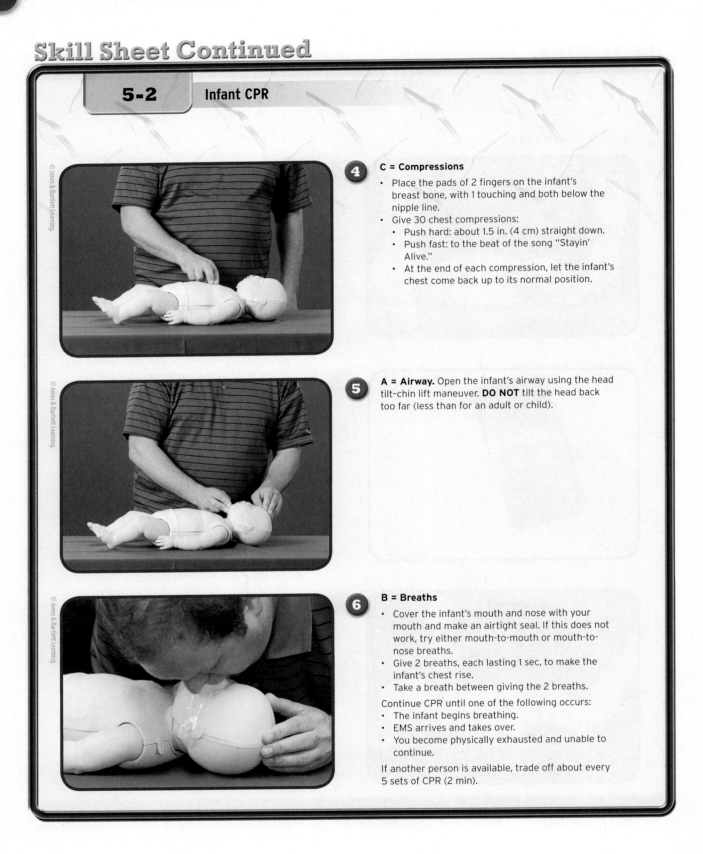

**4**  **C = Compressions**
- Place the pads of 2 fingers on the infant's breast bone, with 1 touching and both below the nipple line.
- Give 30 chest compressions:
  - Push hard: about 1.5 in. (4 cm) straight down.
  - Push fast: to the beat of the song "Stayin' Alive."
  - At the end of each compression, let the infant's chest come back up to its normal position.

**5**  **A = Airway.** Open the infant's airway using the head tilt–chin lift maneuver. **DO NOT** tilt the head back too far (less than for an adult or child).

**6**  **B = Breaths**
- Cover the infant's mouth and nose with your mouth and make an airtight seal. If this does not work, try either mouth-to-mouth or mouth-to-nose breaths.
- Give 2 breaths, each lasting 1 sec, to make the infant's chest rise.
- Take a breath between giving the 2 breaths.

Continue CPR until one of the following occurs:
- The infant begins breathing.
- EMS arrives and takes over.
- You become physically exhausted and unable to continue.

If another person is available, trade off about every 5 sets of CPR (2 min).

## Flowchart 5-2 | Infant CPR

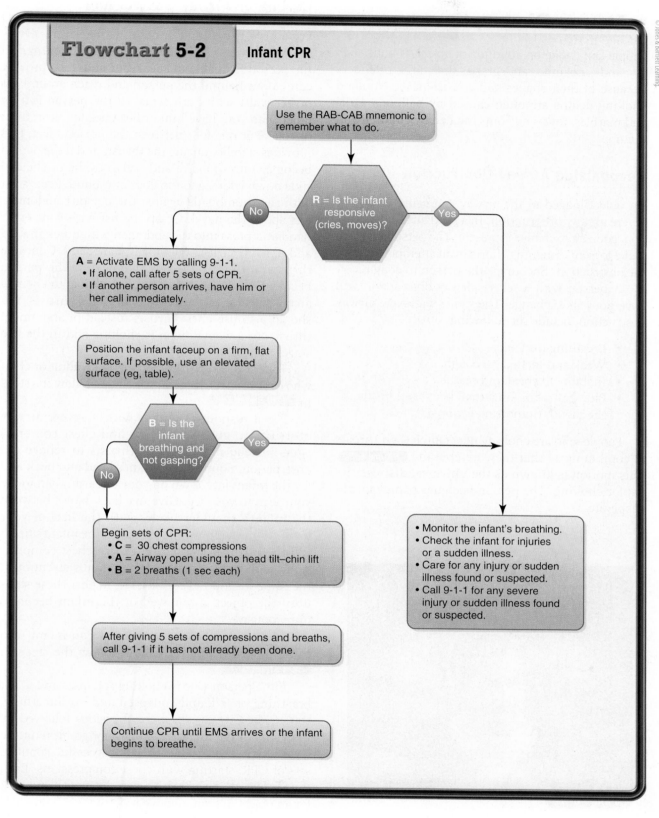

Use the RAB-CAB mnemonic to remember what to do.

**R** = Is the infant responsive (cries, moves)?

No — →

Yes — →

**A** = Activate EMS by calling 9-1-1.
• If alone, call after 5 sets of CPR.
• If another person arrives, have him or her call immediately.

Position the infant faceup on a firm, flat surface. If possible, use an elevated surface (eg, table).

**B** = Is the infant breathing and not gasping?

Yes — →

No

Begin sets of CPR:
• **C** = 30 chest compressions
• **A** = Airway open using the head tilt–chin lift
• **B** = 2 breaths (1 sec each)

After giving 5 sets of compressions and breaths, call 9-1-1 if it has not already been done.

Continue CPR until EMS arrives or the infant begins to breathe.

• Monitor the infant's breathing.
• Check the infant for injuries or a sudden illness.
• Care for any injury or sudden illness found or suspected.
• Call 9-1-1 for any severe injury or sudden illness found or suspected.

# ▶ Airway Obstruction

People can choke on all kinds of objects. Foods such as candy, peanuts, and grapes are major offenders because of their shapes and consistencies. Nonfood choking deaths are often caused by balloons, balls and marbles, toys, and coins inhaled by children and infants.

## Recognizing Airway Obstruction

An object lodged in the airway can cause a mild or severe **airway obstruction**. In a mild airway obstruction, good air exchange is present. The person is able to make forceful coughing efforts in an attempt to relieve the obstruction. Encourage the person to cough.

A person with a severe airway obstruction will have poor air exchange. The signs of a severe airway obstruction include the following:

- Breathing difficulty
- Weak and ineffective cough
- Inability to speak or breathe
- Blue-gray skin, fingernail beds, and inside of the mouth (indicating **cyanosis**)

People who are choking may clutch their throats to communicate that they are choking  Figure 5-5 . This motion is known as the universal distress signal for choking. The person becomes panicked and desperate.

**Figure 5-5**

The universal sign of choking.

## Caring for Airway Obstruction

For a responsive adult or child with a severe airway obstruction, ask the person "Are you choking?" If the person is unable to speak but nods yes, provide care. Move behind the person and reach around his or her waist with both arms. (If the person is a lot taller than you, have him or her kneel or sit in front of you.) Put one foot between the person's feet; this provides stability during the thrusts and if the person becomes unresponsive and collapses, he or she can slide down your leg to the floor or ground. Place a fist with the thumb side against the person's abdomen, just above the navel. Grasp the fist with your other hand and press into the abdomen with quick inward and upward thrusts (Heimlich maneuver). Continue thrusts until the object is removed or the person becomes unresponsive. If you are unable to encircle an obese person's abdomen, apply chest thrusts. You should also use chest thrusts instead of abdominal thrusts for a woman who is choking and in the late stages of pregnancy.

To relieve airway obstruction in an adult or child who cannot speak, breathe, or cough, follow the steps in  Skill Sheet 5-3 .

For a responsive infant with a severe airway obstruction, give back blows and chest compressions instead of abdominal thrusts to relieve the obstruction. Support the infant's head and neck and lay the infant facedown on your forearm, then lower your arm to your leg. Give five back blows between the infant's shoulder blades with the heel of your hand. While supporting the back of the infant's head, roll the infant faceup and give five chest compressions with two fingers on the infant's sternum in the same location used for CPR. Repeat these steps until the object is removed or the infant becomes unresponsive.

To relieve airway obstruction in an infant who cannot cry, breathe, or cough, follow the steps in  Skill Sheet 5-4 .

If the person who is choking collapses and is not breathing or is found collapsed and not breathing, start CPR. Give 30 chest compressions followed by 2 breaths. If the first breath does not go in, retilt the head and try a second breath. If unsuccessful, continue sets of CPR, starting with chest compressions. Each time before giving a breath, open the mouth and look for an object; if seen, remove it.  Table 5-1  provides a review of CPR and AED procedures using the RAB-CAB procedure.

# Skill Sheet

| 5-3 | Adult and Child Choking |

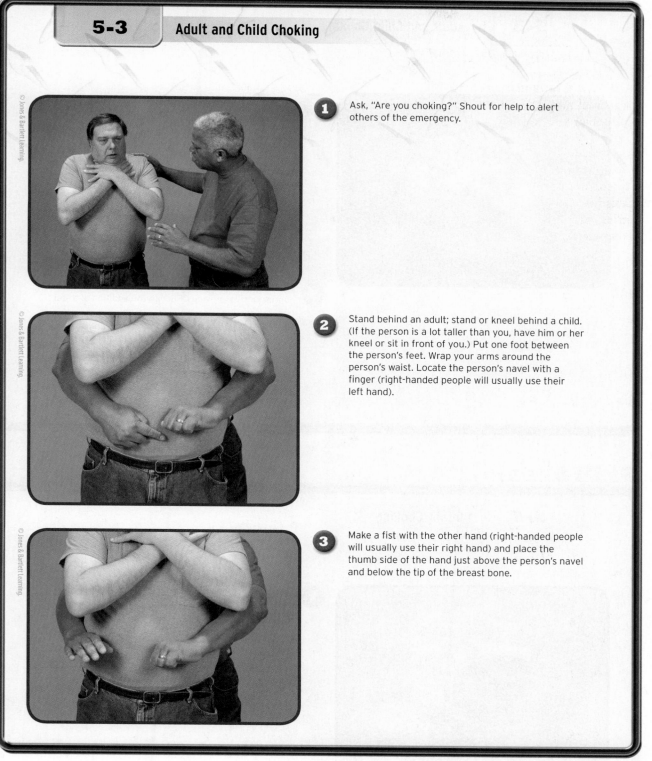

**1** Ask, "Are you choking?" Shout for help to alert others of the emergency.

**2** Stand behind an adult; stand or kneel behind a child. (If the person is a lot taller than you, have him or her kneel or sit in front of you.) Put one foot between the person's feet. Wrap your arms around the person's waist. Locate the person's navel with a finger (right-handed people will usually use their left hand).

**3** Make a fist with the other hand (right-handed people will usually use their right hand) and place the thumb side of the hand just above the person's navel and below the tip of the breast bone.

*(Continues)*

## Skill Sheet Continued

**5-3**    **Adult and Child Choking**

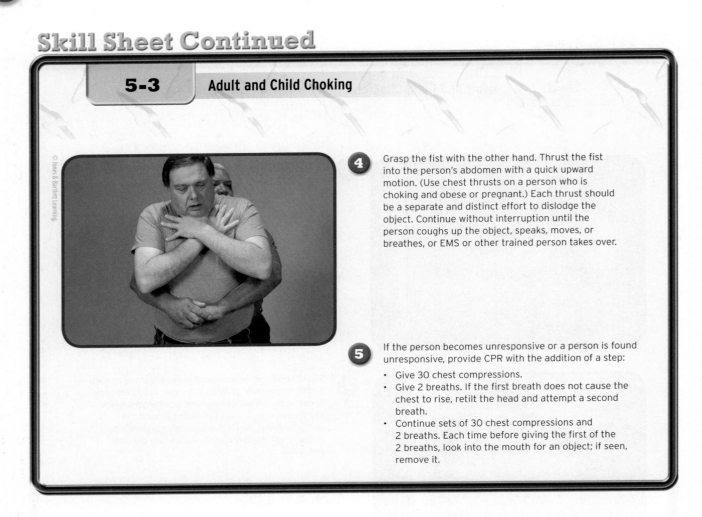

**4** Grasp the fist with the other hand. Thrust the fist into the person's abdomen with a quick upward motion. (Use chest thrusts on a person who is choking and obese or pregnant.) Each thrust should be a separate and distinct effort to dislodge the object. Continue without interruption until the person coughs up the object, speaks, moves, or breathes, or EMS or other trained person takes over.

**5** If the person becomes unresponsive or a person is found unresponsive, provide CPR with the addition of a step:

- Give 30 chest compressions.
- Give 2 breaths. If the first breath does not cause the chest to rise, retilt the head and attempt a second breath.
- Continue sets of 30 chest compressions and 2 breaths. Each time before giving the first of the 2 breaths, look into the mouth for an object; if seen, remove it.

## Skill Sheet

**5-4**    **Infant Choking**

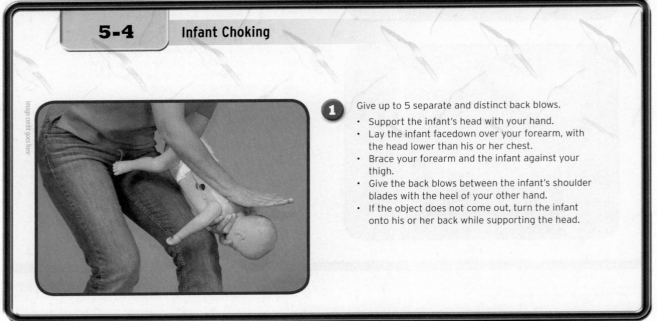

**1** Give up to 5 separate and distinct back blows.

- Support the infant's head with your hand.
- Lay the infant facedown over your forearm, with the head lower than his or her chest.
- Brace your forearm and the infant against your thigh.
- Give the back blows between the infant's shoulder blades with the heel of your other hand.
- If the object does not come out, turn the infant onto his or her back while supporting the head.

# Skill Sheet Continued

## 5-4 Infant Choking

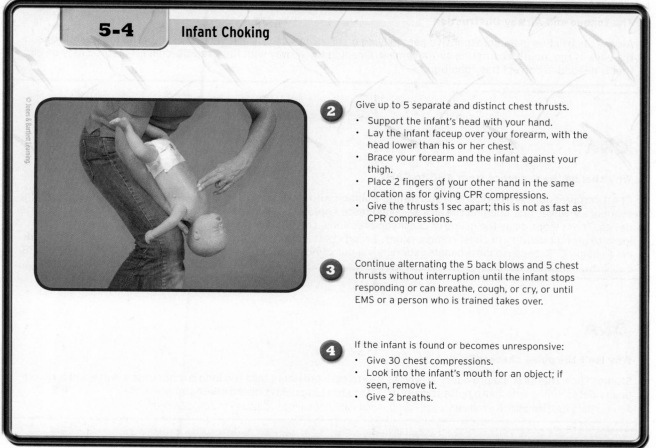

© Jones & Bartlett Learning.

**2** Give up to 5 separate and distinct chest thrusts.

- Support the infant's head with your hand.
- Lay the infant faceup over your forearm, with the head lower than his or her chest.
- Brace your forearm and the infant against your thigh.
- Place 2 fingers of your other hand in the same location as for giving CPR compressions.
- Give the thrusts 1 sec apart; this is not as fast as CPR compressions.

**3** Continue alternating the 5 back blows and 5 chest thrusts without interruption until the infant stops responding or can breathe, cough, or cry, or until EMS or a person who is trained takes over.

**4** If the infant is found or becomes unresponsive:

- Give 30 chest compressions.
- Look into the infant's mouth for an object; if seen, remove it.
- Give 2 breaths.

## Q&A

**What are the types of upper airway obstruction?**

- *Tongue.* Unconsciousness produces relaxation of soft tissues, and the tongue can fall into the airway. Swallowing one's tongue is impossible, but the widespread belief that it can happen is explained by slippage of the relaxed tongue into the airway. The tongue is the most common cause of airway obstruction.
- *Foreign body.* People, especially children, inhale all kinds of objects. Foods such as hot dogs, candy, peanuts, and grapes are major offenders because of their shapes and consistencies. According to the Journal of Forensic Science, meat is the main cause of choking in adults. Coins and toys are the top causes of nonfood choking deaths in children, as reported by the American Academy of Pediatrics. Unconscious people's airways can also be obstructed by a foreign material such as vomit and teeth.
- *Swelling.* Severe allergic reactions (anaphylaxis) and irritants (eg, smoke, chemicals) can cause swelling. Even a nonallergic person who is stung inside the throat by a bee, yellow jacket, or other flying insect can experience swelling in the airway.
- *Spasm.* Water that is suddenly inhaled can cause a spasm in the throat.
- *Vomit.* Many people vomit when they are near death. Whenever performing CPR, expect vomit before or during CPR.

## FYI

### The Tongue and Airway Obstruction

Airway obstruction in an unresponsive person lying on his or her back is usually the result of the tongue relaxing in the back of the mouth, restricting air movement. Opening the airway with the head tilt–chin lift method may be all that is needed to correct this condition.

## Q&A

### Why change the sequence from ABC to CAB?

Chest compressions are critical to resuscitating a person with cardiac arrest. The ABC (airway, breathing, circulation) sequence involves first opening the airway, giving rescue breaths, and perhaps getting and placing a mouth-to-barrier device. These steps delay the giving of chest compressions. The CAB (compressions, airway, breathing) sequence leads to prompt delivery of chest compressions. Giving chest compressions first may also encourage first aid providers to begin CPR, because most people experiencing out-of-hospital cardiac arrest do not receive any bystander CPR.

## Q&A

### Why isn't the pulse checked?

Studies show that first aid providers as well as health care providers take too long to check for a pulse and have difficulty determining whether a pulse is present. Taking too long delays giving chest compressions.
*Source:* Berg RA, Hemphill R, Abella BS, et al. Part 5: Adult basic life support. *Circulation* 2010;122:S689.

### Table 5-1 Quick Review of CPR and AED Procedures Using the RAB-CAB Procedure

| Steps/Action | Adults (at or past puberty) | Child (1 year to puberty) | Infant (younger than 1 year) |
|---|---|---|---|
| **R = Responsive?** | | | |
| Technique | Tap a shoulder and shout, "Are you OK?" A person who is responsive will answer, move, or moan. | | Tap the bottom of a foot and shout his or her name. A responsive infant will cry or move. |
| **A = Activate EMS and get an AED.** (Shout for nearby help and call 9-1-1 or the emergency response number. An AED may or may not be available.) | | | |
| When? | • If you are alone, call 9-1-1 and get an AED. When you return, use the AED.<br>• If another person is with you, send him or her to call and get an AED while you begin CPR immediately. | • If you are alone, and before calling 9-1-1, give 5 sets of 30 chest compressions and 2 breaths (CPR).<br>• After 5 sets of CPR, leave the child or infant to call 9-1-1 and get an AED.<br>• When you return, use the AED on the child as soon as possible. | |
| Whom to call? | Call 9-1-1 or the emergency response number. | | |

## Table 5-1  Quick Review of CPR and AED Procedures Using the RAB-CAB Procedure, (Continued)

| Steps/Action | Adults (at or past puberty) | Child (1 year to puberty) | Infant (younger than 1 year) |
|---|---|---|---|
| **B = Breathing? Check for no breathing or only gasping.** | | | |
| • Place person faceup on a flat, firm surface.<br>• Observe the face and chest movement for breathing. Take 5 sec but no more than 10 sec. | If the person is not breathing or is only occasionally gasping (may sound like a quick inhalation or like a groan/snore), CPR is needed. | | |
| | If the person is breathing but not responding, CPR is not needed; place the person in the recovery position to keep his or her airway clear, and monitor breathing. | | |
| **C = Chest compressions** | | | |
| Where to place person? | Firm, flat surface (eg, floor, ground, sidewalk) | | Can be placed on table or cabinet top |
| Where to place hands? | Center of chest and lower half of breast bone (sternum) | | Pads of 2 fingers in the center of chest on the breast bone with 1 touching and both below the imaginary nipple line |
| | 2 hands:<br><br>• Heel of 1 hand on breast bone; other hand on top<br>• Fingers of both hands interlocked<br>• Arms straight with shoulders directly over the hands | 1 hand for very small child: Heel of 1 hand only<br><br>2 hands:<br><br>• Same as for an adult<br>• Arms straight with shoulders directly over the hands | |
| Depth | At least 2 in. (5 cm) but no more than 2.4 in. (6 cm) | About 2 in. (5 cm) or at least 1/3 depth of the upper body (chest) | About 1.5 in. (4 cm) or at least 1/3 depth of the upper body (chest) |
| | After each compression, allow full recoil of the chest.<br><br>**DO NOT** lean on the chest of an adult or child. | | |
| Rate | 100-120 per minute<br><br>(Follow the beat of the Bee Gees song "Stayin' Alive," the beats from a smartphone application that was previously installed and is quickly accessible, or a dispatcher's directions heard over a cell phone's speaker.) | | |
| Ratio of chest compressions to breaths | 30:2 | | |
| **A = Airway open** | | | |
| Technique | Head tilt-chin lift | | |
| **B = Breaths** | | | |
| Technique | • Pinch the nose shut, and, with your mouth, make an airtight mouth-to-mouth seal. Use a CPR mask or face shield, if available.<br>• Perform the head tilt-chin lift maneuver.<br>• Give 2 breaths:<br>  • Each breath should last 1 sec.<br>  • Blow enough to make the chest rise. | | Perform the head tilt-chin lift maneuver (**DO NOT** tilt the head back too far).<br><br>• Cover the infant's mouth and nose with your mouth, making an airtight seal. If this does not work, try either mouth-to-mouth or mouth-to-nose breaths.<br>• Give 2 breaths:<br>  • Each breath should last 1 sec.<br>  • Blow enough to make the chest rise. |
| | If first breath does not cause chest to rise, retilt head and give second breath. If second breath does not make chest rise, begin CPR (30 compressions and 2 breaths). Each time before giving a breath, open the mouth and look for an object; if seen, remove it. | | |

*(Continues)*

**Table 5-1  Quick Review of CPR and AED Procedures Using the RAB-CAB Procedure, (Continued)**

| Steps/Action | Adults (at or past puberty) | Child (1 year to puberty) | Infant (younger than 1 year) |
|---|---|---|---|

Continue CPR until:

1. The person begins breathing.
2. Other rescuer(s) (ie, trained layperson, EMS personnel) take over.
3. An AED arrives and is used (except for infants).
4. You become physically exhausted and unable to continue.

If a bystander is available, he or she could help by giving chest compressions while you perform rescue breathing, or vice versa.

**Defibrillation**

If available, use an AED as soon as possible. (See Chapter 6, *Automated External Defibrillation*.)

1. Turn on the AED.
2. Attach the pads to the person's bare, dry chest (shown on the pads' diagrams). If needed, plug the cables into the AED. Child-sized pads may be available.
3. Stay clear of the person. Make sure no one, including you, is touching the person. Say, "Clear!"
4. Allow the AED to analyze the heart rhythm (push Analyze button, if necessary). The AED will prompt one of three actions:

   • Stay clear while the AED automatically delivers a shock.
   • Press the shock button.
   • **DO NOT** shock but give CPR, starting with chest compressions with the pads staying in place.

After performing any one of the three actions, give 5 sets of CPR unless the person moves, begins to breathe, or wakes up.

Repeat defibrillation Steps 2 and 3 until the person moves, begins to breathe, or wakes up, or EMS arrives and takes over.

## ▶ Ready for Review

- A heart attack occurs when heart muscle tissue dies because the blood supply is severely reduced or stopped.
- The five links in the chain of survival are recognition and activation of EMS, CPR, defibrillation, advanced care, and post-arrest care.
- CPR consists of moving blood to the heart and brain by giving chest compressions and breathing oxygen into a person's lungs.
- The signs of a severe airway obstruction include difficult breathing, weak and ineffective cough, inability to speak or breathe, and signs of cyanosis.

## ▶ Vital Vocabulary

**airway obstruction** A blockage, often the result of a foreign body, in which airflow to the lungs is reduced or completely blocked.

**cardiac arrest** Stoppage of the heartbeat.

**cardiopulmonary resuscitation (CPR)** The act of providing chest compressions and rescue breaths for a person in cardiac arrest.

**chain of survival** A concept involving five critical links (recognition and activation of EMS, CPR, defibrillation, advanced care, post-arrest care) to help improve survival from cardiac arrest.

**chest compression** The act of depressing the chest and allowing it to return to its normal position as part of CPR.

**cyanosis** A blue-gray skin color that is caused by a reduced level of oxygen in the blood.

**head tilt–chin lift maneuver** A combination of two movements to open the airway by tilting the forehead back and lifting the chin.

**heart attack** Death of a part of the heart muscle.

## ▶ Assessment in Action

You are having dinner in a very crowded restaurant with your family on New Year's Eve. An older man is pushing a piano into the restaurant as part of the entertainment that evening. As he passes your table, he clutches his chest and falls to the floor. He is not moving.

*Directions:* Circle Yes if you agree with the statement; circle No if you disagree.

Yes No 1. If he is not breathing or is breathing abnormally, you should call 9-1-1.

Yes No 2. The man must be choking because he is in a restaurant.

Yes No 3. If the man is choking, you should perform abdominal thrusts.

Yes No 4. If the man is choking, you should perform sets of 30 chest compressions and 2 breaths.

Yes No 5. Check for breathing before giving any breaths to the person.

Yes No 6. Continue CPR until an AED becomes available or EMS personnel arrive.

## ▶ Check Your Knowledge

*Directions:* Circle Yes if you agree with the statement; circle No if you disagree.

Yes No 1. Gasping in an unresponsive person can indicate that the person is not breathing.

Yes No 2. After you determine that an adult is unresponsive, the next step is for someone to call 9-1-1.

Yes No 3. Tilting the head back and lifting the chin helps move the tongue and open the airway.

Yes No 4. If you determine that a person is not breathing, begin chest compressions.

Yes No 5. Do not start chest compressions until you have checked for a pulse.

Yes No 6. For all people (adult, child, infant) needing CPR, give 30 compressions followed by 2 breaths.

Yes No 7. Use two fingers when performing CPR on an infant.

Yes No 8. A sign of choking is that the person is unable to speak or cough.

Yes No 9. To give abdominal thrusts to a responsive choking person, place your fist below the person's navel.

Yes No 10. When giving abdominal thrusts to a responsive choking person, repeat the thrusts until the object is removed or the person becomes unresponsive.

# Automated External Defibrillation

## Public Access Defibrillation

A person's chance of survival dramatically improves through early cardiopulmonary resuscitation (CPR) and early <u>defibrillation</u> with the use of an <u>automated external defibrillator (AED)</u>. To be effective, defibrillation must be used in the first few minutes following cardiac arrest. The implementation of state public access defibrillation (PAD) laws and the Food and Drug Administration's (FDA) approval of home-use AEDs have made this important care step available to many first aid providers in many places, including the following :

- Airports and airplanes
- Stadiums
- Health clubs
- Golf courses
- Schools
- Government buildings
- Offices
- Homes
- Shopping centers/malls

# ▶ How the Heart Works

The heart is an organ with four hollow chambers. The two chambers on the right side receive blood from the body and send it to the lungs for oxygen. The two chambers on the left side receive freshly oxygenated blood from the lungs and send it back out to the body **Figure 6-2**.

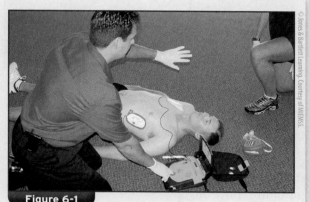

**Figure 6-1**

AEDs are available in many places for use by trained first aid providers.

The heart has a unique electrical system that controls the rate at which the heart beats and the amount of work the heart performs. In the right upper chamber of the heart, there is a collection of special pacemaker cells. These cells emit electrical impulses about 60 to 100 times a minute that cause the other heart muscle cells to contract in a coordinated manner.

Because the heart contracts approximately every second, it needs an abundant supply of oxygen, which it gets through the coronary arteries. These arteries run along the outside of the heart muscle and branch into smaller vessels. These arteries sometimes become diseased (atherosclerosis), resulting in a lack of oxygen to the pacemaker cells, which can cause abnormal electrical activity in the heart.

## When Normal Electrical Activity Is Interrupted

<u>Ventricular fibrillation</u> (also known as *V-fib*) is the most common abnormal heart rhythm in cases of sudden cardiac arrest in adults **Figure 6-3**.

The organized wave of electrical impulses that cause the heart muscle to contract and relax in a regular fashion is lost when the heart is in ventricular

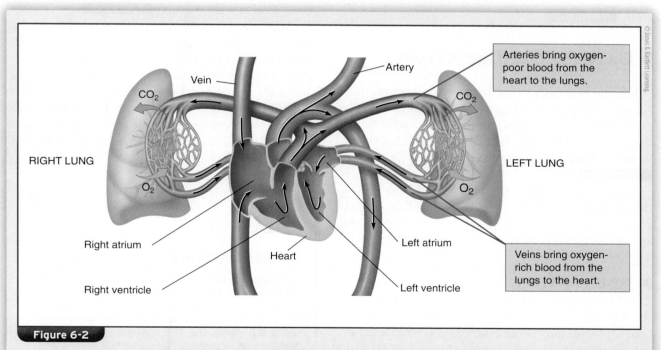

RIGHT LUNG

$CO_2$

$O_2$

Vein

Artery

Arteries bring oxygen-poor blood from the heart to the lungs.

LEFT LUNG

$CO_2$

$O_2$

Right atrium

Heart

Right ventricle

Left atrium

Left ventricle

Veins bring oxygen-rich blood from the lungs to the heart.

**Figure 6-2**

The right side of the heart receives blood from the body and sends it to the lungs. The left side of the heart receives the oxygenated blood and sends it to the body.

Figure 6-3

Ventricular fibrillation is disorganized electrical activity.

Figure 6-4

Ventricular tachycardia is very rapid electrical activity.

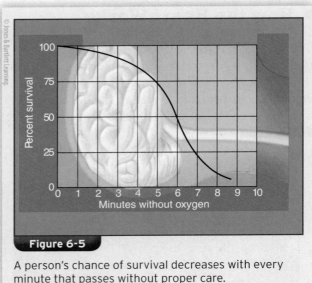

Figure 6-5

A person's chance of survival decreases with every minute that passes without proper care.

fibrillation. As a result, the lower chambers of the heart quiver and cannot pump blood, so circulation is lost (no pulse).

A second, potentially life-threatening, electrical condition is **ventricular tachycardia** (*V-tach*), in which the heart beats too fast to pump blood effectively Figure 6-4 .

## ▶ Care for Cardiac Arrest

When the heart stops beating, the blood stops circulating, cutting off all oxygen and nourishment to the entire body. In this situation, time is a crucial factor. For every minute that defibrillation is delayed, the person's chance of survival decreases by 7% to 10% Figure 6-5 .

CPR is the initial care for cardiac arrest until a defibrillator is available. Perform cycles of chest compressions and breaths until an AED is ready to be connected to the person.

## ▶ About AEDs

An AED is an electronic device that analyzes the heart rhythm and if necessary (such as in cardiac arrest) delivers an electric shock, known as defibrillation, to the heart. The purpose of this shock is to correct one of the abnormal electrical disturbances

previously discussed and to reestablish a heart rhythm that will result in normal electrical and pumping function.

All AEDs are attached to the person by a cable connected to two adhesive pads (electrodes) placed on the person's chest Figure 6-6 . The pad-and-cable system sends the electrical signal from the heart into the device for analysis and delivers the electric shock to the person when needed Figure 6-7 .

AEDs have built-in rhythm analysis systems that determine whether the person needs a shock. This system enables first aid providers and other rescuers to deliver early defibrillation with only minimal training.

AEDs also record the person's heart rhythm (known as an electrocardiogram, or ECG), shock data, and other information about the device's performance (eg, the date, time, and number of shocks supplied) Figure 6-8 .

### Q&A

**How does an AED work?**

A microprocessor inside the defibrillator interprets (analyzes) the person's heart rhythm through adhesive electrodes. The computer analyzes the heart rhythm and advises the rescuer whether a shock is needed. The AED advises a shock only if it detects ventricular fibrillation or fast ventricular tachycardia.

**Figure 6-6**

Two adhesive pads are placed on the person's chest and connected by a cable to the AED.

**Figure 6-8**

AEDs store information, including heart rhythms and shock data.

**Figure 6-7**

The pad-and-cable system sends the electrical signal from the heart into the device for analysis and delivers the electric shock to the person when needed.

## Common Elements of AEDs

Many different AED models exist. The principles for use are the same for each, but the displays, controls, and options vary slightly. You will need to know how to use your specific AED. All AEDs have the following elements in common:

- Power on/off mechanism
- Cable and pads (electrodes)
- Analysis capability
- Defibrillation capability
- Prompts to guide you
- Battery operation for portability

## ▶ Using an AED

Once you have determined the need for the AED (person unresponsive and not breathing), the basic operation of all AED models follows the sequence in **Skill Sheet 6-1**.

1. Some AEDs power on by pressing an on/off button. Others power on when opening the AED case lid. Once the power is on, the AED will quickly go through some internal checks and will then begin to provide voice and screen prompts **(Step 1)**.

2. Expose the person's chest. The skin must be fairly dry so that the pads will adhere and conduct electricity properly. If necessary, dry the skin with a towel. Because excessive chest hair may interfere with adhesion and electrical conduction, you may need to quickly shave the area where the pads are to be placed.

3. Remove the backing from the pads and apply them firmly to the person's bare chest according to the diagram on the pads **(Step 2)**. One pad is placed to the right of the breast bone, just below the collar bone and above the right nipple. The second pad is placed on the left side of the chest, left of the nipple and above the lower rib margin.

## Skill Sheet

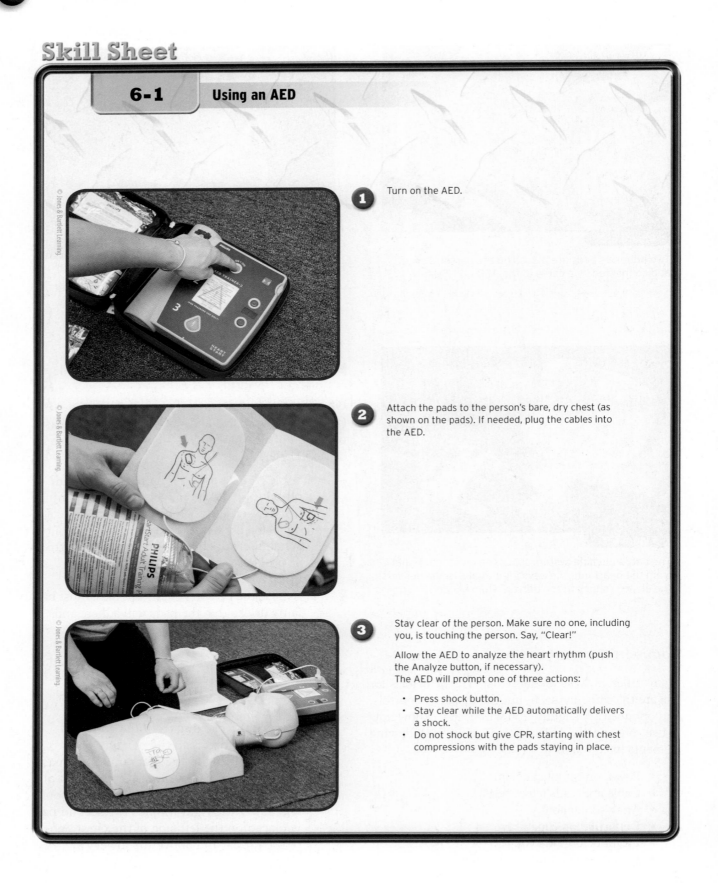

**6-1**    **Using an AED**

**1** Turn on the AED.

**2** Attach the pads to the person's bare, dry chest (as shown on the pads). If needed, plug the cables into the AED.

**3** Stay clear of the person. Make sure no one, including you, is touching the person. Say, "Clear!"

Allow the AED to analyze the heart rhythm (push the Analyze button, if necessary).
The AED will prompt one of three actions:

- Press shock button.
- Stay clear while the AED automatically delivers a shock.
- Do not shock but give CPR, starting with chest compressions with the pads staying in place.

© Jones & Bartlett Learning

## Skill Sheet Continued

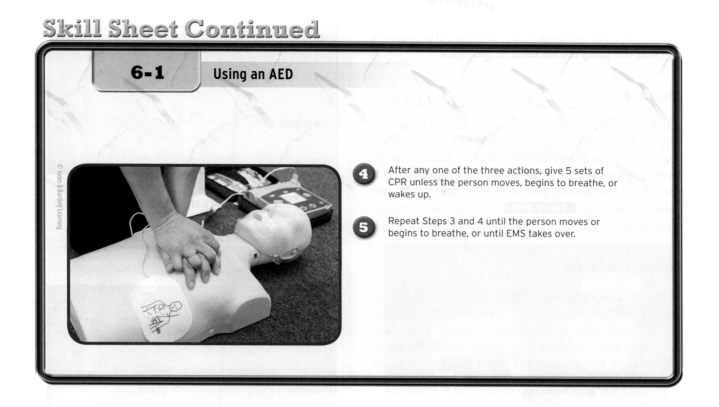

**6-1**    Using an AED

© Jones & Bartlett Learning.

**4** After any one of the three actions, give 5 sets of CPR unless the person moves, begins to breathe, or wakes up.

**5** Repeat Steps 3 and 4 until the person moves or begins to breathe, or until EMS takes over.

4. Stay clear for analysis of the heart's electrical activity (**Step 3**). Make sure no one, including you, is touching the person. Say, "Clear!" The AED will advise of the need to shock and, depending on the device, will either advise you to push a button to administer the shock or will deliver the shock automatically.

5. Begin CPR immediately following the shock, and follow the prompts, which include reanalyzing the rhythm (**Step 4**).

6. If the shock worked, the person may begin to regain signs of life. Continue providing care until the person moves or begins to breathe, or until emergency medical services (EMS) personnel arrive and take over (**Step 5**).

### Q&A

**Will I get zapped if a person is shocked in the rain or near water?**

It is remotely possible to get shocked or to shock bystanders if standing water is present around and under the person. Try to move the person to a dry area and cut off wet clothing. Also be sure that the skin has been dried off so that the electrode pads will stick to the skin. No one should be touching any part of the person while the device emits an electrical current.

## ▶ Special Considerations

There are several special situations that you should be aware of when using an AED. These include the following:

- Water
- Children
- Medication patches
- Implanted devices

### Water

Because water conducts electricity, it may provide an energy pathway between the AED and you or bystanders. Remove the person from free-standing water.

Quickly dry the chest before applying the pads. The risk to you and bystanders is very low if the chest is dry and the pads are secured to the chest.

## Children

Cardiac arrest in children is usually caused by an airway or breathing condition, rather than a primary heart condition as in adults. AEDs can deliver energy levels appropriate for children aged 1 year or older. If your AED has special pediatric pads and cable, use these for the child **Figure 6-9**. If the pediatric equipment is not available, use the adult equipment.

## Medication Patches

Some people wear an adhesive patch containing medication (such as nitroglycerin, nicotine, or pain medication) that is absorbed through the skin. Because these patches may block the delivery of energy from the pads to the heart, they need to be removed and the skin wiped dry before attaching the AED pads **Figure 6-10**.

## Implanted Devices

Implanted pacemakers and defibrillators are small devices placed underneath the skin of people with certain types of heart disease **Figure 6-11**. These devices can often be seen or felt when the chest is exposed. Avoid placing the pads directly over these

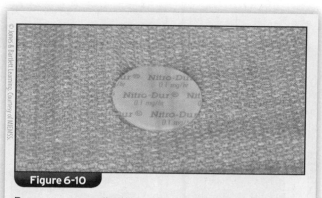

**Figure 6-10**

Remove any medication patches before applying AED pads.

**Figure 6-11**

Implanted defibrillator.

**Figure 6-9**

If your AED has pediatric pads, use them according to the manufacturer's instructions.

devices whenever possible. If an implanted defibrillator is discharging, you may see the person twitching periodically. Allow the implanted unit to stop before using your AED.

## ▶ AED Maintenance

Periodic inspection of your AED ensures that the device has the necessary supplies and is in proper working condition **Figure 6-12**. AEDs conduct automatic internal checks and provide visual indications that the unit is ready and functioning properly. You do not need to turn the device on daily to check it. Doing so will only wear down the battery.

AED supplies should include items such as the following:

- Two sets of electrode pads with expiration dates that are not expired
- An extra battery
- A razor
- A hand towel

Other items that should be considered are a breathing device (eg, a mask or shield) and exam gloves.

## ▶ AED Manufacturers

AED devices and related supplies are available from different manufacturers **Figure 6-13**.

**Figure 6-12**

Periodic inspection of your AED supplies ensures that all items are in working condition.

**Figure 6-13**

Various AED devices.

# prep kit

## ▶ Ready for Review

- A person's chances for survival are dramatically improved through early CPR and early defibrillation.
- Because the heart contracts approximately every second, it needs an abundant supply of oxygen.
- CPR is the initial care for cardiac arrest until a defibrillator is available.
- An AED is an electronic device that analyzes the heart rhythm and delivers an electrical shock to the heart of a person in cardiac arrest.
- There are several special situations to be aware of when using an AED, including water, children, medication patches, and implanted devices.
- Periodic inspection of the AED can ensure that the device has the necessary supplies and is in proper working condition.

## ▶ Vital Vocabulary

**automated external defibrillator (AED)** A device capable of analyzing the heart rhythm and providing a shock.

**defibrillation** The electrical shock administered by an AED to reestablish a normal heart rhythm.

**ventricular fibrillation** A potentially life-threatening electrical condition, in which the heart muscle contracts and relaxes in a disorganized fashion; the lower chambers of the heart quiver and cannot pump blood.

**ventricular tachycardia** A potentially life-threatening electrical condition, in which the heart beats too fast to pump blood effectively.

## ▶ Assessment in Action

Your workplace has recently implemented an AED program. You and several other employees have been trained to locate and use an AED. While at work, a coworker collapses. She is around 50 years old and you know she has a history of heart conditions. You tell a coworker to call 9-1-1 and to bring the AED.

*Directions:* Circle Yes if you agree with the statement; circle No if you disagree.

Yes   No   **1.** You should establish unresponsiveness before starting anything else.

Yes   No   **2.** You should begin chest compressions as soon as possible and stop only to apply the AED pads to the chest or to give two breaths.

Yes   No   **3.** AED pads can be applied over the top of the person's blouse.

Yes   No   **4.** The AED will alert you about improper pad placement.

Yes   No   **5.** You should deliver a shock even if the AED has not alerted you to do so.

## ▶ Check Your Knowledge

*Directions:* Circle Yes if you agree with the statement; circle No if you disagree.

Yes   No   **1.** The earlier defibrillation occurs, the better the person's chance of survival.

Yes   No   **2.** An AED is to be applied only to a person who is unresponsive and not breathing.

Yes   No   **3.** CPR is not needed if you are sure an AED will be available in 3 to 4 minutes.

Yes   No   **4.** AEDs require the operator to know how to interpret heart rhythms.

Yes   No   **5.** Because all AEDs are different, the basic steps of operation are also different.

Yes   No   **6.** The AED pads (electrodes) need to be attached to a dry chest.

Yes   No   **7.** Two electrode pads are placed on the left side of the person's chest.

Yes   No   **8.** Batteries and pads have expiration dates of which you should be aware.

Yes   No   **9.** You can still use an AED if an implanted pacemaker is present.

Yes   No   **10.** You need to turn the AED on daily as part of a routine inspection.

Shock

## Shock

Perfusion is the delivery of blood and oxygen to all of the cells in the body tissues and organs. Shock occurs when the body tissues do not receive enough oxygen-rich blood. Do not confuse this type of shock with electric shock or being shocked, as in being scared or surprised. <u>**Shock**</u> (hypoperfusion) describes a state of collapse and failure of the cardiovascular system in which blood circulation decreases and eventually ceases. Shock can be associated with a wide variety of conditions—from a heart attack to a severe allergic reaction.

## ▶ Causes of Shock

Understanding the basic physiologic causes of shock will better prepare you to treat it. The damage caused by shock depends on which body part is deprived of oxygen and for how long. For example, without oxygen, the brain will be irreparably damaged in 4 to 6 minutes, the abdominal organs in 45 to 90 minutes, and the skin and muscle cells in 3 to 6 hours.

To understand shock, think of the circulatory system as having three components: a working pump (the heart), a network of pipes (the blood vessels), and an adequate amount of fluid (the blood) pumped through the pipes. Damage to any of these components can deprive tissues of blood and produce shock. These three parts can be referred to as the perfusion triangle **Figure 7-1**. When a person is in shock,

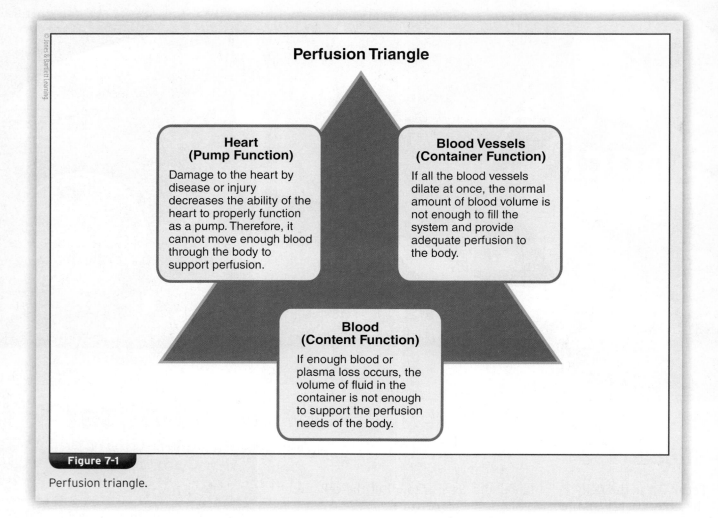

**Figure 7-1**

Perfusion triangle.

one or more of the three sides of the triangle is not working properly.

Causes of shock can be both cardiovascular and noncardiovascular. The noncardiovascular causes of shock are respiratory insufficiency, **psychogenic shock**, and **anaphylaxis**, an extreme allergic reaction to a foreign substance. There are three major cardiovascular causes of shock **Figure 7-2** :

- *Poor pump function*. If damaged by disease or injury, the heart might not generate sufficient energy to move blood through the system (eg, cardiogenic shock).
- *Blood or fluid loss from blood vessels*. If enough blood or plasma loss occurs, the volume of fluid left in the vascular system is inadequate to perfuse all tissues and organs (eg, hemorrhagic shock).
- *Poor vessel function*. With widespread vessel dilation, the normal volume of blood will be

insufficient to fill the system and provide efficient perfusion (eg, **neurogenic shock**).

## Cardiovascular Causes of Shock

- *Pump failure*. Cardiogenic shock is caused by inadequate function of the heart, or pump failure. Circulation requires the constant pumping action of a normal heart muscle. Many diseases can cause destruction or inflammation of this muscle. The heart can adapt somewhat to these conditions, but if too much muscle damage occurs, as sometimes happens in a heart attack, the heart no longer functions well. The major effect is the backup of blood into the lungs. The resulting buildup of fluid in the lungs is called pulmonary edema.

**A. Pump failure**
Causes: Heart attack, trauma to heart, obstructive causes

**B. Low fluid volume**
Causes: Trauma to vessels or tissues, fluid loss from GI tract (vomiting/diarrhea can also lower the fluid component of blood)

**C. Poor vessel function**
Causes: Infection, drug overdose (narcotic), spinal cord injury, anaphylaxis

© Jones & Bartlett Learning

**Figure 7-2**

There are three basic cardiovascular causes of shock and the resulting impaired tissue perfusion. **A.** Pump failure occurs when the heart is damaged by disease, injury, or obstructive causes. The heart may not generate enough energy to move the blood through the system. **B.** Low fluid volume, often a result of bleeding, leads to inadequate perfusion. A common cause of low volume fluid is fluid loss in the gastrointestinal (GI) tract. **C.** The blood vessels can dilate excessively so that the blood within them, even though it is of normal volume, is inadequate to fill the system and provide efficient perfusion.

- *Loss of fluid or blood.* In injuries, shock is most often the result of fluid or blood loss. This type of shock is called hypovolemic (low-volume) shock or hemorrhagic shock. The loss can be due to internal or external bleeding. Hypovolemic shock also occurs with severe thermal burns. Plasma, the fluid portion of the blood, leaks from the circulatory system into burned tissues. Dehydration aggravates shock. In all these circumstances, the common factor is an insufficient volume of blood within the vascular system to provide adequate perfusion to the tissues.

- *Poor vessel function.* Spinal cord damage can injure the part of the nervous system that controls blood vessel size and muscle tone. Neurogenic shock can result. Cut off from their impulses to contract, muscles in the blood vessels dilate (relax) widely, increasing the size and capacity of the vascular system. The blood in the body can no longer fill the enlarged vessels **Figure 7-3** .

- *Combined vessel and content failure.* Septic shock is seen in people who have severe bacterial infections that produce toxins (poisons). The toxins damage the vessel walls, causing them to become leaky and unable to contract. Widespread vessel dilation, combined with the loss of plasma through injured vessel walls, results in shock. Infections that result in septic shock can be associated with serious illness, injury, or surgery.

## Noncardiovascular Causes of Shock

- *Respiratory insufficiency.* A severe chest injury or an airway obstruction can make a person unable to breathe adequately. Insufficient oxygen in the blood can produce shock as rapidly as vascular causes, even when cardiovascular function is normal. Circulation of nonoxygenated blood will not benefit the person.

- *Anaphylactic shock.* Anaphylaxis, or anaphylactic shock, occurs when the immune system reacts violently to a substance to which it has already been sensitized. Severe allergic reactions commonly follow exposure to one of the following:

  - Medications (penicillin and related drugs, aspirin, sulfa drugs)
  - Food (shellfish, nuts—especially peanuts, eggs)
  - Insect stings (honeybee, wasp, yellow jacket, hornet, fire ant)

  Anaphylactic reactions can develop in minutes or even seconds after contact with the substance to which a person is sensitized.

Spinal cord damage

Dilated vessels
Absence of sweating
Loss of body temperature control

Normal vessel        Dilated vessel

**Figure 7-3**

Neurogenic shock.

The signs of such allergic reactions are distinct from those of other forms of shock. Table 7-1 shows the signs and symptoms of anaphylactic shock.

In anaphylactic shock, although there is no loss of blood, no vascular damage, and only a slight possibility of cardiac muscular injury, the widespread vascular dilation causes poor oxygenation and poor perfusion of tissues, which can easily cause death.

- *Psychogenic shock.* Psychogenic shock is a sudden nervous system reaction that produces a temporary vascular dilation, resulting in fainting, or syncope. Blood pools in the dilated vessels, reducing the blood supply to the brain, and the person becomes unresponsive. Causes of fainting (psychogenic shock) include fear, bad news, or unpleasant sights (often the sight of blood).

## Table 7-1 Signs and Symptoms of Anaphylactic Shock

**Skin**
- Flushing, itching, or burning, especially over the face and upper chest
- Hives, which can spread over large areas of the body
- Swelling, especially of the face, tongue, and lips
- Blue discoloration around lips and mouth (cyanosis)

**Circulatory System**
- Weak pulse (you might be barely able to feel it)
- Dizziness
- Fainting and unresponsiveness

**Respiratory System**
- Sneezing or itching in the nostrils
- Tightness in the chest, with a persistent, dry cough
- Breathing difficulty
- Secretions of fluid and mucus into the throat and lungs
- Wheezing
- Breathing stoppage

## ▶ The Progression of Shock

Although shock itself cannot be seen, you can see its signs and symptoms progress Table 7-2. The early stage of shock, when the body can still compensate for blood loss, is called compensated shock. The late stage, when blood pressure is falling, is decompensated shock. The final stage, when shock is terminal, is called irreversible shock. Even transfusion will not save the person's life at this point.

### Table 7-2 Progression of Shock

**Compensated Shock**
- Agitation
- Anxiety
- Restlessness
- Feeling of impending doom
- Altered mental status
- Weak, rapid, or absent pulse
- Clammy (pale, cool, moist) skin
- Paleness, with cyanosis about the lips
- Shallow, rapid breathing
- Shortness of breath
- Nausea or vomiting
- Capillary refill longer than 2 sec in infants and children
- Thirst

**Decompensated Shock**
- Difficulty breathing
- Ashen, mottled, or cyanotic skin
- Dull eyes, dilated pupils

### FYI

**Red Flags for Shock**

Shock is seen in both injured and suddenly ill people. Anticipate and expect shock if a person has any of these conditions:
- Massive external or internal bleeding
- Multiple severe fractures
- An abdominal or chest injury
- A severe infection
- Any signs of a heart attack
- Anaphylaxis

## ▶ General Care for Shock

Automatically treat any injured person for shock, because every injury affects the circulatory system to some degree. Shock is one of the most common causes of death in an injured person. Provide care for shock even if an injured person does not have signs or symptoms of shock. You can prevent shock from getting worse, but you cannot reverse it.

Refer to Flowchart 7-1 for additional information regarding the care of a person in shock.

### What to Look For

- Altered mental status (anxiety and restlessness)
- Pale, cold, and clammy skin
- Pale or cyanotic lips and/or nail beds
- Nausea/vomiting
- Rapid breathing and heart rate
- Unresponsiveness when shock is severe

### What to Do

1. Treat injuries.
2. If responsive and breathing normally, keep the person flat on his or her back. If there is no sign of injury, the feet can be raised 6 to 12 inches (15 to 30 cm) if it does not cause pain Figure 7-4.
3. If unresponsive, roll the person onto his or her side.
4. Prevent the loss of body heat by putting blankets or coats under and over the person.
5. Call 9-1-1.
6. **DO NOT** give anything to eat or drink unless medical help is delayed over 1 hour, in which case, sips of water can be given if fluids do not cause nausea and/or vomiting.

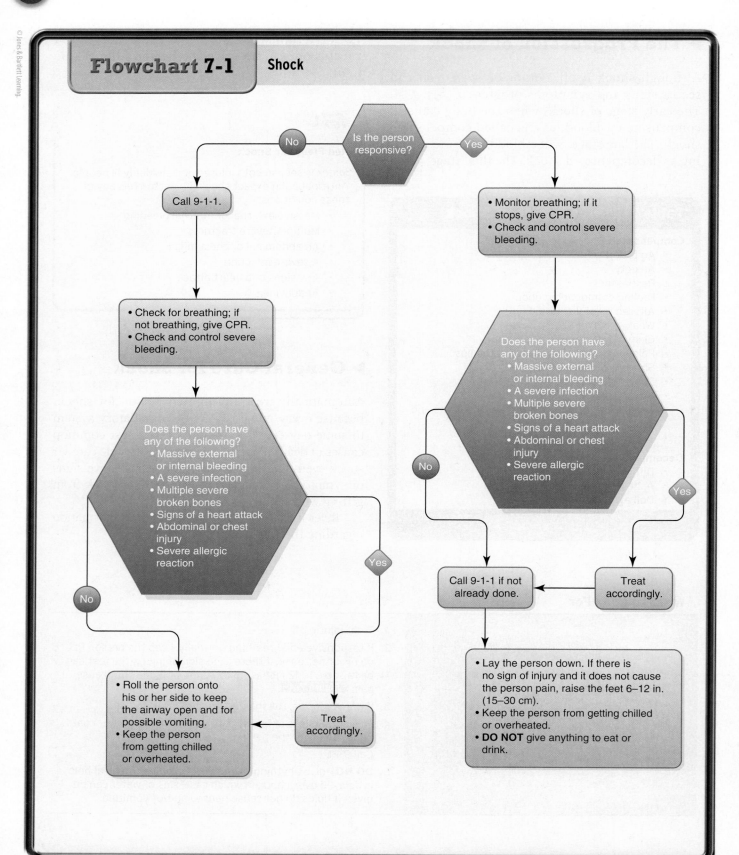

**Flowchart 7-1** | **Shock**

Is the person responsive?

No → Call 9-1-1.
- Check for breathing; if not breathing, give CPR.
- Check and control severe bleeding.

Does the person have any of the following?
- Massive external or internal bleeding
- A severe infection
- Multiple severe broken bones
- Signs of a heart attack
- Abdominal or chest injury
- Severe allergic reaction

No →
- Roll the person onto his or her side to keep the airway open and for possible vomiting.
- Keep the person from getting chilled or overheated.

Yes → Treat accordingly.

Yes →
- Monitor breathing; if it stops, give CPR.
- Check and control severe bleeding.

Does the person have any of the following?
- Massive external or internal bleeding
- A severe infection
- Multiple severe broken bones
- Signs of a heart attack
- Abdominal or chest injury
- Severe allergic reaction

No → Call 9-1-1 if not already done.

Yes → Treat accordingly.

- Lay the person down. If there is no sign of injury and it does not cause the person pain, raise the feet 6–12 in. (15–30 cm).
- Keep the person from getting chilled or overheated.
- **DO NOT** give anything to eat or drink.

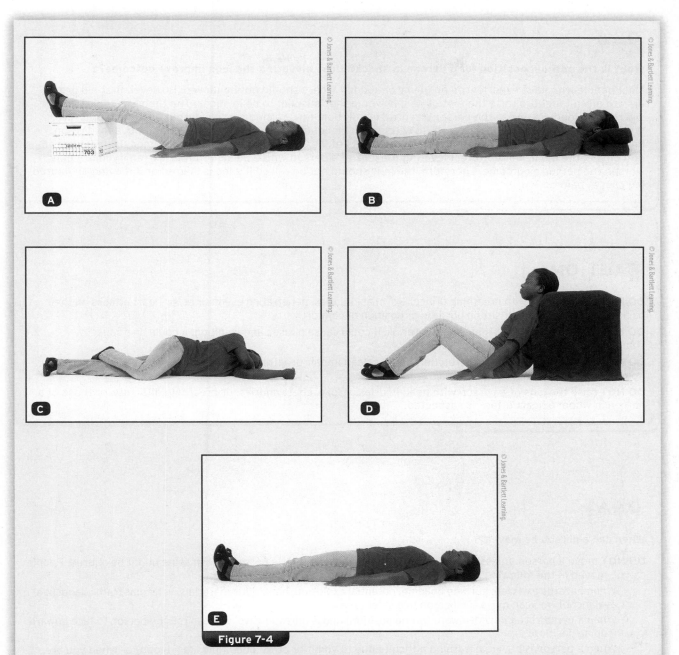

**Figure 7-4**

Shock positions. **A.** Feet can be raised 6 to 12 inches (15 to 30 cm) if it does not cause pain or if the legs or pelvis are not injured. **B.** For a person with head injury, elevate the head (if spinal injury is not suspected). **C.** Position a person who is unresponsive or has experienced a stroke in the recovery position. **D.** Use a half-sitting position for people with breathing difficulties, chest injuries, or a heart attack. **E.** Keep the person flat if a spinal injury or leg fracture is suspected.

## Q&A

**What is the optimal position for a person in shock? Does elevating the legs improve outcome?**

Most people who have experienced an injury or sudden illness should not be moved. However, first aid providers are often taught to raise the feet of people whom they suspect to be in shock. The theory is that doing so will return blood volume to the person's central circulation, thus raising cardiac output and blood pressure. While raising the feet 6 to 12 inches (15 to 30 cm) can be beneficial in some cases (eg, fainting, dehydration, heat exhaustion), the evidence is mixed on the effects of leg elevation, and no studies demonstrate improved outcome in the medical literature. Elevating the legs of a person with a pelvic or lower extremity injury may worsen the person's outcome. Therefore, the legs should not be raised if a leg is injured or if moving an injured leg causes pain.

## CAUTION

**DO NOT** place people with breathing difficulties, chest injuries, penetrating eye injuries, or heart attacks on their backs. Place them in a half-sitting position or position of comfort.

**DO NOT** give the person anything to eat or drink. It could cause nausea and vomiting. It could also cause complications if surgery is needed.

**DO NOT** lift the foot of a bed or stretcher; doing so can impair breathing. Lift only the legs instead, which will help with circulation but will not impair breathing.

**DO NOT** raise the legs of a person with head injuries, stroke, chest injuries, or breathing difficulty, or those of a person in whom a heart attack is suspected.

## Q&A

**When can a person be moved?**

**DO NOT** move a person unless necessary. This is especially true for a person whose spine might be injured. People can be moved in the following circumstances:

- When hazards exist (eg, burning building, potential explosion, hazardous materials, vehicular traffic, landslide, avalanche), you can move the person to a safer area.
- When a person is facing downward (prone position) and is unresponsive, you can roll the person to face upward (supine position).
- When a person is having breathing difficulty due to vomit or other body fluids (eg, blood) or when you are alone and must leave an unresponsive person to get help, you can place the person in the recovery position. Roll the body, as a single unit, until the person is on his or her side. Support the head by resting it on the extended arm.
- When shock becomes apparent, keep the person in a supine position. The feet can be raised about 6 to 12 inches (15 to 30 cm) if there are no injuries. If pain occurs while moving or positioning the person, do not raise the feet.

*Source:* Markenson D, et al. Part 13: First aid: 2010 consensus on first aid science. *Circulation* 2010;122(suppl):S532–S605.

## ▶ Care for Anaphylaxis

| What to Look For | What to Do |
|---|---|
| Severe allergic reaction (anaphylaxis), indicated by:<br>• Shortness of breath<br>• Swelling of tongue, mouth, nose<br>• Intense itching<br>• Flushed skin or swollen face<br>• Sneezing, coughing, wheezing<br>• Tightness and swelling in the throat<br>• Tightness in the chest<br>• Increased heart rate<br>• Blue discoloration around lips and mouth (cyanosis)<br>• Dizziness<br>• A history of previous severe allergic reactions<br>• Medical identification tag | 1. Call 9-1-1.<br>2. Monitor breathing.<br>3. If the person has his or her own physician-prescribed **epinephrine auto-injector**, you may need to get it and help the person self-administer it `Figure 7-5`. If the person is not capable of using it and you are allowed by state law to give an injection, use the person's prescribed epinephrine auto-injector `Skill Sheet 7-1`.<br>  • Find the injection site on the outer midthigh between the knee and the hip. Check for coins, keys, and pant seams, which could obstruct the needle.<br>  • Remove the safety cap.<br>  • Push the auto-injector against the outer midthigh until you hear a click (if necessary, the injection can be done through light clothing).<br>  • Hold in place for 10 seconds.<br>  • Pull the auto-injector straight out from the leg.<br>  • Rub the area for 10 seconds.<br>4. If the first dose does not help and emergency medical services (EMS) arrival will exceed 5 to 10 minutes, consider giving a second dose. About 25% to 35% of people require a second dose.<br>5. If the person can swallow, give an antihistamine. It is not lifesaving, but it can help prevent further reactions. |
| Mild allergic reaction, indicated by:<br>• Red, itchy eyes<br>• Itchy, sneezing, runny nose<br>• Rash on skin, usually on one part of body | Help the person (1) self-administer his or her asthma "rescue" inhaler and/or (2) take an antihistamine. |

Refer to `Flowchart 7-2` for additional information regarding the care of a person with anaphylaxis.

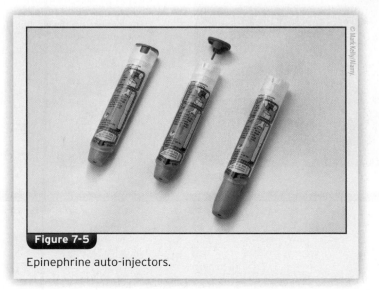

**Figure 7-5**

Epinephrine auto-injectors.

## Skill Sheet

**7-1**    **Using an Epinephrine Auto-injector**

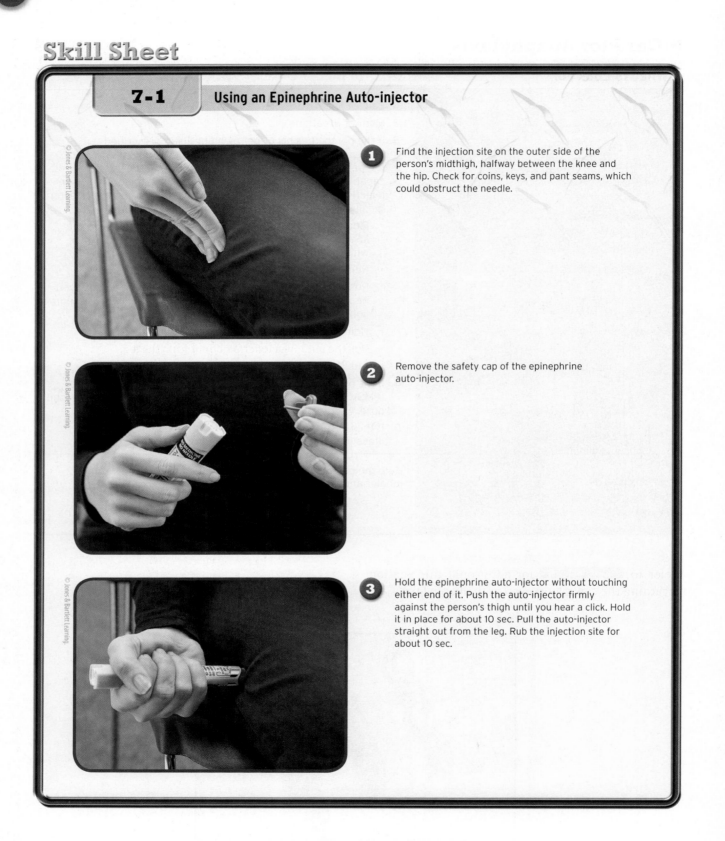

1. Find the injection site on the outer side of the person's midthigh, halfway between the knee and the hip. Check for coins, keys, and pant seams, which could obstruct the needle.

2. Remove the safety cap of the epinephrine auto-injector.

3. Hold the epinephrine auto-injector without touching either end of it. Push the auto-injector firmly against the person's thigh until you hear a click. Hold it in place for about 10 sec. Pull the auto-injector straight out from the leg. Rub the injection site for about 10 sec.

© Jones & Bartlett Learning

# Flowchart 7-2    Anaphylaxis

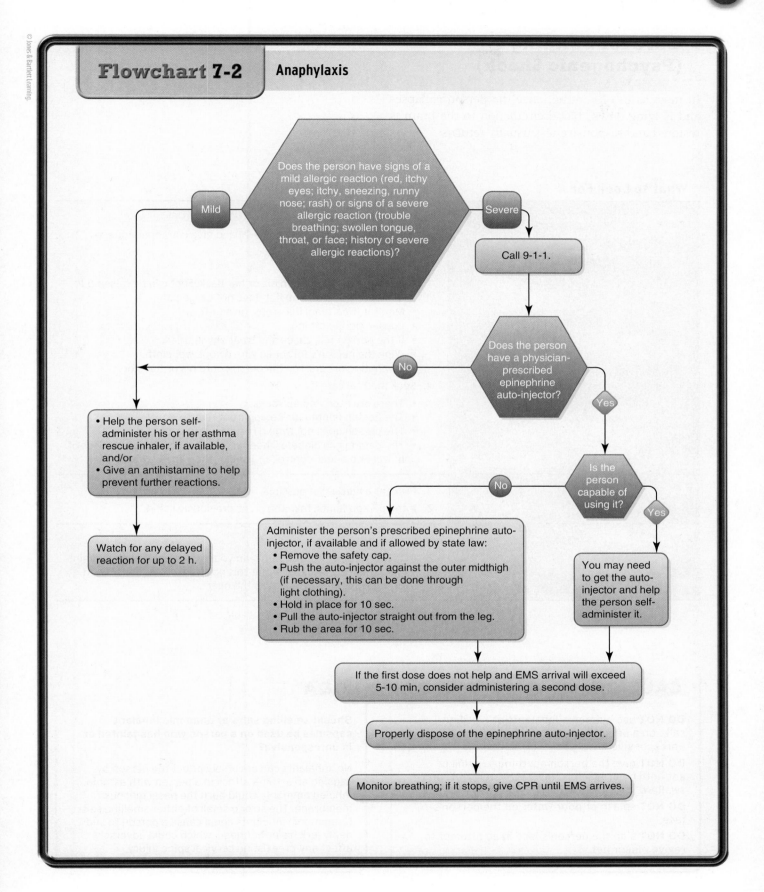

Does the person have signs of a mild allergic reaction (red, itchy eyes; itchy, sneezing, runny nose; rash) or signs of a severe allergic reaction (trouble breathing; swollen tongue, throat, or face; history of severe allergic reactions)?

**Mild**

**Severe**

Call 9-1-1.

- Help the person self-administer his or her asthma rescue inhaler, if available, and/or
- Give an antihistamine to help prevent further reactions.

Does the person have a physician-prescribed epinephrine auto-injector?

**No**

**Yes**

Watch for any delayed reaction for up to 2 h.

Is the person capable of using it?

**No**

**Yes**

Administer the person's prescribed epinephrine auto-injector, if available and if allowed by state law:
- Remove the safety cap.
- Push the auto-injector against the outer midthigh (if necessary, this can be done through light clothing).
- Hold in place for 10 sec.
- Pull the auto-injector straight out from the leg.
- Rub the area for 10 sec.

You may need to get the auto-injector and help the person self-administer it.

If the first dose does not help and EMS arrival will exceed 5-10 min, consider administering a second dose.

Properly dispose of the epinephrine auto-injector.

Monitor breathing; if it stops, give CPR until EMS arrives.

## ▶ Care for Fainting (Psychogenic Shock)

In most cases of fainting, once the person collapses and is lying down, blood circulation to the brain is restored and responsiveness usually returns.

| What to Look For | What to Do |
|---|---|
| • A person that has suddenly collapsed<br>• Pale skin, lips, and nail beds<br>• Clammy, sweaty skin | 1. Check breathing.<br>2. If breathing has stopped, call 9-1-1 and give cardiopulmonary resuscitation (CPR).<br>3. If the person is breathing:<br>  • Keep the person flat on his or her back. Feet can be raised 6 to 12 inches (15 to 30 cm) if it does not cause pain.<br>  • Monitor breathing; if it stops, give CPR.<br>  • Loosen tight clothing.<br>  • If the person fell, check and treat any injuries.<br>  • Wipe the person's forehead with a cool, wet cloth.<br>  • If vomiting occurs, roll the person onto his or her side.<br>4. Seek medical care if:<br>  • There are repeated episodes.<br>  • The person fainted for no apparent reason.<br>  • The person does not regain responsiveness quickly.<br>  • The person has diabetes, has seizures, is pregnant, has a loss of bowel or bladder control, or is older than age 50 years. |
| A person that is about to faint | 1. Prevent a hard fall if possible.<br>2. If the person faints, take the steps previously listed. |
| You feel faint | 1. Lie down or sit down.<br>2. **DO NOT** place your head between your knees because if you faint you may fall. Some believe that this position also inhibits blood flow returning from the legs to the heart. |

## CAUTION

**DO NOT** use ammonia inhalants or smelling salts on a person who has fainted or is unresponsive.

**DO NOT** give the person anything to drink or eat until he or she has fully recovered and can swallow.

**DO NOT** splash or pour water on the person's face.

**DO NOT** slap the person's face in an attempt to revive him or her.

## Q&A

**Should smelling salts or ammonia inhalant capsules be used on a person who has fainted or is unresponsive?**

No. Inhalants can adversely affect the person by causing an asthma attack in a person with asthma. Inhaled ammonia could burn the nasal mucous membrane. The strong smell of either smelling salts or ammonia inhalants could cause a person to suddenly jerk his or her head, which could adversely affect any preexisting cervical spine injury.

# prep kit

## ▶ Ready for Review

- Shock is a state of collapse and failure of the cardiovascular system in which blood circulation decreases and eventually ceases.
- The damage caused by shock depends on which body part is deprived of oxygen and for how long.
- Causes of shock can be both cardiovascular and noncardiovascular.
- Anaphylaxis occurs when the immune system reacts violently to a substance to which it has already been sensitized.
- Although shock itself cannot be seen, you can see the progression of its signs and symptoms.
- First aid providers should automatically treat people for shock.

## ▶ Vital Vocabulary

<u>anaphylaxis</u> A life-threatening allergic reaction.

<u>epinephrine auto-injector</u> Prescribed device used to administer an emergency dose of epinephrine to a person experiencing anaphylaxis.

<u>neurogenic shock</u> Circulatory failure caused by paralysis of the nerves that control the size of the blood vessels, leading to widespread dilation; seen in people with spinal cord injuries.

<u>psychogenic shock</u> A sudden nervous system reaction that produces a temporary vascular dilation, resulting in fainting, or syncope.

<u>shock</u> Inadequate tissue perfusion resulting from serious injury or illness.

## ▶ Assessment in Action

You are walking up a popular canyon trail on a cool fall afternoon. You hear someone call for help farther up the trail, near a cliff. You jog up the trail and find a hiker bent over another person at the base of a cliff. The hiker says the person lying motionless fell about 20 feet (6 m) while climbing the cliff with no ropes or harness. There are no obvious signs of injury. The person appears to be breathing, and no serious bleeding is seen.

*Directions:* Circle Yes if you agree with the statement; circle No if you disagree.

| | | | |
|---|---|---|---|
| Yes | No | **1.** | You should suspect spinal injury. |
| Yes | No | **2.** | You should keep the person flat if a spinal injury is suspected. |
| Yes | No | **3.** | You should offer the person something to eat and drink. |
| Yes | No | **4.** | There is no need to seek medical care for this situation. |

## ▶ Check Your Knowledge

*Directions:* Circle Yes if you agree with the statement; circle No if you disagree.

| | | | |
|---|---|---|---|
| Yes | No | **1.** | Place all people with severe injuries in the recovery position. |
| Yes | No | **2.** | Prevent the loss of body heat by putting blankets under and over the person. |
| Yes | No | **3.** | A person in shock with possible spinal injuries should be placed in a seated position. |
| Yes | No | **4.** | A person in shock with breathing difficulty or chest injury should be placed on his or her back. |
| Yes | No | **5.** | Anxiety and restlessness are signs of shock. |
| Yes | No | **6.** | An epinephrine auto-injector can be used for people experiencing anaphylaxis. |
| Yes | No | **7.** | All people with severe injuries or illnesses should be treated for shock. |
| Yes | No | **8.** | Treat people with severe injuries for shock even if there are no signs of it. |
| Yes | No | **9.** | Anaphylaxis is a life-threatening breathing emergency. |
| Yes | No | **10.** | People in shock have hot skin. |

# Bleeding

## Bleeding

The average-size adult has 5 to 6 quarts (about 5 to 6 L) of blood and can safely donate a half quart (0.5 L). However, rapid blood loss of 1 quart (about 1 L) or more can lead to shock and death. A child who has a loss of a half quart (0.5 L) of blood is in extreme danger.

## ▶ External Bleeding

External bleeding refers to blood coming from an open wound. The term **hemorrhage** refers to a large amount of bleeding in a short time. External bleeding can be classified into three types according to the type of blood vessel that is damaged: an artery, a vein, or a capillary **Figure 8-1**.

In **arterial bleeding**, blood spurts (up to several feet) from the wound. Arterial bleeding is the most serious type of bleeding because a large amount of blood loss can occur in a very short time. This type of bleeding does not clot well because the high flow of the blood reduces the ability of a clot to adhere to the damaged vessel.

In **venous bleeding**, blood from a vein flows steadily or gushes. Venous bleeding is easier to control than arterial bleeding. Even though small cuts bleed a lot at first, by the time you treat a bleeding person, most bleeding will have already slowed or stopped. Most veins collapse when cut. Bleeding from deep veins, however, can be as massive and as hard to control as arterial bleeding.

© E.M. Singleary, M.D. Used with permission.

**Figure 8-1**

Capillary bleeding **(A)**, venous bleeding **(B)**, and arterial bleeding **(C)**.

In **capillary bleeding**, the most common type of bleeding, blood oozes from capillaries. It usually is not serious and can be controlled easily. Quite often, this type of bleeding will clot and stop by itself.

Each type of blood vessel—artery, vein, or capillary—contains blood of a different shade of red. An inexperienced person may have difficulty detecting the color difference but would still be able to identify the type of bleeding by its flow. The body naturally responds to bleeding in the following ways:

- *Blood vessel spasm.* Arteries contain small amounts of muscle tissue in their walls. If a blood vessel is completely severed, it draws back into the tissue, constricts its diameter, and slows the bleeding dramatically. If an artery is only partially cut across its diameter, however, constriction is incomplete. The vessel may not contract and the loss of blood may not slow as dramatically.
- *Clotting.* Special elements in blood, called platelets, form a clot. Clotting serves as a protective covering for a wound until the tissues underneath can repair themselves. In a healthy person, initial clot formation normally takes about 10 minutes. Clotting time is longer in people who have a great deal of blood loss over a prolonged time, are taking aspirin or anticoagulants, are anemic, or have hemophilia or severe liver disease.

An alert and responsive person can often tell and show where he or she is bleeding. Ask the person, "Are you bleeding?" Check wet spots on clothing, which may be blood. Thick clothing may hide visible traces of blood, but severe bleeding can soak through clothing and appear on its surface. For an unresponsive, injured person, you may also need to feel for blood; be sure to wear exam gloves when doing so. Blood's stickiness will differentiate it from other fluids.

## Q&A

**What are the largest artery and the largest vein in the human body?**

The aorta is the largest artery in the human body. In adults, it is about the size of a garden hose. Its internal diameter is 1 inch (2.5 cm) and its wall is 0.0790 inch (0.2 cm) thick.

The largest vein in the human body is the inferior vena cava, the vein that returns blood from the lower half of the body back to the heart.

## CAUTION

**DO NOT** come in contact with blood with your bare hands. Protect yourself with exam gloves, extra gauze pads, or clean cloths, or have the person apply the direct pressure. If you must use your bare hands, do so only as a last resort. After the bleeding has stopped and the wound has been cared for, vigorously wash your hands with soap and water.

**DO NOT** use direct pressure on an eye injury, a wound with an embedded object, or a skull fracture.

**DO NOT** remove a blood-soaked dressing. Doing so can pull off clots that have already formed. Apply another dressing on top and continue putting pressure over the wound.

## Care for External Bleeding

Regardless of the type of bleeding or the type of wound, the first aid is the same. First and foremost, you must control the bleeding **Skill Sheet 8-1** :

1. Protect yourself against disease by wearing exam gloves. If they are not available, use several layers of gauze pads, clean cloths, plastic wrap, a plastic bag, a sanitary napkin, or waterproof material. If those items are unavailable, you can have the person apply pressure on the wound with his or her hand.

2. Expose the wound by removing or cutting the person's clothing to find the source of the bleeding **(Step 1)**.

3. Place a sterile gauze pad or a clean cloth such as a handkerchief, washcloth, or towel over the entire wound and apply direct pressure with your fingers for small wounds and with the palm of your hand for large wounds **(Step 2)**.

4. Hold steady, firm, and uninterrupted pressure on the wound for at least 5 minutes. The gauze or cloth allows you to apply even pressure. Direct pressure stops most bleeding **Figure 8-2** . Applying direct pressure to the wound compresses the sides of the torn vessel and helps the body's natural clotting mechanisms work. Be sure the pressure remains constant, is not too light, and is applied to the bleeding source **(Step 3)**.

5. If the bleeding does not stop within 10 minutes, add more dressings onto the first one and press harder over a wider area. **DO NOT** remove blood-soaked dressings; add new dressings over the old ones so you do not dislodge any clot that has formed **(Step 4)**.

6. To free you to attend to other injuries or people, use a pressure bandage to hold the dressing on the wound. Wrap a roller gauze bandage tightly over the dressing and above and below the wound site **(Step 5)**. **DO NOT** wrap it so tightly that it cuts off circulation.

7. If the bleeding continues, call 9-1-1 if not already done. Consider using a **tourniquet** if severe bleeding (ie, spurting or flowing) from an arm or leg cannot be stopped by direct pressure **(Step 6)**.

8. When bleeding stops, properly dispose of the gloves and wash your hands **(Step 7)**. Use procedures found in Chapter 9, *Wounds*, for wound care.

Some people panic when they see even the smallest amount of blood. The sight of more than a couple of tablespoons of blood generally is enough to frighten an injured person and bystanders. Take time to reassure the person that everything possible is being done, but do not belittle the person's concerns.

## Skill Sheet

### 8-1     Bleeding Control

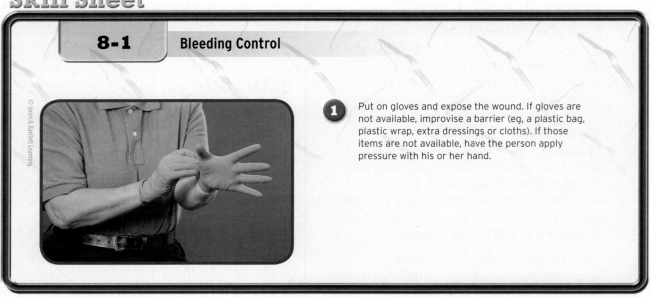

1 Put on gloves and expose the wound. If gloves are not available, improvise a barrier (eg, a plastic bag, plastic wrap, extra dressings or cloths). If those items are not available, have the person apply pressure with his or her hand.

© Jones & Bartlett Learning.

# Skill Sheet Continued

**8-1**    **Bleeding Control**

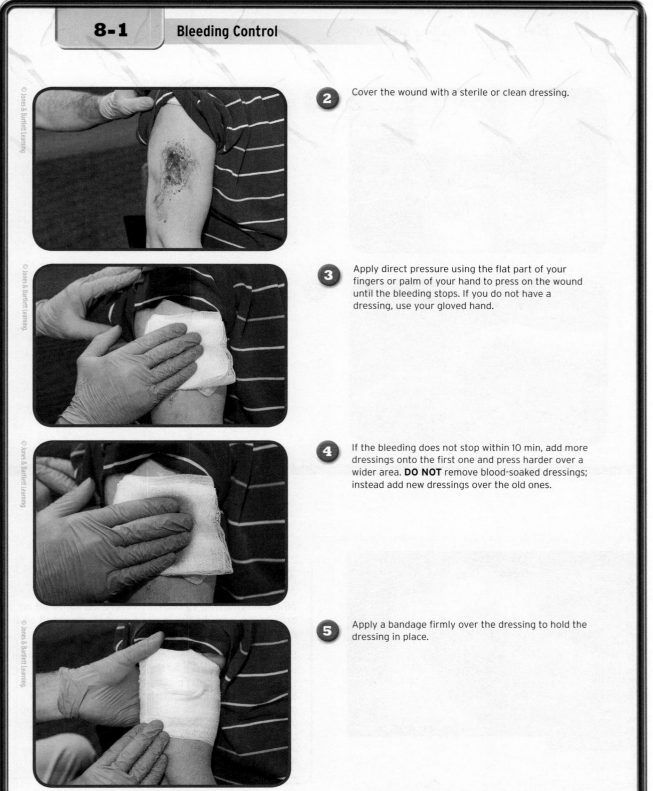

2  Cover the wound with a sterile or clean dressing.

3  Apply direct pressure using the flat part of your fingers or palm of your hand to press on the wound until the bleeding stops. If you do not have a dressing, use your gloved hand.

4  If the bleeding does not stop within 10 min, add more dressings onto the first one and press harder over a wider area. **DO NOT** remove blood-soaked dressings; instead add new dressings over the old ones.

5  Apply a bandage firmly over the dressing to hold the dressing in place.

© Jones & Bartlett Learning.

*(Continues)*

## Skill Sheet Continued

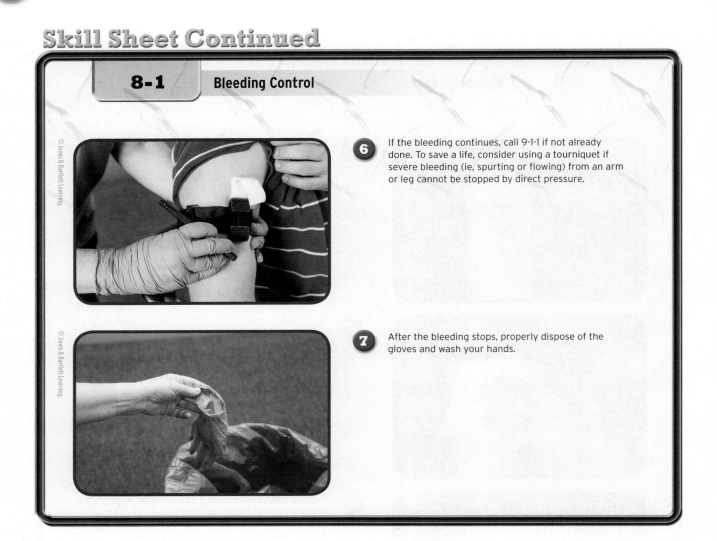

**8-1**    Bleeding Control

6  If the bleeding continues, call 9-1-1 if not already done. To save a life, consider using a tourniquet if severe bleeding (ie, spurting or flowing) from an arm or leg cannot be stopped by direct pressure.

7  After the bleeding stops, properly dispose of the gloves and wash your hands.

**Figure 8-2**

Direct pressure.

### Q&A

**While attempting to control severe bleeding on an arm or leg, should the injured part be elevated and pressure points be used?**

Studies show that bleeding can be stopped by manual (direct) pressure applied over gauze pads. It is the single most effective method for controlling bleeding. Studies found that an elastic bandage applied over gauze pads is best for maintaining a hands-free stoppage of bleeding. No evidence exists that the use of pressure points eliminates distal pulses or that the elevation of a bleeding part has any role in stopping bleeding.

**What to Look For**          **What to Do**

| Bleeding is controlled | 1. Care for the wound. |
| --- | --- |
| | 2. If needed, seek medical care for cleaning, stitches, or a tetanus immunization. |
| **Bleeding continues** | 1. Apply a manufactured tourniquet 2 to 3 inches (5 to 7 cm) above the wound ` Figure 8-3 `. |
| | • Tourniquets are used only on arms and legs. |
| | • Tighten the tourniquet until the bleeding stops, then secure it in place. If bleeding continues, apply a second tourniquet near the first one. |
| | 2. Manufactured tourniquets appear to be better than those that are improvised ` Skill Sheet 8-2 `. If a manufactured tourniquet is not available, an improvised tourniquet can be applied ` Skill Sheet 8-3 `: |
| | • Wrap a band of soft material (eg, folded triangular bandage) twice around the arm or leg and about 2 to 3 inches (5 to 7 cm) above the wound. |
| | • **DO NOT** use narrow materials (eg, belt, rope, or string; tourniquet should be 2 to 4 inches [5 to 10 cm] wide). **DO NOT** use elastic materials or bungee-type devices. |
| | • Tie a half or overhand knot on the arm or leg, and place a short rigid object (eg, stick, screwdriver) over it. Then, tie a square knot over the rigid object. |
| | • Twist the rigid object until the bleeding stops. |
| | • Tie or tape the rigid object in place to keep the tourniquet from unwinding. |
| | 3. **DO NOT** cover, release, or remove a tourniquet. Write "TQ" (for tourniquet) and the time it was applied on a piece of tape, and apply it to the person's forehead. |
| | 4. Call 9-1-1 if it has not already been done, or drive the person to a medical facility. |
| **Bleeding still continues** | 1. Apply a **hemostatic dressing** if: |
| | • Direct pressure is not effective in controlling bleeding. |
| | • A tourniquet is not available, is ineffective, or cannot be applied (ie, wound is on abdomen, chest, back). |
| | 2. Apply a hemostatic dressing in combination with direct pressure, followed by a pressure bandage. Certain hemostatic dressings have been proven to be effective and safe ` Figure 8-4 `. |
| | 3. Call 9-1-1 if it has not already been done, or drive the person to a medical facility |

**Figure 8-3**

A tourniquet is a device wrapped tightly around an extremity to stop blood flow.

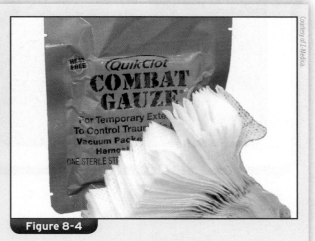

**Figure 8-4**

Hemostatic dressings are gauze-style dressings saturated with an agent that stops bleeding.

## Skill Sheet

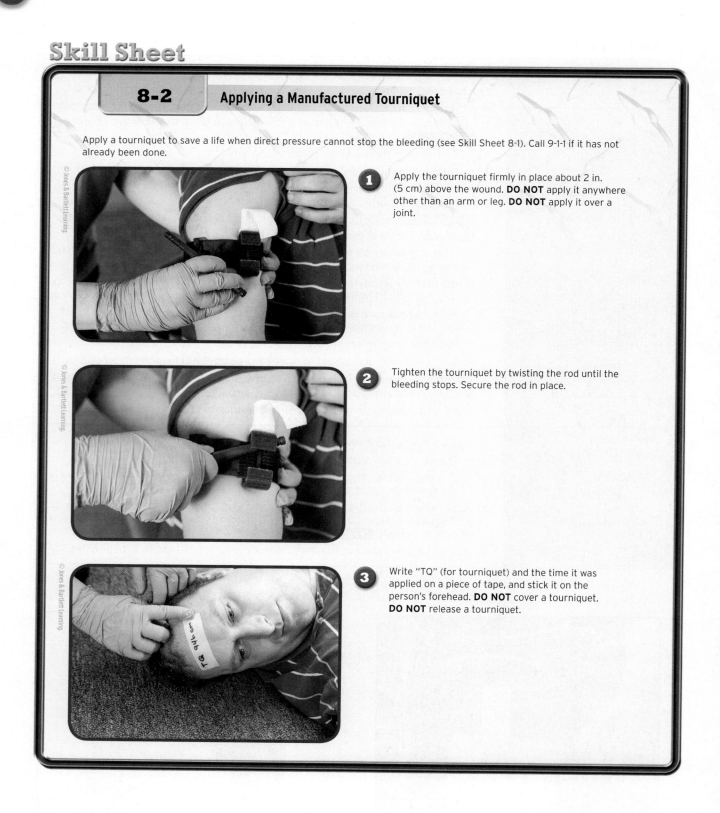

**8-2**    **Applying a Manufactured Tourniquet**

Apply a tourniquet to save a life when direct pressure cannot stop the bleeding (see Skill Sheet 8-1). Call 9-1-1 if it has not already been done.

**1** Apply the tourniquet firmly in place about 2 in. (5 cm) above the wound. **DO NOT** apply it anywhere other than an arm or leg. **DO NOT** apply it over a joint.

**2** Tighten the tourniquet by twisting the rod until the bleeding stops. Secure the rod in place.

**3** Write "TQ" (for tourniquet) and the time it was applied on a piece of tape, and stick it on the person's forehead. **DO NOT** cover a tourniquet. **DO NOT** release a tourniquet.

© Jones & Bartlett Learning

# Skill Sheet

## 8-3    Applying an Improvised Tourniquet

Improvise a tourniquet to save a life when direct pressure cannot stop the bleeding (see Skill Sheet 8-1) and a manufactured tourniquet is not available. Call 9-1-1 if not already done.

**1** Use a folded triangle bandage, wide roller bandage, or similar cloth folded into a long band about 2 in. (5 cm) wide and several layers thick. **DO NOT** use narrow materials (eg, wire, rope, cord).

**2** Wrap the band twice around the arm or leg about 2 in. (5 cm) above the wound and tie a knot (ie, overhand knot). Place padding underneath the band. **DO NOT** apply it anywhere other than the arm or leg. **DO NOT** apply it over a joint.

**3** Place a short (6-8 in. [15-20 cm]) rigid object (eg, stick, screwdriver) onto the knot and then tie a square knot over the rigid object.

(Continues)

## Skill Sheet Continued

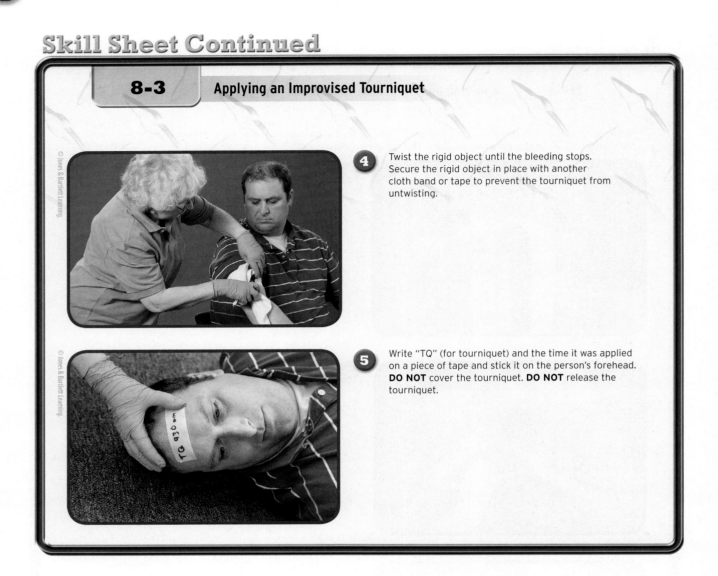

**8-3** Applying an Improvised Tourniquet

**4** Twist the rigid object until the bleeding stops. Secure the rigid object in place with another cloth band or tape to prevent the tourniquet from untwisting.

**5** Write "TQ" (for tourniquet) and the time it was applied on a piece of tape and stick it on the person's forehead. **DO NOT** cover the tourniquet. **DO NOT** release the tourniquet.

**CAUTION**

**DO NOT** touch a surgical wound that is bleeding unless the bleeding is profuse. Applying pressure on a surgical wound may further open the wound by tearing internal or external sutures that have not completely healed. A small amount of bleeding associated with postoperative incisions does not warrant the risk of tissue damage unless the bleeding is truly severe.

**CAUTION**

**DO NOT** apply a pressure bandage so tightly that it cuts off circulation. Check the radial pulse if the bandage is on an arm; for a leg, check the posterior tibial pulse between the medial malleolus (the inner ankle knob) and the Achilles tendon. Pulses are hard to feel. Other signs that the dressing is too tight are increasing pain, numbness or tingling, loss of color in the skin, and loss of muscle function.

FYI

**Application of a Hemostatic Dressing**

A hemostatic dressing is best used when a tourniquet cannot be applied to the body part (ie, back, chest, abdomen), when a tourniquet is not available, or when a tourniquet is unable to stop the bleeding. When applying a hemostatic dressing, it is important to cover the entire bleeding surface, including the deep areas of the wound. Skin tissue may need to be splayed open to place the dressing into a deeper portion of the wound. If blood soaks through the first layer of the dressing, a second layer can be applied. If the wound is deep, place a bulky dressing over the hemostatic dressing.

## ▶ Internal Bleeding

Internal bleeding occurs when the skin is not broken and blood is not seen. It can be difficult to detect and can be life threatening. A person with bleeding stomach ulcers, a lacerated liver, or a ruptured spleen may have a considerable amount of blood loss into the abdomen with no outward sign of bleeding other than the presence of shock (see Chapter 7, *Shock*). Broken bones can also cause serious internal blood loss. A broken femur can easily result in a loss of 1 or more quarts (about 1 L or more) of blood.

Refer to **Flowchart 8-1** for additional information regarding care for bleeding.

### CAUTION

**DO NOT** give the person anything to eat or drink. It could cause nausea and vomiting, which could result in aspiration. Food or liquids could also cause complications if surgery is needed.

| What to Look For | What to Do |
|---|---|
| • Bright red blood from the mouth or rectum, or blood in the urine<br>• Nonmenstrual vaginal bleeding<br>• Vomited blood; may be bright red or dark red, or look like coffee grounds<br>• Black, foul-smelling, tarry stools<br>• Pain, tenderness, bruising, or swelling<br>• Broken ribs, bruises over the lower chest, or a rigid abdomen | 1. Monitor breathing.<br>2. Expect vomiting. If vomiting occurs, keep the person lying on his or her left side to allow drainage and to prevent inhalation (aspiration) of vomitus.<br>3. Treat for shock and cover the person with a coat or blanket for warmth. See Chapter 7, *Shock*, for when to use other body positions.<br>4. Treat suspected internal bleeding in an extremity by applying a splint. (See Chapter 16, *Splinting Extremities*.)<br>5. Seek immediate medical care. |
| Bruises (indicating non–life-threatening internal bleeding) | 1. Apply an ice pack over the injury for 20 minutes.<br>2. If an arm or a leg is involved, apply an elastic bandage for compression. Several layers of gauze pads or other cloth could be placed between the bandage and the injury to concentrate the compression to a specific location. |

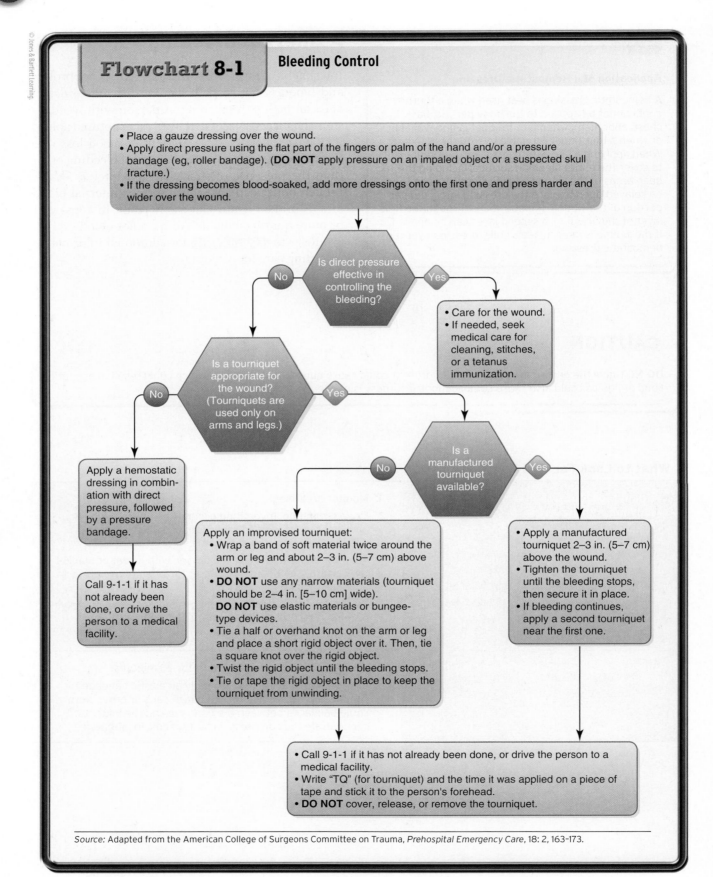

## Flowchart 8-1    Bleeding Control

- Place a gauze dressing over the wound.
- Apply direct pressure using the flat part of the fingers or palm of the hand and/or a pressure bandage (eg, roller bandage). (**DO NOT** apply pressure on an impaled object or a suspected skull fracture.)
- If the dressing becomes blood-soaked, add more dressings onto the first one and press harder and wider over the wound.

**Is direct pressure effective in controlling the bleeding?**

No → **Is a tourniquet appropriate for the wound? (Tourniquets are used only on arms and legs.)**

Yes → • Care for the wound.
- If needed, seek medical care for cleaning, stitches, or a tetanus immunization.

**Is a tourniquet appropriate for the wound? (Tourniquets are used only on arms and legs.)**

No → Apply a hemostatic dressing in combination with direct pressure, followed by a pressure bandage.

→ Call 9-1-1 if it has not already been done, or drive the person to a medical facility.

Yes → **Is a manufactured tourniquet available?**

**Is a manufactured tourniquet available?**

No → Apply an improvised tourniquet:
- Wrap a band of soft material twice around the arm or leg and about 2–3 in. (5–7 cm) above wound.
- **DO NOT** use any narrow materials (tourniquet should be 2–4 in. [5–10 cm] wide). **DO NOT** use elastic materials or bungee-type devices.
- Tie a half or overhand knot on the arm or leg and place a short rigid object over it. Then, tie a square knot over the rigid object.
- Twist the rigid object until the bleeding stops.
- Tie or tape the rigid object in place to keep the tourniquet from unwinding.

Yes → • Apply a manufactured tourniquet 2–3 in. (5–7 cm) above the wound.
- Tighten the tourniquet until the bleeding stops, then secure it in place.
- If bleeding continues, apply a second tourniquet near the first one.

- Call 9-1-1 if it has not already been done, or drive the person to a medical facility.
- Write "TQ" (for tourniquet) and the time it was applied on a piece of tape and stick it to the person's forehead.
- **DO NOT** cover, release, or remove the tourniquet.

*Source:* Adapted from the American College of Surgeons Committee on Trauma, *Prehospital Emergency Care*, 18: 2, 163-173.

# prep kit

## ▶ Ready for Review

- Rapid blood loss of 1 quart (about 1 L) or more can lead to shock and death.
- External bleeding can be classified into three types according to the type of blood vessel that is damaged: artery, vein, or capillary.
- Regardless of the type of bleeding or the type of wound, the first aid is the same. First and foremost, you must control the bleeding.

## ▶ Vital Vocabulary

**arterial bleeding** Bleeding from an artery. This type of bleeding tends to spurt with each heartbeat.

**capillary bleeding** Bleeding that oozes from a wound steadily but slowly.

**hemorrhage** A large amount of bleeding in a short time.

**hemostatic dressing** A gauze-style dressing saturated with an agent that stops bleeding.

**tourniquet** A bleeding control device wrapped tightly around an extremity to stop blood flow from a wound.

**venous bleeding** Bleeding from a vein. This type of bleeding tends to flow steadily.

## ▶ Assessment in Action

You are enjoying a bike ride on a paved trail with your friend. As she rounds the next bend, her bike tires slide out on the gravel and she falls to the ground. She gets up but has a large scrape on her knee and part of her lower leg. Blood is oozing from the wound.

*Directions:* Circle Yes if you agree with the statement; circle No if you disagree.

Yes   No   **1.** This person is experiencing capillary bleeding.

Yes   No   **2.** This type of bleeding is the most common type.

Yes   No   **3.** This type of bleeding is difficult to control and usually does not clot and stop by itself.

Yes   No   **4.** Direct pressure will control this type of bleeding.

## ▶ Check Your Knowledge

*Directions:* Circle Yes if you agree with the statement; circle No if you disagree.

Yes   No   **1.** Most cases of bleeding require more than direct pressure to stop the bleeding.

Yes   No   **2.** Remove any blood-soaked dressings before applying additional ones.

Yes   No   **3.** Applying a pressure bandage over a wound can allow you to attend to another injury or another injured person.

Yes   No   **4.** If a bleeding arm wound is not controlled through direct pressure, apply pressure to the brachial artery.

Yes   No   **5.** Dressings are placed directly on a wound.

Yes   No   **6.** Internal bleeding is normal.

Yes   No   **7.** Dressings should be sterile or as clean as possible.

Yes   No   **8.** Clotting is the body's way of stopping bleeding.

Yes   No   **9.** If the person feels sick to the stomach and may vomit, roll him or her onto the left side.

Yes   No   **10.** When applying a tourniquet to control bleeding, place the tourniquet about 2 to 3 inches above the wound.

# Wounds

**9**

## Chapter at a glance

## ▶ Open Wounds

An open wound is a break in the skin's surface resulting in external bleeding. It may allow bacteria to enter the body, causing an infection. There are several types of open wounds. Recognizing the type of wound helps you give proper first aid. With an <u>abrasion</u>, the top layer of skin is removed, with little or no blood loss **Figure 9-1**. Abrasions tend to be painful because the nerve endings often are abraded along with the skin. Ground-in debris may be present. This type of wound can be serious if it covers a large area or becomes embedded with foreign matter. Other names for an abrasion are *scrape*, *road rash*, and *scuff*.

A <u>laceration</u> is cut skin with jagged, irregular edges **Figure 9-2**. This type of wound is usually caused by a forceful tearing away of skin tissue. <u>Incisions</u> have smooth edges and resemble a surgical or paper cut **Figure 9-3**. The amount of bleeding depends on the depth, the location, and the size of the wound. <u>Punctures</u> are usually deep, narrow wounds in the skin and underlying organs such as a stab wound from a nail or a knife **Figure 9-4**. The entrance is usually small, and the risk of infection is high. The object causing the injury may remain impaled in the wound.

With an <u>avulsion</u>, a piece of skin and possibly underlying tissue is torn loose and is hanging from the body or completely removed **Figure 9-5**. An <u>amputation</u> involves the cutting or tearing off of a body part, such as a finger, toe, hand, foot, arm, or leg.

**Figure 9-1**
Abrasion.

**Figure 9-4**
Puncture.

**Figure 9-2**
Laceration.

**Figure 9-5**
Avulsion.

**Figure 9-3**
Incision.

## Care for Open Wounds

1. Protect yourself against disease by wearing exam gloves. If they are not available, use several layers of gauze pads, clean cloths, plastic wrap or bags, sanitary napkins, or waterproof material. If none of these items are available, you can have the person apply pressure with his or her hand. Your bare hand should be used only as a last resort.
2. Expose the wound by removing or cutting away the clothing to find the source of the bleeding.
3. Control the bleeding by using direct pressure and, if needed, other methods. (See Chapter 8, *Bleeding.*)

## CAUTION

**DO NOT** clean large, extremely dirty, or life-threatening wounds. Let the hospital emergency department personnel do the cleaning.

**DO NOT** scrub a wound. The benefit of scrubbing a wound is debatable, and it can bruise the tissue.

## FYI

**High-Risk Wounds**

The following types of wounds have a high potential for infection:

- Bite wounds
- Very dirty or contaminated wounds
- Crushing, ragged wounds
- Wounds over injured bone, joint, or tendon
- Puncture wounds

## Q&A

**Is a dirty wound the same as a contaminated wound?**

No. For example, road rash, resulting from road gravel, has a low bacterial count. In contrast, wounds that occur in a barnyard or that are exposed to soil contaminated with fecal material have a high bacterial count and are contaminated.

**Figure 9-6**

Irrigate a wound with copious amounts of water.

## Cleaning a Wound

A person's wound should be cleaned to help prevent infection. Wound cleaning usually restarts the bleeding by disturbing the clot, but it should be done anyway for shallow wounds. For wounds with a high risk for infection, leave the pressure bandage in place because medical personnel will clean the wound.

1. Scrub your hands vigorously with soap and water. Put on exam gloves, if available.
2. Expose the wound.
3. Clean the wound.
   - *For a shallow wound:*
     - Wash inside the wound with soap and water.
     - Flush the wound with water (use water that is clean enough to drink) **Figure 9-6**. Run water directly into the wound and allow the water to run over the wound and out, thus carrying the dirty particles away from the wound. Water from a faucet provides sufficient pressure and quantity. Irrigation with water is the most important factor in preventing infection.
   - *For a wound with a high risk for infection* (such as an animal bite, a very dirty or ragged wound, or a puncture), clean the wound and then seek medical care for additional wound cleaning. If you are in a remote setting (more than 1 hour from medical care), clean the wound as best you can.
4. Remove small objects not flushed out with sterile tweezers, if available. A dirty abrasion or other wound that is not properly cleaned will leave a "tattoo" on the person's skin.
5. If bleeding restarts, apply direct pressure over the wound.

## Covering a Wound

Dressings and bandages are two different kinds of first aid supplies. A **dressing** is applied over a wound to control bleeding and prevent contamination. A **bandage** holds the dressing in place. Dressings should be sterile or as clean as possible; bandages need not be.

1. If the wound is small and does not require sutures, cover it with a thin layer of

**FYI**

**Wound Irrigation**

A study compared the effectiveness of tap water with saline solution for irrigating simple skin lacerations to remove bacteria. The results showed no significant difference between bacterial counts in wounds irrigated with normal saline and those irrigated with tap water. The removal of bacteria from a wound depends more on the mechanical effects (speed and pressure) than on the type of solution. Tap water has these advantages over saline: it is readily available; it is more continuous and, therefore, takes less time; it is less expensive; and it does not require other materials such as sterile syringes or splash guards. Other irrigation solutions with antibacterial properties and detergents have an anticellular effect that impairs wound healing and/or resistance to infection. Irrigation pressures above the 20- to 30-psi (138- to 207-kPa) range are discouraged because the higher pressure can damage tissue.

*Source*: Moscati R, Mayrose J, Fincher L, Jehle D. Comparison of normal saline with tap water for wound irrigation. *Am J Emerg Med* 1998;164(4):379-381.

**CAUTION**

**DO NOT** irrigate a wound with full-strength iodine preparations such as povidone iodine (10%) or isopropyl alcohol (70%). They kill body cells as well as bacteria and are painful. Also, some people are allergic to iodine.

**DO NOT** use hydrogen peroxide. It does not kill bacteria well, it adversely affects capillary blood flow, and it extends wound healing.

**DO NOT** use antibiotic ointment on wounds that require sutures or on puncture wounds (the ointment may prevent drainage). Use an antibiotic ointment only on abrasions and shallow wounds.

**DO NOT** soak a wound to clean it. No evidence supports the effectiveness of soaking.

**DO NOT** close gaping wounds with tape such as butterfly tape. Infection is more likely when bacteria are trapped in the wound. If a wound requires closure, this should be done by medical personnel. Extremity wounds are best sutured within 6 hours of the injury.

**DO NOT** breathe or blow on a wound or the dressing.

antibiotic ointment. These ointments can kill many bacteria and rarely cause allergic reactions. No prescription is needed.

2. Cover a small or large wound with a sterile dressing. Do not close gaping or dirty wounds with tape or butterfly bandages. Bacteria may remain, leading to a greater chance of infection. Large, deep, or contaminated wounds should be managed by a medical professional.

3. If a wound bleeds after a dressing has been applied and the dressing becomes stuck, leave it on as long as the wound is healing. Pulling the scab loose to change the dressing retards healing and increases the chance of infection. If you must remove a dressing that is sticking, soak it in warm water to help soften the scab and make removal easier.

4. If a dressing becomes wet or dirty, change it. Dirt and moisture are both breeding grounds for bacteria.

## When to Seek Medical Care

High-risk wounds should receive medical care. Examples of high-risk wounds include those with embedded foreign material (such as gravel), animal and human bites, puncture wounds, and ragged wounds. Large or deep wounds should receive medical care. Any wounds with edges that do not come together spontaneously should receive medical care. Any wounds that have visible bone, joint, muscle, fat, or tendons and wounds that may have entered a joint or body cavity should receive medical care. A particularly high-risk wound is the "fight bite," a wound over the knuckle caused by punching a person in the teeth. Sutures, if needed, are best placed within 6 to 8 hours after the injury. Anyone who has not had a tetanus vaccination within 10 years (5 years in the case of a dirty wound) should seek medical attention within 72 hours to update his or her tetanus inoculation status.

Refer to Flowchart 9-1 for additional information regarding wound care.

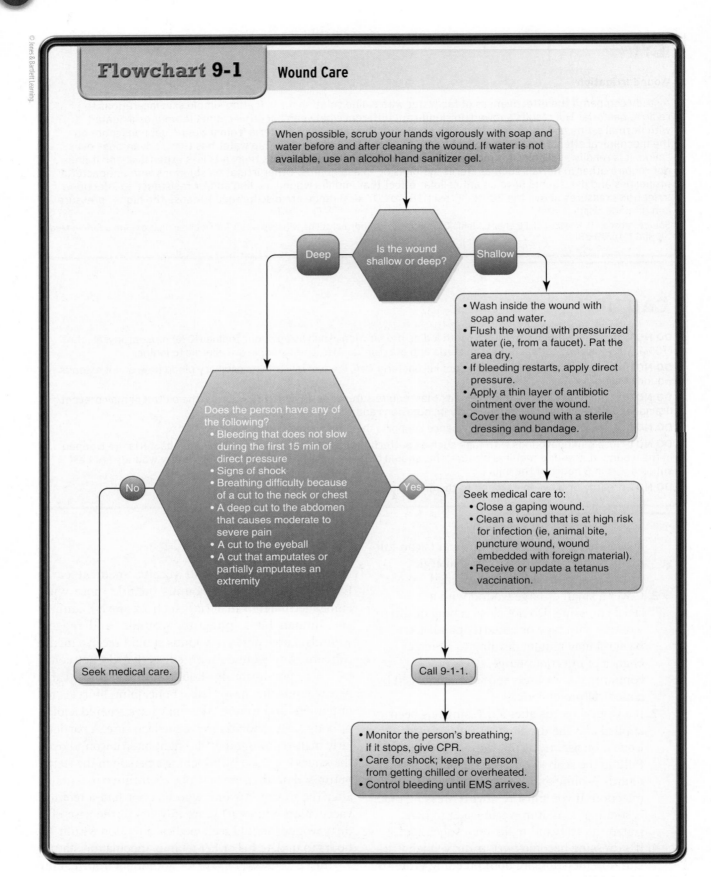

**Flowchart 9-1**     **Wound Care**

When possible, scrub your hands vigorously with soap and water before and after cleaning the wound. If water is not available, use an alcohol hand sanitizer gel.

**Is the wound shallow or deep?**

**Deep** →

**Shallow** →

- Wash inside the wound with soap and water.
- Flush the wound with pressurized water (ie, from a faucet). Pat the area dry.
- If bleeding restarts, apply direct pressure.
- Apply a thin layer of antibiotic ointment over the wound.
- Cover the wound with a sterile dressing and bandage.

**Does the person have any of the following?**
- Bleeding that does not slow during the first 15 min of direct pressure
- Signs of shock
- Breathing difficulty because of a cut to the neck or chest
- A deep cut to the abdomen that causes moderate to severe pain
- A cut to the eyeball
- A cut that amputates or partially amputates an extremity

**No** →

**Yes** →

Seek medical care to:
- Close a gaping wound.
- Clean a wound that is at high risk for infection (ie, animal bite, puncture wound, wound embedded with foreign material).
- Receive or update a tetanus vaccination.

Seek medical care.

Call 9-1-1.

- Monitor the person's breathing; if it stops, give CPR.
- Care for shock; keep the person from getting chilled or overheated.
- Control bleeding until EMS arrives.

## FYI

**Wound Care: What the Medical Literature Says**

- Soaking wounds is not effective and can impair healing.
- The benefit of scrubbing wounds is debatable. Scrubbing can bruise the tissues and skin.
- All wound surfaces should be irrigated; this may require opening wound edges for exposure.
- Wound irrigation is the most important step for optimal wound healing, as long as there is sufficient pressure and volume.
- Irrigating wounds requires a minimum pressure of 5 to 8 psi (34 to 55 kPa) for tissue cleansing.
- Decontamination (brushing off any dry chemicals prior to copious irrigation) is essential.
- Not closing a wound (eg, with butterfly bandages, elastic skin closures), especially a dirty wound, reduces the risk of infection.
- Applying antiseptic solutions such as Merthiolate, Mercurochrome, iodine, isopropyl alcohol, and hydrogen peroxide can injure wounded tissues.
- Applying an antibiotic ointment such as Neosporin or Polysporin reduces the risk of infection in shallow wounds or abrasions.
- A moist wound healing environment helps to promote healing, reduce pain, and improve cosmetic outcome.
- CDC guidelines recommend a tetanus vaccine based on vaccination history and wound severity.
- Sunblock should be used on a new wound for 3 to 6 months.
- You should consider each wound individually to create optimal conditions for wound healing.

*Source:* Howell JM, Chisholm CD. Outpatient wound preparation and care: a national survey. *Ann Emerg Med* 1992;21(8):976–981.; Nicks BA, Ayello EA, Woo K, Nitzki-George D, Sibbald RG. Acute wound management: revisiting the approach to assessment, irrigation, and closure considerations. *Int J Emerg Med* 2010;3:399–407.

## Q&A

**When should wounds be closed by a physician?**

Generally, a wound should be closed by one of several options (eg, sutures, staples, topical skin adhesives) when (1) the edges of the skin do not fall together and/or (2) the cut is more than 1 inch (3 cm) long and is deep. Closing the wound speeds the healing process, lessens the risk of infection, and lessens scarring. If sutures are needed, they should be made by a physician within 6 to 8 hours of the injury.

## FYI

**Myths About Wound Care**

*Myth:* Wounds should be kept dry.
*Fact:* Healing is faster and infection rates are lower when wounds are kept moist. Keep them moist by applying an antibiotic ointment and a dressing.

*Myth:* Redness is a sign of an infected wound.
*Fact:* Although redness *can* signal an infected wound, it does indicate an inflammatory reaction. When you see it, check for the other signs and symptoms of infection: fever and pus coming from the wound.

*Myth:* Saline solution should be used instead of tap water to irrigate a wound.
*Fact:* Saline solution is no more effective in preventing wound infections than is tap water.

*Myth:* A cut should not be covered—it needs to "breathe."
*Fact:* If a cut is not covered, it dries out and scabs over. Keep a cut moist and prevent a scab from forming. Apply an antibiotic ointment and cover with a dressing.

## Infected Wound

Any wound, large or small, can become infected. Once an infection begins, damage can be extensive, so prevention is the best way to avoid infection. A wound should be cleaned using the procedures described earlier in this chapter.

It is important to know how to recognize and treat an infected wound **Figure 9-7**. Factors that increase the likelihood for wound infection include the following:

- Dirty and foreign material left in the wound
- Ragged or crushed tissue
- Injury to an underlying bone, joint, or tendon
- Bite wounds (human or animal)
- Hand and foot wounds
- Puncture wounds or other wounds that cannot drain

## Tetanus

Tetanus is also called *lockjaw* because of its best-known symptom, tightening of the jaw muscles. Tetanus is caused by a toxin produced by a bacterium. The bacterium, which is found throughout the world, forms a spore that can survive for years in a variety of environments. The World Health Organization reports that tetanus causes over 70,000 deaths each year.

Millions of adults in the United States have let their tetanus immunizations lapse; a smaller number have never been vaccinated. In addition, antibody levels in immunized children decline over time. Tetanus is not communicable from one person to another.

The tetanus bacterium by itself does not cause tetanus. When it enters a wound, such as a puncture wound that contains little oxygen, the bacterium can

### What to Look For

- Swelling and redness around wound
- Feeling of increased temperature compared to surrounding area (ie, wound feels warmer)
- Throbbing pain
- Pus discharge
- Fever
- Swelling of lymph nodes
- One or more red streaks leading from the wound toward the heart (this is a serious sign that the infection is spreading and could cause death)

### What to Do

1. Soak the wound in warm water, or apply warm, wet packs over the infected wound. Separate the wound edges to allow pus to escape.
2. Apply an antibiotic ointment.
3. Change the dressings several times a day.
4. Give pain medication.
5. Seek medical care if the infection becomes worse. If chills and fever develop, the infection has reached the circulatory system and immediate medical care is needed.

### FYI

**Using Topical Antibiotics to Improve Wound Healing**

The use of topical triple-antibiotics significantly decreases infection rates in minor wounds that are contaminated. Topical antibiotics are effective for minor wounds but not for major wounds.

Many studies support the use of topical antibiotics on wounds that are clean. Topical bacitracin zinc (Bacitracin); a triple ointment of neomycin sulfate, bacitracin zinc, and polymyxin B sulfate (Neosporin); and silver sulfadiazine (Silvadene) were compared with petrolatum as a control in patients with minor wounds. Wound infection rates were 17.6% for petrolatum, 5.5% for Bacitracin, 4.5% for Neosporin, and 12.1% for Silvadene.
*Source:* Diehr S, Hamp A, Jamieson B, Mendoza M. Clinical inquiries: Do topical antibiotics improve wound healing? *J Fam Pract* 2007;56(2):140-144.

**Figure 9-7**

Infected wound.

produce a powerful, poisonous toxin. The toxin travels through the nervous system to the brain and the spinal cord. It then causes contractions of certain muscle groups, particularly in the jaw. There is no known antidote to the toxin once it enters the nervous system.

It is not just stepping on a rusty nail that can bring on the disease. Tetanus bacteria are commonly found in soil, street dust, organic garden fertilizers, and pet feces, and even minor cuts can introduce them into the bloodstream.

A tetanus vaccination can completely prevent the disease. Everyone needs an initial series of vaccinations to prepare the immune system to defend against the toxin, but then a booster shot only every 5 to 10 years is sufficient to maintain immunity.

The guidelines for tetanus immunization boosters are as follows:

- Anyone with a wound who has never been immunized against tetanus should be given a tetanus vaccine and booster immediately.
- A person who was once immunized but has not received a tetanus booster within the last 10 years should receive a booster.
- A person with a dirty wound who has not had a booster within the past 5 years should receive a booster.
- Tetanus immunization shots must be given within 72 hours of the injury to be effective.

## FYI

**Tetanus Prevalence**

Despite the wide availability of immunization against tetanus in the United States, many people are inadequately protected against this uncommon but often lethal disease. Protection was found in only 72% of people studied, with levels of immunity varying widely. Levels of immunity range from 80 to 90% from age 6 to 39 years and then steadily decrease; by age 70, only 30% of adults have serologic immunity.

About 29 cases of tetanus occur in the United States each year, principally among older people. Adults should have a booster shot for tetanus every 10 years.

*Sources:* McQuillan GM, Kruszon-Moran D, Deforest A, Chu SY, Wharton M. Serologic immunity to diphtheria and tetanus in the United States. *Ann Intern Med* 2002;13(9):660-666.

Centers for Disease Control and Prevention. Tetanus surveillance—United States, 2001-2008. *MMWR* 2011;60(12):365-369.

## ▶ Amputations and Avulsions

In many cases, an amputated extremity can be successfully reattached. It is generally attempted for only upper extremities.

Avulsions most often involve ears, fingers, and hands. This type of wound can bleed heavily. If the flap is still attached, lay it flat and realign it into its normal position.

### Types of Amputations

Amputations usually involve fingers, hands, and arms rather than legs. Amputations are classified according to the type of injury:

- A **clean amputation** is a clean-cut, complete detachment Figure 9-8. Examples would include a finger cut off with an ax or an arm severed with a power tool.
- A **crushing amputation** occurs when an extremity separates by being crushed or mashed off, such as when a hand is caught in a roller machine.
- **Degloving** is when the skin is peeled off, much as you would take off a glove.

In a crushing amputation, the most common type, the chance of reattachment is poor. In a clean amputation, the chance of reattachment is much better because it is clean cut. Many amputations can be reattached by an experienced surgeon, and time is a critical element in success. Function may be nearly normal in some cases.

**Figure 9-8**

Clean amputation.

A complete amputation may not involve heavy blood loss because blood vessels tend to go into spasms, recede into the injured body parts, and shrink in diameter, resulting in a surprisingly small amount of blood loss. More blood is seen in a partial amputation.

Refer to **Flowchart 9-2** for additional information regarding the care of amputations and avulsions.

---

**FYI**

**NEWS: Amputations**

Ronald Malt, MD, performed the first successful reattachment in 1962 on a young boy's severed arm. Today, the reattachment success rate ranges from 80% to 90% due to improved microsurgical techniques and when appropriate actions are taken:

- Minimize the time interval between amputation and replantation.
- Provide hypothermic preservation of the amputated part (39°F [4°C]).
- Avoid freezing and directly immersing the severed part in water.
- Preservation of the amputated part is key to successful replantation.

*Source:* Maricevich M, Carlsen B, Mardini S, Moran S. Upper extremity and digital replantation. *Hand* 2011;6(4):356-363.

---

## What to Look For

## What to Do

| What to Look For | What to Do |
|---|---|
| **Amputation** **Figure 9-9** | 1. Call 9-1-1.<br>2. If a body part is amputated, immediate action is needed for reattachment. Amputated body parts that are left uncooled for more than 6 hours have little chance of survival.<br>3. Control bleeding by using pressure; if unsuccessful, apply a tourniquet or a hemostatic dressing, if available.<br>4. Treat the person for shock.<br>5. Care for the amputated part:<br>  • Wrap the severed part in a sterile gauze or a clean cloth that has been wet with water (make sure the excess water has been squeezed out).<br>  • Put the wrapped part in a waterproof container (eg, plastic bag, plastic wrap) **Figure 9-10** .<br>  • Keep the part cool by placing the wrapped part in a container of ice. **DO NOT** bury the part in the ice or allow the tissue to touch the ice. **DO NOT** submerge it in water.<br>  • Send the part to the medical facility with the injured person.<br>6. If the amputated part was not found, ask others to search for it and, if located, to take it to the medical facility where the person is going. |
| **Avulsion** | 1. Gently move the skin back to its normal position.<br>2. Cover with a sterile or clean dressing and apply pressure.<br>3. If bleeding continues, apply a tourniquet or a hemostatic dressing, if available. |

**Flowchart 9-2**   **Amputations and Avulsions**

- Call 9-1-1.
- Treat for shock by laying the person flat and covering him or her.

**Is the body part torn loose but still attached (avulsion) or completely torn off (amputation)?**

Avulsion — Amputation

- Gently move the skin back to its normal position.
- Cover with a sterile or clean dressing and apply pressure.
- If bleeding continues, apply a tourniquet or a hemostatic dressing, if available.

Control bleeding by using pressure; if unsuccessful, apply a tourniquet or a hemostatic dressing, if available.

**Was the amputated part found?**   No / Yes

Ask others to search for the part and, if located, to take it to the medical facility where the person is going.

- Wrap the part in a sterile gauze or a clean cloth that has been wet with water (make sure the excess water has been squeezed out).
- Put the wrapped part in a waterproof container (eg, plastic bag, plastic wrap).
- Keep the part cool by placing the wrapped part in a container of ice. **DO NOT** bury the part in the ice or allow it to directly touch the ice. **DO NOT** submerge it in water.
- Send the part to the medical facility with the injured person.

**Figure 9-9**

Amputation.

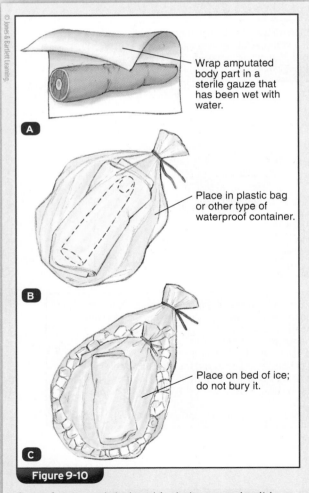

Wrap amputated body part in a sterile gauze that has been wet with water.

**A**

Place in plastic bag or other type of waterproof container.

**B**

Place on bed of ice; do not bury it.

**C**

**Figure 9-10**

Care of an amputated part includes wrapping it in a sterile gauze or a clean cloth **(A)**, placing it in a waterproof container **(B)**, and placing it on ice **(C)**.

## CAUTION

**DO NOT** try to decide whether a body part is salvageable or too small to save. Leave that decision to a physician.

**DO NOT** wrap an amputated part in a soaking wet dressing or cloth. Using a soaking wet wrap on the part can cause waterlogging and tissue softening, which will make reattachment more difficult.

**DO NOT** bury an amputated part in ice; instead, place it on ice. Reattaching frostbitten parts is usually unsuccessful.

**DO NOT** use dry ice.

**DO NOT** cut a skin "bridge," a tendon, or other structure that is connecting a partially attached part to the rest of the body. Instead, reposition the part in the normal position, wrap the part in a dry, sterile dressing or clean cloth, and place an ice pack on it.

## ▶ Blisters

A blister is a collection of fluid in a bubble under the outer layer of skin. (Note: This section applies only to friction blisters and does not apply to blisters from burns, frostbite, drug reactions, insect or snake bites, or contact with a poisonous plant.)

Repeated rubbing of a small area of the skin will produce a blister **Figure 9-11**. Blisters are so common that many people assume they are a fact of life. However, blisters are avoidable, and life for many people could be more comfortable if they knew how to treat and prevent blisters.

Rubbing—as between a sock and a foot—causes stress on the skin's surface because the underlying supporting tissue remains stationary. The stress separates the skin into two layers, and the resulting space fills with fluid. The fluid may collect under or within the skin's outer layer, the epidermis. Because of differences in skin, blister formation varies considerably from person to person.

When caring for a friction blister, try to (1) avoid the risk of infection, (2) minimize the person's pain and discomfort, (3) limit the blister's enlargement when resting is not an option, and (4) promote fast skin healing. The best care for a blister is determined mainly by its size and location.

Refer to **Flowchart 9-3** for additional information regarding the care of friction blisters.

**What to Look For**   **What to Do**

| What to Look For | What to Do |
|---|---|
| **Hot spot (painful, red area caused by rubbing)** | 1. Depending upon availability and the location of the blister, relieve pressure on the area by applying one of the following:<br>• Blister bandage (Blist-O-Ban)<br>• Surgical tape (Micropore paper tape)<br>• Elastic tape (Elastikon)<br>2. Trim and round the edges of the tape to prevent it from peeling off. |
| **Blister that is closed and not very painful** | Depending upon availability and the location of the blister, use the most appropriate method previously discussed. |
| **Blister that is closed and very painful** | 1. Clean the blister and a needle with an alcohol pad.<br>2. Make several small holes at the base of the blister with the needle **Figure 9-12** . **DO NOT** make one large hole. Gently press the fluid out. **DO NOT** remove the blister roof unless it is torn.<br>3. Apply paper tape to protect the blister roof from being torn away when other overlying tape is removed.<br>4. Cover paper tape with elastic or adhesive tape.<br>5. Trim and round the edges of the tape to prevent it from peeling off.<br>6. Watch for signs of an infection. |
| **Blister that is very painful and open or torn** | 1. Use scissors to carefully trim off the dead skin.<br>2. Place a blister pad (Spenco 2nd Skin) over the raw skin.<br>3. Cover the blister pad with paper tape.<br>4. Cover paper tape with elastic or adhesive tape. Trim and round the edges of the tape to prevent it from peeling off.<br>5. Watch for signs of an infection. |

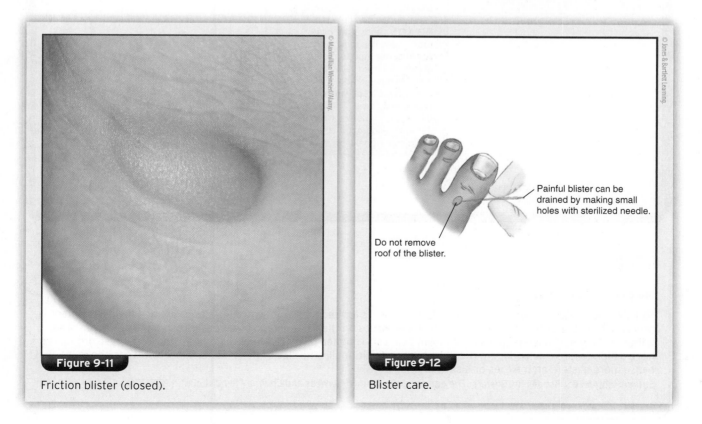

**Figure 9-11**

Friction blister (closed).

Painful blister can be drained by making small holes with sterilized needle.

Do not remove roof of the blister.

**Figure 9-12**

Blister care.

## Flowchart 9-3    Friction Blisters

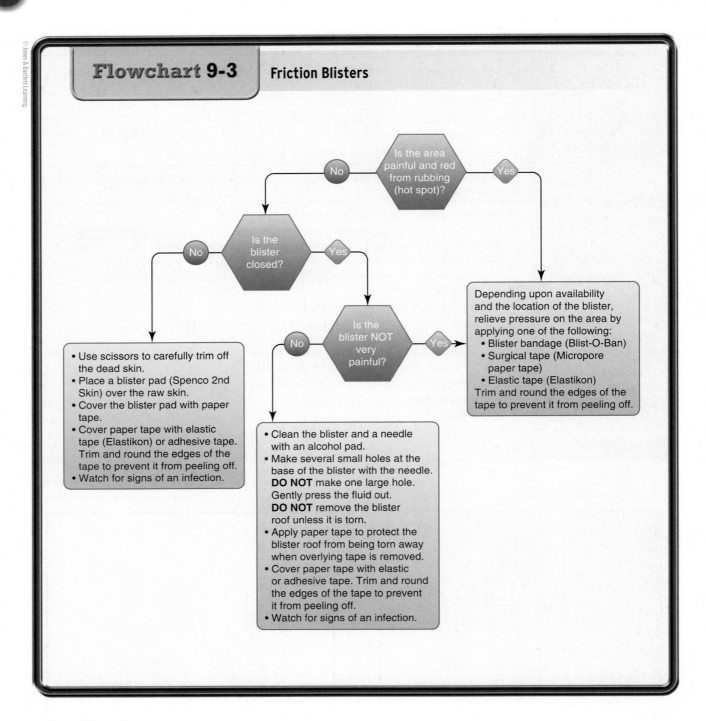

**Is the area painful and red from rubbing (hot spot)?**

No → **Is the blister closed?**

Yes → Depending upon availability and the location of the blister, relieve pressure on the area by applying one of the following:
- Blister bandage (Blist-O-Ban)
- Surgical tape (Micropore paper tape)
- Elastic tape (Elastikon)

Trim and round the edges of the tape to prevent it from peeling off.

**Is the blister closed?**

No →
- Use scissors to carefully trim off the dead skin.
- Place a blister pad (Spenco 2nd Skin) over the raw skin.
- Cover the blister pad with paper tape.
- Cover paper tape with elastic tape (Elastikon) or adhesive tape. Trim and round the edges of the tape to prevent it from peeling off.
- Watch for signs of an infection.

Yes → **Is the blister NOT very painful?**

**Is the blister NOT very painful?**

No →
- Clean the blister and a needle with an alcohol pad.
- Make several small holes at the base of the blister with the needle. **DO NOT** make one large hole. Gently press the fluid out. **DO NOT** remove the blister roof unless it is torn.
- Apply paper tape to protect the blister roof from being torn away when overlying tape is removed.
- Cover paper tape with elastic or adhesive tape. Trim and round the edges of the tape to prevent it from peeling off.
- Watch for signs of an infection.

Yes → Depending upon availability and the location of the blister, relieve pressure on the area by applying one of the following:
- Blister bandage (Blist-O-Ban)
- Surgical tape (Micropore paper tape)
- Elastic tape (Elastikon)

Trim and round the edges of the tape to prevent it from peeling off.

## FYI

### Moleskin for Blisters?

Moleskin has been a fixture in the first aid kits of hikers for decades. Applying a doughnut-shaped moleskin patch around a hot spot or blister places friction and pressure on the surrounding area rather than on the affected area. Large or open heel blisters may benefit from being surrounded by moleskin or molefoam; however, these products have a high failure rate and are difficult to anchor. Additionally, the size of the product in a well-fitted shoe may cause more blisters on the toes or elsewhere.

*Source*: Lipman GS, Scheer BV. Blisters: The enemy of the feet. *Wilderness and Environ Med* 2015;26(2):275-276.

**Preventing Blisters**

Keeping the skin lubricated and protected will reduce the potential for blister formation. Applying paper tape to problem areas, such as around a big toe, can help reduce blister formation by allowing the sock to rub against the tape instead of directly against the skin.

Wearing proper clothing also can prevent blisters. For example, acrylic socks are considered superior to cotton socks in avoiding foot blisters because they are made in layers that are designed to absorb friction. Synthetic socks such as acrylic wick better than cotton. Avoid tube socks made of any material because their less precise fit tends to cause more friction than regular, fitted socks. Wear gloves to protect the skin on your hands.

Anything that can be done to keep the skin dry can also reduce blister formation. Moist skin is more susceptible to blisters than either very dry or very wet skin. One method is to wear socks that wick moisture from the skin. The application of antiperspirants to the feet has been shown to reduce the formation of serious blisters.

# ▶ Impaled (Embedded) Objects

Impaled objects come in all shapes and sizes, from pencils and screwdrivers to knives, glass, steel rods, and fence posts **Figure 9-13**. Proper first aid requires that the impaled object be stabilized because there can be significant internal damage.

**Figure 9-13**

Impaled object.

© American Academy of Orthopaedic Surgeons.

## What to Look For     What to Do

| What to Look For | What to Do |
| --- | --- |
| Sliver (also referred to as a splinter) | 1. Remove with tweezers (may need to use a sterile needle to tease the sliver into a better position for removal).<br>2. Wash the area with soap and water.<br>3. Apply antibiotic ointment.<br>4. Apply an adhesive bandage. |
| Large object (such as a knife, pencil, steel rod) | 1. **DO NOT** remove or move the object.<br>2. Stabilize the object with bulky dressings or padding placed around the base of the object to keep it from moving.<br>3. If bleeding, apply direct pressure around the base of the object. **DO NOT** apply pressure on the object or on the skin next to the sharp edges of the object.<br>4. If necessary, reduce the length or weight of the object by cutting or breaking it.<br>5. Call 9-1-1 if it has not already been done. |
| Impaled object in the cheek | 1. Examine the injury inside the mouth. If the object extends through the cheek and you are more than 1 hour from medical help, consider removing it.<br>2. To remove the object, place two fingers next to the object, straddling it; then gently pull it in the direction from which it entered. If it cannot be removed easily, leave it in place and secure it with bulky dressings.<br>3. Control the bleeding. After you have removed the object, place dressings over the wound inside the mouth between the cheek and the teeth. The dressings will help control the bleeding and will not interfere with the person's airway. Also place a dressing on the outside wound. |
| Impaled object in the eye | 1. **DO NOT** exert any pressure against the eyeball because fluid can be forced out of it, worsening the injury.<br>2. Stabilize the object. Use bulky dressings or clean cloths to stabilize a long, protruding object. You can place a protective paper cup or cardboard folded into a cone over the affected eye to prevent bumping of the object. For short objects, surround the eye—without touching the object—with a doughnut-shaped (ring) pad held in place with a roller bandage. |

*(Continues)*

**What to Look For**    What to Do

| | |
|---|---|
| | 3. Cover the undamaged eye. Most experts suggest that the undamaged eye be covered to prevent sympathetic eye movement (ie, movement of the injured eye when the undamaged eye moves, thus aggravating the injury). Remember that the person is unable to see when both eyes are covered and may be anxious. Make sure you explain to the person everything you are doing.<br>4. Call 9-1-1. |
| **Cactus spines** | Use one of the following methods to remove cactus spines:<br>1. Use tweezers to remove the spines. This method is easy but time consuming because the spines usually are acquired in groupings, are difficult to see, and are designed by nature to resist removal.<br>2. Coat the area with a thin layer of white woodworking glue or rubber cement and allow it to dry for at least 30 minutes. Slowly roll up the dried glue from the margins. Applying the glue in strips rather than puddles will make the rolling procedure go more smoothly. A single layer of gauze gently pressed onto the still-damp glue helps to remove it after it has dried. The combination of using tweezers and glue will remove most of the spines.<br>3. Use adhesive tape, duct tape, or cellophane tape. Although this method is quick and easy, it removes only about 30% of the spines, even after multiple attempts.<br>4. **DO NOT** use super glue (or other similar products) to remove cactus spines. Not only does it fail to roll up when applied to the skin, but it also welds the spines to the skin. In addition, there is the risk that the skin will permanently bond to anything it touches. |
| **Fishhooks**<br>`Figure 9-14` | 1. Tape an embedded fishhook in place and do not try to remove it if injury to a nearby body part (such as the eye or an underlying structure such as a blood vessel or nerve) is possible or if the person (such as a young child) is uncooperative.<br>2. If the point of a fishhook has penetrated the skin but the barb has not, remove the fishhook by backing it out. Then treat the wound like a puncture wound. Seek medical advice for a possible tetanus shot.<br>3. If the hook's barb has entered the skin, follow these procedures:<br>• If medical care is near, transport the person and have a physician remove the hook.<br>• If you are in a remote area, far from medical care, remove the hook using either the pliers method or the string-jerk method.<br><br>*To remove a hook using the pliers method:*<br>1. Use pliers with tempered jaws that can cut through a hook `Figure 9-15`. (Test the pliers by first cutting a similar fishhook.)<br>2. Use an ice pack or use hard pressure around the hook to provide temporary numbness.<br>3. Push the embedded hook further in, in a shallow curve, until the point and the barb come out through the skin. (Use extreme care; pushing the hook into blood vessels, nerves, or tendons can result in severe injury.)<br>4. Cut off the barb, then back the hook out the way it came in.<br>5. After removing the hook, treat the wound and seek medical attention for a possible tetanus shot.<br><br>*To remove a hook using the string-jerk method:*<br>1. Loop a piece of fishing line over the bend or curve of the embedded hook `Figure 9-16`.<br>2. Stabilize the part of the person's body in which the hook is embedded.<br>3. Use an ice pack or use hard pressure around the hook to provide temporary numbness.<br>4. With one hand, press down on the hook's shank and eye while the other hand sharply jerks the fishing line that is over the hook's bend or curve. The jerk movement should be parallel to the skin's surface. The hook will neatly come out of the same hole it entered, causing little pain.<br>5. After removing the hook, care for the wound and seek medical care for a possible tetanus shot. |

**Figure 9-14**

Fishhook.

**Figure 9-16**

Fishhook removal; string-jerk method.

Refer to [Flowchart 9-4] for additional information regarding the care of impaled (embedded) objects.

## ▶ Closed Wounds

A closed wound happens when a blunt object strikes the body. The skin is not broken, but tissue and blood vessels beneath the skin's surface are crushed, causing bleeding within a confined area.

## ▶ Wounds That Require Medical Care

At some point, you will probably have to decide whether medical care is needed for a wounded person. As a guideline, seek medical care for the following conditions, as offered by the American College of Emergency Physicians:

- Long or deep cuts that need stitches
- Cuts over a joint
- Cuts from an animal or human bite
- Cuts that may impair function of a body area, such as an eyelid or lip
- Cuts that remove all the layers of the skin, such as slicing off the tip of a finger
- Cuts caused by metal objects or puncture wounds
- Cuts over a possible broken bone
- Cuts that are deep, jagged, or gaping open

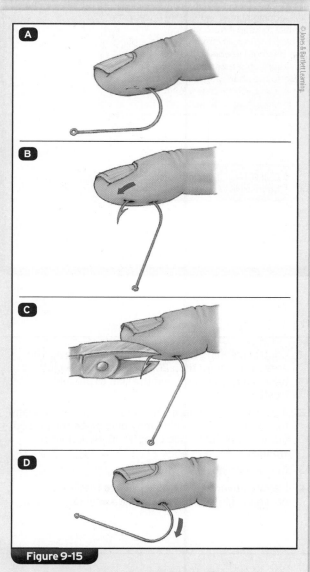

**Figure 9-15**

**A.** The pliers method can be used to remove a fishhook embedded in the skin. **B.** Push the embedded hook further in until the barb comes out through the skin. **C.** Cut off the barb. **D.** Back the hook out the way it came in.

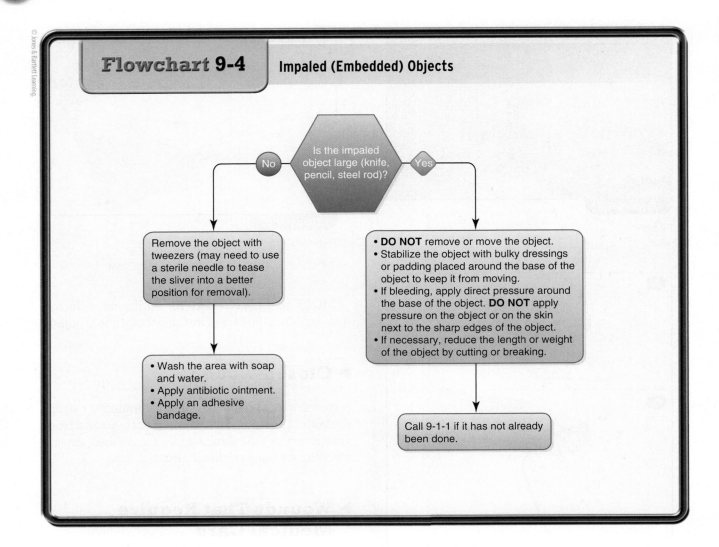

## Flowchart 9-4    Impaled (Embedded) Objects

**Is the impaled object large (knife, pencil, steel rod)?**

No → Remove the object with tweezers (may need to use a sterile needle to tease the sliver into a better position for removal).

- Wash the area with soap and water.
- Apply antibiotic ointment.
- Apply an adhesive bandage.

Yes →
- **DO NOT** remove or move the object.
- Stabilize the object with bulky dressings or padding placed around the base of the object to keep it from moving.
- If bleeding, apply direct pressure around the base of the object. **DO NOT** apply pressure on the object or on the skin next to the sharp edges of the object.
- If necessary, reduce the length or weight of the object by cutting or breaking.

Call 9-1-1 if it has not already been done.

## What to Look For

There are three types of closed wounds:

1. Bruises and contusions occur when blood collects under the skin in the injured area. The person will experience pain and swelling (immediately or within 24 to 48 hours). As blood accumulates, a black-and-blue mark may appear.

2. A hematoma is a clot of blood under the skin. There may be a lump or blue discoloration.

3. Crush injuries are caused by extreme forces, which can injure vital organs and bones without breaking open the skin. Crush injuries may indicate an underlying condition such as a fracture. Signs and symptoms include discoloration, swelling, pain, and loss of use.

## What to Do

1. Control bleeding by applying an ice pack over the area for no more than 20 minutes. Place a cloth between the ice pack and the skin to prevent frostbite.

2. If the injury involves a limb, apply an elastic bandage for compression. A splint may help make the person more comfortable. See Chapter 10, *Bandaging Wounds*.

3. Check for a possible fracture.

4. Elevate an injured extremity above the person's heart level to decrease pain and swelling.

- Cuts that involve damage to underlying nerves, tendons, or joints
- Cuts in which foreign materials, such as dirt, glass, metal, or chemicals, are embedded
- Cuts that show signs of infection, such as fever, swelling, redness, a pungent smell, pus, or fluid draining from the area
- Cuts that include issues with movement or sensation, or increased pain

Call 9-1-1 immediately if:

- Bleeding from a cut does not slow during the first 15 minutes of steady pressure
- Signs of shock occur
- Breathing is difficult because of a cut to the neck or chest
- A deep cut to the abdomen causes moderate to severe pain
- A cut occurs to the eyeball
- A cut amputates or partially amputates an extremity

### Sutures

If sutures (stitches) are needed, they usually should be placed by a physician within 6 to 8 hours of the injury. Suturing wounds allows faster healing, reduces infection, and lessens scarring. Some wounds do not usually require sutures, including:

- Wounds in which the skin's cut edges tend to fall together
- Shallow cuts less than 1 inch (3 cm) long

Rather than close a gaping wound with butterfly bandages or elastic skin closures, cover the wound with sterile gauze. Closing the wound might trap bacteria inside, resulting in an infection. In most cases, a physician can be reached in time for sutures to be placed; if not, a wound without sutures will still heal but with scars. Scar tissue can be attended to later by a plastic surgeon.

## ▶ Gunshot Wounds

Guns are abundant in the United States; it is estimated that about one-half of all American homes have a firearm. Shootings, stabbings, and other penetrating injuries that result from violence represent a major challenge to a first aid provider. Rescuers sometimes take greater than normal risks to help people who have been shot or stabbed. If you are at the scene of an active shooter, you should "run, hide, fight." *Run* when it is safe to run, *hide* where it is safe to hide, and *fight* if you or others around you have no other options.

There are two general types of firearms: low velocity, such as most civilian firearms, and high velocity, such as military weapons. Shotguns have low velocity but create severe tissue damage.

A bullet causes injury in the following ways, depending on its velocity, or speed:

- *Laceration and crushing.* When the bullet penetrates the body, it crushes tissue and forces it apart. That is the main effect of low-velocity bullets. The crushing and laceration caused by the passage of the bullet usually are not life threatening unless vital organs or major blood vessels are injured. The bullet damages only the tissues that it contacts directly, and the wound is comparable to that caused by weapons such as knives.
- *Shock waves and temporary cavitation.* When a bullet penetrates the body, a shock wave exerts outward pressure from the bullet's path. The shock wave pushes tissues away and creates a temporary cavity that can be as much as 30 times the diameter of the bullet. As the cavity forms, a negative pressure develops inside, creating a vacuum. The vacuum then draws debris in with it.

  Temporary cavitation occurs only with high-velocity bullets and is the main reason for their immensely destructive effect. The cavitation lasts only a millisecond but can damage muscles, nerves, blood vessels, and bone.

Bullets sometimes hit hard tissue such as bones and may bounce around in the body cavities, causing a great deal of damage to tissue and organs. Moreover, bone chips can ricochet to other body areas and cause damage. Because a split or misshapen bullet tumbles and exerts its force over a larger area, it does more damage than does a smooth bullet going in a straight line.

## What to Look For

Penetrating wound, indicated by:

- A bullet entry point but no exit
- Little or no external bleeding (The person may still bleed to death because of internal bleeding.)
- Signs and symptoms of shock (ie, diminishing alertness, fainting or near fainting) if the person has significant internal bleeding

Perforating wound, indicated by both entry and exit points

- The exit wound of a high-velocity bullet is usually larger than the entrance wound.
- The exit wound from a low-velocity bullet is about the same size as the entry wound **Figure 9-17** .
- If the bullet was fired at very close range, the entrance wound may be larger than the exit wound because the gases from the gun's muzzle contribute to the surface-tissue damage.

## What to Do

Regardless of the type of gunshot wound, initial care is roughly the same as for any other wound.

1. Monitor the person's breathing.
2. Expose the wound(s). Make sure to look at all the skin, including hidden areas.
3. Control the bleeding with direct pressure.
4. Apply dry, sterile dressings to the wound(s) and bandage them securely in place.
5. Treat the person for shock.
6. Keep the person calm and quiet.
7. Seek immediate medical care.

Figure 9-17

Gunshot wounds. **A.** An entrance wound from a gunshot may have burns around the edges. **B.** An exit wound is sometimes larger and results in greater damage to soft tissues.

## Q&A

**How do the physical characteristics of the bullet affect injury to the person?**

- The larger the size of the bullet, the greater the size of the wound (eg, .22 versus .45 caliber).
- A hollow-point bullet widens when it hits tissues, causing a wider path of destruction.
- A bullet that tumbles around damages more tissue.
- Soft-nose bullets or bullets with vertical cuts in the nose break apart on impact, spreading fragments in a wider path and causing more tissue and organ damage. A shotgun blast also causes fragmentation.

## CAUTION

**DO NOT** try to remove material from a gunshot wound. The hospital emergency department personnel will clean the wound.

## Legal Implications of Gunshot Wounds

Because interactions with people with gunshot wounds will involve contact with law enforcement agencies and will possibly require you to testify in court, carefully observe the scene and the person. Keep an accurate record of your observations. Do not touch or move anything unless absolutely necessary to treat the person. All gunshot wounds must be reported to the police regardless of whether they are intentional (suicide, assault, murder, self-defense) or unintentional.

## ▶ Ready for Review

- An open wound is a break in the skin's surface resulting in external bleeding.
- Knowing what type of open wound the person has will help you in providing first aid.
- In many cases, an amputated extremity can be successfully replanted.
- A blister is a collection of fluid in a bubble under the outer layer of skin.
- Proper first aid of an impaled object requires that the object be stabilized because significant internal damage can occur.
- A closed wound happens when a blunt object strikes the body. Although the skin remains unbroken, the tissue and blood vessels beneath the skin's surface are crushed, causing bleeding within a confined area.
- Wounds that require medical care include:
  - Long or deep cuts that need stitches
  - Cuts over a joint
  - Cuts from an animal or human bite
  - Cuts that may impair function of a body area, such as an eyelid or lip
  - Cuts that remove all the layers of the skin, such as slicing off the tip of a finger
  - Cuts caused by metal objects or puncture wounds
  - Cuts over a possible broken bone
  - Cuts that are deep, jagged, or gaping open
  - Cuts that involve damage to underlying nerves, tendons, or joints
  - Cuts in which foreign materials, such as dirt, glass, metal, or chemicals, are embedded
  - Cuts that show signs of infection, such as fever, swelling, redness, a pungent smell, pus, or fluid draining from the area
  - Cuts that include issues with movement or sensation, or increased pain
- Call 9-1-1 immediately if:
  - Bleeding from a cut does not slow during the first 15 minutes of steady pressure
  - Signs of shock occur
  - Breathing is difficult because of a cut to the neck or chest
  - A deep cut to the abdomen causes moderate to severe pain
  - A cut occurs to the eyeball
  - A cut amputates or partially amputates an extremity
- Regardless of the type of gunshot wound, initial care is roughly the same as for any other wound.

## ▶ Vital Vocabulary

**abrasion** An injury in which a portion of the skin is removed by rubbing or scraping on a hard, rough surface.

**amputation** An injury in which a body part is completely removed.

**avulsion** An injury that leaves a piece of skin or other tissue either partially or completely torn away from the body.

**bandage** A material used to cover a dressing to keep it in place on the wound and to apply pressure to help control bleeding.

**clean amputation** A clean-cut, complete detachment of an extremity.

**crushing amputation** An injury in which an extremity separates by being crushed or mashed off.

**degloving** An injury in which the skin is peeled off the extremity.

**dressing** A sterile gauze pad or clean cloth covering that is placed over an open wound.

**incision** A wound that is usually made deliberately in connection with surgery. The edges are cleanly cut as opposed to a laceration.

**laceration** A wound made by the tearing or cutting of body tissues.

**puncture** A deep, narrow wound in the skin and underlying organs.

# prep kit

## ▶ Assessment in Action

You are helping your mother prepare for a barbeque on a Saturday afternoon. She is slicing tomatoes with a very dull kitchen knife. She is startled by something and cuts into her finger. The wound is bleeding and you can see the bone in the wound.

*Directions:* Circle Yes if you agree with the statement; circle No if you disagree.

Yes    No    **1.** This type of wound is called an avulsion.

Yes    No    **2.** You should not be concerned about infection because she was using a clean knife.

Yes    No    **3.** You should cover the wound with a sterile dressing but should not close the wound with tape or butterfly bandages.

Yes    No    **4.** You decide to take her to the emergency department for possible sutures. Because you and your mother do not want to miss the barbeque, it will be okay to wait until the next day.

## ▶ Check Your Knowledge

*Directions:* Circle Yes if you agree with the statement; circle No if you disagree.

Yes    No    **1.** An open wound may allow bacteria to enter the body, causing an infection.

Yes    No    **2.** A laceration is cut skin with smooth, straight edges.

Yes    No    **3.** A dressing is applied over a wound to control bleeding and prevent contamination.

Yes    No    **4.** A bandage is applied over a wound to hold a dressing in place.

Yes    No    **5.** Any wound can become infected.

Yes    No    **6.** The signs and symptoms of an infection include swelling and redness around the wound, throbbing pain, and a lack of fever.

Yes    No    **7.** A bite wound is more likely to become infected.

Yes    No    **8.** Impaled objects should be removed immediately.

Yes    No    **9.** Tetanus is communicable from one person to another.

Yes    No    **10.** In many cases, an amputated extremity can be successfully reattached.

# Bandaging Wounds

## 10

## ▶ Dressings

A dressing covers an open wound; it touches the wound. Whenever possible, a dressing should be:

- Sterile. If a sterile dressing is not available, use a clean cloth, handkerchief, washcloth, or towel.
- Larger than the wound.
- Thick, soft, and compressible so pressure is evenly distributed over the wound.
- Lint free.

The purposes of using a dressing are to:

- Control bleeding.
- Prevent infection and contamination.
- Absorb blood and wound drainage.
- Protect the wound from further injury.

### Types of Dressings

Use commercial dressings whenever possible. Dressings used in most first aid situations are commercially prepared, but dressings may need to be improvised.

- **Gauze pads** are used for small wounds. They come in separately wrapped packages of various sizes (eg, 2- by 2-inch [5- by 5-cm] squares; 4- by 4-inch [10- by 10-cm] squares) and are sterile, unless the package is broken. Some gauze pads have a special coating to keep them from sticking to the wound and are especially helpful for burns or wounds secreting fluids **Figure 10-1**.

- **Adhesive bandages** are used for small cuts and abrasions and are a combination of a sterile dressing and a bandage **Figure 10-2**.
- **Trauma dressings** are made of large, thick, absorbent, sterile materials. Individually wrapped sanitary napkins can serve as a dressing because of their bulk and absorbency, but they usually are not sterile **Figure 10-3**.

**Figure 10-3**

Trauma dressings.

**Figure 10-1**

Gauze pads.

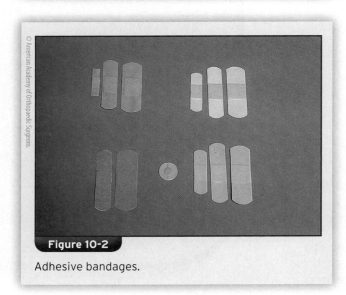

**Figure 10-2**

Adhesive bandages.

- When commercial sterile dressings are not available, an improvised dressing should be as clean, absorbent, soft, and free of lint as possible (eg, a handkerchief or a towel). Use the cleanest cloth available, or, in some conditions and if time allows, sterilize a cloth by ironing it for several minutes.

## CAUTION

**DO NOT** use fluffy cotton or cotton balls as a dressing. Cotton fibers can get in the wound and become difficult to remove.
**DO NOT** remove a blood-soaked dressing until the bleeding stops. Cover it with a new dressing.
**DO NOT** pull off a dressing stuck to a wound. If it needs to be removed, soak it off in warm water.

### Applying a Sterile Dressing

1. If possible, wash your hands and wear exam gloves.
2. Use a dressing large enough to extend beyond the edges of the wound. Hold the dressing by a corner. Place the dressing directly over the wound. **DO NOT** slide it on; doing so can cause pain and dislodge blood clots.
3. Cover the dressing with one of the types of bandages.

## CAUTION

**DO NOT** touch any part of the wound or any part of the dressing that will be in contact with the wound.

# ▶ Bandages

A bandage should be clean but need not be sterile. A bandage can be used to:

- Hold a dressing in place over an open wound.
- Apply direct pressure over a dressing to control bleeding.
- Prevent or reduce swelling.
- Provide support and stability for an extremity or joint.

Remember, bandages should be applied firmly enough to keep dressings and splints in place but not so tightly that they will reinjure the body part or impede blood circulation. The signs that a bandage is too tight include:

- Blue tinge of the fingernails or toenails
- Skin looks blue or pale
- Tingling or loss of sensation
- Coldness of the extremity
- Inability to move the fingers or toes
- A pulse is felt before bandaging, but not after.

A square knot is preferred because it is neat, holds well, and can be easily untied. If the knot or the bandage is likely to cause the person discomfort, a pad should be placed between the knot or bandage and the body.

## CAUTION

**DO NOT** apply a bandage directly over a wound. Put a sterile dressing on first.

**DO NOT** bandage so tightly as to restrict blood circulation. Always check the extremity's pulse. If you cannot feel the pulse, loosen the bandage. Always check for signs that the bandage is too tight.

**DO NOT** bandage so loosely that the dressing will slip. This is the most common bandaging error. Bandages tend to stretch after a short time.

**DO NOT** leave loose ends. They might get caught on something or loosen.

**DO NOT** cover the person's fingers or toes unless they are injured. They need to be observed for color changes that would indicate impaired circulation.

**DO NOT** use elastic bandages over a wound. There is a tendency to apply them too tightly.

**DO NOT** apply a circular bandage around a person's neck; strangulation may occur.

**DO NOT** start a roller bandage above the wound. Instead, start below the wound and work upward.

## Types of Bandages

The following are the basic types of bandages:

- **Roller bandages** come in various widths, lengths, and types of material. For best results, use different widths for different body areas:
  - 1-inch (3-cm) width for fingers
  - 2-inch (5-cm) width for wrists, hands, and feet
  - 3-inch (7-cm) width for ankles, elbows, and arms
  - 4-inch (10-cm) width for knees and legs
- **Self-adhering, conforming bandages** `Figure 10-4` come as rolls of slightly elastic, gauzelike material in various widths. Their self-adherent quality makes them easy to use.
- **Gauze rollers** are cotton and nonelastic. They come in various widths (1, 2, and 3 inches [3, 5, and 7 cm]) and usually are 10 yards (9 m) long. When commercial roller bandages are unavailable, you can improvise bandages from belts, neckties, or strips of cloth torn from a sheet or other similar material.
- **Elastic roller bandages** `Figure 10-5` are used for compression on sprains, strains, and contusions and come in various widths. Elastic bandages are not usually applied over dressings covering a wound.
- **Triangular bandages** `Figure 10-6` are available commercially or can be made from a

**Figure 10-4**

Self-adhering, conforming bandages and gauze bandages of various sizes.

© American Academy of Orthopaedic Surgeons.

**Figure 10-5**

Elastic roller bandages of various sizes.

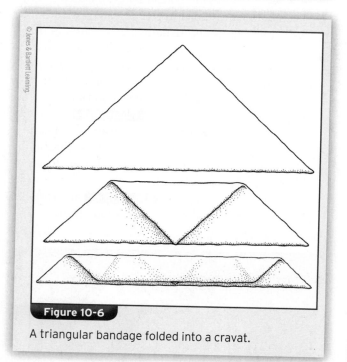

**Figure 10-6**

A triangular bandage folded into a cravat.

square piece of preshrunk cotton muslin measuring 36 to 40 inches (230 to 260 cm²) along each side of the square. Cut the material diagonally from corner to corner to produce two triangular pieces of cloth. The longest side is called the base; the corner directly across from the base is the point; and the other two corners are called ends. A triangular bandage may be applied two ways:

- *Fully opened (not folded)*. Best used for an arm sling. When used to hold dressings in place, fully opened triangular bandages do not apply sufficient pressure on the wound.

- **Cravat** *(folded triangular bandage)*. The point is folded to the center of the base and then the fabric is folded in half again from the top to the base to form a cravat. It is used to hold splints in place, to hold dressings in place, to apply pressure evenly over a dressing, or as a swathe (binder) around the person's body to stabilize an injured arm in an arm sling.
- **Adhesive tape** comes in rolls and in a variety of widths. It is often used to secure roller bandages and small dressings in place. For people allergic to adhesive tape, use paper tape or special dermatologic tape.
- Adhesive bandages are used for small cuts and abrasions and are a combination of a dressing and a bandage.

## Applying a Cravat Bandage

A cravat bandage **Figure 10-6** can be applied on the head, forehead, ear, eyes, arm, leg, or hand. For an injured eye, cover both eyes to prevent the injured eye from moving. Follow the steps in **Skill Sheet 10-1**:

1. Place the middle of the bandage over the dressing covering the wound (or eyes) and wrap the bandage around the head (**Step 1**).

# Skill Sheet

## 10-1  Cravat Method of Bandaging the Head, Forehead, Ear, or Eyes

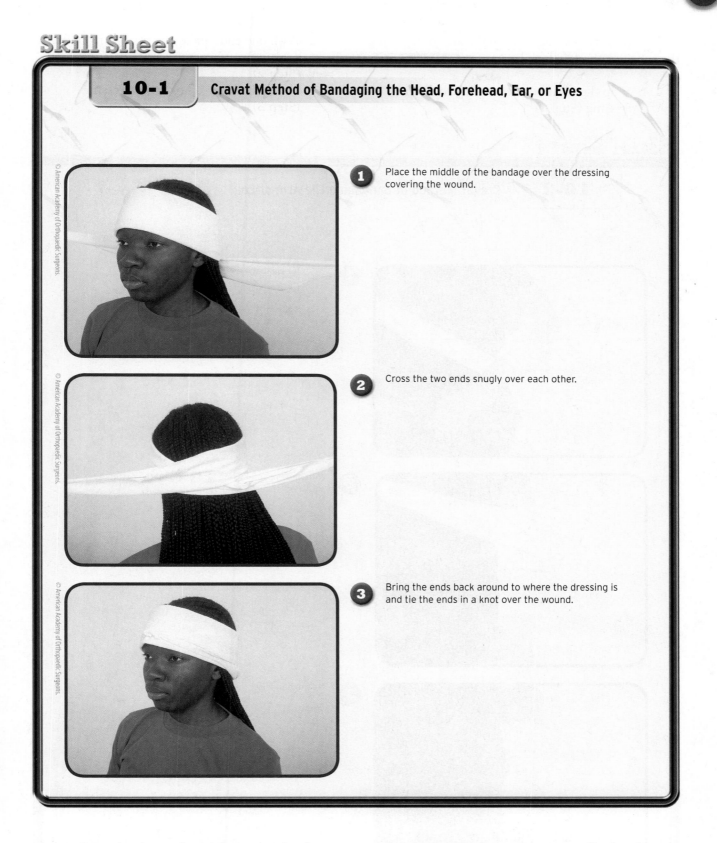

**1** Place the middle of the bandage over the dressing covering the wound.

**2** Cross the two ends snugly over each other.

**3** Bring the ends back around to where the dressing is and tie the ends in a knot over the wound.

**2.** Cross the two ends snugly over each other (**Step 2**).

**3.** Bring the ends back around to where the dressing is and tie the ends in a knot

(**Step 3**). When wrapping a roller bandage around the head, keep the bandage near the eyebrows and low on the back of the head to prevent the bandage from slipping.

To apply a cravat bandage to the arm or leg using the cravat method, follow the steps in Skill Sheet 10-2:

1. Wrap the center of the bandage over the dressing (**Step 1**).

2. With one end, make one turn going up the extremity and another turn going down (**Step 2**).

3. Tie the bandage off over the dressing (**Step 3**).

## Skill Sheet

### 10-2    Cravat Method of Bandaging the Arm or Leg

1 Wrap the bandage over the dressing.

2 With one end, make one turn going up the extremity and another turn going down.

3 Tie the bandage over the dressing.

To apply a bandage to the palm of the hand using the cravat method, follow the steps in **Skill Sheet 10-3** :

1. Fill the palm with a bulky dressing or pad and close the fingers over it (**Step 1**).

2. Wrap one end of the bandage across the fingers and the other around the wrist (**Step 2**).
3. Wrap the bandage crossing over the fingers and around the wrist (**Step 3**).
4. Tie the bandage off at the wrist (**Step 4**).

## Skill Sheet

**10-3**   **Cravat Method for Applying a Bandage to the Palm of the Hand**

**1** Fill the palm with a bulky dressing or pad.

**2** Wrap one end of the bandage around the fingers and the other around the wrist.

**3** Wrap the bandage crossing over the fingers and around the wrist.

© Jones & Bartlett Learning.

*(Continues)*

## Skill Sheet Continued

**10-3**    Cravat Method for Applying a Bandage to the Palm of the Hand

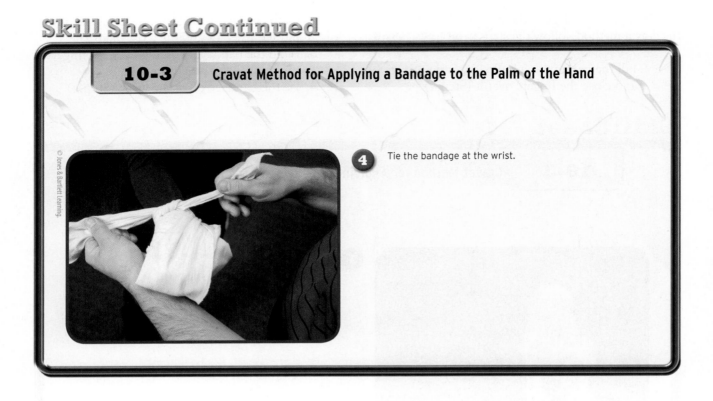

**4** Tie the bandage at the wrist.

© Jones & Bartlett Learning.

### Applying a Roller Bandage

With a little ingenuity, you can apply a roller bandage to almost any body part. Self-adhering, conforming roller bandages eliminate the need for many of the complicated bandaging techniques that standard gauze roller, cravat, and triangular bandages require.

### The Spiral Method

This method employs a 2- or 3-inch (5- or 7-cm) roller bandage for the arm or a 4-inch (10-cm) bandage for the leg. To apply a bandage to the arm or leg using the spiral method, follow the steps in Skill Sheet 10-4:

1. Start at the narrow part of an arm or leg and wrap upward toward the wider part to make the bandage more secure. Start below and at the edge of the dressing.
2. Make two straight anchoring turns with the bandage (**Step 1**).
3. Make a series of turns, progressing up the arm or leg. Each turn should overlap the previous wrap. Wrap with crisscross (figure-eight) turns (**Step 2**).
4. Finish with two straight turns and secure the bandage (**Step 3**).

### The Figure-Eight Method

Use this method of applying a roller bandage to hold dressings or to provide compression at or near a joint such as the ankle. The figure-eight method involves continuous spiral loops of bandage, one up and one down, crossing each other to form an 8. To apply a 4- or 6-inch (10- or 15-cm) roller bandage to the elbow or knee using the figure-eight method, follow the steps in Skill Sheet 10-5:

1. Bend the elbow or knee slightly and make two straight anchoring turns with the bandage over the elbow point or knee cap (**Step 1**).
2. Bring the bandage above the joint to the upper arm or leg, and make one turn, covering one-half to three-fourths of the bandage from the first turn (**Step 2**).
3. Bring the bandage just under the joint and make one turn around the lower arm or leg, covering one-half to three-fourths of the first straight turn (**Step 3**).
4. Continue alternating the turns in a figure-eight maneuver by covering the previous layers (**Step 4**).
5. Finish by making two straight turns, and secure the end (**Step 5**).

# Skill Sheet

## 10-4    Spiral Method of Bandaging a Forearm

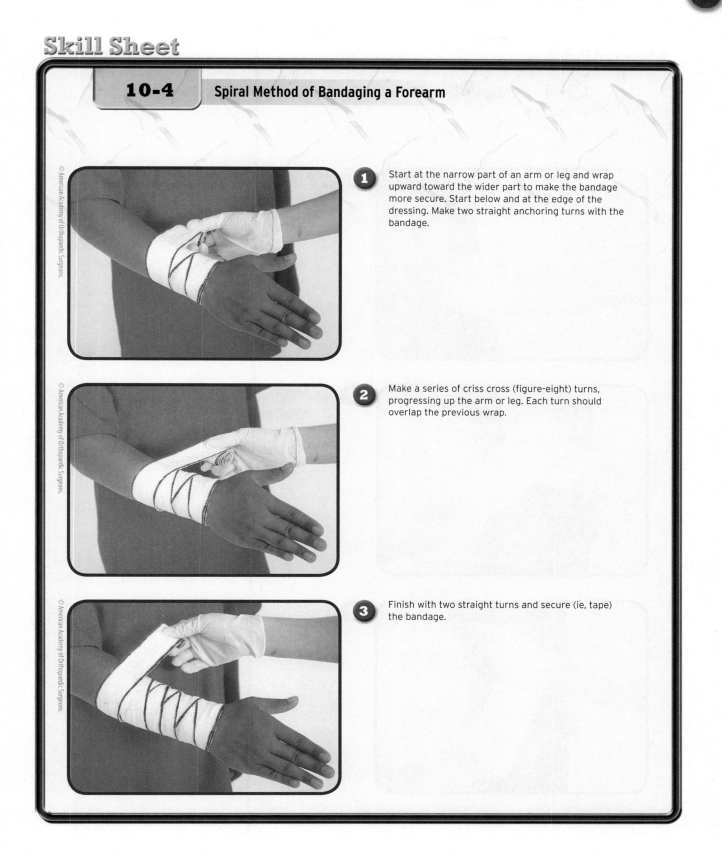

**1** Start at the narrow part of an arm or leg and wrap upward toward the wider part to make the bandage more secure. Start below and at the edge of the dressing. Make two straight anchoring turns with the bandage.

**2** Make a series of criss cross (figure-eight) turns, progressing up the arm or leg. Each turn should overlap the previous wrap.

**3** Finish with two straight turns and secure (ie, tape) the bandage.

© American Academy of Orthopaedic Surgeons.

## Skill Sheet

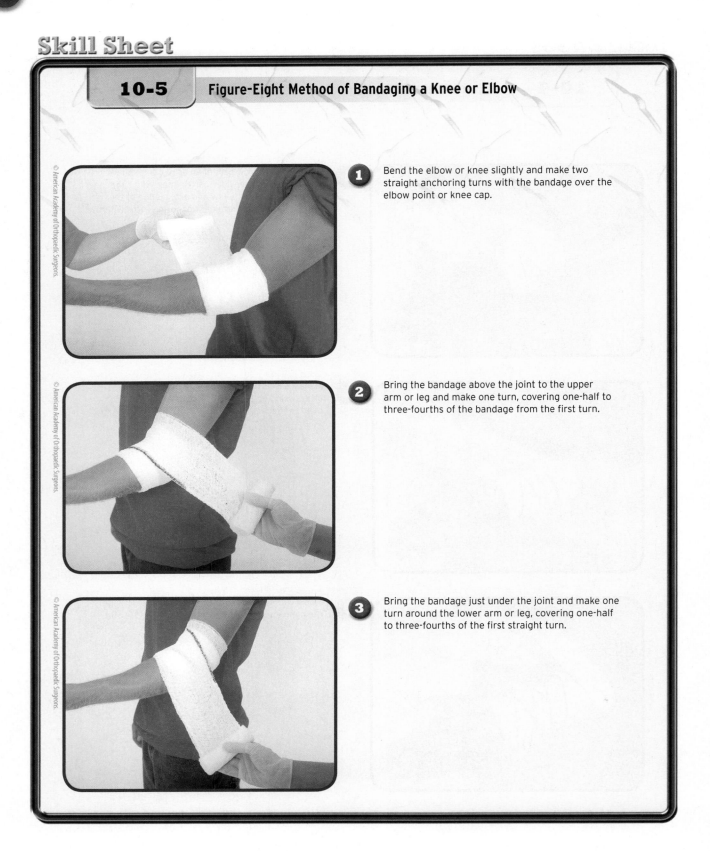

**10-5**    **Figure-Eight Method of Bandaging a Knee or Elbow**

**1** Bend the elbow or knee slightly and make two straight anchoring turns with the bandage over the elbow point or knee cap.

**2** Bring the bandage above the joint to the upper arm or leg and make one turn, covering one-half to three-fourths of the bandage from the first turn.

**3** Bring the bandage just under the joint and make one turn around the lower arm or leg, covering one-half to three-fourths of the first straight turn.

# Skill Sheet Continued

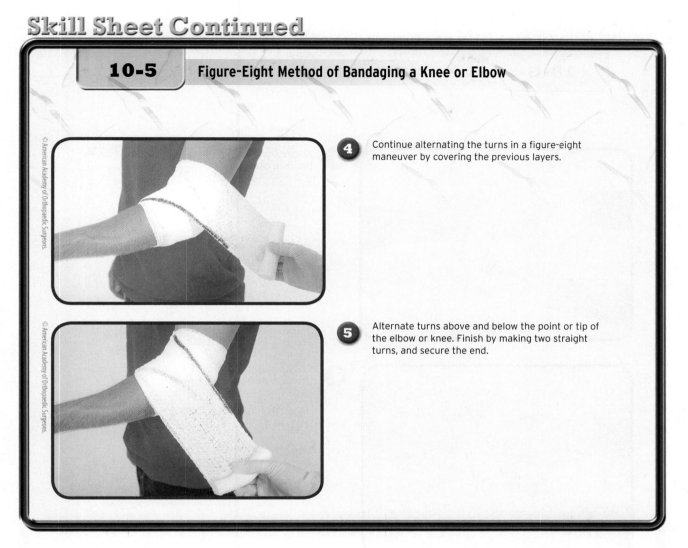

**10-5**   **Figure-Eight Method of Bandaging a Knee or Elbow**

**4** Continue alternating the turns in a figure-eight maneuver by covering the previous layers.

**5** Alternate turns above and below the point or tip of the elbow or knee. Finish by making two straight turns, and secure the end.

To apply a roller bandage to the hand using the figure-eight method, follow the steps in **Skill Sheet 10-6**. This method uses a 2- or 3-inch (5- or 7-cm) roller bandage.

1. Make two straight anchoring turns with the bandage around the palm of the hand **(Step 1)**.
2. Carry the bandage diagonally across the back of the hand and then around the wrist and back across the palm **(Step 2)**.
3. Complete several figure-eight turns, overlapping each by about three-fourths of the previous bandage width. Repeat this figure-eight maneuver as many times as necessary to cover the dressing, overlapping wraps to "stair-step" up the hand **(Step 3)**.
4. Make two straight turns around the wrist, and secure the bandage.

To wrap an ankle or foot using the figure-eight method, follow the steps in **Skill Sheet 10-7**. This wrapping will hold a dressing or apply pressure to treat a sprained ankle. It should not be used to support the ankle and foot during sports activity; that type of bandaging involves additional maneuvers. Either 2- or 3-inch (5- or 7-cm) roller bandages can be used.

1. Make two straight anchoring turns with the bandage around the foot's instep **(Step 1)**.
2. Make a figure-eight turn by taking the bandage diagonally across the front of the foot, around the ankle, and again diagonally across the foot and under the arch **(Step 2)**.
3. Make several of these figure-eight turns, each time overlapping the previous one by about three-fourths the width of the bandage. The bandage advances up the leg **(Step 3)**.
4. Finish with two straight turns around the leg, and secure the bandage.

## Skill Sheet

**10-6**    **Figure-Eight Method of Bandaging a Hand**

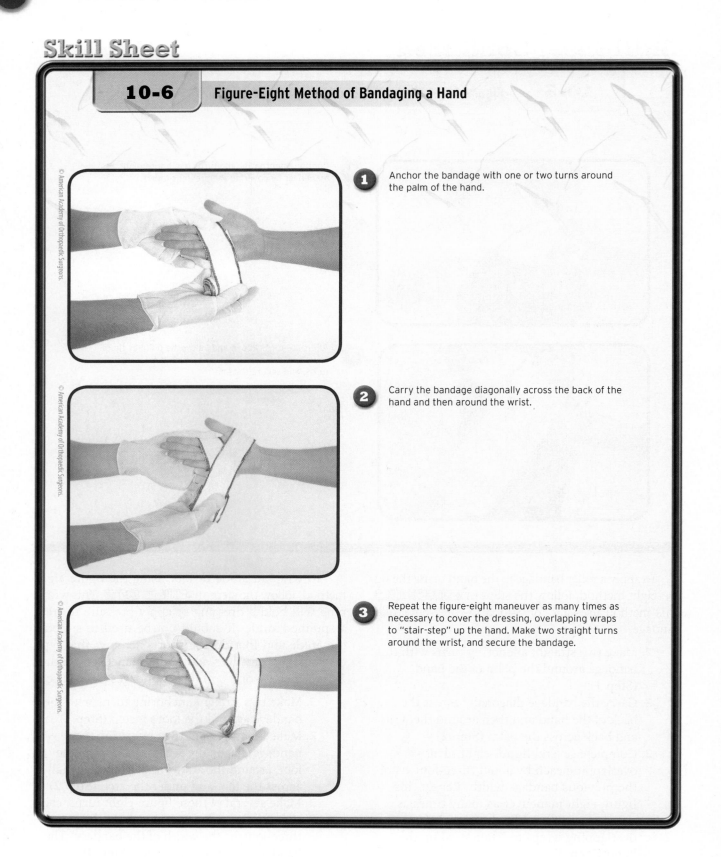

**1**  Anchor the bandage with one or two turns around the palm of the hand.

**2**  Carry the bandage diagonally across the back of the hand and then around the wrist.

**3**  Repeat the figure-eight maneuver as many times as necessary to cover the dressing, overlapping wraps to "stair-step" up the hand. Make two straight turns around the wrist, and secure the bandage.

© American Academy of Orthopaedic Surgeons.

## Skill Sheet

### 10-7    Figure-Eight Method of Bandaging an Ankle or Foot

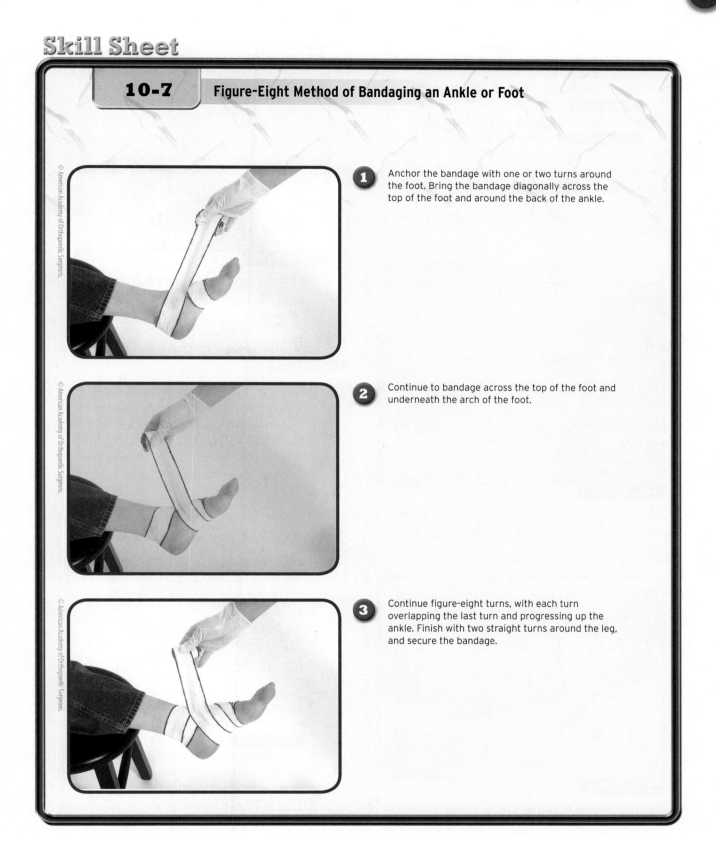

**1** Anchor the bandage with one or two turns around the foot. Bring the bandage diagonally across the top of the foot and around the back of the ankle.

**2** Continue to bandage across the top of the foot and underneath the arch of the foot.

**3** Continue figure-eight turns, with each turn overlapping the last turn and progressing up the ankle. Finish with two straight turns around the leg, and secure the bandage.

## Securing a Roller Bandage

To securely fasten a roller bandage, you can:

- Apply adhesive tape to secure the bandage **Figure 10-7**.
- Use safety pins to secure the bandage **Figure 10-8**. Be very careful with people who may have decreased sensation.
- Use the special clips provided with elastic bandages **Figure 10-9**.

You can also use either the loop or split-tail methods.

**Figure 10-9**

Using special clips to secure an elastic roller bandage.

**Figure 10-7**

Applying adhesive tape to secure a roller bandage.

**Figure 10-8**

Using safety pins to secure a roller bandage.

To perform the loop method, follow the steps in **Skill Sheet 10-8**:

1. Reverse the direction of the bandage by looping it around a thumb or finger and continue back to the opposite side of the body part (**Step 1**).
2. Encircle the part with the looped end and the free end and tie them together (**Step 2**).

To perform the split-tail method of securing a bandage, follow the steps in **Skill Sheet 10-9**:

1. Split the end of the bandage lengthwise for about 12 inches (30 cm), then tie a knot to prevent further splitting (**Step 1**).
2. Pass the ends in opposite directions around the body part and tie (**Step 2**).

## Applying an Adhesive Bandage

1. Remove the wrapping and hold the dressing, pad-side down, by the protective strips **Figure 10-10**.
2. Peel back, but do not remove, the protective strips. Without touching the dressing pad, place it directly onto the wound.
3. Carefully pull away the protective strips. Press the ends and edges down.

# Skill Sheet

## 10-8   Loop Method of Securing Bandages

**1** Reverse the direction of the bandage by looping it around a thumb or finger and continue back to the opposite side of the body part.

**2** Encircle the part with the looped end and the free end and tie them together.

© American Academy of Orthopaedic Surgeons.

**Figure 10-10**

Applying an adhesive dressing.

# Skill Sheet

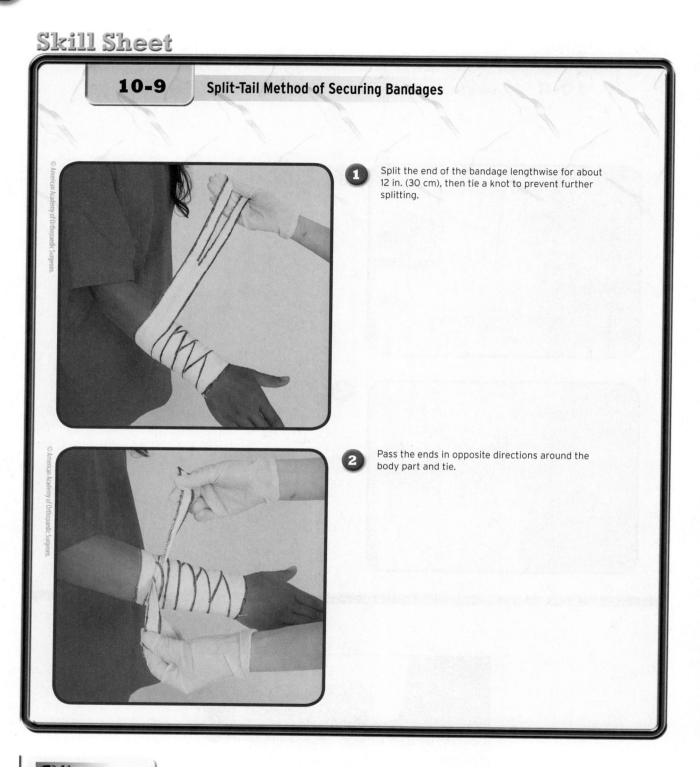

## 10-9    Split-Tail Method of Securing Bandages

**1** Split the end of the bandage lengthwise for about 12 in. (30 cm), then tie a knot to prevent further splitting.

**2** Pass the ends in opposite directions around the body part and tie.

© American Academy of Orthopaedic Surgeons.

© American Academy of Orthopaedic Surgeons.

---

## FYI

### Adhesive Bandage

To make an adhesive bandage snug on a chin, knee, or elbow, first cut the adhesive parts of the bandage lengthwise, but do not cut into the pad. Place the pad horizontally over the cut or wound. Then bring the bottom strips of the adhesive bandage up and smooth them on the skin. Bring the top parts of the adhesive bandage down and smooth them on the skin. Result: An adhesive bandage that contours to the wound.

## ▶ Ready for Review

- A dressing covers an open wound; it touches the wound.
- Dressings used in most first aid situations are commercially prepared, but dressings may need to be improvised.
- A bandage should be clean but need not be sterile.
- The basic types of bandages are roller bandages; self-adhering, conforming bandages; gauze rollers; elastic roller bandages; triangular bandages; adhesive tape; and adhesive bandages.
- With a little ingenuity, you can apply a roller bandage to almost any body part.

## ▶ Vital Vocabulary

<u>adhesive bandage</u> A combination of both a sterile dressing and a bandage.

<u>adhesive tape</u> Tape used to secure bandages and dressings; available in rolls and in a variety of widths.

<u>cravat</u> A folded triangular bandage used to hold splints and dressings in place, to apply pressure evenly over a dressing, or as a swathe (binder) for an injured arm in an arm sling.

<u>elastic roller bandage</u> A type of bandage used for compression on sprains, strains, and contusions; available in various widths.

<u>gauze pad</u> A type of sterile dressing used for small wounds; available in separately wrapped packages of various sizes. Some have a special coating to keep them from sticking to the wound.

<u>gauze roller</u> A type of bandage that is cotton and non-elastic, and used to wrap or bind various body parts; available in various widths.

<u>roller bandage</u> A type of bandage used to wrap or bind various body parts; available in various widths, lengths, and types of material.

<u>self-adhering, conforming bandage</u> A type of bandage that bonds to itself as it is wrapped, helping to secure itself in place; available as rolls of slightly elastic, gauzelike material in various widths.

<u>trauma dressing</u> A type of dressing made of large, thick, absorbent, sterile materials.

<u>triangular bandage</u> A type of bandage available commercially or can be made from a square piece of preshrunk cotton muslin measuring 36 to 40 inches (230 to 260 cm$^2$) along each side of the square.

## ▶ Assessment in Action

You are enjoying a fly-fishing trip along a popular trout fishing river. It is a Saturday and there are several others fishing the same area. You and your friend decide to descend a steep riverbank to access a less crowded spot. Your friend slips down the river bank. You hurry down the bank and find her clutching her arm, which is bleeding. Another bystander arrives with a first aid kit.

*Directions:* Circle Yes if you agree with the statement; circle No if you disagree.

Yes No **1.** You should wash your hands with sanitizer and apply exam gloves from the first aid kit.

Yes No **2.** A dressing goes directly on the wound.

Yes No **3.** You can apply a roller bandage on the arm using spiral turns.

Yes No **4.** You should start bandaging from the upper part of the arm and progress down to the wrist.

Yes No **5.** After applying the bandage, you see that your friend's fingers look blue. This is a sign that the bandage is too tight.

## ▶ Check Your Knowledge

*Directions:* Circle Yes if you agree with the statement; circle No if you disagree.

Yes No **1.** A dressing does not touch an open wound.

Yes No **2.** Adhesive bandages are used for small cuts and abrasions.

**prep kit**

Yes    No    **3.** A bandage should be clean but need not be sterile.

Yes    No    **4.** Roller bandages come in only one size.

Yes    No    **5.** Roller bandages can be used only on the arm.

Yes    No    **6.** A square knot is the preferred knot for bandages.

Yes    No    **7.** Check the person's lips for signs a bandage is too tight.

Yes    No    **8.** If the person can wiggle his or her fingers, the bandage is not on correctly.

Yes    No    **9.** Elastic roller bandages are used for compression on sprains, strains, and contusions.

Yes    No    **10.** The figure-eight method is used to apply a roller bandage to hold dressings or to provide compression at or near a joint.

# Burns

## Burns

Each year, approximately 486,000 people are treated for burns, and over 3,000 people die from exposure to fire or smoke in the United States, according to the American Burn Association. <u>Burns</u> occur in every age group, across all socioeconomic levels, at home and in the workplace, and in urban, suburban, and rural settings. It has been estimated that about 80% of all burn injuries occur in the home, with house fires responsible for the majority of fire deaths. Most people with burns are injured as a result of their own actions.

The highest-risk age groups for burn injuries are children younger than 5 years and adults older than 55 years. Both groups may have limited ability to recognize and escape from a fire or burn incident. In addition, their relatively thinner skin predisposes them to more serious injuries. Death and complications increase dramatically for people older than 55 years owing to the likelihood of preexisting health conditions and their immune systems' decreased ability to fight infection.

Skin death and injury occur as the applied heat exceeds the body's ability to disperse the heat; that point starts at about 113°F (45°C). The amount and depth of skin damage depend on the heat's intensity, the duration of contact, and the skin's thickness.

Burn injuries can be classified as thermal (heat), chemical, or electrical.

- **Thermal (heat) burns**. Not all thermal burns are caused by flames. Contact with hot objects, flammable vapor that ignites and causes a flash or an explosion, and steam and hot liquid are other common causes of burns. Just 3 seconds of exposure to water at 140°F (60°C) can cause a full-thickness (third-degree) burn in an adult. At 156°F (69°C), the same burn occurs in 1 second.
- **Chemical burns**. A wide range of chemical agents can cause tissue damage and death on contact with the skin. As with thermal burns, the amount of tissue damage depends on the duration of contact, the skin thickness in the area of exposure, and the strength of the chemical agent. Chemicals will continue to cause tissue destruction until the chemical agent is removed. Three types of chemicals—acids, alkalis, and organic compounds—are responsible for most chemical burns. Alkalis produce deeper, more extensive burns than do acids.
- **Electrical burns**. The injury severity from contact with electric current depends on the type of current (direct or alternating), the voltage, the area of the body exposed, and the duration of contact. Electricity can induce ventricular fibrillation (a type of cardiac arrest), cause respiratory arrest, or "freeze" the person to the electrical contact point with powerful muscle spasms that increase the length of exposure. People with low-voltage electrical injuries may have no skin burns at all but might still experience cardiac or respiratory arrest.

## ▶ Thermal Burns

Evaluate a thermal burn using the following steps. Each step provides valuable information about the type and severity of injury the person has sustained. Insights gained can determine the immediate action you must take in caring for the person. Taken together, the steps will prepare you to effectively determine the burn's severity, which is the basis for treatment of thermal burns.

1. *Determine the depth (degree) of the burn.* Historically, burns have been described as first-degree, second-degree, and third-degree injuries. The terms *superficial*, *partial thickness*, and *full thickness* are often used by burn-care professionals because they are more descriptive of the tissue damage.
- **First-degree (superficial) burns** affect the skin's outer layer (epidermis) **Figure 11-1**. Signs and symptoms include redness, mild swelling, tenderness, and pain. Healing occurs without scarring, usually within a week. The outer edges of deeper burns often are first-degree burns.
- **Second-degree (partial-thickness) burns** extend through the entire outer layer and into the inner skin layer **Figure 11-2**. Signs and symptoms include blisters, swelling, weeping of fluids, and severe pain. The signs occur because the capillary blood vessels in the dermis are damaged and give up

**Figure 11-1**

First-degree burn.

fluid into surrounding tissues. Intact blisters provide a sterile, waterproof covering. Once a blister breaks, a weeping wound results, and the risk of infection increases.

- **Third-degree (full-thickness) burns** are severe burns that penetrate all the skin layers into the underlying fat and muscle **Figure 11-3** . Signs and symptoms include leathery, waxy, or pearly gray skin that is sometimes charred. The skin has a dry appearance because capillary blood vessels have been destroyed and no more fluid is brought to the area. The skin does not blanch after being pressed because the area is dead. The person feels no pain from a third-degree burn because the nerve endings have been damaged or destroyed. Any pain felt is from surrounding burns of lesser degrees. A third-degree burn

**Figure 11-2**

Second-degree burn blisters.

*© American Academy of Orthopaedic Surgeons*

**Figure 11-3**

Third-degree burn.

*© American Academy of Orthopaedic Surgeons*

requires medical care and the removal of dead tissue and often a skin graft to heal properly.

2. *Determine the extent of the burn.* Skin will not ignite unless heated to thousands of degrees. However, if clothing ignites or skin is kept in contact with a heat source, such as scalding water, large areas of the skin will be injured. Determining the extent of a burn means estimating how much body surface area the burn covers.

   A rough guide known as the rule of nines assigns a percentage value of total body surface area (BSA) to each part of an adult's body **Figure 11-4** . The entire head is 9%, one complete arm is 9%, the front torso is 18%, the complete back is 18%, and each leg is 18%. The rule of nines must be modified for small children to take into account the different proportions of their bodies. In small children and infants, the head accounts for 18%, and each leg is 14%.

   For small or scattered burns, use the rule of the hand **Figure 11-5** . The person's hand, including the fingers and the thumb held together, represents about 1% of his or her BSA. For a very large burn, estimate the unburned area in number of hands and subtract from 100%. Although the exact percentage is nearly impossible to accurately determine at the scene, attempt to get as close as possible.

3. *Determine which parts of the body are burned.* Burns on the face, hands, feet, and genitals are more severe than those on other body parts. A circumferential burn (one that goes around a finger, toe, arm, leg, neck, or chest) is considered more severe than a

## Q&A

**What is the rule of the palm?**

The rule of the palm says that a person's palm surface represents 1% of the BSA, but in actuality, it represents about 0.4%. The entire hand including the closed fingers and thumb represents about 0.8%. This text suggests using the rule of the hand—using the entire hand, including the closed fingers and thumb—as an easy method to estimate the extent of a burned area.

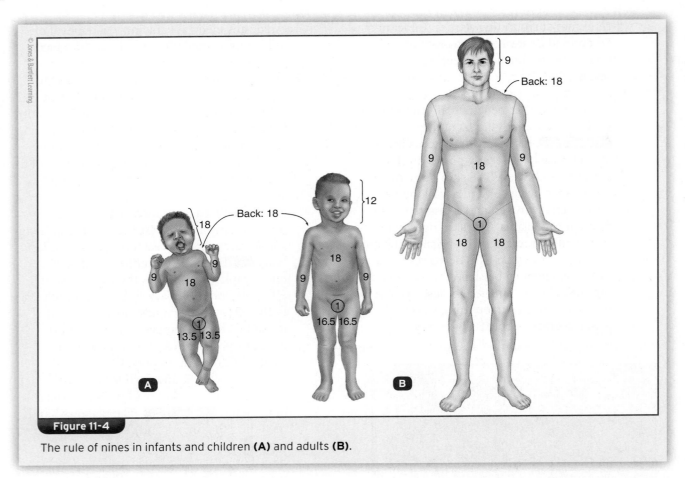

**Figure 11-4**

The rule of nines in infants and children **(A)** and adults **(B)**.

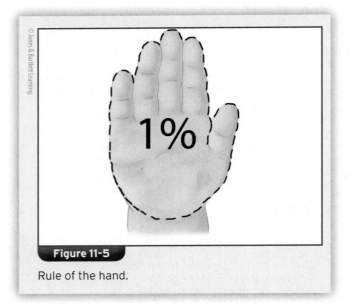

**Figure 11-5**

Rule of the hand.

noncircumferential one because of the possible constriction and tourniquet effect on circulation and, in some cases, breathing. All of these burns require medical care.

4. *Determine respiratory involvement.* Respiratory tract damage caused by heat associated with a burn can cause death after a person is hospitalized. Respiratory damage may result from breathing heat or the products of combustion, from being burned by a flame while in a closed space, or from being in an explosion. In these cases, even with no burn injury to the skin, there may be respiratory damage. Super-heated air is absorbed by the upper respiratory tract (the area from the nose to the trachea), resulting in inflammation. Swelling occurs in 2 to 24 hours, restricting or completely shutting off the airway so that air cannot reach the lungs. All respiratory injuries must receive medical care. The following are signs and symptoms of respiratory injury:

- Burns around the nose or mouth
- Breathing difficulty
- Hoarseness, wheezing, coughing
- Coughing that expels sooty substance
- Soot on face
- Swollen nostrils or throat
- A person who is rescued from a burning building

5. *Determine whether other injuries or preexisting medical conditions exist or whether the person is older than 55 years or younger than 5 years.* Having a medical condition or being in one of the sensitive age groups increases a burn's severity. Burns can aggravate existing medical conditions such as diabetes, heart disease, and lung disease, as well as other medical conditions. Concurrent injuries such as fractures, internal injuries, and open wounds increase the severity of a burn.

6. *Determine the burn's severity.* How you care for the burned person depends on the burn's severity. Most burns are minor, occur at home, and can be managed outside a medical setting. Seek medical care for all moderate and severe burns, as classified by the American Burn Association ( Table 11-1 ), or if any of the following conditions applies:

- The person has difficulty breathing.
- Other injuries exist.
- An electrical injury exists.
- The face, hands, feet, or genitals are burned.
- Child abuse is suspected.
- The surface area of a second-degree burn is greater than 10% of the BSA.
- The burn is third degree.

| What to Look For | What to Do |
|---|---|
| **First-degree (superficial) burn, indicated by:**<br>• Redness<br>• Mild swelling<br>• Tenderness<br>• Pain | 1. Immerse the burned area in cool or cold water, place it under running cold water, or apply a wet, cool or cold compress for at least 10 minutes as soon as possible ( Figure 11-6 ). If cold water is unavailable, use any available cold liquid.<br>2. Give ibuprofen to relieve pain and inflammation.<br>3. Keep a burned arm or leg raised to reduce swelling and pain.<br>4. Have the person drink water.<br>5. After the burn has been cooled, apply an aloe vera gel or an inexpensive skin moisturizer lotion to keep the skin moistened and to reduce itching and peeling. Use a lotion that does not have alcohols or strong fragrances. Lotions with glycerin and mineral oil are best. Aloe vera has antimicrobial and anti-inflammatory properties and is a mild analgesic. |
| **Small (<20% BSA) second-degree (partial-thickness) burn, indicated by:**<br>• Blisters<br>• Swelling<br>• Weeping of fluids<br>• Severe pain | Follow Steps 1 through 3 for first-degree burns, with the following additions:<br>1. After the burn has been cooled, apply a thin layer of an antibacterial ointment.<br>2. Cover the burn with a loose, dry, nonstick, sterile or clean dressing. Covering the burn reduces the amount of pain by keeping air from the exposed nerve endings. The main purpose of a dressing over a burn is to keep the burn clean, prevent evaporative moisture loss, and reduce pain. If fingers or toes have been burned, place dry dressings between them and seek medical care.<br>3. Have the person drink water only if he or she does not need medical care. |
| **Large (>20% BSA) second-degree (partial thickness) burn** | Follow Steps 1 through 3 for first-degree burns, with the following additions:<br>1. Apply cold, but monitor the person for hypothermia (eg, shivering, cold skin on unburned areas).<br>2. Call 9-1-1. |
| **Third-degree (full thickness) burn, indicated by:**<br>• Dry, leathery, gray colored, or charred skin | 1. Cover the burn with a dry, nonstick, sterile or clean dressing.<br>2. Call 9-1-1. |

## Table 11-1 Burn Severity

**Minor Burns**
- First-degree burn covering less than 50% BSA in adults (face, hands, feet, and genitals not burned)*
- Second-degree burn covering less than 10% BSA in adults
- Second-degree burn covering less than 10% BSA in children and older adults

**Moderate Burns**
- First-degree burn covering more than 50% BSA in adults
- Second-degree burn covering 15% to 30% BSA in adults*
- Second-degree burn covering 10% to 20% BSA in children and older adults
- Third-degree burn covering up to 10% BSA in adults (face, hands, and feet not burned)

**Critical Burns**
- Second-degree burn covering more than 30% BSA in adults
- Second-degree burn covering more than 20% BSA in children and older adults
- Third-degree burn covering more than 10% BSA in adults
- Third-degree burn covering more than 2% BSA in children and older adults
- Third-degree burn of hands, face, eyes, feet, or genitalia; also most inhalation injuries, electrical injuries, and burns accompanied by major trauma or significant preexisting conditions

*Criteria for children have not been established. If in doubt, consult a medical professional.

*Source*: Adapted from the American Burn Association.

Cool burn with cold water until pain is relieved.

Cooling usually takes 10–45 minutes.

**Figure 11-6**

Immerse the burn. Cool the burn with cold water until pain is relieved. Cooling usually takes 10 to 45 minutes.

## Later Care for Thermal Burns

For after-thermal burn care, follow a physician's recommendations, if a physician has been consulted (many burns are never seen by a physician). The following suggestions may apply:

- Wash hands thoroughly before changing any dressing.

## CAUTION

**DO NOT** remove clothing stuck to the skin. Cut around the areas where clothing sticks to the skin.

**DO NOT** pull on stuck clothing; pulling will further damage the skin.

## CAUTION

**DO NOT** apply cold over a large burn for a prolonged time because it can produce hypothermia.

**DO NOT** use an ice pack or ice water unless it is the only source of cold available. If you must use it, apply it for only 10 to 15 minutes.

**DO NOT** apply grease, butter, cream, or a home remedy. Such coatings are unsterile and can lead to infection. They also can seal in heat, causing further damage.

**DO NOT** cover a first-degree burn.

- Leave unbroken blisters intact.
- Change dressings once or twice a day unless a physician instructs otherwise.

To change a dressing:

1. Remove the old dressing. If a dressing sticks, soak it off with cool, clean water.
2. Cleanse the area gently with mild soap and water.
3. Pat the area dry with a clean cloth.

4. Apply a thin layer of antibiotic ointment to the burn.
5. Apply a nonstick sterile dressing.

Watch for signs of infection. Call a physician if any of the following appear:

- Increased redness, pain, tenderness, swelling, or red streaks near the burn
- Pus
- Elevated temperature (fever)

Keep the area and dressing as clean and dry as possible. Elevate the burned area, if possible, for the first 24 hours. Give pain medication, if necessary.

## Scald Burns

Scald burns are the result of contact with hot liquids. Scald burns can be divided into two types: immersion burns and spill burns. An immersion burn results when an area of the body is fully immersed in a hot liquid. It generally has definite demarcations between healthy and injured tissue. This type of burn tends to be deep and is often full thickness. This type of injury is generally caused by abuse and is seen most often in children.

A spill burn occurs when a liquid spills, drops, or is thrown on a person. The pattern of this type of burn generally is irregular and may be scattered across large body areas. A spill burn usually is not as deep as an immersion burn.

Neglect and lack of supervision of children in the kitchen and the bathtub are frequent causes of spill burns. Scalds in adults occur more often in the older population, who generally have decreased sensation. As a result, many older people are scalded in the bath.

## Sunburn

Sunburn is the skin's response to the trauma of ultraviolet (UV) radiation. Sunburn may be the most common burn sustained by humans, and probably all people have had one at some time . True sunburn reaction begins 2 to 8 hours after UV radiation exposure. The amount of UV light the skin has received is difficult to gauge accurately. Not until after exposure (4 to 12 hours later) does the redness, tenderness, and discomfort of sunburned skin confirm the overexposure. Painful blistering and swelling peak about 24 hours later.

Sunburn results in first- or second-degree burns. A third-degree burn can occur from a sunburn, but it is rare. The redness of a sunburn is caused by the dilation of the small blood vessels. Blister formation comes from plasma leakage.

Human skin displays marked differences in its response to UV radiation exposure. Some people always burn and never tan, while others rarely experience a painful sunburn. The variability is largely attributed to the degree of pigmentation (melanin) that the skin contains. Darker-hued people generally are more resistant to the sun's rays than are those with light complexions, but all people eventually will burn if exposed to enough UV. Other variables that contribute to individual sensitivity include the area of the body exposed, the underlying condition of the skin, the degree of tanning, and the role of various photosensitizing medicines (such as certain antibiotics).

Various skin types respond differently to UV light:

- Type I skin always burns easily and never tans. A person with type I skin normally has blue eyes, red hair, and freckles.

- Type II skin burns easily and tans slightly. A person with type II skin normally has fair skin and blue eyes.
- Type III skin sometimes burns, but always tans gradually and moderately. An example of people with type III skin is Caucasians.
- Type IV skin minimally burns and always tans well. Examples of people with type IV skin are people of Hispanic or Asian descent.
- Type V skin rarely burns and tans deeply. Examples of people with type V skin are Middle Easterners and Indians (heavily pigmented).
- Type VI skin does not burn (although it can be damaged with significant exposure). An example of people with type VI skin is people of African descent (deeply pigmented).

## Care for Sunburns

1. Cool compresses for up to 45 minutes are quite soothing to sunburned skin. Frequent cool showers or soaking in a tub may provide remarkable relief. Some experts advise against the use of topical analgesics, sprays, or lotions, especially those containing benzocaine. Benzocaine may sensitize the skin, resulting in contact dermatitis that compounds the original condition. Topical anesthetic sprays or lotions may provide temporary relief, but they are expensive and generally ineffective. Over-the-counter (OTC) analgesics such as ibuprofen should suffice in most cases because they reduce pain and inflammation. Drinking a lot of water is also suggested.
2. First- and second-degree sunburns can be quite painful. When a large area of skin is involved, the person may feel ill and have chills and fever. After the pain of a first-degree sunburn has subsided, the use of aloe vera or another body lotion can keep the skin moist. Do not use butter or petroleum jelly.

## Sunburn Aftercare

For aftercare of a second-degree sunburn, apply antibiotic ointment (available as an OTC medication) in a thin layer. It is inexpensive, antimicrobial, widely available, and easily applied, and it adheres even to exposed areas such as the face. If blisters break, gently wash the area twice daily with soap

**Figure 11-7**

Sunburn.

and water and then cover with an antibiotic ointment and sterile gauze to prevent infection. If the burn becomes infected, seek medical care. If the eyes are affected, seek medical care.

Refer to **Flowchart 11-1** for additional information regarding the care of thermal burns.

**Windburn Prevention**

Windburn resembles a first-degree sunburn. A greasy sunscreen can be used to prevent and treat it.

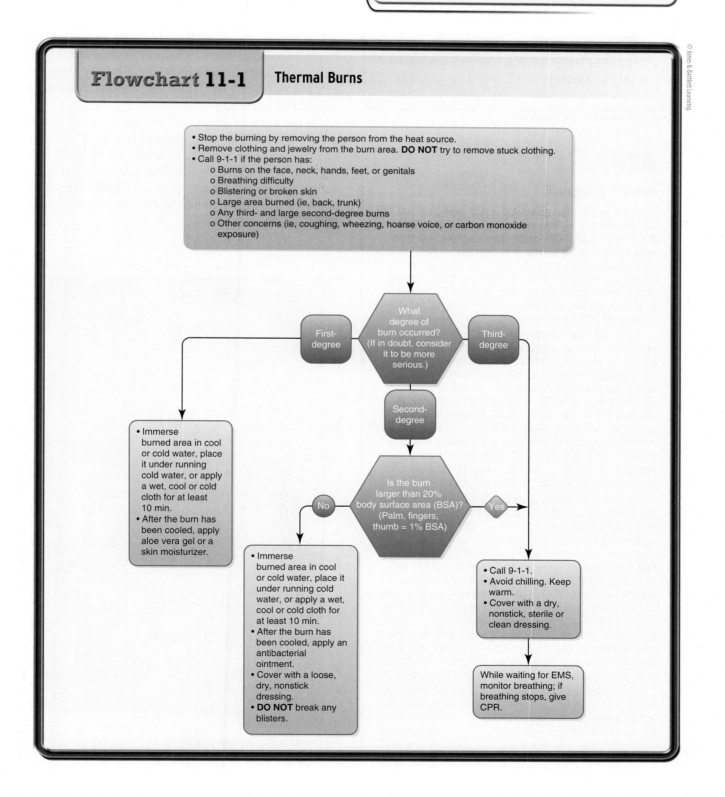

**Flowchart 11-1** | **Thermal Burns**

- Stop the burning by removing the person from the heat source.
- Remove clothing and jewelry from the burn area. **DO NOT** try to remove stuck clothing.
- Call 9-1-1 if the person has:
  - o Burns on the face, neck, hands, feet, or genitals
  - o Breathing difficulty
  - o Blistering or broken skin
  - o Large area burned (ie, back, trunk)
  - o Any third- and large second-degree burns
  - o Other concerns (ie, coughing, wheezing, hoarse voice, or carbon monoxide exposure)

What degree of burn occurred? (If in doubt, consider it to be more serious.)

First-degree

Third-degree

Second-degree

Is the burn larger than 20% body surface area (BSA)? (Palm, fingers, thumb = 1% BSA)

No

Yes

First-degree:
- Immerse burned area in cool or cold water, place it under running cold water, or apply a wet, cool or cold cloth for at least 10 min.
- After the burn has been cooled, apply aloe vera gel or a skin moisturizer.

Second-degree (No):
- Immerse burned area in cool or cold water, place it under running cold water, or apply a wet, cool or cold cloth for at least 10 min.
- After the burn has been cooled, apply an antibacterial ointment.
- Cover with a loose, dry, nonstick dressing.
- **DO NOT** break any blisters.

Third-degree / Yes:
- Call 9-1-1.
- Avoid chilling. Keep warm.
- Cover with a dry, nonstick, sterile or clean dressing.

While waiting for EMS, monitor breathing; if breathing stops, give CPR.

© Jones & Bartlett Learning

## CAUTION

**DO NOT** use topical OTC burn ointments or sprays or anesthetic sprays because:

- Some products may cause allergic reactions.
- Most do not contain enough benzocaine or lidocaine to suppress pain.
- The duration of any possible relief is relatively short (30 to 40 minutes). More than three or four applications per day of products containing local anesthetics is discouraged because toxic effects can occur if the agents are used too frequently.
- They seal in the heat.
- They are expensive.

## FYI

### Sunburn Prevention

The best protection against the damaging effects of UV radiation is to limit exposure to sunlight. That is done most easily with protective clothing, such as hats, long-sleeved shirts, and long pants. Wet, white cotton will transmit UV radiation, so people can be sunburned while wearing such clothing. People should avoid prolonged exposure during times of the day when radiation is most intense (usually between 1000 and 1400 hours) and apply effective sunscreens.

Sunscreens are readily available and offer the best protection against sunburn, skin cancers, and other long-term skin injury. The proper use of sunscreens will protect a person from the harmful effects of the sun. Sunscreens must be applied correctly, which generally means applying the sunscreen at least 20 minutes before sun exposure, so it will bond to your skin, and reapplying it every few hours. Use waterproof sunscreen if you sweat a lot or if you will be in and out of the water. It is important to note that sunscreens do not promote tanning; they do, however, allow the user to tan gradually without serious burning.

To help consumers select an effective sunscreen, the system of rating products by the skin protection factor (SPF) has been developed. The higher the SPF number, the greater the protection against sunburn. However, a sunscreen that has an SPF of 30 is not twice as good as one with an SPF of 15. An SPF of 15 blocks out 95% of the most harmful rays; a sunscreen with an SPF of 30 gives you only another 3% of protection. Because most people usually use only half the amount of sunscreen that is effective, using a sunscreen with an SPF of 15 probably affords protection equivalent to a sunscreen with an SPF of 7.5. If they use a sunscreen with a 30 SPF, they are probably getting the protection of a 15 SPF sunscreen.

Many suntan lotions have no sunscreen effect and serve only to keep the skin moist. Products such as baby oil and cocoa butter offer no protection against serious sunburn and may actually enhance burning.

## ▶ Chemical Burns

A chemical burn is the result of an acid or an alkali substance touching the skin **Figure 11-8**. Because chemicals continue to burn as long as they are in contact with the skin, they should be removed from the person as rapidly as possible.

First aid is the same for all chemical burns. Alkalis such as drain cleaners cause more serious burns than acids such as battery acid because they penetrate deeper and remain active longer. Organic compounds such as petroleum products are also capable of burning.

If the burn occurred at a workplace, send someone to check the **safety data sheet (SDS)** for the hazardous materials used at the worksite. SDSs include first aid procedures. The Occupational Safety and Health Administration (OSHA) requires employers to identify chemical hazards using labels **Figure 11-9**.

© American Academy of Orthopaedic Surgeons.

**Figure 11-8**

Chemical burn from sulfuric acid.

## Q&A

**How can you determine how deep a burn is?**

There are two layers of skin: the epidermis and the dermis. The epidermis, the outer layer of skin, serves primarily as a barrier between the body and the environment. The dermis has blood vessels and contains nerves, sweat glands, sebaceous glands, and hair roots.

The individual layers of skin are not visible to the naked eye, so when determining depth of a burn, it is helpful to remember that the dermis is the layer that will bleed. Full-thickness burns do not bleed because the blood vessels have been destroyed.

| What to Look For | What to Do |
|---|---|
| • Pain<br>• Burning<br>• Breathing difficulty<br>• Eye pain or vision changes | First aid is the same for most chemical burns. Once the area is safe:<br>1. Brush a dry or powder chemical off the skin with a gloved hand or piece of cloth before flushing with water.<br>2. Flush the burn immediately with large amounts of cool running water for at least 20 minutes or until EMS arrives **Figure 11-10**. Clothing can be removed while flushing.<br>3. Call 9-1-1 immediately for all chemical burns.<br>4. For a chemical in an eye: Tip the head so the affected eye is below the nose, and wash the eye with warm water (which is tolerated in the eye better than cold water) from nose out to side of face for at least 20 minutes. |

## CAUTION

**DO NOT** waste time! A chemical burn is an emergency!

**DO NOT** apply water under high pressure; it will drive the chemical deeper into the tissue.

**DO NOT** try to neutralize a chemical even if you know which chemical is involved; heat may be produced, resulting in more damage. Some product labels for neutralizing may be wrong. Save the container or the label for the chemical's name.

**Figure 11-9**

This pictogram is displayed on the packaging of corrosive chemicals.

**Figure 11-10**

Flushing a chemical burn.

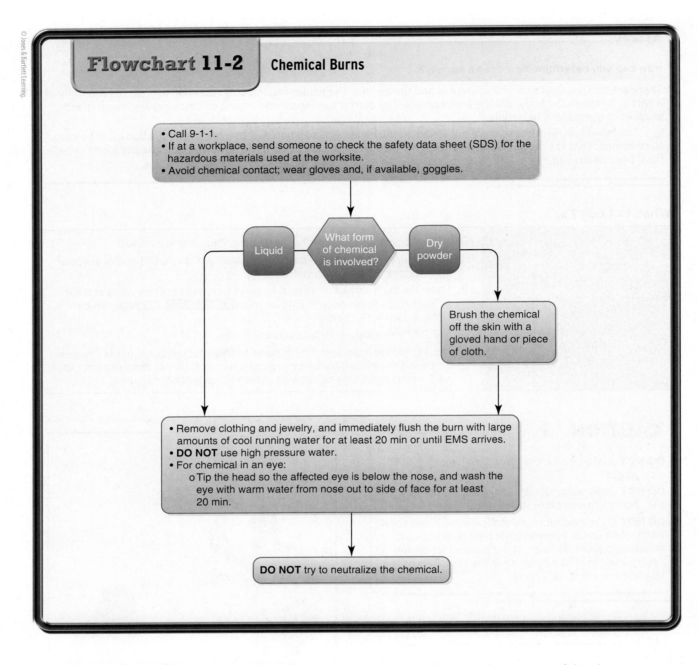

**Flowchart 11-2** | **Chemical Burns**

- Call 9-1-1.
- If at a workplace, send someone to check the safety data sheet (SDS) for the hazardous materials used at the worksite.
- Avoid chemical contact; wear gloves and, if available, goggles.

What form of chemical is involved?

Liquid

Dry powder

Brush the chemical off the skin with a gloved hand or piece of cloth.

- Remove clothing and jewelry, and immediately flush the burn with large amounts of cool running water for at least 20 min or until EMS arrives.
- **DO NOT** use high pressure water.
- For chemical in an eye:
  o Tip the head so the affected eye is below the nose, and wash the eye with warm water from nose out to side of face for at least 20 min.

**DO NOT** try to neutralize the chemical.

Refer to **Flowchart 11-2** for additional information regarding the care of chemical burns.

## ▶ Electrical Burns

Even a mild electrical shock can cause serious internal injuries **Figure 11-11**. There are three types of electrical injuries: thermal burn (flame), arc burn (flash), and true electrical injury (contact). A thermal burn (flame) results when clothing or objects in direct contact with the skin are ignited by an electric current. These injuries are caused by the flames produced by the electric current and not by the passage of the electric current or arc.

An arc burn (flash) occurs when electricity jumps, or arcs, from one spot to another and not from the passage of an electric current through the body. Although the duration of the flash may be brief, it usually causes extensive superficial injuries.

A true electrical injury (contact) happens when an electric current passes directly through the body. This type of injury is characterized by an entrance wound and an exit wound. The important factor with this type of injury is that the surface injury may be just

**Figure 11-11**

Electrical burns. **A.** Exit wound on a foot. **B.** Electrical burn caused by chewing through an electrical cord.

the tip of the iceberg. High-voltage electric currents passing through the body may disrupt the normal heart rhythm and cause cardiac arrest, internal burns, and other injuries.

During an electrical shock, electricity enters the body at the point of contact and travels along the path of least resistance (nerves and blood vessels). Although the entrance burn may appear small, major damage may occur inside the body. Usually, the electricity exits where the body is touching a surface or is in contact with a ground (eg, a metal object). The exit wound can be extensive. Sometimes, a person has more than one exit site.

## Contact With an Outdoor Power Line

If the electrical shock is from contact with a downed power line, the power must be turned off before a first aid provider approaches anyone who may be in contact with the wire. If a power line falls across a vehicle containing a person, tell the person to stay in the vehicle until the power can be shut off. The only exception is if fire threatens the vehicle. In that case, tell the person to jump out of the vehicle without making contact with the vehicle or the wire.

If you feel a tingling sensation in your legs and lower body as you approach a person, stop. The sensation signals that you are on energized ground and that an electric current is entering through one foot, passing through your lower body, and leaving through the other foot. Raise one foot off the ground, turn around, and hop to a safe place.

If you can safely reach the person, do not attempt to move any wires, even with wooden poles, tools with wood handles, or tree branches. Wood can conduct electricity and the first aid provider will be electrocuted. **DO NOT** attempt to move downed wires unless you are trained and equipped with tools able to handle the high voltage. Wait until trained personnel with the proper equipment can cut the wires or disconnect them. Prevent bystanders from entering the danger area.

## Contact Inside Buildings

Most electrical burns that occur indoors are caused by faulty electrical equipment or careless use of electrical appliances. Turn off the electricity at the circuit breaker, fuse box, or outside switch box, or unplug the appliance if the plug is undamaged. Do not touch the appliance or the person until the current is off.

Once there is no danger to first aid providers, first aid can begin. Electric current flows quickly into the body's tissues and then exits. The surface injuries of the skin involve small surface areas (entrance and exit points); the major damage occurs deep under the skin **Figure 11-12** . See Chapter 24, *Wilderness First Aid*, for lightning burns and their care.

Refer to **Flowchart 11-3** for additional information regarding the care of electrical burns.

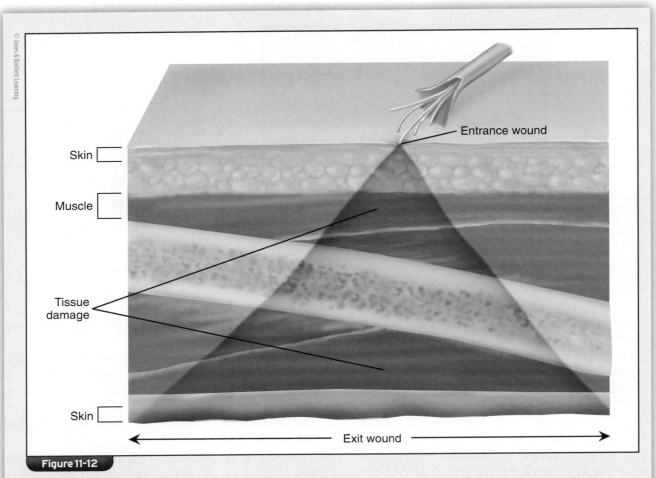

Skin

Muscle

Tissue damage

Skin

Entrance wound

Exit wound

**Figure 11-12**

The external signs of an electrical burn may be deceiving. The entrance wound may be a small burn, while the damage to deeper tissue may be massive.

## What to Look For

- Burn wound, which might appear small
- Entrance and exit wounds (Usually, the electricity exits where the body is touching a surface or is in contact with a ground [ie, a metal object]; this is often the hand or foot.)
- Multiple burns (Most electrical burns are third-degree burns.)
- Absent breathing/pulse (Electricity can cause a person's breathing or heart to stop.)

## What to Do

Once the area is safe:

1. Check breathing and, if absent, begin CPR.
2. Call 9-1-1 immediately. Every person who has been electrocuted needs medical care.
3. If the person fell, check for broken bones and a spinal injury.
4. Most electrical burns are third-degree burns, so cover all burn wounds with sterile dressings.

## Flowchart 11-3    Electrical Burns

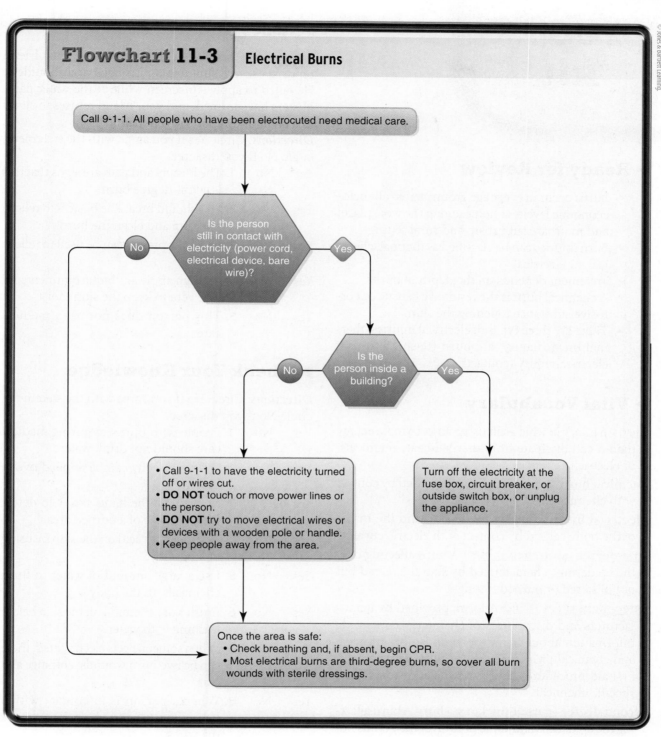

Call 9-1-1. All people who have been electrocuted need medical care.

Is the person still in contact with electricity (power cord, electrical device, bare wire)?

No

Yes

Is the person inside a building?

No

Yes

- Call 9-1-1 to have the electricity turned off or wires cut.
- **DO NOT** touch or move power lines or the person.
- **DO NOT** try to move electrical wires or devices with a wooden pole or handle.
- Keep people away from the area.

Turn off the electricity at the fuse box, circuit breaker, or outside switch box, or unplug the appliance.

Once the area is safe:
- Check breathing and, if absent, begin CPR.
- Most electrical burns are third-degree burns, so cover all burn wounds with sterile dressings.

# prep kit

## ▶ Ready for Review

- Burns occur in every age group; across all socio-economic levels; at home and in the workplace; and in urban, suburban, and rural settings.
- Burn injuries can be classified as thermal, chemical, or electrical.
- Treatment depends on the depth of burns.
- A chemical burn is the result of a caustic or corrosive substance touching the skin.
- There are three types of electrical injuries: thermal burn (flame), arc burn (flash), and true electrical injury (contact).

## ▶ Vital Vocabulary

<u>burn</u> An injury in which soft tissue absorbs more energy than it can dissipate from thermal heat, chemicals, or electricity.

<u>chemical burn</u> An injury to the skin caused by contact with chemicals.

<u>electrical burn</u> An injury to the skin and the inside of the body caused by contact with electric current.

<u>first-degree (superficial) burn</u> A burn affecting only the epidermis; characterized by skin that is red but not blistered or burned through.

<u>safety data sheet (SDS)</u> A form, provided by manufacturers and distributors of chemicals, containing information about chemical composition, physical and chemical properties, health and safety hazards, first aid procedures, and handling and storage of a specific chemical.

<u>second-degree (partial-thickness) burn</u> A burn affecting the epidermis and some portion of the dermis but not the subcutaneous tissue; characterized by blisters and skin that is white to red and moist.

<u>thermal (heat) burn</u> Damage to the skin caused by contact with hot objects, flammable vapor, steam, hot liquid, or flames.

<u>third-degree (full-thickness) burn</u> A burn that affects all skin layers and possibly the subcutaneous layers, muscle, bone, and internal organs, leaving the area dry, leathery, and white, dark brown, or charred.

## ▶ Assessment in Action

After a long, hot day at the water park, your friend reports a severe sunburn on his back and shoulders. He failed to apply sunscreen while at the water park. Blisters have formed, and your friend refuses to sit up in a chair and reports severe pain.

*Directions:* Circle Yes if you agree with the statement; circle No if you disagree.

Yes  No  1. The blisters and pain are signs that this is a first-degree burn.

Yes  No  2. You should break the blisters to relieve pressure and clean the burn.

Yes  No  3. Cool compresses can be used to relieve pain.

Yes  No  4. You can apply antibiotic ointment and aloe vera to keep the skin moist.

Yes  No  5. This person does not need medical care.

## ▶ Check Your Knowledge

*Directions:* Circle Yes if you agree with the statement; circle No if you disagree.

Yes  No  1. People with burns requiring medical care should not drink water.

Yes  No  2. Petroleum jelly can be applied over a burn.

Yes  No  3. The rule of the hand can help determine the size of a burned area.

Yes  No  4. Neutralize an acid on the skin by using baking soda.

Yes  No  5. Use a large amount of water to flush chemicals off the body.

Yes  No  6. Brush a dry chemical off the skin before flushing with water.

Yes  No  7. When someone gets electrocuted, there can be two burn wounds: entrance and exit.

Yes  No  8. When a person is in contact with a power line, use a tree branch to remove the wires.

Yes  No  9. Ibuprofen helps relieve pain and swelling.

Yes  No  10. Cold water can be used, in moderation, on any burn of any size.

# Head and Spinal Injuries

**12**

## Head Injuries

Any head injury is potentially serious. If not properly treated, injuries that seem minor could become life threatening. Head injuries include scalp wounds, skull fractures, and brain injuries. Spinal injuries (that is, neck and back injuries) can also be present in people with a head injury.

## ▶ Scalp Wounds

Scalp wounds bleed profusely because the scalp has many blood vessels. A bleeding scalp wound does not affect the blood supply to the brain. The brain obtains its blood supply from arteries in the neck, not the scalp. A concussion, skull fracture, impaled object, brain injury, or spinal injury may accompany a severe scalp wound.

| What to Look For | What to Do |
|---|---|
| Scalp wound | 1. Control bleeding by pressing on the wound **Figure 12-1**. Replace any skin flap to its original position and apply pressure. Another option is applying an ice pack or instant cold pack to control bleeding.<br>2. If you suspect a skull fracture, **DO NOT** apply excessive pressure; doing so may push bone pieces into the brain. Press on the edges of the wound to help control bleeding **Figure 12-2**.<br>3. Apply a dry, sterile or clean dressing.<br>4. Keep the head and shoulders raised if no spinal injury is suspected.<br>5. If bleeding continues, **DO NOT** remove the first blood-soaked dressing; instead, add another dressing over it.<br>6. Call 9-1-1 if the following occur:<br>  &bull; The wound is extensive.<br>  &bull; There is significant facial damage.<br>  &bull; Signs of concussion occur (eg, nausea and vomiting, headache, drowsiness). |

**Figure 12-2**

Apply pressure around the edges of the wound to control bleeding from a suspected skull fracture.

## ▶ Skull Fracture

A <u>skull fracture</u>; is a break or a crack in the cranium (bony case surrounding the brain). Skull fractures may be open (with an accompanying scalp laceration) or closed (without an accompanying scalp laceration).

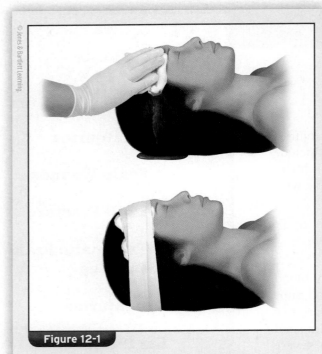

**Figure 12-1**

Apply direct pressure with a dry, sterile dressing to control the bleeding.

## What to Look For

- Pain
- Skull deformity
- Bleeding from an ear or the nose
- Leakage of **cerebrospinal fluid (CSF)** (clear or pink-tinged, watery fluid from an ear or the nose)
- Discoloration around the eyes **Figure 12-3** or behind the ears, known as **Battle sign** **Figure 12-4**, that appears several hours after the injury
- Unequal-sized pupils of the eye
- Heavy scalp bleeding (skull and/or brain tissue may be exposed)
- Penetrating or impaled object

## What to Do

1. Apply a sterile or clean dressing over the wound and hold it in place with gentle pressure. Harder pressure can be applied on the edges of the wound to avoid pressing bone pieces into the brain.
2. Control bleeding by pressing on the edges of the wound and gently on the center of it. A doughnut-shaped pad is useful in applying pressure around the edges of a suspected skull fracture **Figure 12-5**.
3. Call 9-1-1.

**Figure 12-3**

Discoloration around the eyes.

**Figure 12-4**

Battle sign.

**Figure 12-5**

Make a doughnut for skull fracture-related bleeding and to surround an eye for protection when a short object is embedded in an eye. **A.** Using a cravat bandage or strip of cloth, wrap about half the length into a circle large enough to surround the injured area. **B.** Pass the tail thorough the hole repeatedly to form a circle. **C.** The completed dressing should have a hole large enough to surround the injury.

**CAUTION**

**DO NOT** stop the flow of blood or CSF from an ear or nose. Blocking the flow could increase pressure within the skull.

**DO NOT** remove an impaled object from the head. Stabilize it in place with bulky dressings.

**DO NOT** clean an open skull fracture; infection of the brain could result.

**DO NOT** press on the fractured area.

## ▶ Traumatic Brain Injuries

It is not injury to the head, per se, that causes most short- and long-term conditions, but injuries to the brain itself. Most head injuries are a result of motor vehicle crashes, sports injuries, and falls. Many of these injuries are minor—shallow lacerations or localized bruising and swelling. However, according to the Centers for Disease Control and Prevention (CDC), over 50,000 people die each year in the United States from head trauma, and twice that many have brain injuries that leave them with permanent damage.

The brain is a delicate organ. When the head is struck with sufficient force, the brain bounces against the inside of the skull. Brain injuries can be serious and difficult first aid emergencies to handle. The person is often confused or unresponsive, making assessment difficult. Many brain injuries are life threatening. Mishandling a person with a brain injury could result in permanent damage or death.

The brain, like other body tissues, will swell from bleeding when it is injured. Unlike other tissues, however, the brain is confined in the skull, where there is little room for swelling. Any swelling of brain tissue or accumulation of blood inside the skull compresses the brain and increases the pressure inside the skull, which interferes with brain functioning. Furthermore, because the skull is hard, the brain and its surface blood vessels may be damaged if they strike the inside of the skull, which can occur when the head is struck directly or is rapidly accelerated or decelerated (such as in a vehicle crash). The phenomenon of a person "seeing stars" when struck on the back of the head results because the occipital lobe of the brain (the part that controls vision) strikes the back of the skull.

The nerve cells of the brain and the spinal cord, unlike most other cells in the body, are unable to regenerate. When those cells die, they are lost forever and cannot be replaced. Injuries to the brain can be caused by a penetrating foreign object, by bony fragments from a skull fracture, or by the brain striking the inside of the skull after a person's head has hit a stationary object (such as the ground)—a deceleration injury—or has been hit by something like a baseball bat or a teammate's knee—an acceleration injury. Sometimes there will be two points of injury: one at the point of impact and one where the brain rebounds off the skull on the opposite side.

All brain injuries are unique. The brain can sustain several types of injuries depending on the type and amount of force that impacts the head. The type of injury may affect just one functional area of the brain, various areas, or even the entire brain.

The following sections on traumatic brain injury are adapted from the Centers for Disease Control and Prevention.

### Concussion

A **concussion** is considered a mild traumatic brain injury (MTBI) and occurs when a blow to the head alters the function of the brain Table 12-1 .

Recovery from a concussion can last anywhere from several minutes to days, weeks, months, or even longer. Children, adolescents, and older adults tend to take longer to recover than do adults. A person with a concussion who has experienced previous concussions may need increased recovery time as well. Although most people with a concussion make a full recovery, it is possible for people to experience postconcussion syndrome, in which concussion symptoms last longer than 3 months.

**FYI**

**Suspect a Concussion (MTBI)**

- High-speed activities (motor vehicle crashes, bicycle riding, skateboarding)
- Sports and recreation activities
- Falls (including those among older adults), especially from a significant distance (eg, off a ladder, from a tree)
- Suspected child maltreatment (eg, shaking, hitting, throwing)
- Exposure to blasts (including military personnel returning from war zones)
- Injuries to the external parts of the head and/or scalp (eg, lacerations) and orthopedic injuries (eg, fractures, dislocations)

*Source:* Centers for Disease Control and Prevention, US Department of Health and Human Services. Heads Up: Facts for Physicians About Mild Traumatic Brain Injury (MTBI). http://www.brainlinemilitary.org/concussion_course/course_content/pdfs/mtbi.pdf.

## Table 12-1 Symptoms of Concussion or MTBI

| Thinking/ Remembering | Physical | Emotional/ Mood | Sleep Disturbance |
|---|---|---|---|
| • Difficulty thinking clearly<br>• Feeling slowed down<br>• Difficulty concentrating<br>• Difficulty remembering new information | • Headache<br>• Nausea or vomiting (early on)<br>• Balance problems<br>• Dizziness<br>• Fuzzy or blurry vision<br>• Feeling tired, having no energy<br>• Sensitivity to noise or light | • Irritability<br>• Sadness<br>• More emotional<br>• Nervousness or anxiety | • Sleeping more than usual<br>• Sleeping less than usual<br>• Trouble falling asleep |

*Source:* Data from Centers for Disease Control and Prevention, National Center for Injury Prevention and Control.

### Other Traumatic Brain Injuries

Other types of traumatic brain injuries include the following:

- **Contusion**. A direct blow to the head can cause a bruise to the brain.
- **Coup-contrecoup**. In this injury, a blow to the head is strong enough to cause a contusion at the site of impact, as well as move the brain, causing it to hit the opposite side of the skull. This second hit causes a second contusion.
- **Diffuse axonal**. Shaking or strong rotation of the head causes this tearing injury. One example of diffuse axonal injury is shaken baby syndrome.
- *Penetration*. In this injury, an object such as a bullet, knife, or other sharp object enters the

brain. The wound is then contaminated by hair, skin, bone, and pieces of the penetrating object. These contaminants may not be retrievable.

### Q&A

**How does blunt head trauma cause death?**

Blunt trauma can cause bleeding into or around the brain, or can lead to swelling of the brain (called edema). The skull is a rigid capsule that protects the brain. Bleeding in or around the brain causes a rapid rise of pressure within the rigid skull. The only escape route for this excess pressure is through the foramen magnum, an opening at the base of the skull through which the brain stem and spinal cord exit. The pushing of brain material through this opening compresses the brain stem, resulting in the cessation of breathing, followed by death.

| What to Look For | What to Do |
|---|---|
| • The following signs or symptoms may worsen over minutes or hours:<br>  • Behavior or personality changes<br>  • Blank stare/dazed look<br>  • Changes to balance, coordination, and reaction time<br>  • Delayed or slowed spoken or physical responses<br>  • Disorientation, memory loss (confused about date/location) | 1. If unresponsive, check for breathing. If breathing stops, call 9-1-1 and give cardiopulmonary resuscitation (CPR).<br>2. If a neck injury is suspected, or if the person is unresponsive:<br>  • **DO NOT** move the head, neck, or spine.<br>  • Call 9-1-1. |

*(Continues)*

| What to Look For | What to Do |
|---|---|
| <br>• Loss of responsiveness (occurs in fewer than 10% of concussions)<br>• Slurred/unclear speech<br>• Difficulty controlling emotions<br>• Vomiting<br>• Headache<br>• Fuzzy or blurry vision<br>• Nausea<br>• Dizziness<br>• Sensitivity to noise or light<br>• Difficulty remembering new information | 3. If the person is wearing a helmet, such as a motorcycle or football helmet, **DO NOT** remove it unless:<br>  • You suspect an obstructed airway.<br>  • The helmet is so loose that you cannot stabilize the spine.<br>If the helmet must be removed to provide life-saving care of an airway condition, make sure to stabilize the head and neck as the helmet is carefully removed.<br>4. Seek medical care as soon as possible if the person:<br>  • Looks very drowsy or cannot be awakened<br>  • Has one pupil (the black part in the middle of the eye) that is larger than the other<br>  • Has a seizure<br>  • Cannot recognize people or places<br>  • Becomes more and more confused, restless, or agitated<br>  • Exhibits unusual behavior<br>  • Becomes unresponsive<br>  • Has a headache that gets worse and/or does not go away<br>  • Has repeated vomiting or nausea<br>  • Has slurred speech<br>5. Following the injury, the person should:<br>  • Get plenty of sleep at night and rest during the day.<br>  • Avoid visual and sensory stimuli, including video games and loud music.<br>  • Ease into normal activities slowly, not all at once.<br>  • Avoid strenuous physical activities that increase the heart rate or require a lot of concentration.<br>  • Avoid driving, cycling, operating machinery, or playing sports until assessed by a health care provider.<br>  • Avoid anything that could cause another blow to the head or body.<br>  • **DO NOT** use aspirin or anti-inflammatory medications such as ibuprofen or naproxen because of the risk of bleeding. (Acetaminophen can be used for postconcussion headaches.) |

## Further Care of Head Injury

Several signs appearing within 48 hours of a head injury indicate the need to seek medical care. A person who has a concussion and experiences any of the following signs and symptoms may have a blood clot that is pushing the brain against the skull:

• *Headache.* Expect a headache. If it lasts more than 1 or 2 days or increases in severity, seek medical advice.

• *Nausea, vomiting.* If nausea lasts more than 2 hours, seek medical advice. Vomiting once or twice, especially in children, may be expected after a head injury. Vomiting does not indicate the severity of the injury. However, if vomiting begins again hours after the initial episodes have ceased, seek medical care.

• *Drowsiness.* Allow the person to sleep, but wake the person at least every 2 hours to check the state of consciousness and sense of orientation by asking his or her name and testing information-processing skills (eg, "Recite the months of the year backward."). If the person cannot respond or appears confused or disoriented, seek medical advice.

- *Vision impairment.* If the person "sees double," if the eyes do not move together, or if one pupil appears to be larger than the other, seek medical advice.
- *Mobility impairment.* If the person cannot use his or her arms or legs as well as previously or is unsteady when walking, seek medical care.
- *Speech impairment.* If the person has slurred speech or is unable to talk, seek medical care.
- *Seizures (convulsions).* If the person has a violent involuntary contraction (spasm) or series of contractions of the skeletal muscles, seek medical care.

Refer to **Flowchart 12-1** for additional information regarding the care of head injuries.

# Eye Injuries

Significant eye injuries are rare. However, of all the parts of the human body, an injured eye probably causes the most anxiety and concern in a person. The eyes—arguably the most important human sense organs—are easily damaged by trauma. A very slight penetration by a metal fragment, for example, means hospitalization. Medical care may include surgery; despite technical advances, blindness or the loss of an eye remains a possibility whenever there is an eye injury. Have an ophthalmologist or other physician examine the eye as soon as possible, even if an injury seems minor at first.

**FYI**

**Blows to the Eye**

A direct blow or a flying object that lands against the eye or pierces it can potentially cause a severe injury. The chance of partial or complete vision loss is especially high if the injury involves leakage of either of the fluids inside the eyeball. These fluids, vitreous humor and aqueous humor, give the eyeball its shape and grapelike compressibility. When injured, it may be difficult for the first aid provider to determine whether the eye fluid is leaking. Do not touch the area to find out. The fluid could be the result of an allergy or infection.

| What to Look For | What to Do |
|---|---|
| Blow to the eye (ranging in severity from minor to sight threatening), indicated by:<br>• A shiner or black eye, occurring when some of the many delicate blood vessels around the eye rupture **Figure 12-6**<br>• Person reports being hit by a fist, ball, or other blunt object<br>• Broken bone around the eyeball indicated by double vision and the inability to look upward | 1. Apply an ice or cold pack around the eye for 15 minutes. **DO NOT** place the pack on the eye.<br>2. Have the person keep the eyes closed.<br>3. Seek medical care. |
| Loose object in the eye, indicated by:<br>• Severe pain<br>• Tearing (the body's way of trying to remove the object) | Try, in order, each of the following methods:<br>1. Have the person blink the eye several times.<br>2. Pull the upper eyelid out and over the lower lid. This allows the lower lashes to brush the object off the inside of the upper lid. Have the person blink a few times and let the eye move the object out.<br>3. Gently irrigate the eye with clean, warm water. Hold the eyelid open and tell the person to move the eye as it is rinsed.<br>4. Examine the lower lid by pulling it down gently. If you see the object, remove it with a moistened gauze pad **Figure 12-7**.<br>5. Lift the upper eyelid up and over a cotton swab. Many foreign bodies lodge under the upper eyelid; if the object is seen, remove it with the corner of a wet gauze pad.<br>6. If any of the previously discussed methods are successful, medical care is usually not needed unless there is continued pain or itching to the eye. |

*(Continues)*

| What to Look For | What to Do |
|---|---|
| Penetrating eye injury, indicated by lid laceration or cut | 1. **DO NOT** remove the object.<br>2. For a long object, place padding around the object to stabilize against movement, and place a paper cup or similar object over the object for protection **Figure 12-8**.<br>3. For a short object, place a doughnut-shaped pad (formed from a roller gauze bandage or a cravat bandage made from a triangular bandage) around the eye, and wrap a bandage around the head to hold the pad in place.<br>4. Cover both eyes; movement of the uninjured eye will cause movement of the injured eye.<br>5. Keep the person flat on his or her back.<br>6. Call 9-1-1. |
| Cut on the eyeball **Figure 12-9**, indicated by:<br>• Cut appearance of the cornea (clear part of the eye) or sclera (white part of eye)<br>• Inner liquid filling of the eye coming out through the wound<br>• Cut lid | 1. **DO NOT** apply pressure to the eye.<br>2. Cover both eyes with gauze pads, and lightly wrap a bandage around the head to hold the pads in place.<br>3. Call 9-1-1 or drive the person to a medical facility as soon as possible. |
| Chemical, smoke, or other irritant in eye | Chemicals in the eyes can threaten sight, with alkalis causing greater damage than acids. Because damage can occur in 1 to 5 minutes, the chemical must be removed immediately. First aid may determine the fate of the eye and vision.<br>1. Hold the eye wide open; flush with warm water for at least 15 minutes or until emergency medical services (EMS) arrives **Figure 12-10**. If tap water is not available, normal saline or other eye irrigation solution may be used.<br>  • Irrigate from the nose side of the eye toward the outside to avoid flushing the material into the other eye.<br>  • Tell the person to roll the eye as much as possible to help wash out the eye.<br>2. Loosely bandage the eye(s) if necessary.<br>3. For a chemical eye injury, contact the poison control center (1-800-222-1222). If not available, seek medical care as soon as possible or call 9-1-1. |
| Eye avulsion, indicated by:<br>• Eye knocked out from its socket | 1. Cover the eye loosely with a sterile or clean dressing that has been moistened with clean water. Do not try to push the eyeball back into the socket.<br>2. Protect the injured eye with a paper cup, a piece of cardboard folded into a cone, or a doughnut-shaped pad made from a roller gauze bandage or a cravat bandage.<br>3. Cover the undamaged eye with a patch to stop movement of the damaged eye.<br>4. Call 9-1-1. |
| Burns caused by light, indicated by:<br>• Person reports looking at a source of ultraviolet light such as sunlight, arc welding, bright snow, or tanning lamps<br>• Severe pain occurring 1 to 6 hours after exposure | 1. Cover both eyes with moist, cool cloths.<br>2. Give pain medication if needed.<br>3. Seek medical advice. |

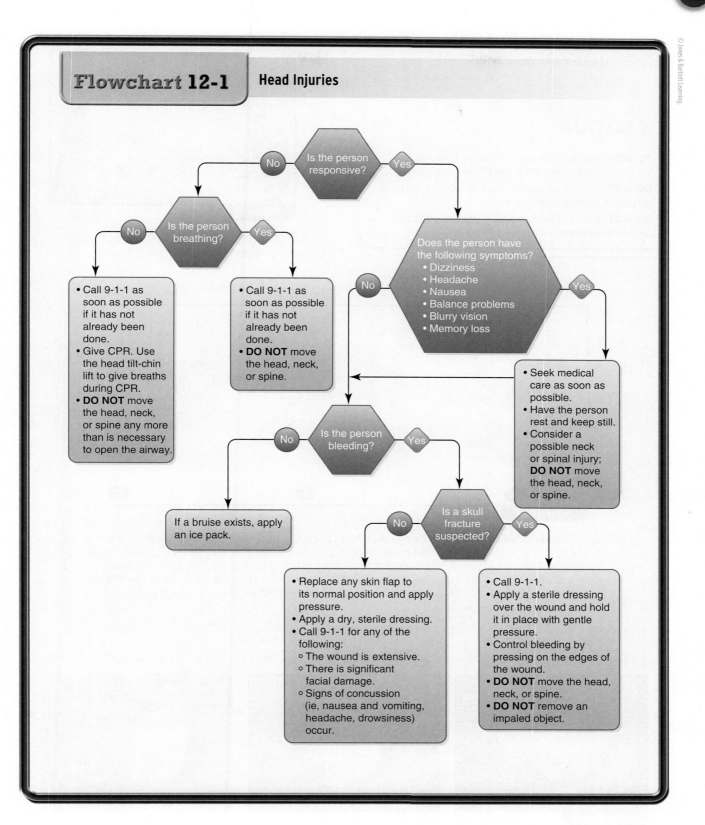

## Flowchart 12-1    Head Injuries

**Is the person responsive?**
- No
- Yes

**Is the person breathing?** (from No)
- No
- Yes

**No (breathing):**
- Call 9-1-1 as soon as possible if it has not already been done.
- Give CPR. Use the head tilt-chin lift to give breaths during CPR.
- **DO NOT** move the head, neck, or spine any more than is necessary to open the airway.

**Yes (breathing):**
- Call 9-1-1 as soon as possible if it has not already been done.
- **DO NOT** move the head, neck, or spine.

**Does the person have the following symptoms?** (from Yes responsive)
- Dizziness
- Headache
- Nausea
- Balance problems
- Blurry vision
- Memory loss

With branches: No / Yes

**Yes (symptoms):**
- Seek medical care as soon as possible.
- Have the person rest and keep still.
- Consider a possible neck or spinal injury; **DO NOT** move the head, neck, or spine.

**Is the person bleeding?** (from No symptoms)
- No
- Yes

**No (bleeding):**
If a bruise exists, apply an ice pack.

**Is a skull fracture suspected?** (from Yes bleeding)
- No
- Yes

**No (skull fracture):**
- Replace any skin flap to its normal position and apply pressure.
- Apply a dry, sterile dressing.
- Call 9-1-1 for any of the following:
  ○ The wound is extensive.
  ○ There is significant facial damage.
  ○ Signs of concussion (ie, nausea and vomiting, headache, drowsiness) occur.

**Yes (skull fracture):**
- Call 9-1-1.
- Apply a sterile dressing over the wound and hold it in place with gentle pressure.
- Control bleeding by pressing on the edges of the wound.
- **DO NOT** move the head, neck, or spine.
- **DO NOT** remove an impaled object.

Refer to Flowchart 12-2 for additional information regarding the care of eye injuries.

**Figure 12-6**

Blow to the eye.

**CAUTION**

**DO NOT** assume that any eye injury is minor. When in doubt, seek medical care immediately.

**DO NOT** remove an object stuck in the eye or try to wash out an object with water.

**DO NOT** exert pressure on an injured eyeball or a penetrating object.

**Figure 12-7**

Removing loose objects from the eye. **A.** If tears or gentle flushing do not remove the object, gently pull down the lower lid. Remove an object by gently flushing with lukewarm water or by using wet, sterile gauze. **B.** If unsuccessful, tell the person to look down. Pull gently downward on the upper eyelashes. Lay a swab or matchstick across the top of the lid. **C.** Next, fold the lid over the swab or matchstick. Remove an object by gently flushing with lukewarm water or by using wet, sterile gauze.

**Figure 12-8**

Stabilize a long penetrating object against movement. **A.** Place padding around the object. **B.** Place a shield (ie, paper cup or similar object) over, but not touching, the penetrating object to protect the object from being hit. **C.** Cover both eyes to prevent the uninjured eye from moving with the injured eye.

**Figure 12-9**

Lacerated eyelid.

**Figure 12-10**

Flushing the eye to treat a chemical burn.

## Q&A

**What causes a black eye?**

A black eye is a bruise (contusion) caused by the leakage of blood from the small capillary blood vessels that have been injured. The extent of a blue-black discoloration depends on how much blood seeps from the damaged vessels, and it varies in different areas of the body. The tissues around the eyes have a lot of blood vessels. As a result, they bruise easily. The discoloration appearing in this area is more pronounced and prolonged than a contusion of the leg or arm.

## CAUTION

**DO NOT** try to neutralize a chemical in the eye. Water usually is readily available for eye irrigation.

**DO NOT** use an eye cup for a chemical burn.

**DO NOT** bandage an eye tightly.

**DO NOT** try to remove an object stuck in the eye.

**DO NOT** allow the person to rub an injured eye.

**DO NOT** try to remove an embedded foreign object in the eye.

**DO NOT** use dry cotton (cotton balls or cotton-tipped swabs) or instruments such as tweezers to remove an object from the surface of an eye.

## FYI

**Sympathetic Eye Movement**

Eyes move in the same direction together, focusing on the same object. This is known as sympathetic eye movement. Therefore, when the uninjured eye moves, the injured eye moves as well. This movement may aggravate an injury.

To lessen movement in an injured eye:

- Tell the person to keep the uninjured eye closed.
- Cover the undamaged eye with a cravat or roller bandage.

The person may become anxious if both eyes are covered and he or she cannot see. Help overcome anxiety by:

- Explaining everything that you are doing.
- Leaving a small peephole at the bottom of the bandage for the uninjured eye to see through. This keeps the person's eyes still by allowing the eyes to look in only one direction.

## FYI

**An Unresponsive Person's Eyes**

An unconscious person may lose the reflexes that protect the eye, such as blinking. If the eyes do not stay closed, keep them closed by covering them with moist dressings.

## FYI

**Contact Lenses**

Determine whether a person is wearing contact lenses by asking, by checking a driver's license, or by looking for them on the eyeball, using a light shining on the eye from the side. In cases of chemicals in the eye, lenses should be removed immediately. Usually the person can remove the lenses.

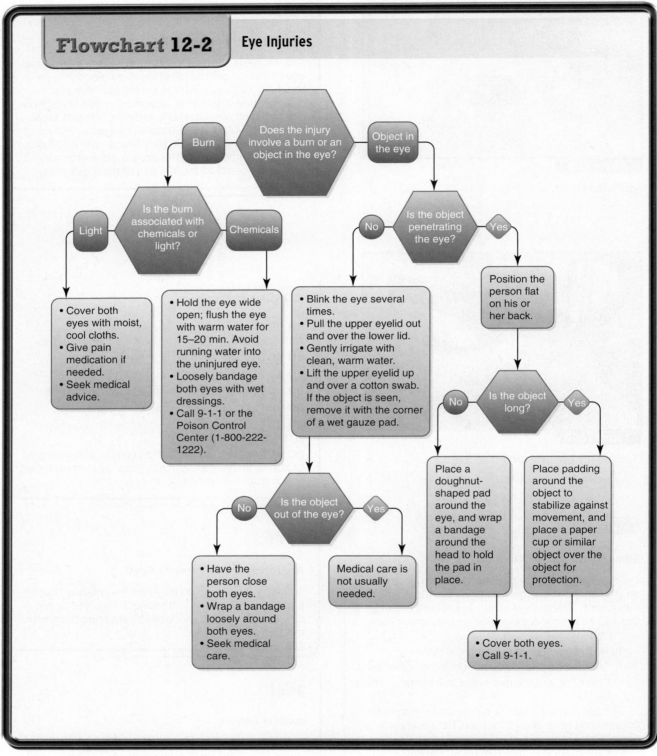

## Flowchart 12-2 — Eye Injuries

Does the injury involve a burn or an object in the eye?

**Burn** → Is the burn associated with chemicals or light?

- **Light:**
  - Cover both eyes with moist, cool cloths.
  - Give pain medication if needed.
  - Seek medical advice.

- **Chemicals:**
  - Hold the eye wide open; flush the eye with warm water for 15–20 min. Avoid running water into the uninjured eye.
  - Loosely bandage both eyes with wet dressings.
  - Call 9-1-1 or the Poison Control Center (1-800-222-1222).

**Object in the eye** → Is the object penetrating the eye?

- **No:**
  - Blink the eye several times.
  - Pull the upper eyelid out and over the lower lid.
  - Gently irrigate with clean, warm water.
  - Lift the upper eyelid up and over a cotton swab. If the object is seen, remove it with the corner of a wet gauze pad.

  Is the object out of the eye?
  - **No:**
    - Have the person close both eyes.
    - Wrap a bandage loosely around both eyes.
    - Seek medical care.
  - **Yes:** Medical care is not usually needed.

- **Yes:** Position the person flat on his or her back.

  Is the object long?
  - **No:** Place a doughnut-shaped pad around the eye, and wrap a bandage around the head to hold the pad in place.
  - **Yes:** Place padding around the object to stabilize against movement, and place a paper cup or similar object over the object for protection.

  - Cover both eyes.
  - Call 9-1-1.

# Ear Injuries

Most ear conditions are not life threatening. Fast action may be needed, however, to relieve pain and to prevent or reverse hearing loss. Head trauma may involve the ear. Foreign bodies in the ear canal usually produce overzealous removal attempts. Except for disk batteries (which damage moist tissue by creating a current) and live insects, few foreign bodies must be extracted immediately. Seek medical care for the person; attempts to remove a foreign body from the ear can rupture the eardrum or lacerate the ear canal.

Children insert all sorts of things into their ears that may be impossible for you to remove safely. If the object is visible near the ear canal opening and you feel it is safe, cautiously try to remove the object with tweezers. Small objects can sometimes be removed by irrigating the ear with warm water. Do not try irrigation if the object blocks the entire ear canal or if the object is vegetable matter such as a kernel of corn or a bean, which will swell when wet.

| What to Look For | What to Do |
| --- | --- |
| Objects stuck in an ear | 1. **DO NOT** use tweezers or try to pry an object out unless the object can be seen near the ear canal opening. <br> 2. Seek medical care to remove the object. Except for disk batteries and live insects, few foreign bodies must be removed immediately. <br> 3. For a live insect in the ear canal, shine a small light into the ear. The insect may crawl out toward the light; if it does not, pour warm water into the ear and then drain it. This may drown the insect; regardless of whether it is dead or alive, it should wash out. When draining the water, turn the head to the side. If the insect cannot be removed, seek medical care. |
| Fluids coming from the ear (blood or clear fluid draining from the ear may indicate a skull fracture) | 1. **DO NOT** attempt to stop bleeding or clear fluid (CSF) with or without blood coming from an ear. Doing so could increase pressure on the brain, causing permanent damage. <br> 2. Place a sterile gauze dressing over the ear and loosely bandage it in place to prevent bacteria getting into the brain. <br> 3. Stabilize the head and neck against movement. Have the person remain as still as possible. <br> 4. Call 9-1-1. |

# Nose Injuries

A severe nose injury frightens the injured person and often challenges the first aid provider's skill. Most nosebleeds are self-limiting and do not require medical attention. In cases of accompanying head or neck injuries, stabilize the head and neck for protection. In some cases, loss of blood could cause shock.

| What to Look For | What to Do |
| --- | --- |
| Broken nose, indicated by: <br> • Pain, swelling, and a possible crooked appearance <br> • Bleeding and difficulty breathing through the nostrils <br> • Black eyes appearing 1 to 2 days after the injury | 1. If bleeding, provide care as you would for a nosebleed. <br> 2. Apply an ice or cold pack for 15 minutes. <br> 3. Medical care can be delayed. <br> 4. **DO NOT** try to straighten a crooked nose. |

*(Continues)*

**What to Look For**

**What to Do**

| | |
|---|---|
| Nosebleed<br><br>• The <u>anterior nosebleed</u> (front of nose) is the most common type (90%). Blood flows from the nose through one nostril.<br><br>• The <u>posterior nosebleed</u> (back of nose) may involve massive bleeding, usually backward into the mouth or down the back of the throat. A posterior nosebleed is serious and requires medical care. | 1. If the nose was hit, suspect a broken nose.<br>2. Have the person sit leaning slightly forward. **DO NOT** tilt the head back or lie the person down.<br>3. Pinch the nostrils shut constantly for 10 minutes **Figure 12-11**. Tell the person to breathe through the mouth and not swallow any blood.<br>4. If bleeding has not stopped, have the person gently blow his or her nose to get rid of ineffective blood clots. Pinch the nostrils shut again for 10 minutes.<br>5. If bleeding continues, try other methods in addition to nose pinching, such as applying an ice pack or spraying nasal decongestant spray into the nostrils.<br>6. Medical care is not usually needed. If bleeding reoccurs or if the nose is broken, seek medical care.<br>7. After a nosebleed has stopped, suggest that the person:<br><br>  • Sneeze through an open mouth, if he or she needs to sneeze.<br>  • Avoid bending over and participating in too much physical exertion.<br>  • Elevate the head with two pillows when lying down.<br>  • Keep the nostrils moist by applying a little petroleum jelly just inside the nostril for 1 week; increase the humidity in the bedroom during the winter months by using a cold-mist humidifier.<br>  • Avoid picking or rubbing the nose. |
| Foreign object in the nose (a medical condition mainly occurring to small children, who often put peanuts, beans, raisins, and other similar objects into their nostrils) | Try one or more of the following methods to remove the object:<br>1. Have the person gently blow his or her nose while compressing the opposite nostril.<br>2. If an object is visible, pull it out with tweezers. **DO NOT** push the object deeper.<br>3. Seek medical care if the object cannot be removed. |

Refer to **Flowchart 12-3** for additional information regarding the care of nosebleeds.

**CAUTION**

**DO NOT** allow the person to tilt the head backward.
**DO NOT** probe the nose with a cotton-tipped swab.
**DO NOT** move the person's head and neck if a spinal injury is suspected.

*© American Academy of Orthopaedic Surgeons.*

**Figure 12-11**

Control bleeding from the nose by pinching the nostrils together.

# Tooth Injuries

Because dental emergencies generally cause considerable pain and anxiety, managing them promptly can provide great relief to the person.

## Flowchart 12-3    Nosebleeds

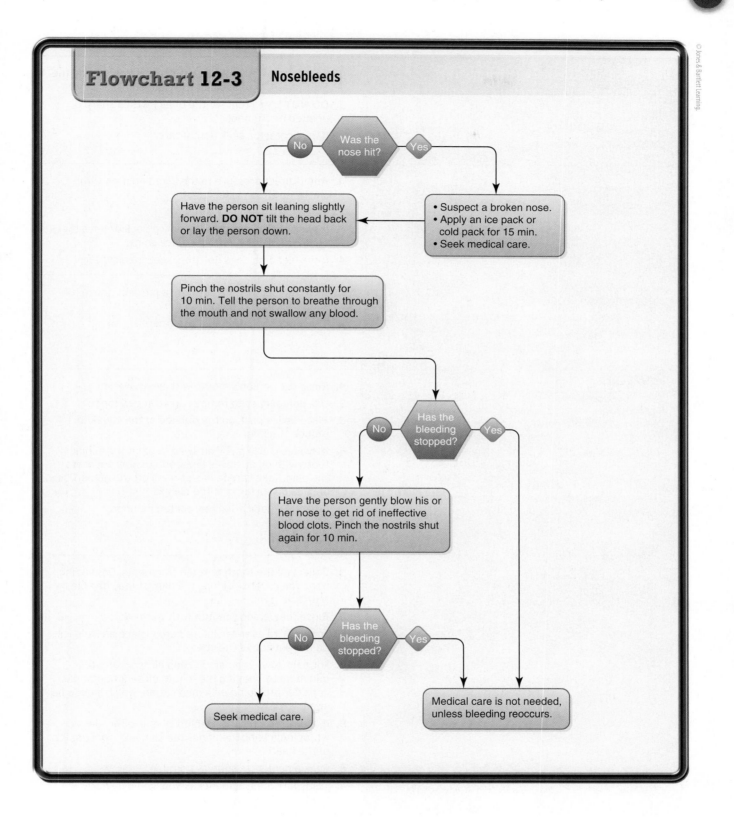

| What to Look For | What to Do |
|---|---|
| Object caught between teeth, indicated by:<br>• Person reports that something is caught between his or her teeth<br>• An object that may or may not be seen (Even with the use of a flashlight, it is still difficult to see a small object.) | 1. Try to remove the object with dental floss. Guide the floss carefully to avoid cutting the gums.<br>2. **DO NOT** try to remove the object with a sharp or pointed instrument.<br>3. If unsuccessful, seek dental care. |
| Bitten lip or tongue, indicated by:<br>• Immediate pain<br>• Bleeding<br>• Swelling | 1. Apply direct pressure to the bleeding area with sterile gauze or a clean cloth.<br>2. Clean the area with a cloth.<br>3. If swelling is present, apply an ice pack or have the person suck on a Popsicle or ice chips.<br>4. If the bleeding does not stop, seek medical care. |
| Loosened tooth<br>• Apply pressure on either side of each tooth with the fingers to determine looseness.<br>• Any tooth movement, even if it is barely felt, indicates a possibly loose tooth. | 1. Have the person bite down on a piece of gauze to keep the tooth in place.<br>2. Consult a dentist or an oral surgeon. |
| Toothache, indicated by:<br>• Person reports pain limited to one area of the mouth (although it can be more widespread); pain can also affect the ear, eye, neck, or even the opposite side of the jaw<br>• Person reports a tooth that is sensitive to heat and cold<br>• Dental decay (identified by tapping the area with a spoon handle or similar object; a diseased tooth will hurt.) | 1. Rinse the person's mouth with warm water.<br>2. Use dental floss to remove any trapped food.<br>3. Place an ice pack on the outside of the cheek to reduce swelling.<br>4. If available, use a cotton swab to paint the aching tooth with oil of cloves (eugenol) to help suppress the pain. Take care to keep the oil off the gums, lips, and inside surfaces of the cheeks.<br>5. Give pain medication (eg, acetaminophen, ibuprofen).<br>6. Seek a dentist. |
| Broken tooth  **Figure 12-12** | 1. Collect all the tooth or teeth fragments. Depending upon the severity of injury, a dentist may be able to reattach them.<br>2. Rinse the person's mouth with warm water.<br>3. For swelling over the injured area, place an ice pack on the outside of the cheek.<br>4. For pain, have the person keep air exposure to a minimum by keeping the mouth closed. Additionally, consider providing pain medication, which should be swallowed.<br>5. If a jaw fracture is suspected, stabilize the jaw by wrapping a bandage under the chin and over the top of the head.<br>6. Seek a dentist as soon as possible.<br>7. Transport the fragments as you would a knocked-out tooth. |

## What to Look For

## What to Do

| What to Look For | What to Do |
|---|---|
| Knocked-out (avulsed) tooth **Figure 12-13** | 1. Attempt to reimplant the tooth (only if it is a permanent [adult] tooth): <br>  • Hold the tooth by the crown (tooth part normally seen when looking into a mouth). <br>  • If the tooth is dirty, rinse it in a bowl of warm water. <br>  • Gently push the tooth down into the socket so the top is even with adjacent teeth. The person can bite down gently on gauze or a handkerchief placed between the teeth. <br> 2. If unable to reimplant the tooth, keep the knocked-out tooth viable by storing it in a solution (listed in order of preference): <br>  • Hank's Balanced Salt Solution <br>  • Egg white <br>  • Coconut water <br>  • Whole milk <br>  • If none of these is available, have the person spit saliva into a small container into which the tooth can be placed. <br> 3. Seek a dentist as soon as possible. |
| Infected or abscessed tooth, indicated by: <br> • Swelling of the gums around the affected tooth <br> • Foul breath <br> • Pain that is increased by tapping the tooth with something metal (eg, spoon handle) | 1. Have the person rinse his or her mouth several times a day with warm water. <br> 2. Give pain medication. **DO NOT** have the person suck an aspirin, and **DO NOT** place an aspirin on the tooth or gum tissue. <br> 3. An ice pack on the cheek may help. <br> 4. Use dental floss to remove any trapped food. <br> 5. Seek a dentist. |
| Cavity—caused by decay or lost filling—indicated by: <br> • Sensitivity to heat, cold, or sweets <br> • Sensitivity to touch (Tap the tooth gently with something metal [eg, spoon handle] on the top and side. This increases the pain in the affected tooth.) | 1. Have the person rinse his or her mouth with warm water. <br> 2. Apply oil of cloves (eugenol) with a cotton swab to the cavity to deaden the pain. **DO NOT** apply any on the gums or lips, or inside the cheeks. <br> 3. If available, apply a temporary filling with cavity dental filling paste. Other options include sugarless chewing gum, candle wax, or ski wax. <br> 4. Seek a dentist. |
| Bleeding from mouth | 1. Allow blood to drain out of the mouth. <br> 2. For a bleeding tongue, put a dressing on the wound and apply pressure. <br> 3. For a cut through a lip, place a rolled dressing between the lip and gum and press another dressing against the outer lip. <br> 4. Seek medical care. |

**Figure 12-12**

Broken teeth.

**Figure 12-13**

Knocked-out tooth.

## CAUTION

**DO NOT** touch the root of a knocked-out tooth.

**DO NOT** handle a knocked-out tooth roughly.

**DO NOT** put a knocked-out tooth in water, mouthwash, alcohol, or povidone iodine (Betadine).

**DO NOT** put a knocked-out tooth in skim milk, reconstituted powdered milk, or milk by-products such as yogurt.

**DO NOT** rinse a knocked-out tooth unless you are reinserting it in the socket.

**DO NOT** place a knocked-out tooth in anything that can dry or crush the outside of the tooth.

**DO NOT** scrub a knocked-out tooth or remove any attached tissue fragments.

**DO NOT** remove a partially extracted tooth. Push it back into place and seek a dentist so the loose tooth can be stabilized.

**Dental First Aid**

If you are in a remote area with no dentist nearby, you can make a temporary cap from melted candle wax or paraffin and a few strands of cotton. When the wax begins to harden but can still be molded, press a wad of it onto the tooth. Other improvisations include using ski wax or chewing gum (preferably sugarless).

## CAUTION

**DO NOT** place pain medication (such as aspirin, acetaminophen, or ibuprofen) on the aching tooth or gum tissues or allow them to dissolve in the mouth. A serious acid burn can result.

**DO NOT** cover a cavity with cotton if there is any pus discharge or facial swelling. See a dentist immediately.

Refer to **Flowchart 12-4** for additional information regarding the care of tooth injuries.

# Spinal Injuries

The *spine* is a column of **vertebrae** stacked on one another from the tailbone to the base of the skull. Each vertebra has a hollow center through which the spinal cord passes. The spinal cord consists of long tracts of nerves that join the brain with all other body organs and parts.

If a broken vertebra pinches spinal nerves, paralysis can result. All unresponsive people with an injury should be treated as though they have a spinal injury. Suspect a possible spinal injury any time one of the following are encountered **Figure 12-14**:

- Motor vehicle crashes (includes motorcycles, snowmobiles, and all-terrain vehicles)
- Pedestrian-motor vehicle crashes
- Falls from heights
- Penetrating injury to the head, neck, back, or torso
- Violent assaults and direct blows
- Diving incidents
- Sports injuries

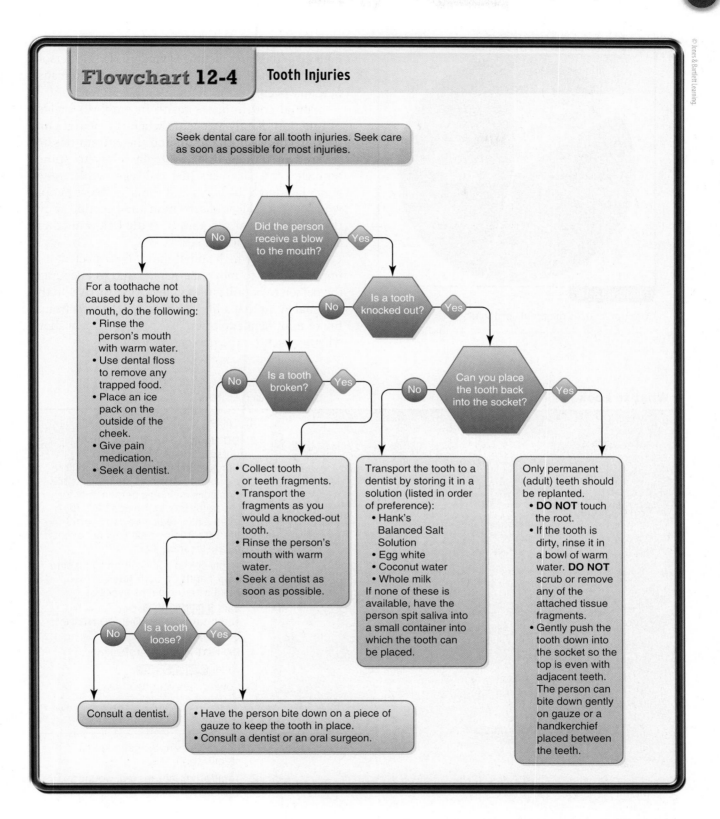

**Flowchart 12-4**   **Tooth Injuries**

Seek dental care for all tooth injuries. Seek care as soon as possible for most injuries.

**Did the person receive a blow to the mouth?**

**No** → For a toothache not caused by a blow to the mouth, do the following:
- Rinse the person's mouth with warm water.
- Use dental floss to remove any trapped food.
- Place an ice pack on the outside of the cheek.
- Give pain medication.
- Seek a dentist.

**Yes** → **Is a tooth knocked out?**

**No** → **Is a tooth broken?**

**No** → **Is a tooth loose?**

**No** → Consult a dentist.

**Yes** →
- Have the person bite down on a piece of gauze to keep the tooth in place.
- Consult a dentist or an oral surgeon.

**Is a tooth broken? — Yes** →
- Collect tooth or teeth fragments.
- Transport the fragments as you would a knocked-out tooth.
- Rinse the person's mouth with warm water.
- Seek a dentist as soon as possible.

**Is a tooth knocked out? — Yes** → **Can you place the tooth back into the socket?**

**No** → Transport the tooth to a dentist by storing it in a solution (listed in order of preference):
- Hank's Balanced Salt Solution
- Egg white
- Coconut water
- Whole milk

If none of these is available, have the person spit saliva into a small container into which the tooth can be placed.

**Yes** → Only permanent (adult) teeth should be replanted.
- **DO NOT** touch the root.
- If the tooth is dirty, rinse it in a bowl of warm water. **DO NOT** scrub or remove any of the attached tissue fragments.
- Gently push the tooth down into the socket so the top is even with adjacent teeth. The person can bite down gently on gauze or a handkerchief placed between the teeth.

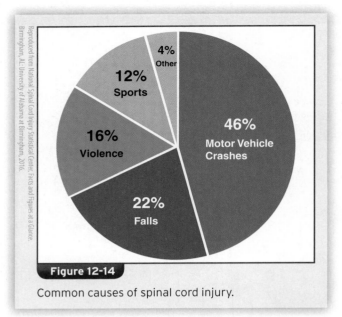

**4%** Other

**12%** Sports

**16%** Violence

**46%** Motor Vehicle Crashes

**22%** Falls

**Figure 12-14**

Common causes of spinal cord injury.

A mistake in the handling of a person with a spinal injury could mean a lifetime of paralysis for the person. Suspect a spinal injury whenever a significant cause of injury occurs.

Spinal cord injuries result in paralysis or loss of function. Paralysis occurs when the neural connections between the brain and the extremities are severed or damaged. <u>Paraplegia</u> refers to spinal damage that paralyzes just the legs, while <u>quadriplegia</u> affects the arms and the legs. Most people who suffer total loss of sensation and function above the third cervical vertebra (C3) die before medical care can be provided.

In cases in which spinal injury is suspected, it is important not to move the person and to encourage the person to be still and wait for EMS to arrive. In the unusual event that a life is threatened, such as from a fire or imminent explosion, use good judgment about whether to move the person.

## What to Look For

| What to Look For | What to Do |
|---|---|
| A reliable (alert, calm, cooperative, lacking distracting injuries, not intoxicated by drugs or alcohol) person with signs of spinal injury **Skill Sheet 12-1**, indicated by:<br>• Reports of back pain and leg numbness and tingling<br>• Tenderness/pain when you run fingers all the way down spine (if possible). (Press each bump of vertebrae and press on depressions produced on each side when you touch or push on the spine bones.)<br>• Failure of the following tests for sensation and movement (test all four extremities):<br>  • Upper body:<br>    – Pinch several fingers while the person has his or her eyes closed, and ask, "Can you feel this?" and "Which finger am I touching?"<br>    – Ask, "Can you wiggle your fingers?"<br>    – Have the person squeeze your hand.<br>  • Lower body:<br>    – Pinch toes while the person has his or her eyes closed, and ask, "Can you feel this?" and "Which toes am I touching?"<br>    – Ask, "Can you wiggle your toes?"<br>    – Have the person push and pull a foot against your hand. | 1. Call 9-1-1.<br>2. **DO NOT** attempt to move the person. Leave the person in the position in which found. Tell the person to remain as still as possible. Consider moving a person only for the following: to provide CPR, to open a blocked airway, to control life-threatening bleeding, or to reach a safe location.<br>3. Apply spinal stabilization by placing your hands on both sides of the head with the palms over the ears **Figure 12-15**. Once spinal stabilization is applied, **DO NOT** let go until EMS arrives.<br>4. **DO NOT** apply a cervical (neck) collar **Figure 12-16**.<br>5. Cover to prevent heat loss. |
| A reliable person without signs of a spinal injury, indicated by:<br>• Alert, not intoxicated, and no distracting injuries<br>• No report of neck pain or neurologic symptoms (eg, tingling, numbness)<br>• No neck tenderness when felt, no loss of sensation when fingers and toes are pinched, and able to move the fingers and toes | 1. Person does not require spinal stabilization.<br>2. Treat other injuries (eg, wounds, bruises, fractures). |
| An unreliable person (altered mental status, intoxicated by drugs or alcohol, combative, confused, painful distracting injury) with signs of a spinal injury (see examples previously discussed) | 1. Assume a spinal injury exists.<br>2. Use the methods previously discussed to stabilize the person. |

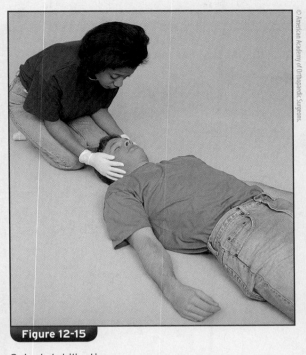

Figure 12-15

Spinal stabilization.

Refer to Flowchart 12-5 for additional information regarding the care of spinal injuries.

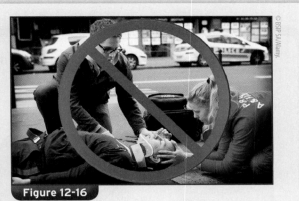

Figure 12-16

Do not place a cervical (neck) collar on a person with a suspected spinal injury.

## CAUTION

**DO NOT** move the person with a suspected spinal injury, even if the person is in water, unless the person's location puts him or her in additional danger. (For a water-related rescue, manually stabilize the person while keeping the injured person floating on the water's surface. Only perform a water rescue if you are properly trained.) Wait for EMS personnel to arrive; they have the proper training and equipment to safely move the injured person.

# Skill Sheet

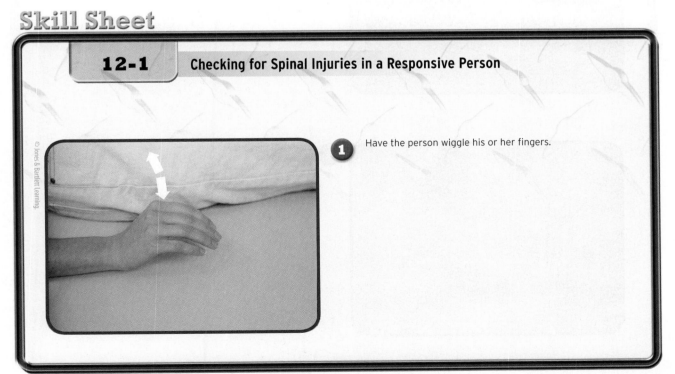

### 12-1   Checking for Spinal Injuries in a Responsive Person

1. Have the person wiggle his or her fingers.

*(Continues)*

## Skill Sheet Continued

| 12-1 | Checking for Spinal Injuries in a Responsive Person |

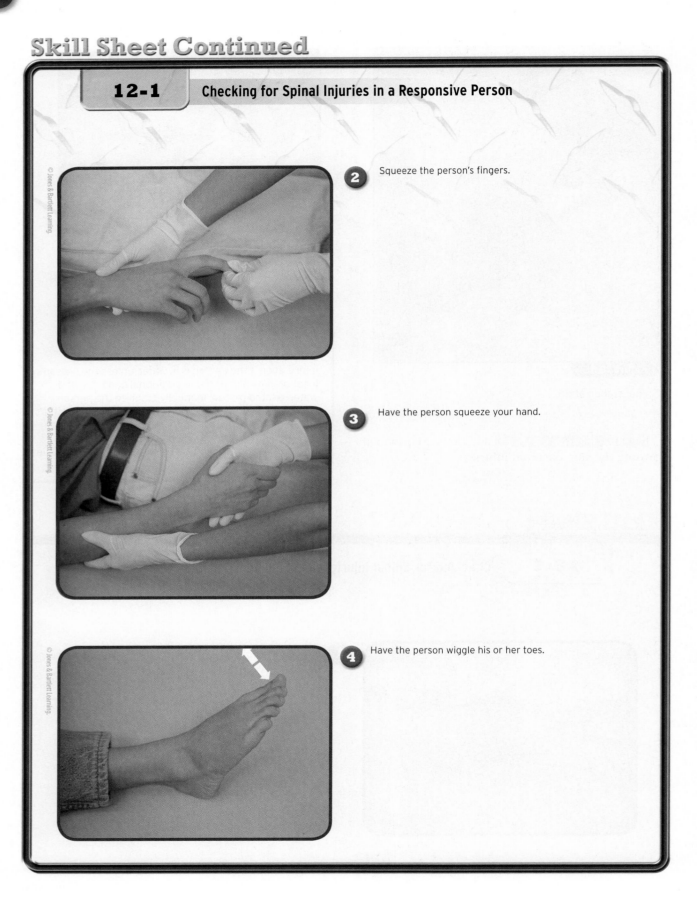

© Jones & Bartlett Learning

2 Squeeze the person's fingers.

© Jones & Bartlett Learning

3 Have the person squeeze your hand.

© Jones & Bartlett Learning

4 Have the person wiggle his or her toes.

# Skill Sheet Continued

**12-1**     **Checking for Spinal Injuries in a Responsive Person**

**5** Squeeze the person's toes.

**6** Have the person push his or her foot against your hand.

© Jones & Bartlett Learning.

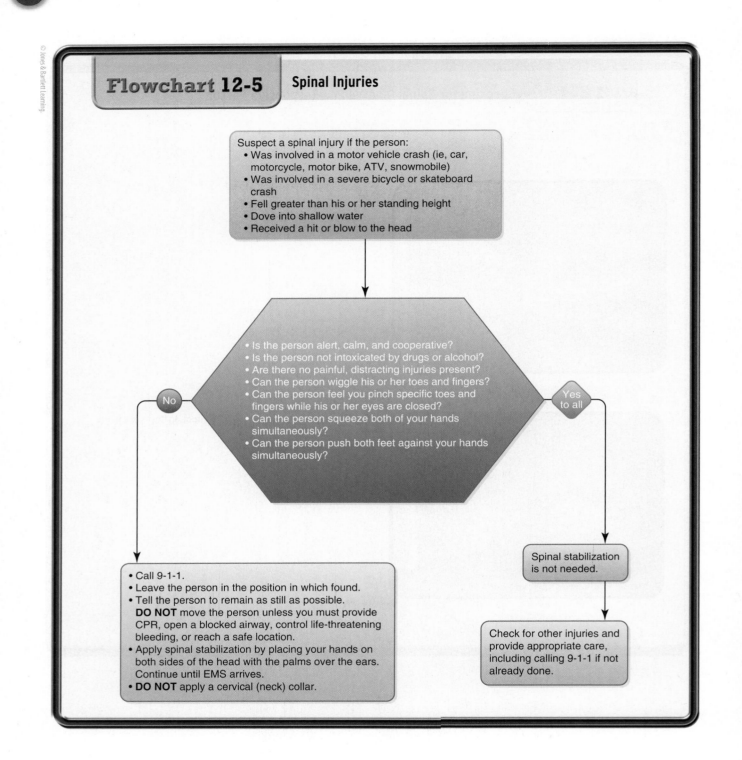

**Flowchart 12-5**    **Spinal Injuries**

Suspect a spinal injury if the person:
- Was involved in a motor vehicle crash (ie, car, motorcycle, motor bike, ATV, snowmobile)
- Was involved in a severe bicycle or skateboard crash
- Fell greater than his or her standing height
- Dove into shallow water
- Received a hit or blow to the head

- Is the person alert, calm, and cooperative?
- Is the person not intoxicated by drugs or alcohol?
- Are there no painful, distracting injuries present?
- Can the person wiggle his or her toes and fingers?
- Can the person feel you pinch specific toes and fingers while his or her eyes are closed?
- Can the person squeeze both of your hands simultaneously?
- Can the person push both feet against your hands simultaneously?

No

Yes to all

- Call 9-1-1.
- Leave the person in the position in which found.
- Tell the person to remain as still as possible. **DO NOT** move the person unless you must provide CPR, open a blocked airway, control life-threatening bleeding, or reach a safe location.
- Apply spinal stabilization by placing your hands on both sides of the head with the palms over the ears. Continue until EMS arrives.
- **DO NOT** apply a cervical (neck) collar.

Spinal stabilization is not needed.

Check for other injuries and provide appropriate care, including calling 9-1-1 if not already done.

# prep kit

## ▶ Ready for Review

- Any head injury is potentially serious. If not properly treated, injuries that seem minor could become life threatening.
- Scalp wounds bleed profusely because the scalp has a rich supply of blood.
- A skull fracture is a break or crack in the cranium. Skull fractures may be open or closed.
- Injuries to the brain cause short- and long-term conditions.
- An injured eye probably causes the most anxiety and concern in a person.
- Penetrating eye injuries are severe injuries that result when a sharp object penetrates the eye.
- Blows to the eye can range in severity from minor to sight threatening.
- Cuts of the eye or lid require medical care.
- Chemicals in the eyes can threaten sight.
- A blow to the eye can knock it from its socket.
- Loose objects in the eye are the most frequent eye injury and can be very painful.
- Burns to the eye can result if a person looks at a source of ultraviolet light.
- Most ear injuries are not life threatening, but fast action may be needed to relieve pain or to prevent or reverse hearing loss.
- Most nosebleeds are self-limiting and seldom require medical attention.
- A foreign object in the nose is a condition mainly among small children who put small objects up their nostrils.
- Because dental emergencies generally cause considerable pain and anxiety, managing them promptly can provide great relief to the person.
- Trauma can cause teeth to become loosened in their sockets.
- A knocked-out tooth is a dental emergency.
- The front teeth are frequently broken by falls or direct blows.
- The most common reason for toothaches is dental decay.
- A mistake in the handling of a person with a spinal injury could mean a lifetime of paralysis for the person.

## ▶ Vital Vocabulary

**anterior nosebleed** Bleeding from the front of the nose.

**Battle sign** A contusion on the mastoid area of either ear; sign of a basilar skull fracture.

**cerebrospinal fluid (CSF)** A clear, watery solution similar to blood plasma.

**concussion** A temporary disturbance of brain activity caused by a blow to the head; also known as mild traumatic brain injury.

**contusion** A bruise; an injury that causes a hemorrhage in or beneath the skin but does not break the skin.

**coup-contrecoup** Dual impacting of the brain into the skull; coup injury occurs at the site of impact; contrecoup injury occurs on the opposite side of impact, as the brain rebounds.

**diffuse axonal** Tearing brain injury caused by shaking or strong rotation of the head.

**paraplegia** Paralysis of the legs caused by damage to the spine.

**posterior nosebleed** Bleeding from the back of the nose, which may flow out of the nostrils and into the mouth or throat.

**quadriplegia** Paralysis of the arms and legs caused by damage to the spine.

**skull fracture** A break or a crack in the cranium (bony case surrounding the brain).

**vertebrae** The 33 bones that make up the spinal column.

## ▶ Assessment in Action

While working at a construction site, you witness a fellow worker fall to the ground after being struck by a piece of wood thrown by a table saw. He was not wearing his safety glasses and you see a cut to his eyeball and eyelid.

# prep kit

**Directions:** Circle Yes if you agree with the statement; circle No if you disagree.

Yes   No   **1.** Apply pressure immediately to the injured eyeball.

Yes   No   **2.** Tell the person to keep both eyes closed. Both eyes can be covered with a cravat or roller bandage.

Yes   No   **3.** Position the person with his head elevated.

Yes   No   **4.** Medical care is not necessary in this case.

## ▶ Check Your Knowledge

**Directions:** Circle Yes if you agree with the statement; circle No if you disagree.

Yes   No   **1.** Remove objects embedded in an eyeball.

Yes   No   **2.** Scalp wounds produce very little bleeding.

Yes   No   **3.** Scrub and rinse the roots of a knocked-out tooth.

Yes   No   **4.** After a blow to the area around an eye, apply a cold pack.

Yes   No   **5.** Tears are sufficient to flush a chemical from the eye.

Yes   No   **6.** Use clean, damp gauze to remove an object from the eyelid's surface.

Yes   No   **7.** Preserve a knocked-out tooth in mouthwash.

Yes   No   **8.** Do not move a person with a suspected spinal injury.

Yes   No   **9.** Inability to move the hands or feet, or both, may indicate a spinal injury.

Yes   No   **10.** To care for a nosebleed, have the injured person sit down and tilt his or her head back.

# Chest, Abdominal, and Pelvic Injuries

## Chest Injuries

Chest injuries fall into two categories: open or closed. In an open chest injury, the chest wall is penetrated by some object (eg, knife, bullet). In a closed chest injury, the skin is not broken. The injury is caused by blunt trauma (eg, falling object, motor vehicle crash, struck during a fight or assault).

Check and recheck the airway, breathing, and circulation of all people with chest injuries. A responsive person with a chest injury should usually sit up in a comfortable position or, if the injury is on a side, be placed with the injured side down. This position prevents blood inside the chest cavity from seeping into the uninjured side and allows the uninjured side to expand.

### ▶ Closed Chest Injuries

As mentioned, in a **closed chest injury**, the skin is not broken. Closed chest injuries include rib fractures and flail chest.

#### Rib Fractures

The upper four ribs are rarely fractured because they are protected by the collar bone and the shoulder blades. The upper four ribs are so enmeshed with the muscles that they rarely need to be splinted or realigned like other broken bones. The lower two ribs are difficult to fracture because they are attached on only one end and have the freedom to move, which is why they are called *floating ribs*. Broken ribs usually occur along the side of the chest. The main symptom of a rib fracture is pain at the injured rib site; pain when the person breathes, coughs, or moves; or pain when the area is touched.

| **What to Look For** | **What to Do** |
|---|---|
| • Sharp pain when the person takes deep breaths, coughs, or moves<br>• Guarding (tensing the muscles around the injury to help to protect the area)<br>• Tenderness<br>• Shallow breathing due to pain that occurs from normal or deep breathing<br>• Bruising of skin over the injury (usually occurs along the side of the chest) | 1. Help the person find a comfortable position.<br>2. Stabilize the chest **Figure 13-1** by:<br>  • Having the person hold a pillow or other similarly soft material against the area, or<br>  • Placing the arm on the injured side in a sling and binder (swathe) if necessary to control pain.<br>3. **DO NOT** apply constrictive bandages around the chest.<br>4. Give pain medication.<br>5. Tell the person to take very deep, slow breaths every few breaths.<br>6. Call 9-1-1. |

© American Academy of Orthopaedic Surgeons.

**A**    **B**

**Figure 13-1**

Stabilize the ribs by holding **(A)** or tying in place **(B)** a soft object such as a pillow, coat, or blanket. Tell the person to take very deep, slow breaths every few breaths.

## Q&A

**How could broken ribs become life threatening?**

A rib fracture is extremely painful, especially because it cannot be stabilized while it heals. Inhaling air causes the muscles between the ribs to expand the chest and move a fractured rib, making it a very painful process. In an attempt to avoid the pain, a person may develop shallow breathing, which does not fully inflate the small air sacs (alveoli) in the lungs. As a result, fluid may accumulate in the alveoli, leading to pneumonia.

The pain is usually localized to the area of the fracture. If the sharp end of the broken rib protrudes into the chest cavity, it may puncture the lung, causing it to collapse and allow air between the lung and the chest wall (known as a **pneumothorax**). A life-threatening condition known as tension pneumothorax occurs when air progressively accumulates in the space between the lung and the chest wall (known as the pleural space) during inhalation and cannot escape during exhalation. This accumulation compresses the heart, uninjured lung, aorta, and vena cava, causing a decrease in blood return to the heart and thereby decreasing cardiac output.

**Rib Fractures**

Fractured ribs are a common injury and most frequently occur between ribs 4 and 10. The location for most fractures is on the sides of the body. The first three pairs of ribs are protected by the clavicles, whereas the last two pairs move freely and give with impact. Little can be done to assist the healing of broken ribs. Tightly binding the chest limits breathing, and because inhalation is inadequate, fluid accumulates in the air sacs (alveoli) and can result in pneumonia. This relationship between broken ribs and fluid accumulation in the lungs often explains pneumonia deaths.

## Flail Chest

A <u>flail chest</u> is a serious injury that involves several ribs in the same area broken in more than one place.

The area over the injury may move in a direction opposite to that of the rest of the chest wall during breathing (known as **paradoxical movement**). This injury is very painful and makes breathing difficult.

### What to Look For

- Area over the injury moving in a direction opposite to that of the rest of the chest wall during breathing
- Very painful and difficult breathing
- Bruising of skin over the injury
- Same signs as for rib fractures

### What to Do

1. **DO NOT** apply constrictive bandages around the chest.
2. Call 9-1-1.

## ▶ Open Chest Injuries

In an <u>open chest injury</u>, the skin has been broken and the chest wall is penetrated by an object such as a knife or bullet.

### Sucking Chest Wound

A <u>sucking chest wound</u> results when a chest wound allows air to pass into and out of the chest with each breath. Bubbles may be seen at the wound during exhalations and a sucking sound heard during inhalations.

### What to Look For

- Blood bubbling out of a chest wound during exhalation
- Sucking sound heard during inhalations

### What to Do

1. Leave the wound exposed to air without a dressing or any airtight material.
2. **DO NOT** cover an open chest wound unless using direct pressure and a dry gauze dressing to control bleeding. If the dressing becomes blood-soaked, replace it to avoid trapping air in the chest, which may result in death.
3. Call 9-1-1.

## Penetrating (Impaled, Embedded) Object in the Chest

If an object penetrates the chest wall, air and blood escape into the space between the lungs and the chest wall. The air and blood cause the lung to collapse. Lung collapse can lead to shock and death.

Refer to Flowchart 13-1 for additional information regarding the care of chest injuries.

## Flowchart 13-1 | Chest Injuries

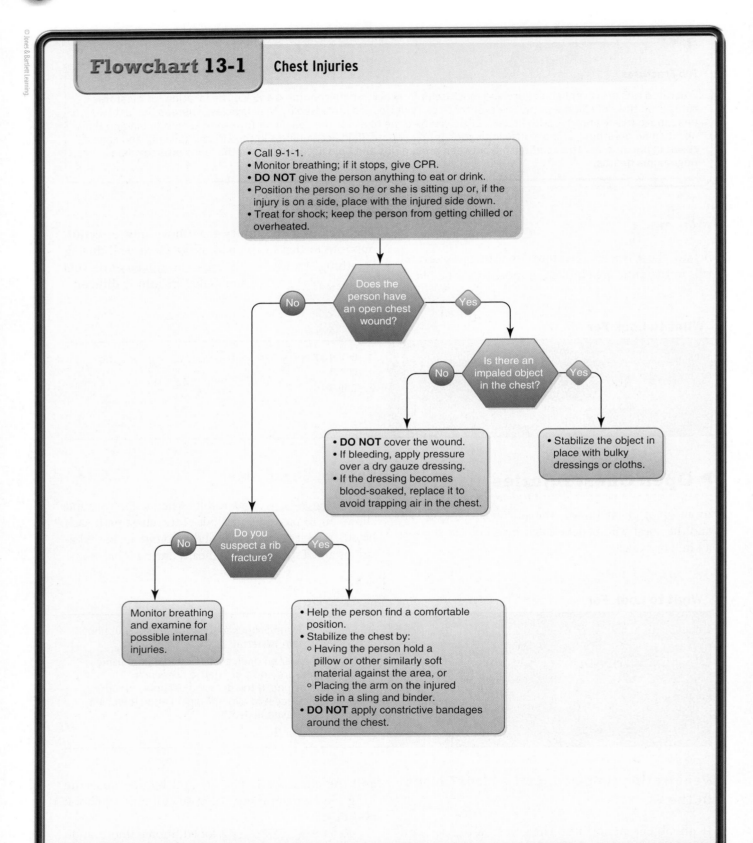

- Call 9-1-1.
- Monitor breathing; if it stops, give CPR.
- **DO NOT** give the person anything to eat or drink.
- Position the person so he or she is sitting up or, if the injury is on a side, place with the injured side down.
- Treat for shock; keep the person from getting chilled or overheated.

**Does the person have an open chest wound?**

No → 

Yes → **Is there an impaled object in the chest?**

No → 
- **DO NOT** cover the wound.
- If bleeding, apply pressure over a dry gauze dressing.
- If the dressing becomes blood-soaked, replace it to avoid trapping air in the chest.

Yes → 
- Stabilize the object in place with bulky dressings or cloths.

**Do you suspect a rib fracture?**

No → Monitor breathing and examine for possible internal injuries.

Yes → 
- Help the person find a comfortable position.
- Stabilize the chest by:
  ○ Having the person hold a pillow or other similarly soft material against the area, or
  ○ Placing the arm on the injured side in a sling and binder.
- **DO NOT** apply constrictive bandages around the chest.

## What to Look For

An impaled object is usually easily recognized. However, in some cases the object may be below the skin surface and is difficult to see. Carefully look at wounds that could be hiding the object that caused the damage.

## What to Do

1. Stabilize the object in place with bulky dressings or clothes **Figure 13-2**. **DO NOT** try to remove the object.
2. Call 9-1-1.

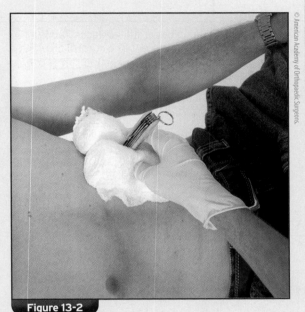

**Figure 13-2**

Stabilize a penetrating object with bulky padding. Secure the padding and object.

# Abdominal Injuries

Injuries to the abdomen are either open or closed and can involve hollow and/or solid organs. A closed abdominal injury is one of the most frequently unrecognized injuries; when missed, it becomes one of the main causes of death. A hollow organ rupture (eg, of the stomach or intestines) spills the contents of the organ into the abdominal cavity, causing inflammation. Solid organ rupture (eg, of the liver or spleen) results in severe internal bleeding.

## ▶ Closed Abdominal Injury

Closed abdominal injuries occur when the internal abdominal tissues are damaged but the skin is unbroken. These are also known as blunt injuries. Such an injury might result from striking the handlebar of a bicycle or the steering wheel of a car, or from being struck by a board or baseball bat.

Bruising and damage to internal organs can result from a severe blow to the abdomen. Examine the abdomen by gently pressing all four quadrants of the abdomen with your fingertips **Figure 13-3**. A normal abdomen is soft and not tender when pressed.

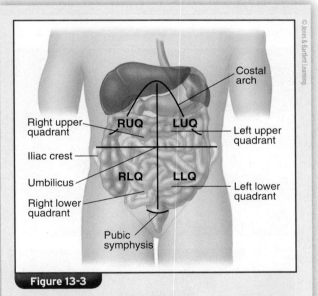

**Figure 13-3**

The four quadrants of the abdomen: left upper, right upper, right lower, and left lower.

## What to Look For

- Bruises or other marks
- Pain, tenderness, muscle tightness, or rigidity
- Distention (swelling)

## What to Do

1. If unresponsive, place the person in the recovery position with the legs bent (ie, the fetal position).
2. If responsive, place the person in a comfortable, side-lying position with the legs slightly bent. Be prepared for potential vomiting.
3. Call 9-1-1.

## ▶ Open Abdominal Injury

<u>Open abdominal injuries</u> are those in which the skin has been broken. These injuries are also known as penetrating injuries. Examples include stab wounds and gunshot wounds. It is difficult to know whether a penetrating injury involves more than just the abdominal wall. Always assume the worst—that internal organs have been damaged. A <u>**protruding organ injury**</u> (evisceration) refers to a severe injury to the abdomen in which internal organs escape or protrude from the wound.

Refer to Flowchart 13-2 for additional information regarding the care of abdominal injuries.

| What to Look For | What to Do |
|---|---|
| Penetrating object such as a knife or other sharp object | 1. If the penetrating object is still in place, stabilize the object against movement and control bleeding by placing bulky dressings around it Figure 13-4 . DO NOT remove the object.<br>2. Call 9-1-1. |
| Internal organs escaping or protruding from the wound Figure 13-5 | 1. Tell the person to stay in a comfortable position (usually lying down) with the legs pulled up toward the abdomen.<br>2. Cover the organs with a moist, clean dressing Figure 13-6 . Place a loose plastic wrap or occlusive dressing, if available, over the dressing. Loosely tape the plastic wrap or occlusive dressing in place.<br>3. Call 9-1-1. |

**Figure 13-5**

Protruding organs.

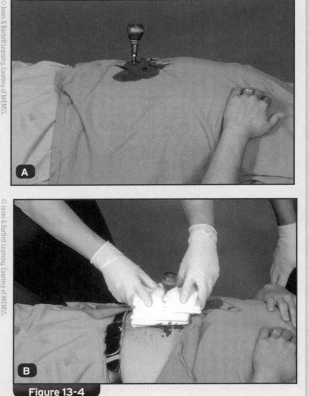

**Figure 13-4**

Stabilize a penetrating object against movement **(A)** and control bleeding by placing bulky dressings around it **(B)**.

## CAUTION

**DO NOT** try to reinsert protruding organs into the abdomen; you could introduce infection or damage the intestines.

**DO NOT** cover the organs tightly.

**DO NOT** cover the organs with any material that clings or disintegrates when wet.

**DO NOT** give anything by mouth.

**DO NOT** touch the organs.

## Flowchart 13-2   Abdominal Injuries

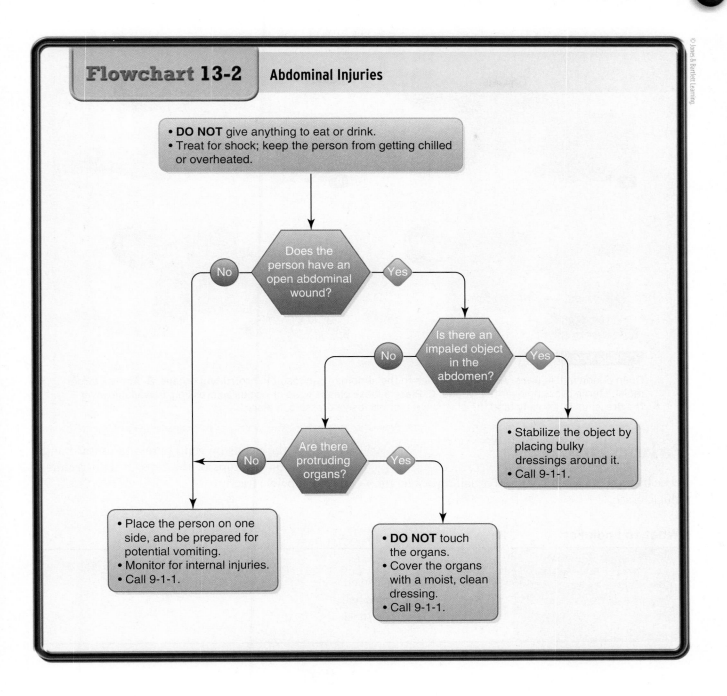

- **DO NOT** give anything to eat or drink.
- Treat for shock; keep the person from getting chilled or overheated.

Does the person have an open abdominal wound?

No → Yes

Is there an impaled object in the abdomen?

No → Yes

Are there protruding organs?

No → Yes

- Stabilize the object by placing bulky dressings around it.
- Call 9-1-1.

- Place the person on one side, and be prepared for potential vomiting.
- Monitor for internal injuries.
- Call 9-1-1.

- **DO NOT** touch the organs.
- Cover the organs with a moist, clean dressing.
- Call 9-1-1.

**Figure 13-6**

Open abdominal injuries. **A.** Severe injuries to the abdomen can result in protruding organs. **B.** Apply a large moist, sterile dressing over the wound. **C.** Place a loose plastic wrap or occlusive dressing, if available, over the dressing. **D.** Loosely tape the plastic wrap or occlusive dressing in place.

# Pelvic Injuries

Pelvic fractures are usually caused by falling or a motor vehicle crash.

Check the pelvis by gently pressing inward and downward on the tops of the hips. If pain results, suspect a pelvic fracture.

| What to Look For | What to Do |
|---|---|
| • Pain in the hip, groin, or back that increases with movement<br>• Inability to stand or walk<br>• Signs of shock | 1. Call 9-1-1.<br>2. **DO NOT** move the person.<br>3. Keep the person lying flat.<br>4. Treat the person for shock. |

## CAUTION

**DO NOT** roll the person; additional internal damage could result.

**DO NOT** move the person. Whenever possible, wait for trained emergency medical services (EMS) personnel with their ambulance, backboard, and other specialized equipment.

## FYI

### Pelvic Fractures

A pelvic fracture should be suspected in anyone with pelvic pain on movement or with squeezing and/or pushing of the pelvis. Motor vehicle crashes, being struck by a motor vehicle, falls, and bicycle and motorcycle crashes are common causes of pelvic injury. It is important to suspect pelvic injuries because they can result in massive blood loss. Unstable pelvic bones can cause continued arterial and venous bleeding that can go unnoticed. Splinting is necessary. Laypeople should stabilize the person and wait for trained EMS personnel and their equipment to transport the person to a hospital emergency department.

## ▶ Ready for Review

- Chest injuries fall into two categories: open or closed.
- Closed chest injuries include rib fractures and flail chest.
- In an open chest injury, the skin has been broken and the chest wall is penetrated by an object such as a knife or bullet.
- Injuries to the abdomen are either open or closed and can involve hollow and/or solid organs.
- Closed abdominal injuries occur when the internal abdominal tissues are damaged but the skin is unbroken.
- Open abdominal injuries are those in which the skin has been broken and the abdominal wall penetrated.
- Pelvic fractures are usually caused by falling or a motor vehicle crash.

## ▶ Vital Vocabulary

**closed abdominal injury** An injury to the abdomen that occurs as a result of a direct blow from a blunt object. There is no break in the skin.

**closed chest injury** An injury to the chest in which the skin is not broken; usually due to blunt trauma.

**flail chest** A condition that occurs when several ribs in the same area are broken in more than one place.

**open abdominal injury** An injury to the abdomen in which the skin is broken; can involve a penetrating wound or protruding organs.

**open chest injury** An injury to the chest in which the chest wall itself is penetrated by an external object such as a bullet or knife.

**paradoxical movement** The movement of the portion of the chest wall that is detached in a flail chest; the movement (in during inhalation, out during exhalation) is the opposite of normal chest wall movement during breathing.

**pneumothorax** Accumulation of air in the pleural space.

**protruding organ injury** A severe injury to the abdomen in which the internal organs escape or protrude from the wound; also known as evisceration.

**sucking chest wound** A chest wound that allows air to pass into the chest cavity with each breath.

## ▶ Assessment in Action

You are on the first aid team at a local scout camp. The scout leaders are conducting a funny skit on a stage at the main lodge. One of the scouts in the skit jumps in the air and lands on his side. As he runs off the stage toward you, he is in obvious pain and is clutching his side. He lies down and a knife falls to the ground. You hear a sucking sound coming from the wound on his side whenever he inhales.

*Directions:* Circle Yes if you agree with the statement; circle No if you disagree.

Yes   No   **1.** You should check the person's breathing and treat accordingly.

Yes   No   **2.** Blood bubbling out of the wound during breathing is a sign of a sucking chest wound.

Yes   No   **3.** The wound should be covered tightly to prevent air from escaping.

Yes   No   **4.** If the person develops breathing difficulty, remove any dressing in order to allow trapped air to escape.

Yes   No   **5.** This is a medical emergency and 9-1-1 should be called immediately.

## ▶ Check Your Knowledge

*Directions:* Circle Yes if you agree with the statement; circle No if you disagree.

Yes   No   **1.** Stabilize a broken rib with a soft object, such as a pillow or blanket, tied to the chest.

Yes   No   **2.** For suspected rib fractures, apply tight bandages around the chest.

Yes   No   **3.** Remove a penetrating or impaled object from the chest or the abdomen.

Yes   No   **4.** A flail chest refers to a single broken rib.

Yes   No   **5.** Keep the person with a broken pelvis still.

Yes   No   **6.** Sharp pain while breathing can be a sign of a rib fracture.

Yes   No   **7.** Rib fractures should be treated by tightly taping the chest.

Yes   No   **8.** Most people with abdominal injuries are more comfortable with their knees bent.

Yes   No   **9.** Leave a chest wound uncovered if you hear air being sucked in and out.

Yes   No   **10.** A broken pelvis can threaten life because of the large amount of blood loss.

# Bone, Joint, and Muscle Injuries

**14**

## Bone Injuries

Bone, joint, and muscle injuries are among the most common reasons for seeking medical care. Although rarely fatal, they often result in short- or long-term disability. Of these injuries, bone fractures and dislocations can be very distressing. They are typically associated with a forceful cause of injury and may present with obvious disfigurement. If not properly cared for, both at the time of injury and during the subsequent healing process, these injuries can result in long-term disability. As a first aid provider, your role is to help manage the person's pain and distress and to ensure no further damage is done before the person can receive proper medical care.

### ▶ Fractures

The real issue is not the broken bones themselves but the potential injury to the vital organs next to them. People usually do not die of broken bones. They die of airway obstruction, blood loss, and brain injury. However, broken bones can be painful and debilitating and can cause lifelong aggravation, disability, and deformity.

The terms <u>fracture</u> and *broken bone* have the same meaning: a break or crack in a bone. There are two categories of fractures **Figure 14-1** :

- **<u>Closed fracture</u>**. The skin is intact, and no wound exists anywhere near the fracture site.
- **<u>Open fracture</u>**. The skin over the fracture has been broken. The wound may result from the bone protruding through the skin or from a direct blow that cut the skin at the time of the fracture. The bone may not always be visible in the wound.

It is not possible to determine the exact nature of a broken bone outside a medical facility. Nonetheless, it may be helpful for first aid providers to be familiar with the terminology that physicians use to describe fractures **Figure 14-2** .

Greenstick fractures are incomplete fractures that commonly occur in children, whose bones (like

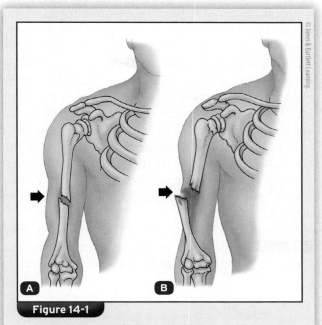

**Figure 14-1**

**A.** Closed fracture. **B.** Open fracture.

**Figure 14-2**

Types of fractures.

Greenstick    Transverse    Oblique    Comminuted    Impacted green sticks) are pliable. A transverse fracture cuts across the bone at right angles to its long axis and is often caused by direct injury. The fracture line of an oblique fracture crosses the bone in a slanting direction (or at an oblique angle, thus the name). A comminuted fracture is one in which the bone is fragmented into more than two pieces (that is, splintered or crushed). In an impacted fracture, the broken ends of the bone are jammed together and the bone may function as if no fracture were present. A spiral fracture usually results from a twisting injury, and the fracture line has the appearance of a spring.

It may be difficult to tell if a bone is broken **Figure 14-3**. When in doubt, treat the injury as a fracture. A quick nerve and pulse check is extremely important. The most serious complication of a fracture is inadequate blood flow in an extremity. The major blood vessels of an extremity tend to run close to the bones, which means that any time a bone is broken, the adjacent blood vessels are at risk of being torn by bone fragments or pinched off between the ends of the broken bone. The tissues of the arms and legs cannot survive for more than about 3 hours without a continuing blood supply. If you note any disruption in the nerve or blood supply, seek immediate medical care. Major nerve pathways also travel close to bones and may be torn or pinched off between the ends of the broken bone.

Refer to **Flowchart 14-1** for additional information regarding the care of bone injuries.

**Figure 14-3**

**A.** Forearm fracture. **B.** X-rays of a forearm fracture before setting.

## Q&A

**Which bone is the most frequently fractured bone in the body?**

Due to its vulnerable position and its relative thinness, the clavicle (collar bone) is the most frequently fractured bone in the body. Fractured clavicles are caused by either a direct blow or a transmitted force resulting from a fall on the outstretched arm.

**Flowchart 14-1** | **Bone Injuries**

Suspect a broken bone if one or more of the following exist:
- D = Deformity
- O = Open wound
- T = Tenderness
- S = Swelling

- Call 9-1-1 if the extremity looks blue or extremely pale.
- **DO NOT** move or try to straighten the injured extremity.

Is there bleeding from an open wound at the injured site?

No / Yes

- Apply pressure on the edges of the wound.
- **DO NOT** push on the bone.
- Cover the wound and exposed bone with a dressing.

Will emergency medical services (EMS) arrive soon?

No / Yes

If EMS will be delayed or if you are transporting the person, use the RICE procedure.
- R = Rest
- I = Ice
- C = Compression
- E = Elevate

If necessary, either you or the person may hold the injured part until EMS arrives.

- Stabilize the injured part with a splint in the position it was found.
- Check for circulation, sensation, and movement (CSM) before and after splinting to avoid tightness.

## Q&A

**How strong is bone?**

Bone is one of the strongest materials found in nature. One cubic inch of bone can withstand loads of at least 19,000 pounds (8,618 kg), which is about the weight of five standard-size pickup trucks. This is roughly four times the strength of concrete. Bone's resistance to load is equal to that of aluminum and light steel. Ounce for ounce, bone is actually stronger than steel and reinforced concrete, because steel bars of comparable size would weigh four or five times as much as bone.

## What to Look For

Use the mnemonic DOTS to assess for an injury:

- *Deformity*, such as:
  - Shortening or severe deformity (angulation) between the joints or deformity around the joints
  - Shortening of the extremity
  - Rotation of the extremity when compared with the opposite extremity
- *Open wound*. Lacerations or small puncture wounds near the site of a bone fracture are considered open fractures.
- *Tenderness and pain*. A useful technique for detecting a fracture is to gently feel, touch, or press along the length of the bone; a person's report of tenderness or pain can indicate a fracture.
- *Swelling* that happens rapidly

Additional signs and symptoms include:

- Loss of function of the injured part
- Guarding (the person refuses to use the injured part when motion produces pain)
- Crepitus (a grating sensation felt and sometimes even heard when the ends of a broken bone rub together). **DO NOT** move the injured extremity in an attempt to detect it.
- Person reports a history of injury that includes a serious incident, or having heard or felt the bone snap

## What to Do

1. Check for life-threatening conditions. A fracture, even an open fracture, seldom presents an immediate threat to life unless it has severed an artery or large vein. Only when all life-threatening conditions have been dealt with is it appropriate to identify and stabilize fractures.
2. Gently remove clothing covering the injured body part. Cut away clothing at the seams if necessary.
3. Examine the area by looking and feeling for DOTS.
4. Check the pulse and nerves. Check CSM. Follow the steps in [ Skill Sheet 14-1 ] for checking CSM in an upper extremity and [ Skill Sheet 14-2 ] for a lower extremity.
   - *Circulation*. A pulseless arm or leg is a significant emergency requiring immediate surgical care. If there is no pulse, **DO NOT** move or try to straighten the injured extremity, unless the person is in a remote location or wilderness setting distant from EMS. Some recommend the capillary refill test. Press on a fingernail or toenail, then release it. If circulation is normal, the nail bed should return to its normal color within 2 seconds. Performing the capillary refill test in the dark or in the cold or on tobacco smokers may limit its accuracy. It tends to be more accurate in children.
   - *Sensation*. This is the most useful early sign. Loss of sensation is an early sign of nerve damage, which can accompany some fractures.
   - *Movement*. Inability to move develops later. If the toes or fingers are injured, **DO NOT** have the person attempt to move them.

   If you note any disruption in the nerve or blood supply, seek immediate medical care.

5. Stabilize the injured part against movement.
   - If EMS will arrive soon, stabilize the injured part with your hands until they arrive.
   - If EMS will be delayed or if you are transporting the person to medical care, stabilize the injured part with a splint.
6. If the injury is an open fracture, **DO NOT** push on any protruding bones [ Figure 14-4 ]. Cover the wound and exposed bones with a dressing. Place rolls of gauze around the bone and bandage the injury without applying pressure on the bone.
7. Call 9-1-1 for any open fractures or large-bone (ie, femur) fractures or when transporting the person would be difficult or would aggravate the injury.
8. Call 9-1-1 if the extremity looks blue or extremely pale.
9. Generally, first aid providers should not move or straighten an injured extremity. However, if there is no pulse in an extremity and the person is in a remote location or wilderness setting distant from EMS, you may need to gently realign the injured extremity to restore blood flow or to transport the person. In this situation:
   - Use the RICE procedure. An ice pack helps reduce swelling and pain.
   - Stabilize the part against movement. Doing so limits pain and reduces the chance for further injury.

# Skill Sheet

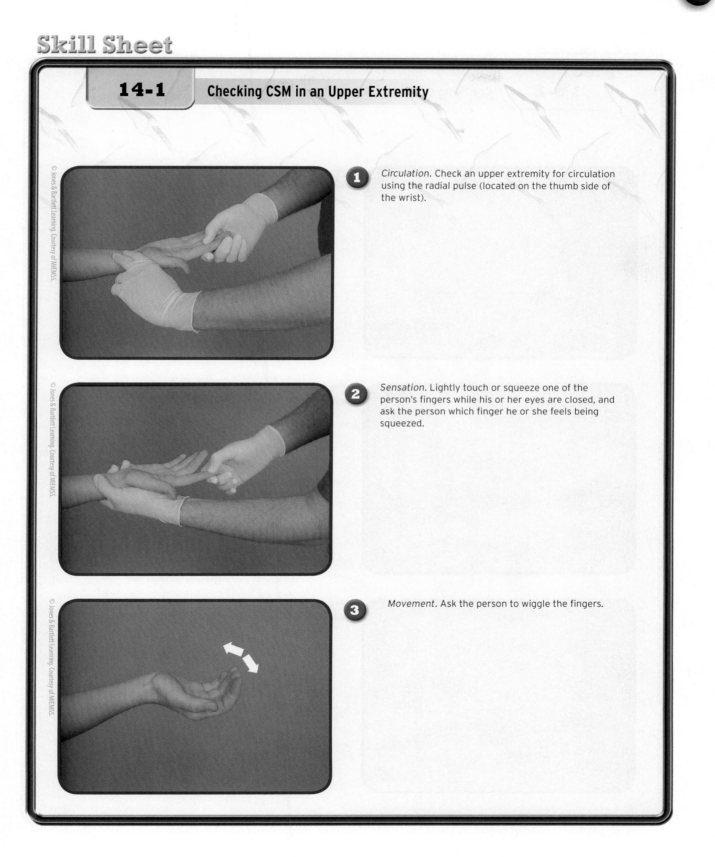

**14-1**   **Checking CSM in an Upper Extremity**

**1** *Circulation.* Check an upper extremity for circulation using the radial pulse (located on the thumb side of the wrist).

**2** *Sensation.* Lightly touch or squeeze one of the person's fingers while his or her eyes are closed, and ask the person which finger he or she feels being squeezed.

**3** *Movement.* Ask the person to wiggle the fingers.

© Jones & Bartlett Learning. Courtesy of MIEMSS.

## Skill Sheet

**14-2**    Checking CSM in a Lower Extremity

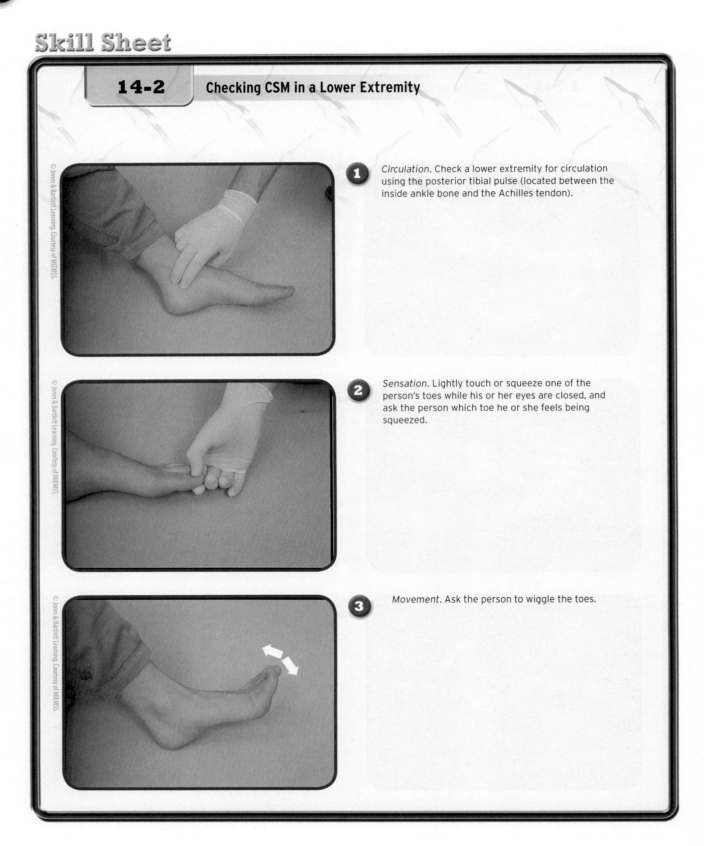

1. *Circulation.* Check a lower extremity for circulation using the posterior tibial pulse (located between the inside ankle bone and the Achilles tendon).

2. *Sensation.* Lightly touch or squeeze one of the person's toes while his or her eyes are closed, and ask the person which toe he or she feels being squeezed.

3. *Movement.* Ask the person to wiggle the toes.

**Figure 14-4**

Open tibia, fibula fracture of the leg.

**Figure 14-5**

Dislocation of the elbow.

# Joint Injuries

A joint is where two or more bones come together.

## ▶ Dislocations

A <u>dislocation</u> occurs when a joint comes apart and stays apart, with the bone ends no longer in contact.

The shoulders, elbows, fingers, hips, knee caps (patellas), and ankles are the joints most frequently affected.

Dislocations cause signs and symptoms similar to those of fractures: deformity, severe pain, swelling, and inability of the person to move the injured joint. The main sign of a dislocation is deformity. Its appearance will be different from that of an uninjured joint **Figure 14-5**.

**What to Look For**

- Obvious deformity compared with the opposite, uninjured joint
- Tenderness
- Severe pain
- Swelling
- Inability to move the injured part
- Numbness or impaired circulation of the extremity

**What to Do**

1. Call 9-1-1 for the following:
   - Extremity looks blue or extremely pale
   - Transport of the person would be difficult or might aggravate the injury
2. Check the CMS, as previously described. If the end of the dislocated bone is pressing on nerves or blood vessels, numbness or paralysis may exist below the dislocation. If there is no pulse in the injured extremity, transport the person to a medical facility immediately.
3. If EMS has been called and will arrive soon, either you or the person may hold the injured part to stabilize it against movement until EMS arrives.
4. If EMS will be delayed or you are transporting the person to distant medical care, use the RICE procedure.
5. **DO NOT** try to reduce a dislocation by putting the displaced part back into its normal position because nerve and blood vessel damage could result. Wilderness medical experts have identified easy and safe ways to reduce knee cap, finger, and anterior shoulder dislocations when medical help is more than 1 hour away. (See Chapter 24, *Wilderness First Aid*.)

## ▶ Sprains

A **sprain** occurs when a joint is twisted or stretched beyond its normal range of motion. Bones are held together at joints by tough bands of tissue called ligaments. When a joint is sprained, the ligaments are either partially or completely torn. There are different degrees of sprains, but it is difficult for a first aid provider to classify the degree of a sprain **Figure 14-6**. Sprains most often occur in the knee and the ankle, but can occur in any joint.

Ankle sprains most often occur when the foot turns inward and stress is placed on the outside (lateral side) of the ankle. A severe lateral ankle sprain, if not correctly treated, can result in a chronically unstable ankle that is prone to sprains. Any ligament or bone injury on the inner side of the ankle usually represents a serious condition and requires medical care.

Refer to **Flowchart 14-2** for additional information regarding the care of joint injuries.

**Figure 14-6**

Sprain.

| What to Look For | What to Do |
|---|---|
| It is often difficult to distinguish between a severe sprain and a fracture because their signs and symptoms are similar.<br><br>• Severe pain, which may prevent the person from moving or using the joint<br>• Swelling<br>• Discolored skin around the joint resulting from bleeding from torn blood vessels | 1. Most sprains do not require medical care. If recuperation seems long, consult a physician.<br>2. Use the RICE procedure:<br>  • *Rest.* Remove weight from and avoid movement of the injured joint.<br>  • *Ice.* Apply an ice pack for about 20 minutes; an elastic bandage can be applied to keep the ice pack in place.<br>  • *Compression.* After the 20 minutes, apply compression with an elastic bandage for 3 to 4 hours.<br>  • Repeat the cycles of an ice pack for 20 minutes and compression for 3 to 4 hours.<br>  • *Elevate.* Raise the injured part to reduce swelling of the injured part. |

# Muscle Injuries

Although muscle injuries pose no real emergency, first aid providers have ample opportunities to care for them.

## ▶ Strains

A muscle **strain**, also known as a muscle pull, occurs when a muscle is torn as a result of stretching beyond its normal range of motion. There are different degrees of strains, but it is difficult for a first aid provider to classify the degree of a strain. When muscle fibers tear, fluid from nearby tissues leaks out and starts to build up near the injury. The area becomes inflamed, swollen, and tender. Inflammation begins immediately after an injury, but it can take 24 to 72 hours for enough tissue fluid to build up to cause pain and stiffness.

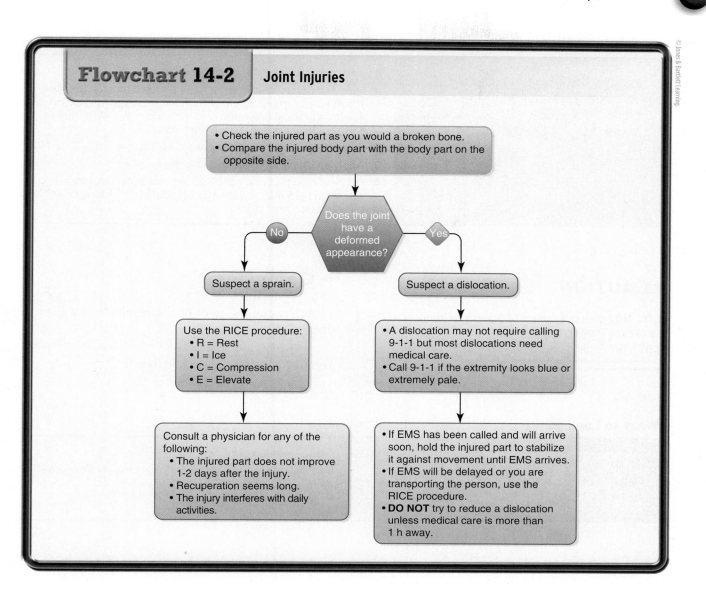

**Flowchart 14-2** | Joint Injuries

- Check the injured part as you would a broken bone.
- Compare the injured body part with the body part on the opposite side.

Does the joint have a deformed appearance?

**No** → Suspect a sprain.

**Yes** → Suspect a dislocation.

Use the RICE procedure:
- R = Rest
- I = Ice
- C = Compression
- E = Elevate

- A dislocation may not require calling 9-1-1 but most dislocations need medical care.
- Call 9-1-1 if the extremity looks blue or extremely pale.

Consult a physician for any of the following:
- The injured part does not improve 1-2 days after the injury.
- Recuperation seems long.
- The injury interferes with daily activities.

- If EMS has been called and will arrive soon, hold the injured part to stabilize it against movement until EMS arrives.
- If EMS will be delayed or you are transporting the person, use the RICE procedure.
- **DO NOT** try to reduce a dislocation unless medical care is more than 1 h away.

| What to Look For | What to Do |
|---|---|
| • Occurs during physical activity<br>• Sharp pain<br>• Extreme tenderness<br>• Inability to use injured part<br>• Stiffness and pain when muscle is used | To care for strains, follow the RICE procedure. |

## ▶ Cramps

A <u>cramp</u> occurs when a muscle goes into an uncontrolled spasm and contraction. Although scientific literature has yet to confirm the causes of muscle cramps, several factors are associated with them. For example, muscle cramping is associated with certain diseases such as diabetes and atherosclerosis (hardening of the arteries). Muscle cramps are often associated with physical activity. Roughly, muscle cramps can be divided into two categories: night cramps, which include any cramp occurring at night or while a person is at rest, and heat cramps, which are related to dehydration and electrolyte imbalance. (The electrolytes potassium and sodium carry an electric charge that helps trigger muscles to contract and relax.)

| **What to Look For** | **What to Do** |
|---|---|
| • Sudden severe muscle pain<br>• A muscle, often the calf muscle, that feels hard because of muscle contraction<br>• Residual discomfort, which may last for a few hours | Try one or more of these methods to relax the muscle:<br>1. Have the person gently stretch the affected muscle. Because the muscle cramp is an uncontrolled muscle contraction or spasm, a gradual extension of the muscle may help lengthen the muscle fibers and relieve the cramp.<br>2. Relax the muscle by pressing and massaging it.<br>3. Apply an ice pack (unless in a cold environment).<br>4. For heat cramps, drink lightly salted cool water (one-fourth teaspoon [1.25 mL] salt in 1 quart [about 1 L] of water) or a commercial sports drink. |

**CAUTION**

**DO NOT** give salt tablets to a person with muscle cramps. They can cause stomach irritation, nausea, and vomiting.

## ▶ Contusions

A muscle **contusion** or bruise results from a blow to the muscle.

Refer to **Flowchart 14-3** for additional information regarding the care of muscle injuries.

| **What to Look For** | **What to Do** |
|---|---|
| • Person reports blow to a muscle<br>• Swelling<br>• Tenderness and pain<br>• Black and blue mark appearing hours later | 1. Use the RICE procedure.<br>2. Seek medical care for any contusion larger than the person's palm. |

## Flowchart 14-3 | Muscle Injuries

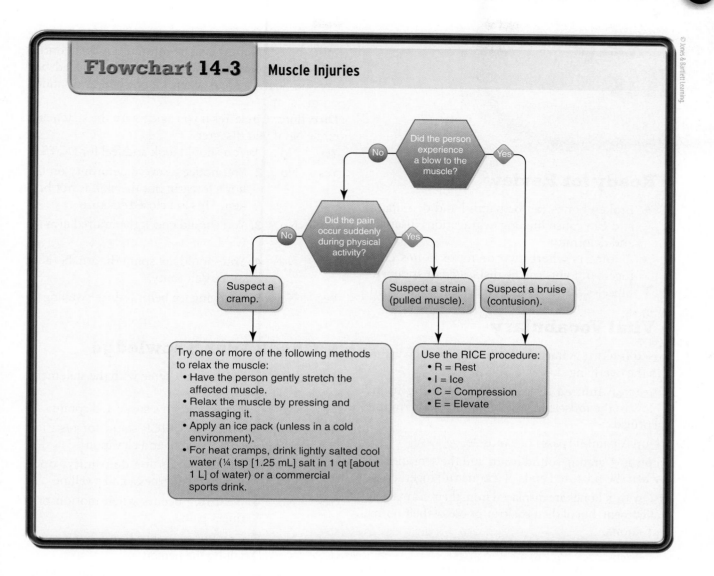

Did the person experience a blow to the muscle?

No → Did the pain occur suddenly during physical activity?

Yes → Suspect a bruise (contusion).

No → Suspect a cramp.

Yes → Suspect a strain (pulled muscle).

**Try one or more of the following methods to relax the muscle:**
- Have the person gently stretch the affected muscle.
- Relax the muscle by pressing and massaging it.
- Apply an ice pack (unless in a cold environment).
- For heat cramps, drink lightly salted cool water (¼ tsp [1.25 mL] salt in 1 qt [about 1 L] of water) or a commercial sports drink.

**Use the RICE procedure:**
- R = Rest
- I = Ice
- C = Compression
- E = Elevate

# Prep Kit

## ▶ Ready for Review

- Broken bones can be painful and debilitating and can cause lifelong aggravation, disability, and deformity.
- A joint is where two or more bones come together. Joints can be dislocated or sprained.
- Muscles can be strained, bruised, or cramped.

## ▶ Vital Vocabulary

**closed fracture** A fracture in which there is no wound in the overlying skin.

**contusion** Injured tissue or skin resulting from a blow to the muscle in which blood vessels rupture; a bruise.

**cramp** A painful spasm of a muscle.

**crepitus** A grating sound heard and the sensation felt when the fractured ends of a bone rub together.

**dislocation** Bones are displaced from their normal joint alignment, out of their sockets, or out of their normal positions.

**fracture** A break or rupture in a bone.

**open fracture** A fracture exposed to the exterior; an open wound lies over the fracture.

**sprain** A trauma to a joint that injures the ligaments.

**strain** A tearing of muscle that occurs when the muscle is stretched beyond its normal range of motion.

## ▶ Assessment in Action

While walking through your neighborhood, you see two boys yelling for help on the sidewalk. One is on the ground in pain and clutching his arm. The other boy explains that the injured boy lost control while skateboarding and crashed. The injured boy says he heard a snap when he crashed and landed on his arm.

*Directions:* Circle Yes if you agree with the statement; circle No if you disagree.

Yes   No   **1.** You should look and feel for DOTS.

Yes   No   **2.** You notice a severe deformity on the boy's forearm but the skin is not broken. This is a closed fracture.

Yes   No   **3.** You should check the injured arm for CSM.

Yes   No   **4.** You should not splint the arm because of the deformity.

Yes   No   **5.** Applying ice helps reduce swelling.

## ▶ Check Your Knowledge

*Directions:* Circle Yes if you agree with the statement; circle No if you disagree.

Yes   No   **1.** Apply cold on a suspected sprain.

Yes   No   **2.** The letters RICE stand for rest, ice, compression, and elevation.

Yes   No   **3.** DOTS stands for deformity, open wound, tenderness, and swelling.

Yes   No   **4.** Guarding occurs when motion produces pain.

Yes   No   **5.** Crepitus cannot be heard, but it can be felt by the person.

Yes   No   **6.** A dislocation is cared for much differently than a fracture.

Yes   No   **7.** Check a suspected fracture by having the person move the extremity.

Yes   No   **8.** Treat a muscle cramp by stretching the affected muscle.

Yes   No   **9.** CSM stands for cold, swelling, and motion.

Yes   No   **10.** Do not push on a protruding bone.

# Extremity Injuries

## 15

## Extremity Injuries

Injuries to the extremities are common because people are involved in active lifestyles that include sports and wilderness activities. This chapter focuses on bone, joint, and muscle injuries of the extremities; bleeding, wounds, and other soft-tissue injuries are covered elsewhere. Most of the conditions discussed result from sudden trauma, although some chronic injuries incurred over time, such as tennis elbow, are included.

## ▶ Assessment

Use these guidelines to assess injuries to the extremities:

1. Look for signs and symptoms of fractures and dislocations.
2. Examine the extremities, using the mnemonic DOTS (Deformity, Open wound, Tenderness, Swelling). Look at and gently feel the extremity, starting at the distal end (fingers or toes) and working upward.
3. Compare one extremity with the other to determine size and shape differences.
4. Use the rule of thirds for extremity injuries. Imagine each long bone as being divided into thirds. If deformity, tenderness, or swelling is located in the upper or lower third of a long bone, assume that the nearest joint is injured.

## Chapter
### at a glance

- ▶ **Extremity Injuries**
- ▶ **RICE Procedure for Bone, Joint, and Muscle Injuries**
- ▶ **Shoulder Injuries**
- ▶ **Elbow Injuries**
- ▶ **Hand Injuries**
- ▶ **Finger Injuries**
- ▶ **Hip Joint Injuries**
- ▶ **Thigh Injuries**
- ▶ **Knee Injuries**
- ▶ **Lower Leg Injuries**

5. Consider the cause of injury when evaluating the possibility of a fracture and its location. Forces that cause musculoskeletal injuries are direct forces (eg, a car bumper striking a pedestrian's leg), indirect forces along the long axis of bones (eg, a person falling onto an outstretched hand and fracturing the collar bone), and twisting forces (eg, a person's foot being fixed in one spot and the leg suddenly twisting).

6. Use the mnemonic CSM as a reminder to check the extremity for circulation, sensation, and movement of fingers or toes.

## ▶ Types of Injuries

Types of injuries to the extremities range from simple contusions to complex open fractures:

1. <u>Contusions</u>, or bruising of the tissue
2. <u>Strains</u>, in which muscles are stretched or torn
3. <u>Sprains</u>, which involve the tearing or stretching of the joints, causing mild to severe damage to the ligaments and joint capsules
4. <u>Tendinitis</u>, which is inflammation of a tendon (cord that attaches muscle to bone) caused by overuse
5. <u>Dislocations</u>, in which bones are displaced from their normal joint alignment, out of their sockets, or out of their normal positions
6. <u>Fractures</u>, which are breaks in bones that may or may not be accompanied by open wounds

# RICE Procedure for Bone, Joint, and Muscle Injuries

RICE is the acronym for rest, ice, compression, and elevation—the recommended immediate treatment for bone, joint, and muscle injuries. The steps during the first 48 to 72 hours after an injury can do a lot to relieve—even prevent—aches and pains. Treat all extremity bone, joint, and muscle injuries with the RICE procedure. In addition to RICE, fractures and dislocations should be splinted to stabilize the injured area.

## ▶ R = Rest

Injuries heal faster if rested. *Rest* means the person does not use or move the injured part. Using any part of the body increases the blood circulation to that area, which can cause more swelling of an injured part. Crutches may be used to rest leg injuries.

## ▶ I = Ice

An ice pack should be applied to the injured area as soon as possible after the injury for about 20 minutes (or 10 minutes if uncomfortable) every 3 to 4 hours while awake, during the first 24 to 48 hours. Never apply ice directly to the skin. Skin treated with cold passes through four stages: cold, burning, aching, and numbness. When the skin becomes numb, usually in 20 minutes, remove the ice pack. After removing the ice pack, compress the injured part with an elastic bandage and keep it elevated (the "C" and "E" of RICE).

Cold constricts the blood vessels to and in the injured area, which helps reduce the swelling and inflammation, and it dulls the pain and relieves muscle spasms. Cold should be applied as soon as possible after the injury; healing time often is directly related to the amount of swelling that occurs. Heat has the opposite effect when applied to fresh injuries: It increases circulation to the area and increases the swelling and the pain.

Use either of the following methods to apply cold to an injury:

1. Put crushed ice (or cubes) into a double plastic bag or commercial ice bag, and place a layer of cloth between the bag of ice and the skin. Alternatively, a wet towel or cloth can be used to hold the ice. Secure the ice in place with an elastic bandage for about 20 minutes. Crushed ice offers the advantage of conforming to the body's contours.
2. Use a chemical snap pack, a sealed pouch that contains two chemical envelopes. Squeezing the pack mixes the chemicals, producing a chemical reaction that has a cooling effect. Although they do not cool as well as other methods, they are convenient to use when ice is not readily available.

They lose their cooling power quickly, however, and can be used only once. Also, they may be impractical because they are expensive.

## CAUTION

**DO NOT** apply an ice pack for more than 20 minutes at a time. Frostbite or nerve damage can result.

**DO NOT** apply an ice pack on the back outside part of the knee. Nerve damage can occur.

**DO NOT** apply cold if the person has a history of circulatory disease, Raynaud disease (spasms in the arteries of the extremities that reduce circulation), or abnormal sensitivity to cold, or if the injured part has been frostbitten previously.

**DO NOT** stop using an ice pack too soon. A common mistake is the early use of heat, which may result in swelling and pain. Use an ice pack three to four times a day for the first 24 hours, preferably up to 48 hours, before applying any heat. For severe injuries, using ice on and off for up to 72 hours is recommended.

## FYI

### Heat and Cold: When to Use Which?

Many people use heat devices or ice packs to speed recovery from sports injuries—but when is the right time to use each technique? Apply cold immediately after an acute injury, such as an ankle sprain. Icing reduces pain, swelling, and muscle spasm immediately after injury, but its use should be discontinued after 2 or 3 days. Heat applications (heat packs, radiant heat, or whirlpool baths) can then be used to reduce muscle spasms and pain. In addition, heat increases blood flow and joint flexibility. Use vigorous heat to treat chronic injuries, but mild heat to reduce muscle spasm. Heat is also effective for acute back pain, but ice massage is preferred if the back pain persists for 2 weeks or more.

*Source:* Kaul MP, Herring SA. Superficial heat and cold. *Phys Sportsmed.* 1994;22(12):65-74.

## FYI

### Homemade Ice Packs

- Ice bags kept in a freezer freeze solid and cannot be shaped to fit the injured area. One part isopropyl (rubbing) alcohol to three parts water prevents freezing, and the ice bag can be easily molded. Bags can be reused for months.
- An unopened bag of frozen vegetables is inexpensive, keeps its basic shape (unlike ice chips, which melt), molds to the shape of the injured area, is reusable, and is packaged in a fairly puncture-resistant, watertight bag.
- For cold therapy over a fairly large area, soak a face towel in cold water, wring it out, fold it, and place it in a large self-sealing plastic bag. Store the bag in the freezer. To use the cold pack, wrap it in a light cotton towel and apply for 20 minutes, after which it can be refrozen. A washcloth in a smaller bag can be used to treat a smaller area.
- Fill a plastic bag with snow.
- Fill a polystyrene plastic cup with water and freeze it. When you need an ice pack, peel the cup to below ice level; the remaining part of the cup forms a cold-resistant handle. Rub the ice over the injured area (movement is necessary to prevent skin damage). These ice packs are inexpensive and convenient and take up little space.
- To make a funnel for filling an ice bag, push out the bottom of a paper cup and fit it into the neck of the ice bag. The ice will slide through the cup and into the bag.

## ▶ C = Compression

Compressing the injured area squeezes fluid out of the injury site. Compression limits the ability of the skin and other tissues to expand and reduces internal bleeding. Apply an elastic bandage to the injured area, especially the foot, ankle, knee, thigh, hand, or elbow. Fill the hollow areas with padding such as a sock or washcloth before applying the elastic bandage.

Elastic bandages come in various sizes for different body areas:

1. 2-inch (5-cm) width for the wrist, hand, and foot
2. 3-inch (8-cm) width for the elbow and arm
3. 4-inch (10-cm) width for the ankle, knee, and leg

Start the elastic bandage several inches below the injury and wrap in an upward, overlapping (about one-half to three-fourths of the bandage's width) spiral, starting with even and somewhat tight pressure, then gradually wrapping more loosely above the injury. Stretch the elastic bandage no more than one-third its ability to stretch.

Applying compression may be the most important step in preventing swelling. The person should wear the elastic bandage continuously for the first 18 to 24 hours (except when cold is applied). At night, have the person loosen but not remove the elastic bandage.

For an ankle injury, place a horseshoe-shaped pad around the ankle knob and secure it with the elastic bandage **Figure 15-1**. The pad can be made from various materials (eg, a twisted wash cloth, socks). The pad will compress the soft tissues and the bones. Wrap the bandage tightest nearest the toes and loosest above the ankle. It should be tight enough to decrease swelling but not tight enough to inhibit blood flow. For a contusion or a strain, place a pad between the injury and the elastic bandage.

**Figure 15-1**

**A.** Place a horseshoe-shaped pad around the ankle knob. **B.** Secure the pad with an elastic bandage.

## ▶ E = Elevation

Gravity slows the return of blood to the heart from the lower parts of the body. Once fluids get to the hands or feet, they have nowhere else to go, and those parts of the body swell. Elevating the injured area, in combination with ice and compression, limits circulation to that area, which in turn helps limit internal bleeding and minimize swelling.

It is simple to prop up an injured leg or arm to limit bleeding. Whenever possible, elevate the injured part above the level of the heart for the first 24 hours after an injury. If a fracture is suspected, do not elevate an extremity until it has been stabilized with a splint. Along with the use of the RICE procedure, fractures and dislocations can be splinted unless emergency medical services (EMS) will soon arrive. In this case, the person can hold the injured part.

## CAUTION

**DO NOT** apply an elastic bandage too tightly. If applied too tightly, elastic bandages will restrict circulation. Stretch a new elastic bandage to about one-third its maximum length for adequate compression. Leave fingers and toes exposed so possible color change can be easily observed. Compare the toes or fingers of the injured extremity with those on the uninjured one. Pale skin, pain, numbness, and tingling are signs that the bandage is too tight. If any of these symptoms appears, immediately remove the elastic bandage. Leave the elastic bandage off until all the symptoms disappear, then rewrap the area less tightly. Always wrap from below the injury and move toward the heart.

To perform the RICE procedure, follow the steps in **Skill Sheet 15-1**:

1. R = Rest. Stop using the injured area (**Step 1**).
2. I = Ice. Place an ice pack on the injured area. Use an elastic bandage to hold the ice pack in place for 20 minutes (**Step 2**).
3. C = Compression. Remove the ice, apply a compression bandage, and leave in place for 3 to 4 hours (**Step 3**).
4. E = Elevation. Raise the injured area higher than the heart, when possible (**Step 4**).

## Skill Sheet

### 15-1    RICE Procedure for Bone, Joint, and Muscle Injuries

**1   R = Rest**
DO NOT use or move the body part.

**2   I = Ice**
Apply cold for 20 min (or 10 min if uncomfortable) every 3-4 h during the first 24-48 h. Put crushed or cubed ice in a plastic bag and place a paper towel or thin cloth between the ice pack and skin for protection, or wrap ice in a damp towel. An elastic bandage can be used to hold the ice pack in place.

**3   C = Compression**
Apply an elastic bandage when not applying ice.

© Jones & Bartlett Learning.

## Skill Sheet Continued

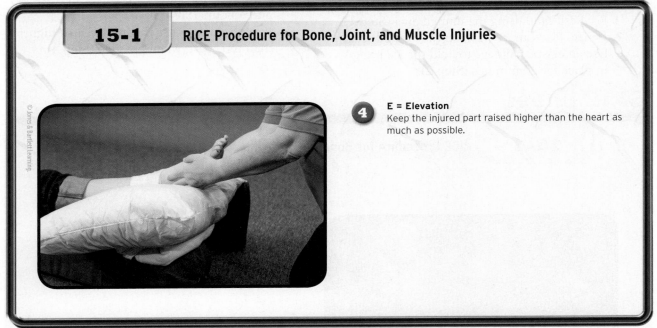

**15-1**    RICE Procedure for Bone, Joint, and Muscle Injuries

**4**  **E = Elevation**
Keep the injured part raised higher than the heart as much as possible.

© Jones & Bartlett Learning.

# Shoulder Injuries

## ▶ Shoulder Dislocation

Three bones come together at the shoulder: the **scapula** (shoulder blade), the **clavicle** (collar bone), and the **humerus** (upper arm bone). The shoulder is the most freely movable joint in the body. The extreme range of its possible movements makes the shoulder joint highly susceptible to dislocation (separation). A dislocation of the shoulder occurs when the bones of the shoulder come apart as a result of a blow or a particular movement. Shoulder dislocation is second in frequency only to finger dislocations.

### What to Look For

- Person holds the upper arm away from the body, supported by the uninjured arm (occurs in about 95% of shoulder dislocations; this position differentiates a dislocation from a fracture of the humerus, in which the person holds the arm against the chest)
- The dislocated arm cannot be brought across the chest wall to touch the opposite shoulder (ie, the sling position)
- Extreme pain in the shoulder area
- Shoulder looks squared off, rather than rounded **Figure 15-2**
- Complete loss of shoulder function
- Reported history of previous dislocations
- Numbness or paralysis in the arm from pressure, pinching blood vessels or nerves

### What to Do

1. **DO NOT** try to force, twist, or pull the shoulder back in place because doing so may cause bone, nerve, or blood vessel injury.
2. Place a folded or rolled blanket or a pillow between the upper arm and the chest to support the arm.
3. Apply an arm sling and swathe (binder) to stabilize and rest the arm. (See Chapter 16, *Splinting Extremities*, for more details.)
4. Apply an ice pack for 20 minutes.
5. Seek immediate medical care.

**Figure 15-2**

Shoulder dislocation. Note the absence of the normal rounded appearance of the shoulder.

# ▶ Clavicle Fracture

Fractures of the clavicle (collar bone) are common and usually are the result of falling directly on the shoulder or on an outstretched arm. They can also be the result of a direct blow to the clavicle that occurs during a fall or a motor vehicle crash. Most clavicle fractures (80%) occur in the middle third of the bone.

## What to Look For

Person reports one of the following:

- Falling directly on the shoulder or on an outstretched arm
- Receiving a direct blow to the clavicle or shoulder
- Severe pain over the injured area
- Person holds the injured arm against the chest with the uninjured arm to stabilize the injury
- Person does not move the arm because of the pain
- Swelling
- Visible deformity
- Tenderness
- Dropped or drooped shoulder
- Bruising

## What to Do

1. Treat for shock.
2. Apply an arm sling and swathe (binder) to stabilize and rest the arm.
3. Apply an ice pack to the area for 20 minutes, three to four times during the next 24 hours.
4. Seek immediate medical care.

# ▶ Contusions

Direct blows to the shoulder resulting in contusions, or bruises, are often called shoulder pointers. Contusions of this type may cause severe discomfort.

## What to Look For

- Swelling
- Pain at the injury site
- Feeling of firmness when pressure is exerted on the shoulder
- Tenderness
- Discoloration under the skin (black and blue)

## What to Do

1. Apply an ice pack to the area for 20 minutes, three to four times during the first 24 hours.
2. Place the arm in a sling and swathe (binder) to stabilize and rest the arm.

## ▶ Tendinitis

The general cause of tendinitis (inflammation) in the shoulder is continuous overuse or unusual use. Repeated arm movement often results in painful shoulders. These injuries are often seen in athletes engaged in the throwing sports (eg, baseball pitcher, football quarterback) and in other sports in which the shoulder is used extensively (eg, swimming).

| What to Look For | What to Do |
|---|---|
| • Constant pain or pain with motion of the shoulder<br>• Limited motion of the shoulder<br>• Crackling sound when the joint is moved<br>• Tenderness over the area | 1. Use an ice massage for 10 minutes after exercise. Fill a Styrofoam cup with water and freeze. Tear a small amount of foam from the top so ice protrudes. Massage firmly over the injured area in a circle about the size of a baseball.<br>2. Use a sling and swathe (binder) to rest the shoulder.<br>3. Use pain medication such as ibuprofen.<br>4. Seek medical advice if needed. |

## ▶ Humerus Fracture

The shaft of the humerus (upper arm) can be felt throughout its entire length along the inner side of the upper arm. Gently pushing on the bone may reveal pain indicating a fracture.

| What to Look For | What to Do |
|---|---|
| • The person reports having one of the following:<br>  • Direct blow to the area<br>  • Twist or fall on the outstretched arm<br>  • Severe pain<br>• Swelling<br>  • Visible deformity (The deformity may be hidden by swelling or by the large muscles surrounding the upper part of the arm.)<br>  • Tenderness if pressed or pushed<br>  • Inability to move the arm<br>  • Person holds the arm against the chest for comfort | 1. Assess and treat for shock if indicated.<br>2. Apply an ice pack for 20 minutes.<br>3. Stabilize the arm by applying one rigid splint on the part of the arm away from the body. Apply an arm sling and swathe (binder).<br>4. Seek immediate medical care. |

# Elbow Injuries

## ▶ Elbow Fractures and Dislocations

All elbow fractures and dislocations should be considered serious and treated with extreme care. Inappropriate care can result in injury to the nearby nerves and blood vessels.

| What to Look For | What to Do |
|---|---|
| • Immediate swelling<br>• Severe pain<br>• Possible visible deformity; compare it with the uninjured elbow<br>• Restricted, painful motion<br>• Numbness or coldness of the hand and fingers below the elbow | 1. **DO NOT** move the elbow.<br>2. Splint the elbow in the position found to prevent nerve and blood vessel damage:<br>   • If straight, keep the splinted elbow straight.<br>   • If bent, keep the elbow bent.<br>3. Apply an ice pack for 20 minutes.<br>4. Seek immediate medical care. |

## ▶ Tennis Elbow

Tennis elbow results from sharp, quick twists of the wrist. Despite its name, it does not occur exclusively from playing tennis. The muscles that bend the wrist back and straighten the fingers all begin in one spot, no bigger than a dime, on the outside bony prominence (protrusion) of the elbow. Tennis elbow, which is an inflammation of the tendons on this outer side of the elbow, can be very painful whenever the wrist and the elbow are used.

| What to Look For | What to Do |
|---|---|
| • Pain that increases while using the arm<br>• Gradual grip weakness<br>• The injured elbow fatigues quicker than normal<br>• Very tender on outer protrusion of elbow | 1. Apply heat before an activity; the person might wear a brace or rubber sleeve on the sore elbow.<br>2. Apply an ice pack for 20 minutes after completion of the activity.<br>3. Seek medical advice for an appropriate rehabilitation program. |

## ▶ Golfer's Elbow

Repetitive motion produces pain. Golfer's elbow is the equivalent of the more common tennis elbow but with pain on the inside of the elbow. It is tendinitis affecting the tendons attached to the bony protrusion on the inside of the elbow.

| What to Look For | What to Do |
|---|---|
| • Pain that increases while using the arm<br>• Gradual grip weakness<br>• The injured elbow fatigues quicker than normal | 1. Apply heat before an activity; the person might wear a brace or rubber sleeve on the tender elbow.<br>2. Apply an ice pack for 20 minutes after completion of an activity.<br>3. Seek medical advice for an appropriate rehabilitation program. |

## ▶ Radius and Ulna Fracture

There are two large bones (<u>radius</u> and <u>ulna</u>) in the forearm, and either or both bones may be broken. When only one bone is broken, the other acts as a splint and there may be little or no deformity. However, a marked deformity may be present in a fracture near the wrist. When both bones are broken, the arm usually appears deformed.

| What to Look For | What to Do |
|---|---|
| Person reports having pain in the forearm or wrist from one of the following:<br>• A direct blow<br>• Falling on an outstretched hand<br>• Visible deformity<br>• Severe pain radiating up and down from the injury site<br>• An inability to move the wrist or pain when moving the wrist | 1. Assess and treat for shock if indicated.<br>2. Apply an ice pack to the area for 20 minutes.<br>3. Do one of the following:<br>  • Keeping the hand and fingers in the position of function (cupping shape as though holding a baseball) with extra padding in the palm, apply a rigid splint against the forearm.<br>  • Apply two rigid splints on both sides of the arm from the tip of the elbow to the fingers.<br>4. Place the arm in a sling and swathe (binder) with the hand in a thumb-up position.<br>5. Seek medical care. |

## ▶ Wrist Fracture

The wrist usually is broken when the person falls with the arm and hand outstretched.

| What to Look For | What to Do |
|---|---|
| • Injury to the wrist associated with a snapping or popping sensation within the wrist<br>• Pain in the wrist that is aggravated by movement<br>• Tenderness<br>• Swelling<br>• Inability or unwillingness to move the wrist<br>• Lumplike deformity on the back of the wrist | 1. Use the RICE procedure (with the exception of compression).<br>2. Stabilize the wrist with a splint.<br>3. Seek medical care. |

# Hand Injuries

## ▶ Crushed Hand

The hand may be fractured by a direct blow or by a crushing injury.

| What to Look For | What to Do |
|---|---|
| • Pain<br>• Swelling<br>• Loss of motion<br>• Open wounds<br>• Broken bones | 1. Control any bleeding<br>2. Cover wounds with a dressing.<br>3. Depending upon the situation, apply an ice pack for no longer than 20 minutes; doing so should not delay seeking medical care.<br>4. Seek medical care. While transporting to medical care, prop the person's hand on a pillow or on his or her chest, or splint the person's hand as you would for a radius and ulna fracture. |

# Finger Injuries

The three bones that make up each finger are the most commonly broken bones in the body. Many of the tendons attached to the finger bones can tear with or without a fracture, and the three joints—the distal interphalangeal, the proximal interphalangeal, and the metacarpal phalangeal—can also be injured.

A so-called finger sprain may be a complicated fracture or dislocation.

## ▶ Finger Fracture

Contrary to popular belief, broken bones—especially the fingers—can move when they are broken.

**What to Look For**

The finger or thumb has:

- A visible deformity; finger has a twisted look
- Immediate pain; hurts with or without movement
- Numbness
- Swelling
- Pinpointed tenderness that usually indicates a fracture

**What to Do**

1. Test for a finger fracture:
   - If possible, straighten the fingers and place them on a hard surface.
   - Tap the tip of the injured finger toward the hand. Pain lower down in the finger or into the hand can indicate a fracture.
2. **DO NOT** try to realign the finger.
3. Gently apply an ice pack.
4. Splint the finger using one of the following methods:
   - Buddy tape the fractured finger to another for support. For a thumb, tape it with three to four figure-eight patterns around the joint. Monitor the finger for swelling and circulation issues.
   - Keep the hand and fingers in the position of function (cupping shape as though holding a baseball) with extra padding in the palm. Secure the hand, fingers, and arm to a rigid splint.
5. Seek medical care.

## ▶ Finger Dislocation

Finger dislocations are common. The same causes of fractured fingers can also cause a dislocated finger.

**What to Look For**

- The finger or thumb has:
  - A visible deformity **Figure 15-3**
  - Immediate pain
  - Swelling
- Shortening of the finger
- May be unable to bend the finger in the injured area; motion is impossible

**What to Do**

1. **DO NOT** try to realign the dislocation.
2. Apply an ice pack for 20 minutes.
3. If possible, splint the finger using one of the following methods:
   - Buddy tape the finger for support. For a thumb, tape it with three to four figure-eight patterns around the joint. Monitor the finger for swelling and circulation issues.
   - Keep the hand and fingers in the position of function (cupping shape as though holding a baseball) with extra padding in the palm. Secure the hand, fingers, and arm to a rigid splint.
4. Seek medical care.

**Figure 15-3**

Finger dislocation.

## ▶ Sprained Finger

The distal joints of the fingers have a ligament on each side of the joint.

**What to Look For**

**What to Do**

- The finger or thumb has been:
  - Jammed or compressed
  - Stepped on
  - Forced or twisted sideways
- Pain and swelling over a joint (especially tenderness on both sides of a joint)
- Inability to make a fist
- Weakness while curling the injured finger alone
- Weakness or pain when gripping

1. Apply an ice pack for 20 minutes.
2. Reevaluate after the ice pack application and seek medical care if pain and weakness exist.
3. Tape fingers with buddy taping for support. Tape thumb with three to four figure-eight patterns around joint.

## ▶ Nail Avulsion

A person may have had a blow to the nail, the nail may have been torn away by a piece of machinery, or a long toenail may have caught on a loop of carpet or other fixed object. An injury in which a nail is partly or completely torn loose is known as a nail avulsion **Figure 15-4**.

**What to Look For**

**What to Do**

The nail may be completely detached or partially held in place by the skin.

1. Secure the damaged nail in place with an adhesive bandage.
2. **DO NOT** trim away the loose nail.
3. Consult a physician for further advice.

**Figure 15-4**

Relieve pain by releasing the blood under a nail.

## ▶ Splinters

Sharp splinters (usually wooden) can be impaled into the skin or under a fingernail or toenail.

| What to Look For | What to Do |
|---|---|
| • A small puncture wound<br>• The sliver may be seen, or in other cases, neither seen nor felt. | 1. If embedded in the skin, use tweezers to remove it. In some cases, you may need to tease it out with a sterile needle until the end can be grasped with tweezers or fingers. Clean the wound with soap and water.<br>2. If the splinter is impaled under a fingernail or toenail and breaks off flush, cut a V-shaped notch in the nail to gain access to the splinter. Remove the embedded splinter by grasping its end with tweezers. |

## ▶ Blood Under a Nail

Blood collects under a fingernail when underlying tissues are bruised (eg, finger struck by a hammer or caught between a door and its frame).

| What to Look For | What to Do |
|---|---|
| • Excruciating pain, because of the pressure of the blood pushing against the nail<br>• Pain that does not disappear until the collection of blood is drained | 1. Immerse the finger in ice water or apply an ice pack with the hand elevated to reduce pain and swelling.<br>2. Relieve the pressure under the injured nail:<br>  • Using a knife, sewing needle, or small drill bit (**DO NOT** use a drill), slowly and gently rotate the sharp point of the object through the nail.<br>3. Apply a dressing to absorb the draining blood and to protect the injured nail.<br>4. If necessary, seek medical care. |

## ▶ Ring Strangulation

Ring strangulation can be a serious condition if it cuts off the blood supply long enough. Permanent damage may result within 4 or 5 hours.

| What to Look For | What to Do |
|---|---|
| The ring has become tight on the finger after an injury or after some other cause of swelling, such as a local reaction to a bee sting. | Try one or more of the following methods to remove a ring:<br>1. Lubricate the finger with soap and water, grease, oil, butter, petroleum jelly, or some other slippery substance, and then try to remove the ring.<br>2. Immerse the finger in cold water or apply an ice pack for several minutes to reduce the swelling.<br>3. Liberally spray window or glass cleaner onto the finger, and then try to slide off the ring.<br>4. Massage the finger from the tip toward the hand to move the swelling; lubricate the finger again and try removing the ring.<br>5. Wind thread around the finger, starting about an inch from the ring edge and going toward the ring, keeping each round of thread touching the next. Wind smoothly and tightly right up to the edge of the ring. This action will push the swelling toward the hand. Slip the end of the thread under the ring with a matchstick or toothpick, then slowly unwind the thread on the hand side of the ring. You should be able to twist the ring gently over the thread and off the finger. |

### FYI

**Ring Removal From an Extremely Swollen Finger**

Rings on swollen fingers are not uncommon, but they must be removed or serious conditions can result. Generally, the removal method is simply to cut the ring off the finger or to use one of several nondestructive removal methods using string or a rubber band. A simple method that eliminates the swelling and permits the removal of a ring involves wrapping the entire finger starting at the nail and wrapping toward the ring with a tight, elastic band, which reduces the swelling and frees the ring.

*Source:* Cresap CR. Removal of a hardened steel ring from an extremely swollen finger. *Am J Emerg Med.* 1995 May;13(3):318-20.

## Hip Joint Injuries

### ▶ Hip Dislocation

A hip can be dislocated by a fall, a blow to the thigh, or direct force to the foot or knee. The hip joint is a stable ball-and-socket joint that requires great force to dislocate. Often a hip is dislocated when the knee strikes the dashboard during a motor vehicle crash. It is difficult to differentiate a hip dislocation from a hip fracture.

| What to Look For | What to Do |
|---|---|
| • Severe pain at the injury site<br>• Swelling at the injury site<br>• Hip is flexed and the knee bent and rotated inward toward the opposite hip<br>• Visible injury | 1. Assess and treat for shock if indicated.<br>2. Stabilize the injury.<br>3. Check for an ankle pulse (posterior tibial).<br>4. Seek medical care. This injury is best transported by EMS personnel. |

## ▶ Hip Fracture

A hip fracture is a fracture of the upper end of the <u>femur</u> (thigh bone), not the pelvis. A fractured hip usually is caused by a fall. Older people, especially women, are susceptible to this type of injury because of brittle bones (osteoporosis). Occasionally, the bone actually fractures while the person is walking, resulting in a fall (rather than the fall causing the fracture).

| What to Look For | What to Do |
|---|---|
| • Severe pain in the groin area<br>• Inability to lift the injured leg<br>• Leg may appear shortened and be rotated with the toes pointing abnormally outward or inward | 1. Treat for shock.<br>2. Stabilize the injured leg against movement.<br>3. Monitor the ankle pulse (posterior tibial).<br>4. Seek immediate medical care. This injury is best transported by EMS personnel. |

# Thigh Injuries

## ▶ Femur Fracture

Because the femur is the largest bone in the body, considerable force is required to break it. Femur injuries can occur in any part of the femur, from the hip to just above the knee joint. A fracture of the femur usually is caused by a fall or a direct blow.

Femur fractures often include open wounds, and external bleeding may be severe. If the blood vessels are damaged, the person may have 1 or 2 quarts (1 to 2 L) of blood loss into the thigh. There may be loss of blood circulation to the lower part of the extremity or nerve damage, especially with lower third femur fractures.

| What to Look For | What to Do |
|---|---|
| • Severe pain at the injury site<br>• Deformity; the leg may appear shorter<br>• Swelling, resulting from severe damage to blood vessels<br>• Person reports having heard or felt a severe pop or snap at the time of injury | 1. Assess and treat for shock if indicated.<br>2. Cover a wound with a sterile dressing.<br>3. Stabilize the injured leg against movement.<br>4. Monitor the ankle pulse (posterior tibial).<br>5. Seek immediate medical care. This injury is best transported by EMS personnel. |

## ▶ Muscle Contusion

The muscle group on the front of the thigh, the quadriceps group, often gets bruised. Depending on the force of impact and the muscles involved, the contusion may be of varying degrees of severity.

| What to Look For | What to Do |
|---|---|
| The person received a direct hit producing:<br>• Swelling<br>• Pain and tenderness<br>• Tightness or firmness of the site when pressed<br>• Visible bruise that may appear hours later | 1. Follow the RICE procedure. Apply an ice pack for 20 minutes, three to four times daily for the next 48 hours.<br>2. Stretch the muscle by bending the knee toward the person's chest. |

## ▶ Muscle Strain

When a muscle is overstretched, it can result in a tear, called a strain. Different degrees of strains occur, but first aid providers will be unable to determine their degree.

| What to Look For | What to Do |
|---|---|
| • Person reports feeling a pop or pulling sensation while running or jumping<br>• Tenderness<br>• Stiffness and pain during movement<br>• Swelling<br>• A visible bruise appearing days later | 1. Follow the RICE procedure. Apply an ice pack for 20 minutes, three to four times daily for the next 48 hours.<br>2. Stretch the muscle, but **DO NOT** force stretching. |

# Knee Injuries

Knee injuries, of which there are many types, are among the most serious joint injuries. Their severity is difficult to determine, thus medical care is necessary if the injury is from being hit or twisted and not from overuse. You probably have seen a physician or an athletic trainer performing stress tests on a player's knee on the sidelines at a football game. Controversy exists about the exact meaning and interpretation of many of the ligament stress tests. First aid providers should not perform such tests.

## ▶ Knee Fracture

A fracture of the knee generally occurs as a result of a fall or a direct blow. Fractures about the knee may occur at the end of the femur, at the end of the tibia, or in the patella (knee cap).

| What to Look For | What to Do |
|---|---|
| Determining whether a fracture exists is difficult. Some fractured knees may look like a dislocation. Other signs include:<br>• Deformity<br>• Tenderness<br>• Swelling | 1. If a pulse can be felt in the ankle (posterior tibial) with no deformity, splint the leg with the knee straight.<br>2. If a pulse can be felt in the ankle with significant deformity, splint the knee in the position found.<br>3. Seek medical care. If a pulse is absent in the ankle, immediately seek medical care. |

## ▶ Knee Dislocation

A knee dislocation is a serious injury. Do not confuse a knee dislocation with a patella dislocation, which is a much less serious injury.

| What to Look For | What to Do |
|---|---|
| • Excruciating pain<br>• Grotesque deformity<br>• Absent pulse in the ankle (posterior tibial) | 1. Stabilize the knee in the position found.<br>2. Seek medical care immediately. |

## ▶ Patella Dislocation

A dislocated patella can be a very painful injury and must be treated immediately. Some people have repeated knee cap dislocations, just as others have a tendency for shoulder dislocations. A dislocated patella most commonly occurs in teenagers and young adults who are engaged in athletic activities.

### What to Look For

- A blow or twisting causes the knee cap to be moved to the outside of the knee joint
- Possible swelling
- Inability to bend or straighten the knee
- Pain
- Deformity compared with the other knee cap
  **Figure 15-5**

### What to Do

1. Follow the RICE procedure (except compression).
2. **DO NOT** try to relocate a dislocated knee cap (sometimes the knee cap replaces itself).
3. Splint the knee in the position found.
4. Seek medical care.

**Figure 15-5**

Patella dislocation.

## ▶ Knee Sprain

Ligament injuries occur most often in sports. The knee is very prone to ligament injury, ranging from mild sprains to complete tearing. The knee will be swollen and painful and usually cannot be used normally.

### What to Look For

At the time of injury, the following signs and symptoms may be present:
- Severe pain
- A pop or snap feeling
- A locking sensation
- Inability to walk without limping
- Inability to bend or straighten the knee

Later, there may be:
- Swelling in the knee
- Bruising

### What to Do

1. Follow the RICE procedure.
2. Seek medical care.

## ▶ Knee Contusion

Contusions of the knee are caused by a direct blow or by falling on the knee.

| What to Look For | What to Do |
|---|---|
| After a direct blow to the knee cap, the person has:<br>• Pain<br>• Swelling<br>• Tenderness<br>• Bruise marks (black-and-blue discoloration) | Follow the RICE procedure. |

# Lower Leg Injuries

## ▶ Tibia and Fibula Fractures

Tibia and <u>fibula</u> injuries can occur at any place between the knee joint and the ankle joint. When both bones are broken, there may be marked deformity of the leg.

When only one bone is broken, the other acts as a splint, and little deformity may be present. Some people with a fibula fracture can walk on the injured leg. When the tibia is broken, an open fracture and severe deformity may exist. Injuries to the blood vessels, caused by the extreme deformity, are common with injuries of the tibia and the fibula, and the pain usually is severe.

| What to Look For | What to Do |
|---|---|
| A direct blow or twisting force produces:<br>• Severe pain<br>• Swelling<br>• Visible deformity<br>• Tenderness when touched | 1. Stabilize the leg using a splint, either improvised by tying the legs together or a rigid splint (two boards or two SAM splints—one on each side to prevent rotation of the lower leg bones). (See Chapter 16, *Splinting Extremities*.)<br>2. Apply an ice pack.<br>3. Seek medical care. |

## ▶ Tibia and Fibula Contusion

Many contusions simply cause a black-and-blue mark and some soreness, then clear up with little attention.

| What to Look For | What to Do |
|---|---|
| • Person received a hit directly on the shin<br>• Tenderness when touched<br>• Sharp pain<br>• The following signs and symptoms appear later:<br>  • Discoloration (black-and-blue mark)<br>  • Difficulty moving ankle up and down<br>  • Numbness or coldness in toes or foot | 1. Expose the injury.<br>2. Apply the RICE procedure. Use an ice pack for 20 minutes, three to four times daily, for the first 48 hours.<br>3. If numbness or tingling exists, seek medical care. |

## ▶ Muscle Cramp

Muscle spasm or cramping usually occurs in the calf and sometimes in the thigh or hamstring. It is a temporary condition of little consequence.

| What to Look For | What to Do |
| --- | --- |
| • Occurs during or after intense exercise sessions<br>• Painful, muscle contraction or spasm that disables the person | There are many treatments for cramps. Try one or more of the following:<br>1. Have the person gently stretch the affected muscle. Because a muscle cramp is an uncontrolled muscle contraction or spasm, a gradual extension of the muscle may help lengthen the muscle fibers and relieve the cramp.<br>2. Relax the muscle by applying pressure to it.<br>3. Apply ice to the cramped muscle to make it relax (unless you are in a cold environment).<br>4. If the cramp is due to exertion in hot conditions, drink lightly salted, cool water (dissolve 1/4 teaspoon [1.25 mL] salt in 1 quart [about 1 L] of water) or a commercial sports drink. |

## ▶ Shin Splints

Shin splints is a term that describes pain in the front of the lower leg, also called the shin. Shin splints are caused by repetitive stress in the leg, such as that caused by running and extensive walking.

| What to Look For | What to Do |
| --- | --- |
| • Ache that occurs during activity but subsides significantly after activity stops<br>• Ache that is a result of an increase in the workout routine (eg, running longer, running on hills)<br>• Chronic condition that gets worse | 1. Apply an ice pack before an activity. Heat can be applied later, when the person is well on the way to recovery.<br>2. Apply pressure with a 3-inch (8-cm) elastic bandage over the sorest point (start below the sore area and spiral wrap up and around the leg).<br>3. Apply an ice pack for 20 minutes after the activity.<br>4. Curtail activity until the shin is pain free.<br>5. Pain medications that are anti-inflammatory drugs may be taken. Use ibuprofen or naproxen. |

## ▶ Ankle and Foot Injuries

The ankle and the foot frequently are injured, mainly by twisting, which stretches or tears the supporting ligaments. Incorrect treatment can have consequences that include lifelong disability. In some cases, the damage requires surgical correction. Most ankle injuries are sprains; about 85% of sprains involve the outside (lateral) ligaments and are caused by the ankle turning or twisting inward **Figure 15-6** .

© American Academy of Orthopaedic Surgeons.

**Figure 15-6**

Sprained ankle.

**What to Look For**

**What to Do**

- Pain and/or a popping or tearing sensation that occurs at the time of the injury
- Swelling and complete loss of function of the ankle that develops minutes after the injury
- Tenderness or pain above, below, and to the sides of the injury when pressed

1. Take off the person's shoe and sock. **DO NOT** move the ankle.
2. Follow the RICE procedure. (**DO NOT** apply heat to the injury.) A horseshoe or "U"-shaped pad kept in place by an elastic bandage reduces fluid in the joint.
3. The amount of swelling and pain does not indicate the severity of the injury. If there is any question about the severity of the injury, splint and seek medical care.

## FYI

**Ankle and Foot Injuries: Is Something Broken?**

Two symptoms were 95% accurate in predicting a broken ankle bone: (1) inability to bear weight and take four steps immediately after the injury and (2) tenderness at the back edge or tip of either malleolus bone (the projections on each side of the ankle). Similar symptoms predicted whether a foot bone was broken: (1) pain in the midfoot or tenderness at the base of the fifth metatarsal bone at the outer edge of the foot or at the navicular bone at the inner edge plus (2) inability to take four steps.

*Source:* Stiell IG, Greenberg GH, McKnight RD, et al. Implementation of the Otawa Ankle Rules. *JAMA.* 1994;271(11):827-832.

## ▶ Toe Injuries

The toes can be injured in various ways. The toes can be stepped on or the foot may kick a hard object, resulting in torn-off nails, hematoma (blood clot) formation under the nails, dislocations, or fractures.

**What to Look For**

**What to Do**

- Pain and swelling
- Deformity

For nail avulsions, splinters, blood under a nail, dislocations, and fractures, refer to the appropriate sections under finger injuries.

# prep kit

## ▶ Ready for Review

- Injuries to the extremities are common.
- There are many types of injuries to the extremities, ranging from simple contusions to complex open fractures.
- RICE is the acronym for Rest, Ice, Compression, and Elevation.
- Shoulder injuries include:
  - Shoulder dislocation
  - Clavicle fracture
  - Contusion
  - Tendinitis
- Elbow injuries include:
  - Elbow fracture and dislocation
  - Tennis elbow
  - Golfer's elbow
- Hand injuries include:
  - Crushed hand
- Finger injuries include:
  - Finger fracture
  - Finger dislocation
  - Sprained finger
  - Nail avulsion
  - Splinters
  - Blood under a nail
  - Ring strangulation
- Hip joint injuries include:
  - Hip dislocation
  - Hip fracture
- Thigh injuries include:
  - Femur fracture
  - Muscle contusion
  - Muscle strain
- Knee injuries include:
  - Knee fracture
  - Knee dislocation
  - Patella dislocation
  - Knee sprain
  - Knee contusion
- Lower leg injuries include:
  - Tibia and fibula fracture
  - Tibia and fibula contusion
  - Muscle cramp
  - Shin splints
  - Ankle and foot injuries
  - Toe injuries

## ▶ Vital Vocabulary

<u>clavicle</u> The collar bone.

<u>contusion</u> A bruise; an injury that causes a hemorrhage in or beneath the skin but does not break the skin.

<u>dislocation</u> The displacement of a bone from its normal joint alignment, out of its socket, or out of its normal position.

<u>femur</u> The thigh bone; the longest and one of the strongest bones in the body.

<u>fibula</u> The smaller of the two bones of the lower leg.

<u>fracture</u> A break or crack in the bone.

<u>humerus</u> The supporting bone of the upper arm.

<u>patella</u> The knee cap; a specialized bone that lies within the tendon of the quadriceps muscle.

<u>radius</u> The bone on the thumb side of the forearm.

<u>scapula</u> The shoulder blade.

<u>sprain</u> A trauma to the joint that injures the ligaments.

<u>strain</u> An injury to a muscle caused by a violent contraction or an excessive, forcible stretching.

<u>tendinitis</u> Inflammation of a tendon caused by overuse.

<u>tibia</u> The shin bone; the larger of the two bones of the lower leg.

<u>ulna</u> The inner bone of the forearm, on the side opposite the thumb.

## ▶ Assessment in Action

During a flag football game at a neighborhood park, your teammate is going back for a sure interception. He jumps for the ball, catches it, and comes down, twisting his ankle in a small hole on the field. Your teammate is in pain and is feeling nauseous.

# prep kit

**Directions:** Circle Yes if you agree with the statement; circle No if you disagree.

Yes　No　**1.** It is difficult to distinguish between a severely sprained ankle and a fractured ankle.

Yes　No　**2.** Use the RICE procedure, regardless of whether the ankle is sprained or fractured.

Yes　No　**3.** Heat should be applied immediately to a sprained ankle to increase blood flow and decrease pain.

Yes　No　**4.** If you are unsure about the injury's severity, you should seek medical care.

## ▶ Check Your Knowledge

**Directions:** Circle Yes if you agree with the statement; circle No if you disagree.

Yes　No　**1.** Injuries heal faster if rested.

Yes　No　**2.** Compression increases internal bleeding, helping the injury to heal faster.

Yes　No　**3.** Tennis elbow results from sharp, quick twists of the wrist.

Yes　No　**4.** The three bones in the fingers are very strong and do not break easily.

Yes　No　**5.** The hip joint is easily dislocated.

Yes　No　**6.** Considerable force is required to break the femur.

Yes　No　**7.** A strain is actually a tear in the muscle.

Yes　No　**8.** Knee injuries are not serious.

Yes　No　**9.** Shin splints are a pain that runs down the back of the leg.

Yes　No　**10.** Most ankle injuries are not fractures.

# Splinting Extremities

## Splinting Extremities

First aid providers usually do not need to splint broken bones. The best first aid for most fractures, whether obvious or not, is non-movement and comfort until emergency medical services (EMS) arrive; however, splinting is advantageous when EMS is delayed or the person is being transported by a first aid provider.

Injured extremities should be stabilized by splinting the extremity in the position in which it was found. To **stabilize** means to minimize further injury by holding a body part to prevent movement. All fractures should be stabilized before a person is moved. The reasons for splinting to stabilize an injured area are to:

- Reduce pain
- Prevent damage to muscles, nerves, and blood vessels
- Prevent a closed fracture from becoming an open fracture
- Reduce bleeding and swelling

All fractures are complicated to some degree by damage to the soft tissue and structures surrounding the bone. The major cause of tissue damage at a fracture site is movement by the end of the broken bone. The end of a broken bone is sharp, and it is important to prevent a fractured bone from moving into soft tissues.

## ▶ Types of Splints

A **splint** is any device used to stabilize a fracture or a dislocation. Such a device can be improvised (eg, a folded newspaper), or it can be one of several commercially available splints (eg, SAM splint). Lack of a commercial splint should never prevent you from properly stabilizing an injured extremity. Splinting sometimes requires improvisation.

A rigid splint is an inflexible device attached to an extremity to maintain stability. It can be a padded board, a piece of heavy cardboard, or a SAM splint molded to fit the extremity. Whatever its construction, a rigid splint must be long enough to be secured well above and below the fracture site. A soft splint, such as a pillow, is useful mainly for stabilizing fractures of the lower leg or the forearm **Figure 16-1** .

A self-splint, or anatomic splint, is almost always available because it uses the body itself as the splint. A self-splint is one in which the injured extremity is tied to an uninjured part (eg, an injured finger to the adjacent finger, the legs together, or an injured arm to the chest).

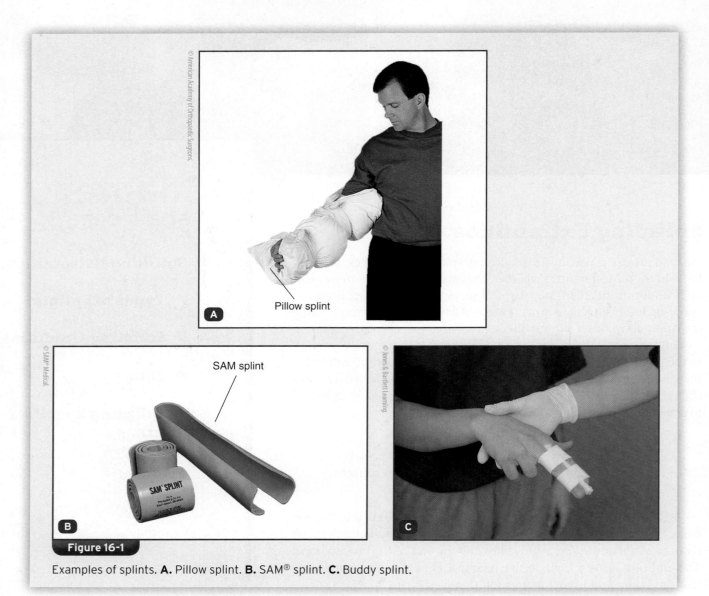

Pillow splint

SAM splint

**A**

**B**

**C**

**Figure 16-1**

Examples of splints. **A.** Pillow splint. **B.** SAM® splint. **C.** Buddy splint.

# ▶ Splinting Guidelines

All fractures and dislocations should be stabilized before the person is moved. When in doubt, apply a splint. To apply a splint:

1. Cover any open wounds with a sterile dressing before applying a splint.

2. Check the CSM (circulation, sensation, movement) in the extremity. If pulses are absent and medical help is hours away, gently line up a fracture or a dislocation to restore blood flow. Support the limb and move it gently to line up the parts. Joints may be left in a position of comfort. Line up the limb above and below the joint; **DO NOT** force anything into position. Any movement of a fracture is expected to cause pain; you should be aware of this and warn the person. You do not have to align the limb perfectly; just align it enough to allow the return of circulation.

3. Determine what to splint by using the **rule of thirds**. Imagine each long bone as being divided into thirds. If the injury is located in the upper or lower third of a bone, assume that the nearest joint is injured. Therefore, the splint should extend to stabilize the bones above and below the unstable joint. For example, for a fracture of the upper third of the tibia (shin bone), the splint must extend above the knee to include the upper leg, as well as the lower leg, because the knee is unstable. For a fracture of the middle third of a bone, stabilize the joints above and below the fracture (eg, the wrist and elbow for a fractured radius or ulna; the shoulder and elbow for a fractured humerus; the knee and ankle for a fractured tibia or fibula). In addition to splinting an upper extremity fracture, place the injured arm in an arm sling and a swathe (binder).

4. If two first aid providers are present, one should support the injury site and minimize movement of the extremity until splinting is completed.

5. When possible, place splint materials on both sides of the injured part, especially when two bones are involved, such as the radius and ulna in the lower arm or the tibia and fibula in the lower leg. This sandwich splint prevents the injured extremity from rotating and keeps the two bones from touching. With rigid splints, use extra padding in natural body hollows and around any deformities.

6. Apply splints firmly but not so tightly that blood flow into an extremity is affected. Check the CSM before and periodically after the splint is applied. If the pulse disappears, loosen the splint enough so you can feel the pulse. Leave the fingers or toes exposed so the CSM can be checked easily.

7. Use the RICE (rest, ice, compression, and elevation) procedure on the injured part. When practical, elevate the injured extremity after it is stabilized to promote drainage and reduce swelling. **DO NOT**, however, apply ice packs if a pulse is absent.

If you suspect a spinal injury, have the person remain as still as possible. **DO NOT** apply a cervical collar. Wait for trained EMS providers to arrive with the proper equipment.

Most fractures do not require rapid transportation. An exception is an arm or a leg without a pulse, which means there is insufficient blood flow to the injured extremity. In that case, immediate medical care is necessary.

Seek medical care for the following injuries or situations:

- Any open fracture
- Any dislocation (injury that causes joint deformity)
- Any joint injury with moderate to severe swelling
- Any injury in which there is deformity, tenderness, or swelling over the bone
- If the person is unable to walk or bear weight after a lower extremity injury
- If a snap, crackle, or pop was heard at the time of injury
- If the injured area, especially a joint, becomes hot, tender, swollen, or painful
- If you are unsure whether a bone was broken
- If the injury does not improve rapidly, especially over the first few days

**CAUTION**

**DO NOT** straighten dislocations or fractures of the spine, elbow, wrist, hip, or knee because of the proximity of major nerves and arteries. Instead, if the CSM assessment findings are normal, splint joint injuries in the position in which you find them.
**DO NOT** apply traction on open fractures. Instead, cover the wound with a sterile dressing and apply a splint.

## ▶ Slings

An open triangular bandage can be used as a **sling**. A folded triangular bandage known as a cravat can be used as a **swathe** (binder) in conjunction with a sling. A cravat can be used instead of a sling when splints on the arm are too large for a sling to fit. Loop the cravat around the wrist and around the neck to support the forearm. To apply an arm sling to the upper arm, forearm, or hand/wrist injuries, follow the steps in **Skill Sheet 16-1**:

1. Hold the person's arm slightly away from the chest, with the wrist and hand slightly higher (about 4 inches [10 cm]) than the tip of the elbow. Place a triangular bandage between the forearm and the chest, with the point of the triangular bandage toward the elbow, and stretch the bandage well beyond the elbow. Pull the upper end of the bandage over the uninjured shoulder (**Step 1**).

2. Bring the lower end of the bandage over the forearm (**Step 2**).

3. Bring the end of the bandage around the neck to the uninjured side and tie to the other end at the hollow above the clavicle on the uninjured side (**Step 3**).

4. If possible, secure the point of the bandage at the elbow with a safety pin or twist it into a pigtail, which can be tied into a knot or tucked inside the sling. Place a swathe (binder) around the upper arm and body. The center of the swathe (binder) should be placed over the arm. The hand should be in thumb-up position within the sling and slightly above the level of the elbow (about 4 inches [10 cm]). Place padding underneath both knots for comfort. Adjust the sling to support the hand and wrist; only the fingers should be exposed (**Step 4**).

If bandages or other resources are unavailable, you may need to improvise a sling **Figure 16-2**.

## Skill Sheet

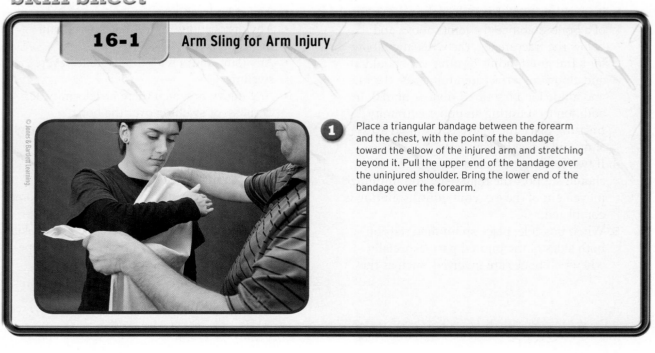

| 16-1 | Arm Sling for Arm Injury |

**1** Place a triangular bandage between the forearm and the chest, with the point of the bandage toward the elbow of the injured arm and stretching beyond it. Pull the upper end of the bandage over the uninjured shoulder. Bring the lower end of the bandage over the forearm.

© Jones & Bartlett Learning

# Skill Sheet Continued

### 16-1    Arm Sling for Arm Injury

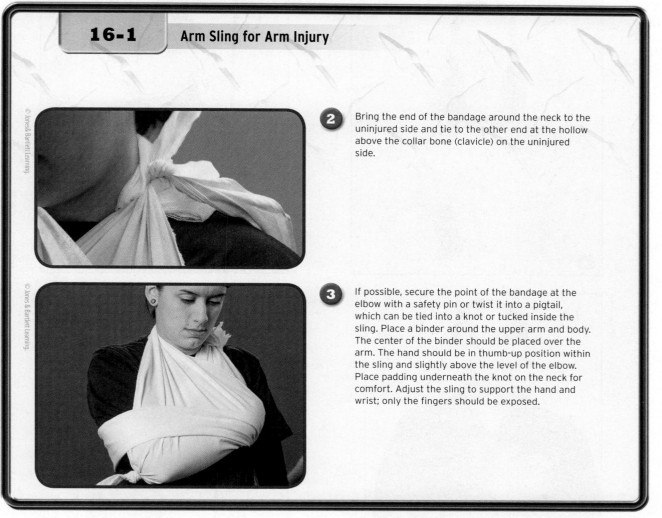

© Jones & Bartlett Learning.

**2** Bring the end of the bandage around the neck to the uninjured side and tie to the other end at the hollow above the collar bone (clavicle) on the uninjured side.

**3** If possible, secure the point of the bandage at the elbow with a safety pin or twist it into a pigtail, which can be tied into a knot or tucked inside the sling. Place a binder around the upper arm and body. The center of the binder should be placed over the arm. The hand should be in thumb-up position within the sling and slightly above the level of the elbow. Place padding underneath the knot on the neck for comfort. Adjust the sling to support the hand and wrist; only the fingers should be exposed.

- Place the hand inside a buttoned jacket.
- Use a belt, necktie, or other clothing item looped around the neck and the injured arm.
- Pin the sleeve of the shirt or jacket to the clothing in the desired position.
- Turn up the lower edge of the person's jacket or shirt over the injured arm and pin it to the upper part of the jacket or shirt.

## ▶ Splinting Specific Areas

### Shoulder

Shoulder injuries involve the clavicle (collar bone), the scapula (shoulder blade), or the head of the humerus (upper arm). To stabilize the shoulder and upper arm against movement, apply an arm sling by following these steps:

1. Support the injured arm slightly away from the chest, with the wrist and hand higher than the elbow.
2. Place an open triangular bandage between the forearm and the chest, with the point stretching well beyond the elbow.
3. Pull the upper end of the bandage over the shoulder on the uninjured side.
4. Bring the lower end of the bandage over the forearm and around the neck to the uninjured side. Tie the end to the other end at the hollow above the clavicle on the uninjured side.
5. Check the pulse and fingernail color for signs of circulation loss. (See Chapter 4, *Finding Out What is Wrong.*)
6. The hand should be in a thumb-up position in the sling and slightly above the level of the elbow.

**Figure 16-2**

Improvised slings. **A.** A buttoned jacket. **B.** A belt, necktie, or other clothing item looped around the neck and the injured arm. **C.** Sleeve of the jacket or shirt pinned to the clothing. **D.** Lower edge of the person's jacket or shirt pinned up over the injured arm.

To further stabilize the arm, fold another triangular bandage to make a swathe that measures 3 to 4 inches (8 to 10 cm) wide. Tie one or two swathes (binders) around the upper arm and chest of the person. This stabilizes the clavicle (collar bone) and most shoulder injuries, as well as upper humerus (upper arm) fractures.

Most shoulder dislocations (about 95%) are anterior, meaning that the top of the humerus pops out in front of the shoulder joint. The person will hold the arm in a fixed position away from the chest wall. In these cases, the most comfortable splinting method is to place a pillow or rolled blanket between the involved arm and the chest. This fills the space created; you can then use cravats or a roller bandage to secure the arm against the chest. If the injury occurs in a remote setting (hours from medical care), use one of the methods described in Chapter 24, *Wilderness First Aid*, to reduce an anterior shoulder dislocation.

## Humerus (Upper Arm)

Fractures of the humerus (upper arm) should be stabilized with a rigid splint. Extend the splint along the outside of the humerus. Then apply a sling and a swathe over the rigid splint, using the chest wall as an additional splint **Skill Sheet 16-2**.

1. Gently place the injured arm across the chest. If available, tie a rigid splint to the outside of the arm (**Step 1**). If a rigid splint is not available, go to Step 2.

2. Loop a cravat bandage or strap around the wrist and neck to allow the arm to hang in the sling position. Gravity will then provide gentle traction (**Step 2**).

3. Secure the arm to the chest with a swathe (folded triangular bandage) (**Step 3**).

## Skill Sheet

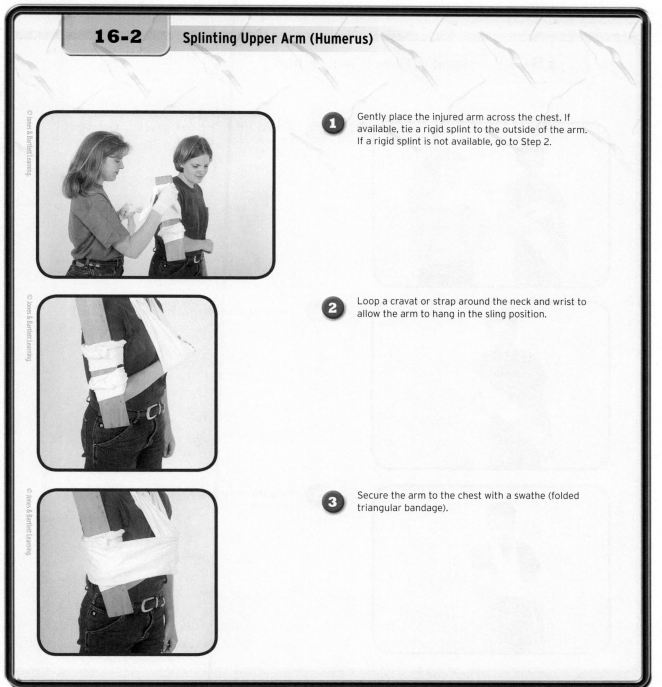

### 16-2    Splinting Upper Arm (Humerus)

**1** Gently place the injured arm across the chest. If available, tie a rigid splint to the outside of the arm. If a rigid splint is not available, go to Step 2.

**2** Loop a cravat or strap around the neck and wrist to allow the arm to hang in the sling position.

**3** Secure the arm to the chest with a swathe (folded triangular bandage).

© Jones & Bartlett Learning.

## Elbow

An elbow must be stabilized in the position in which it is found—if bent, splint it bent; if straight, splint it straight. If the injured elbow is straight, place a rigid splint along the inside of the arm from the hand to the armpit. Secure the splint with a roller bandage or several cravat bandages. For a bent elbow, apply a rigid splint diagonally, so that it extends from the humerus (near the armpit) to the wrist, to prevent motion of the elbow. Depending on how bent the elbow is, you can also use a sling and a swathe (binder) for a bent elbow.

To splint an elbow in the bent position, follow the steps in **Skill Sheet 16-3** :

1. If the injured elbow is bent, place a rigid splint from the upper arm to the wrist (**Step 1**).
2. Tie a rigid splint onto the arm with cravat bandages (**Step 2**).
3. Place the arm in a sling, and check CSM (**Step 3**).

## Skill Sheet

**16-3**    **Splinting Elbow in Bent Position**

1. If the injured elbow is bent, place a rigid splint from the upper arm to the wrist.

2. Tie a rigid splint onto the arm with cravat bandages.

3. Place the arm in a sling, and check CSM (circulation, sensation, movement).

© Jones & Bartlett Learning. Courtesy of MIEMSS.

To splint an elbow in the straight position, follow the steps in **Skill Sheet 16-4**:

1. If the injured elbow is straight, place a rigid splint along the inside of the arm from the hand to the armpit **(Step 1)**.

2. Secure with a roller bandage or several cravat bandages **(Step 2)**.
3. Check CSM **(Step 3)**.

# Skill Sheet

## 16-4    Splinting Elbow in Straight Position

**1** If the injured elbow is straight, place a rigid splint along the inside of the arm from the hand to the armpit.

**2** Secure with a roller bandage or several cravat bandages.

**3** Check CSM (circulation, sensation, movement).

© Jones & Bartlett Learning. Courtesy of MIEMSS.

## Forearm

To stabilize a forearm fracture, place the hand of the injured arm in the position of function (hand looks like it is holding a baseball) by placing a rolled pair of socks or a roller bandage in the palm. Then attach a rigid splint that extends past the tips of the fingers along the forearm. An option is to place splints on both sides of the injured part to keep the forearm from twisting or rotating **Figure 16-3**.

Keep the person's thumb in an upright position so that the two bones in the forearm (the radius and the ulna) do not touch each other. Secure the splint with a roller bandage or several cravats. A pillow or a rolled, folded blanket also can be secured to the arm. Put the arm in a sling and secure it with a swathe (binder) around the body **Figure 16-4**.

To splint the forearm, follow the steps in **Skill Sheet 16-5** and **Skill Sheet 16-6**:

1. Place a rigid splint on the forearm. (You may also consider placing two rigid splints on both sides of the forearm.) **(Step 1)**
2. Secure the splint onto the arm by using either a roller bandage or folded triangular bandages (known as cravat bandages) **(Step 2)**.
3. Place the arm in a sling. A binder or swathe around the body is recommended. Keep the thumb in the upright position **(Step 3)**.

## Wrist, Hand, and Fingers

To stabilize the wrist, hand, and fingers, use one of the following three methods:

- Place the injured hand in the position of function (hand looks like it is holding a baseball) by placing a rolled pair of socks or a roller bandage in the palm. Then attach a rigid splint that extends past the tips of the fingers along the forearm **Figure 16-5**.
- Place the hand in the position of function, mold a pillow around the hand and forearm, and tie the pillow in place with cravats or a roller bandage. Then place the arm in a sling and a swathe (binder), with the thumb in an upright position.
- Splint fingers by taping them together (buddy taping), with gauze separating the fingers.

## Pelvis and Hip

If you suspect a pelvis or hip fracture, stabilize the person as you found him or her. Treat the person for shock, **DO NOT** lift the legs, and wait for EMS to arrive. Pelvis and hip fractures require a long backboard (spine board).

Keep thumb upright.

Rigid splint from palm out past elbow.

**A**

Splints should be on both sides to prevent rotation (shows use of cardboard).

**B**

© American Academy of Orthopaedic Surgeons.

**Figure 16-3**

Splinting a forearm fracture. Attach a rigid splint that extends along the forearm **(A)**. An option is to place splints on both sides of the injured part **(B)**.

**Figure 16-4**

An arm sling with a swathe (binder) helps stabilize upper extremity injuries.

**Figure 16-5**

Splinting a wrist, hand, or finger fracture.

## Skill Sheet

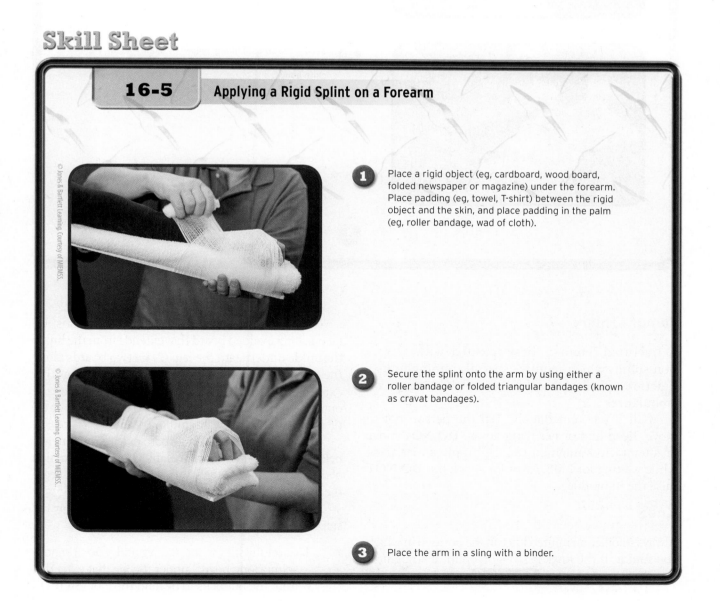

### 16-5   Applying a Rigid Splint on a Forearm

**1** Place a rigid object (eg, cardboard, wood board, folded newspaper or magazine) under the forearm. Place padding (eg, towel, T-shirt) between the rigid object and the skin, and place padding in the palm (eg, roller bandage, wad of cloth).

**2** Secure the splint onto the arm by using either a roller bandage or folded triangular bandages (known as cravat bandages).

**3** Place the arm in a sling with a binder.

## Skill Sheet

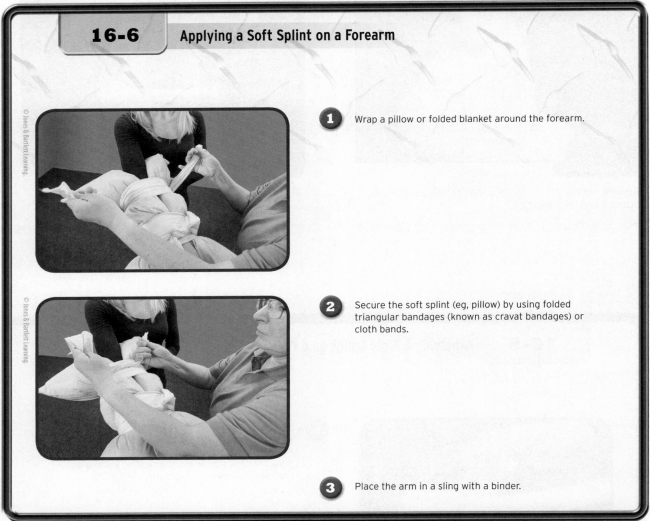

**16-6**    **Applying a Soft Splint on a Forearm**

**1** Wrap a pillow or folded blanket around the forearm.

**2** Secure the soft splint (eg, pillow) by using folded triangular bandages (known as cravat bandages) or cloth bands.

**3** Place the arm in a sling with a binder.

### Femur (Thigh)

A fractured femur is best splinted with a traction splint, which requires special training to use. Traction splints are seldom available except on ambulances.

Call 9-1-1 immediately. Tell the person not to move. Keep him or her lying down. **DO NOT** move or attempt to straighten the leg. Apply an ice pack while waiting for EMS. Treat for shock but **DO NOT** raise the injured leg.

### Knee

Always stabilize an injured knee in the position in which you find it. If the knee is straight, splint it straight; if it is bent, splint it bent **Figure 16-6** .

For a straight knee, there are three options: (1) tie one long, padded board that extends from the hip to the ankle underneath the leg; (2) tie two boards along the sides of the leg, one between the person's legs that extends from the groin to the foot and the other on the outer side that extends from the hip to the foot; or (3) tie the injured leg to the uninjured one.

For a bent knee, tie a long board extending from just below the hip to just above the ankle to prevent motion of the knee. Or, place a pillow or a rolled blanket beneath the knee and tie the injured leg to the uninjured leg.

To splint a knee in the straight position, follow the steps in **Skill Sheet 16-7** :

1. Carefully lift the injured leg and place a rigid splint (long board) under the leg that extends from the buttocks to beyond the foot (**Step 1**).

# Skill Sheet

**16-7** **Splinting a Knee in the Straight Position**

**1** Lift the injured leg and place a rigid splint (long board) under the leg. The splint should extend from the buttocks to beyond the foot.

**2** Place cravat bandages under the rigid splint and place soft padding under the knee and ankle.

**3** Tie the cravat bandages. **DO NOT** tie the knots over the injured area.

2. Place cravat bandages under the rigid splint and place soft padding under the knee and ankle (**Step 2**).

3. Tie the cravat bandages. **DO NOT** tie the knots over the injured area (**Step 3**).

To splint a knee in the bent position, follow the steps in **Skill Sheet 16-8**:

1. Place a rigid splint (long board) against the injured leg. **DO NOT** place the splint against the knee (**Step 1**).

**Figure 16-6**

Splint knee in position found. **A.** If the knee is bent, splint it bent. **B.** If the knee is straight, splint it straight.

## Skill Sheet

### 16-8    Splinting a Knee in the Bent Position

**1** Place a rigid splint (long board) against the injured leg. **DO NOT** place the splint against the knee.

**2** Tie a cravat bandage around the splint and lower leg.

# Skill Sheet Continued

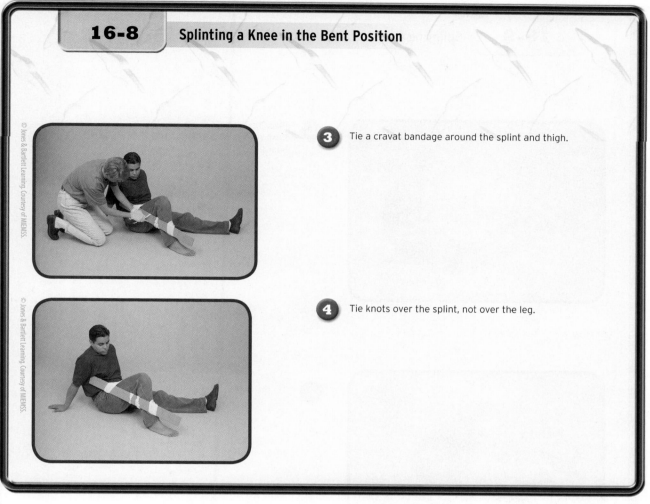

**16-8** Splinting a Knee in the Bent Position

**3** Tie a cravat bandage around the splint and thigh.

**4** Tie knots over the splint, not over the leg.

2. Tie a cravat bandage around the splint and lower leg (**Step 2**).
3. Tie a cravat bandage around the splint and thigh (**Step 3**).
4. Tie knots over the splint, not over the leg (**Step 4**).

## Lower Leg

Stabilize the lower leg with two boards that extend from the upper thigh to the bottom of the foot. Or, place a folded blanket or pillow between the person's legs for padding, and then tie the injured leg to the uninjured leg with several swathes, cravats, or bandages.

To splint the lower leg using the self-splint method, follow the steps in **Skill Sheet 16-9**:

1. Place padding (such as a folded blanket) between the legs. Push the cravat bandages under the leg with a thin board (**Step 1**).
2. Tie the legs together (**Step 2**).
3. Tie knots between the legs, over the padding (folded blanket) (**Step 3**).

## Skill Sheet

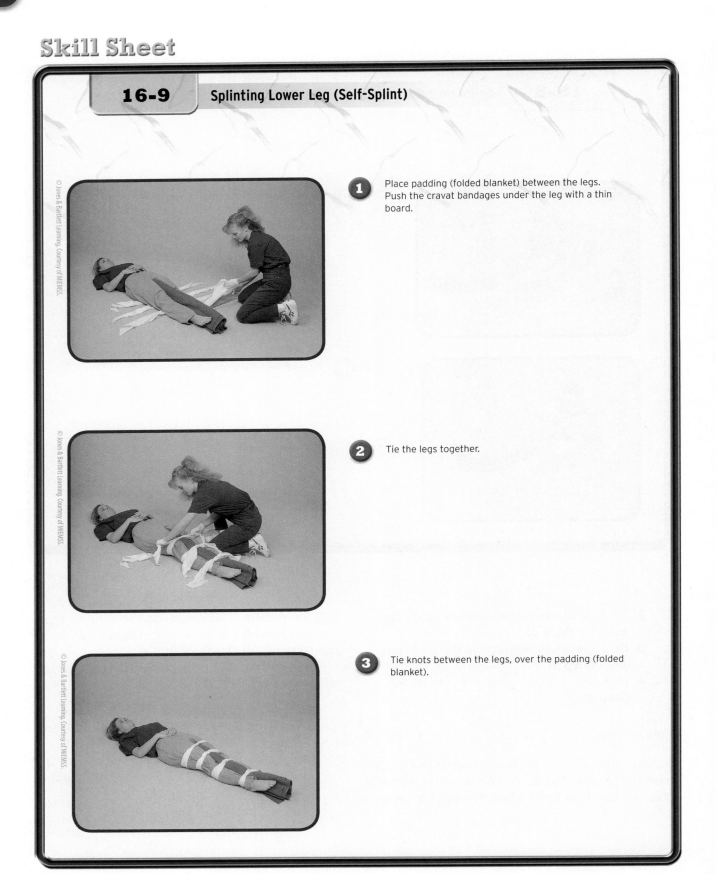

**16-9** | **Splinting Lower Leg (Self-Splint)**

**1** Place padding (folded blanket) between the legs. Push the cravat bandages under the leg with a thin board.

**2** Tie the legs together.

**3** Tie knots between the legs, over the padding (folded blanket).

© Jones & Bartlett Learning, Courtesy of MIEMSS.

To splint the leg using rigid splints, follow the steps in **Skill Sheet 16-10**:

1. Place one rigid splint (board) on the outside (lateral) and another inside (medial). Push the cravat bandages under the leg and splints with a thin board **(Step 1)**.
2. Tie both splints and leg together with cravat bandages **(Step 2)**.
3. Tie knots on top of the splint (board) **(Step 3)**.

## Ankle and Foot

Treat ankle and foot injuries with the RICE procedure. To further stabilize an ankle, wrap a pillow or folded blanket around the ankle and foot and tie with cravats **Figure 16-7**.

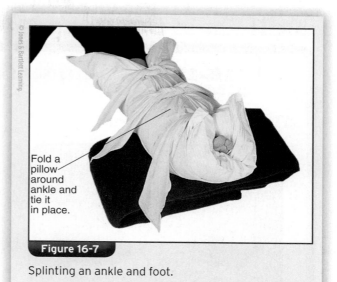

Fold a pillow around ankle and tie it in place.

**Figure 16-7**

Splinting an ankle and foot.

# Skill Sheet

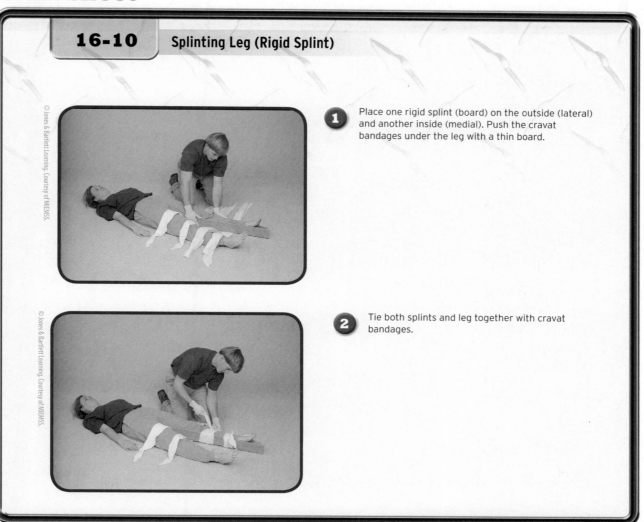

## 16-10   Splinting Leg (Rigid Splint)

**1** Place one rigid splint (board) on the outside (lateral) and another inside (medial). Push the cravat bandages under the leg with a thin board.

**2** Tie both splints and leg together with cravat bandages.

*(Continues)*

## Skill Sheet Continued

**16-10**     Splinting Leg (Rigid Splint)

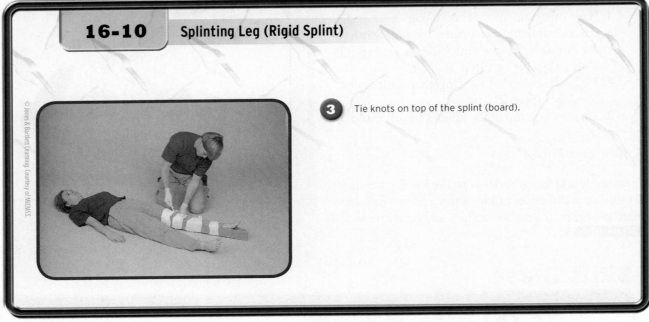

**3** Tie knots on top of the splint (board).

## ▶ Ready for Review

- Until medical care is available, stabilize the injury by splinting the extremity in the position found.
- A splint is any device used to stabilize a fracture or dislocation.
- When in doubt, apply a splint.
- A sling is any bandage or material that helps support the weight of an injured area.

## ▶ Vital Vocabulary

**rule of thirds** A system that divides each long bone into thirds to determine which section(s) of an injured bone should be splinted.

**sling** A triangular bandage applied around the neck to support an injured upper extremity; any material long enough to suspend an upper extremity by passing the material around the neck; used to support and protect an injury of the arm, shoulder, or clavicle.

**splint** Any support used to stabilize a fracture or to restrict movement of a part.

**stabilize** To minimize further injury by holding a body part to prevent movement.

**swathe** A cravat tied around the body to decrease movement of a part.

## ▶ Assessment in Action

You are out with your best friend at a dog park, walking her Irish wolfhound. Your friend is animated and engrossed in your conversation. Suddenly, a rabbit leaps out of the hedges and the dog lurches forward, pulling your friend and causing her to trip and let go of the leash. After you regain control of the dog, your friend complains about pain in one of her fingers, which appears to be deformed.

*Directions:* Circle Yes if you agree with the statement; circle No if you disagree.

Yes    No    **1.** You should stabilize the finger until medical care becomes available.

Yes    No    **2.** You should splint the finger to prevent a possible closed fracture from becoming an open fracture.

Yes    No    **3.** Splinting increases blood flow to the fracture, thus speeding up the healing process.

Yes    No    **4.** If you do not have a commercial splint, you could improvise one.

## ▶ Check Your Knowledge

*Directions:* Circle Yes if you agree with the statement; circle No if you disagree.

Yes    No    **1.** All fractures are complicated to some degree by damage to the soft tissue and structures surrounding the bone.

Yes    No    **2.** A rigid splint should never be used on an extremity.

Yes    No    **3.** All fractures and dislocations should be stabilized before the person is moved.

Yes    No    **4.** Always check the CSM in the extremity.

Yes    No    **5.** Shoulder injuries can involve the clavicle, the scapula, and the tibia.

Yes    No    **6.** An elbow must be stabilized in the position in which it is found.

Yes    No    **7.** Always straighten an injured knee before splinting it.

Yes    No    **8.** First aid providers should always use traction splints on leg fractures.

Yes    No    **9.** Buddy taping is when you tape two fingers together with gauze separating the fingers.

Yes    No    **10.** You can make a temporary sling by pinning a shirt or coat sleeve to the front of the coat or shirt.

# Sudden Illness

**17**

## Chapter
### at a glance

## ▶ Unexplained Change in Responsiveness

People can be fully alert (responsive), can be completely unresponsive, or can range anywhere between these two. Not all responsive people are fully alert, and they may respond to different levels of stimulation; for example a person who does not respond to your voice may react when you squeeze his or her shoulder muscle. The level of responsiveness and mental status indicate how well the brain is functioning.

The main causes for a decrease in a person's alertness and responsiveness are brain injury and lack of either oxygen or glucose reaching the brain. The mnemonic STOP offers clues to the cause(s) of changes in responsiveness Table 17-1 .

## ▶ Heart Attack

Heart muscle needs oxygen to survive. The coronary arteries are the vessels that supply blood and oxygen to the heart muscle, the myocardium. When the blood supply is cut off, a **heart attack**, or myocardial infarction (MI), results. Blockage of blood flow occurs as the vessel walls slowly become thicker and harder due to the buildup of plaque (mainly cholesterol). This slow process is known as atherosclerosis

**Figure 17-1** . If part of the plaque breaks open, a clot can form over it, causing a sudden, complete blockage of the artery, which results in a heart attack.

Heart and blood vessel disease is America's number one killer. About half of the deaths from heart and blood vessel disease are from impairment of blood flow to the heart, known as coronary heart disease, which includes heart attack. The Centers for Disease Control and Prevention (CDC) report over 610,000 people a year die from heart disease. Over 325,000 people a year experience an out-of-hospital cardiac arrest, according to the American Heart Association.

## Table 17-1   Causes of Changes in Responsiveness: STOP Mnemonic

| S | Sugar<br>Seizures<br>Stroke<br>Shock | Blood glucose too low (insulin reaction) or too high (diabetic coma) |
|---|---|---|
| T | Temperature | Too high (heat stroke) or too low (hypothermia) |
| O | Oxygen | Inadequate oxygen |
| P | Poisoning<br>Pressure on brain | Drug/alcohol overdose; carbon monoxide poisoning<br>Head injury |

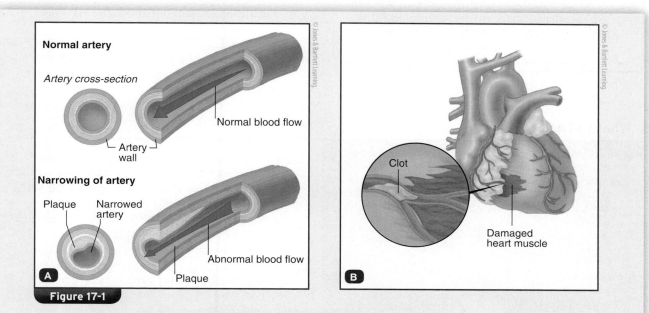

**Figure 17-1**

**A.** A normal artery with normal blood flow and an artery with plaque buildup. **B.** A heart attack occurs when a clot prevents blood from flowing to a part of the heart.

## FYI

**Risk Factors for Heart Disease**
Several factors contribute to an increased risk of heart attack and stroke. The more risk factors present, the greater the possibility that a person will develop heart disease.

**Risk Factors You Cannot Change**
- *Heredity.* Tendencies appear in family lines.
- *Sex.* Men have a greater risk, although heart attack is still the leading cause of death among women.
- *Age.* Most people who experience a heart attack are 65 years or older.

**Risk Factors You Can Change or Control**
- *Cigarette smoking.* Smokers have more than twice the risk of heart attack as nonsmokers.
- *High blood pressure.* This condition adds to the heart's workload.
- *High blood cholesterol level.* Too much cholesterol in the blood can cause a buildup on the walls of the arteries.
- *Diabetes.* This condition affects the blood's cholesterol and triglyceride levels.
- *Obesity.* Being overweight influences blood pressure and blood cholesterol, can result in diabetes, and can place added strain on the heart.
- *Physical inactivity.* Inactive people have twice the risk of heart attack as active people.
- *Stress.* All people feel stress but react in different ways. Excessive, long-term stress can lead to physical conditions in some people.

## Difference Between Heart Attack and Cardiac Arrest

The conditions *heart attack* and *cardiac arrest* confuse many people. The two are very different, and so is the first aid and emergency care for them.

- *Heart attack.* When one or more of the arteries delivering blood to the heart becomes blocked, a heart attack results. Oxygen-rich blood cannot reach the heart muscle, and the heart muscle becomes damaged. This damage to the heart muscle can lead to disturbances of the heart's electrical system and can lead to cardiac arrest.
- *Cardiac arrest.* Cardiac arrest occurs either when the heart stops beating (asystole) or when the heart's lower chambers (ventricles) suddenly develop a rapid irregular rhythm (ventricular fibrillation), causing the ventricles to quiver rather than contract. The quivering motion of the ventricles renders the heart an ineffective pump that can no longer supply the body and brain with oxygen-rich blood. Within seconds, the person becomes unresponsive and has no pulse. Only immediate action such as cardiopulmonary resuscitation (CPR) and external defibrillation can offer hope of survival.

Refer to **Flowchart 17-1** for additional information regarding the care of a person with a heart attack.

### What to Look For

- Chest pain that feels like pressure, squeezing, or fullness, usually in the center of the chest. It may also be felt in the jaw, shoulder, arms, or back; back or jaw pain is more common in women. The pain may last for more than 5 minutes, or it may come and go.
- Sweating or cold sweats
- Light-headedness or dizziness
- Nausea or vomiting (more common in women)
- Numbness, aching, or tingling in the arm (usually the left arm)
- Shortness of breath (more common in women)
- Weakness or fatigue, especially in older adults

### What to Do

1. Have the person sit, with knees raised, and lean against a stable support (ie, fence post, tree trunk) **Figure 17-2**. Try to keep the person calm. **DO NOT** allow the person to walk.
2. Call 9-1-1 immediately. **DO NOT** drive the person to a medical facility; wait for EMS to arrive.
3. Loosen any tight clothing.
4. Ask if the person takes any chest pain medication, such as nitroglycerin, for a known heart condition, and, if so, help him or her take it.
5. If the person is alert, able to swallow, and not allergic to aspirin, help the person take one adult aspirin (325 mg) or two to four baby aspirins (81 mg each). Pulverize or have the person crunch them with his or her teeth before swallowing for faster results.
6. Monitor breathing. If the person becomes unresponsive and stops breathing, begin CPR. (See Chapter 5, *CPR*.)

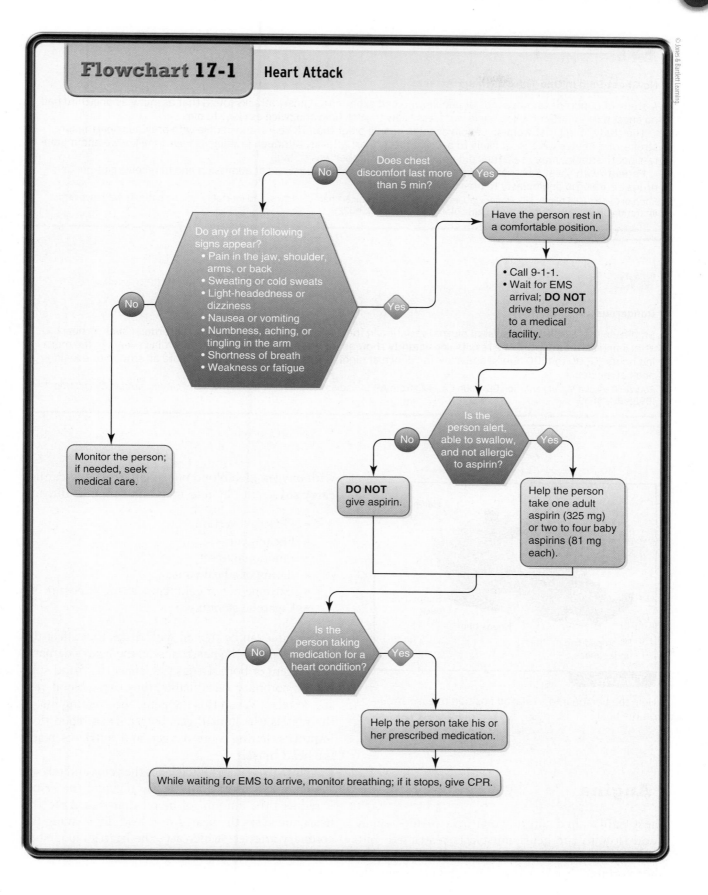

**Flowchart 17-1**   **Heart Attack**

Does chest discomfort last more than 5 min?

No → Do any of the following signs appear?
- Pain in the jaw, shoulder, arms, or back
- Sweating or cold sweats
- Light-headedness or dizziness
- Nausea or vomiting
- Numbness, aching, or tingling in the arm
- Shortness of breath
- Weakness or fatigue

No → Monitor the person; if needed, seek medical care.

Yes / Yes → Have the person rest in a comfortable position.

- Call 9-1-1.
- Wait for EMS arrival; **DO NOT** drive the person to a medical facility.

Is the person alert, able to swallow, and not allergic to aspirin?

No → **DO NOT** give aspirin.

Yes → Help the person take one adult aspirin (325 mg) or two to four baby aspirins (81 mg each).

Is the person taking medication for a heart condition?

No

Yes → Help the person take his or her prescribed medication.

While waiting for EMS to arrive, monitor breathing; if it stops, give CPR.

**No Chest Pain in One-Third of Heart Attacks**

A study of hundreds of thousands of people who had experienced heart attacks found that as many as one-third had no chest pain and that these people were less likely to seek help and twice as likely to die.

The study found that women, people of color, people older than 75 years, and people with previous heart failure, stroke, or diabetes were most likely to have painless heart attacks. Although physicians have long known about painless heart attacks, many said they did not realize the number was so high.

Patients with chest pain were more than twice as likely to be diagnosed at admission and to receive clot-busting drugs or undergo angioplasty to open clogged arteries.

*Source:* Canto JG, Shlipak MG, Rogers WJ, et al. Prevalence, clinical characteristics, and mortality among patients with myocardial infarction presenting without chest pain. *JAMA* 2000;283:3223-3229.

**Dangerous Morning Hours**

Studies in the 1990s demonstrated diurnal variation in the onset of acute cardiovascular disorders (such as heart attack and cardiac death). The results consistently show an increased incidence of acute cardiac events in the morning hours (0600 to 1200 hours) and a low incidence at night. Some data suggest another late afternoon or evening peak of incidence.

*Source:* Peckova M, Fahrenbruch CE, Cobb LA, Hallstrom AP. Circadian variation in the occurrence of cardiac arrests. *Circulation* 1998;98(1):31-39.

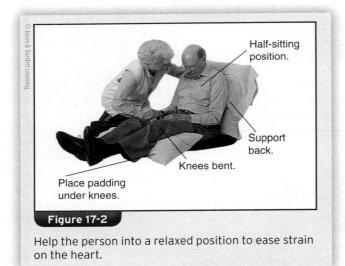

Half-sitting position.

Support back.

Knees bent.

Place padding under knees.

**Figure 17-2**

Help the person into a relaxed position to ease strain on the heart.

## ▶ Angina

Chest pain called **angina pectoris** results when blood flow to the heart muscle is restricted, but not completely blocked **Table 17-2**. Angina occurs when coronary arteries supplying the heart muscle with oxygen-rich blood become narrow and cannot carry sufficient blood to meet the demands during:

- Physical exertion
- Excitement
- Emotional upset
- Eating of a heavy meal
- Extreme hot or cold temperature exposure
- Cigarette smoking

Angina can be treated with drugs that affect the blood supply to the heart muscle, the heart's demand for oxygen, or both. Drugs that affect the blood supply are coronary vasodilators; they cause blood vessels to relax. When this happens, the opening inside the vessels (the lumen) gets bigger. Then blood flow improves, letting more oxygen and nutrients reach the heart muscle.

Nitroglycerin mainly relaxes the veins and relaxes the coronary arteries a little. By relaxing the veins, it reduces the amount of blood that returns to the heart and eases the heart's workload. By relaxing the coronary arteries, it increases the heart's blood supply. Physicians often prescribe nitroglycerin for those with angina.

## What to Look For

It can be difficult to differentiate a heart attack from angina, even for physicians. Differentiate angina from a heart attack by these signs and symptoms:

- Chest pain is described as crushing, squeezing, or like somebody standing on the person's chest.
- Pain can spread to the jaw, the arms (frequently the left arm), and the midback.
- Pain usually lasts from 3 to 10 minutes, but rarely longer than 10 minutes.
- The pain is almost always relieved by the person's prescribed nitroglycerin.
- Pain can be associated with shortness of breath, nausea, or sweating.
- Person feels anxious.

## What to Do

1. Have the person stop what he or she is doing and sit down. Keep bystanders away. Provide calm reassurance to help reduce the person's anxiety.
2. If the person has medically prescribed nitroglycerin, either tablets or a spray, let the person use it. Follow the prescription label's directions. If necessary, help him or her use it.
3. If the chest pain or discomfort does not improve within 5 minutes after taking one dose of nitro-glycerin, call 9-1-1. Previously, people were told to take up to three nitroglycerin tablets, 5 minutes apart, when they had chest pain or discomfort. This procedure has been changed so that if there is no improvement within 5 minutes after taking one dose, 9-1-1 should be called.

### Table 17-2  Chest Pain

| Cause of Pain | Characteristics | Care |
|---|---|---|
| Muscle or rib pain from exercise or injury | Reproduced by movement<br>Tender spot when pressed | Rest<br>Aspirin or ibuprofen |
| Respiratory infection (eg, pneumonia, bronchitis, pleuritis) | Cough<br>Fever<br>Sore throat<br>Production of sputum (mucus) | Antibiotics |
| Indigestion | Belching<br>Heartburn<br>Nausea<br>Sour taste | Antacids |
| Angina pectoris | Lasts less than 10 min (but pain is similar to that of a heart attack) | Rest<br>Prescribed medication |
| Heart attack (myocardial infarction) | Lasts more than 10 min<br>Pressure, squeezing, or pain near center of the chest<br>Pain spreads to shoulders, neck, or arms<br>Light-headedness, fainting, sweating, nausea, shortness of breath | Call 9-1-1<br>Check breathing<br>Resting position<br>Prescribed medication |

## FYI

### Other Causes of Chest Pain

Not all causes of chest pain relate to the heart, including:

- Muscle or rib pain due to exercise, excessive coughing, or injury. The person can reproduce the pain by movement, and often the area of complaint is tender when pressed. Rest and aspirin or ibuprofen relieves the pain.
- Respiratory infections such as pneumonia, bronchitis, pleuritis, or lung injury. Chest pain due to these conditions usually worsens when the person coughs or breathes deeply. Fever and colored sputum might be present. The person needs medical care and may require prescribed medications.
- Indigestion, usually accompanied by belching, heartburn, nausea, and a sour taste in the mouth. This type of pain is relieved by antacids.

**Figure 17-3**

Severe brain hemorrhage causing a stroke.

**Figure 17-4**

A blood clot can block the brain's blood supply.

## ▶ Stroke (Cerebral Vascular Accident)

A **stroke**, also known as a cerebral vascular accident (CVA), occurs when there is a sudden interruption of blood flow to the brain. When arteries in the brain rupture **Figure 17-3** or become blocked **Figure 17-4**, part of the brain does not receive the blood flow it needs. Deprived of oxygen-rich blood, nerve cells in the affected area of the brain cannot function and die within minutes. Because dead brain cells are not replaced, the devastating effects of strokes often are permanent. When nerve cells do not function, the part of the body they control cannot function either. Stroke occurs mostly in older people; however, it is not limited to older people.

Strokes are classified as ischemic or hemorrhagic:

- *Ischemic stroke.* This type of stroke occurs when blood vessels to the brain become narrowed or clogged with fatty deposits called plaque, cutting off blood flow to brain cells. High blood pressure is the most important risk factor for ischemic stroke and can be controlled. Ischemic strokes are the most common type of stroke and account for about 85% of all strokes. Ischemic strokes usually occur at night or first thing in the morning.

Because tissue plasminogen activators (tPA) and other clot-busting drugs must be given as soon as possible after stroke onset

## Table 17-3  Cincinnati Prehospital Stroke Scale

| Test | Normal | Abnormal |
|------|--------|----------|
| *Facial droop* **Figure 17-5**. Ask the person to show his or her teeth or to smile. | Both sides of face move equally well. | One side of the face does not move as well as the other. |
| *Arm drift* **Figure 17-6**. Ask the person to close his or her eyes and hold out both arms with palms up. | Both arms move the same, or both arms do not move. | One arm does not move, or one arm drifts down compared with the other side. |
| *Speech*. Ask the person to say, "The sky is blue in Cincinnati." | The person uses correct words with no slurring. | The person slurs words, uses inappropriate words, or is unable to speak. |

**Figure 17-5**

Facial droop.

A **transient ischemic attack** (TIA; also commonly known as a "little stroke") is a form of stroke that occurs when a part of the brain is deprived of oxygen-rich blood long enough to cause symptoms but not long enough to cause permanent damage. The person may have similar signs and symptoms of a CVA, but the episode resolves completely within 12 hours.

Immediately seek medical care if there is a possibility of stroke. Any or all of the following procedures might be needed:

- Medication to control high blood pressure
- Medication to reduce brain swelling
- Surgery to repair an aneurysm or remove a blood clot

See  **Table 17-3** for help determining whether a person may be experiencing a stroke.

### FYI

Women especially need to know the warning signs of stroke, because they account for over 60% of the deaths from stroke. The most effective treatments for stroke are only available if the stroke is recognized within three hours of symptom onset.

Source: National Stroke Association. "Women and Stroke." http://www.stroke.org/understand-stroke/impact-stroke/women-and-stroke

(within 3 hours), it is important to recognize a stroke and to seek immediate medical care.

- *Hemorrhagic stroke*. About 15% of all strokes happen when a blood vessel ruptures in or near the brain. This kind of stroke is often associated with a very severe headache, nausea, and vomiting. Usually the symptoms appear suddenly.

Refer to **Flowchart 17-2** for additional information regarding the care of a person who is having a stroke.

**Figure 17-6**

**A.** Normal arm position. **B.** Arm droop.

## What to Look For

The acronym FAST acts as an assessment tool to help determine if a stroke may have occurred:

- **F** = *Face*. Ask the person to smile. It is abnormal for one side of the face not to move well compared with the other side.
- **A** = *Arms*. Ask the person to close his or her eyes and raise both arms with the palms up. It is abnormal if one arm drifts downward when held extended.
- **S** = *Speech*. Ask the person to repeat a simple phrase (eg, "The sky is blue."). It is abnormal if the person slurs words, uses the wrong words, or cannot speak at all.
- **T** = *Time*. Seek medical help if any of the preceding signs occur. The presence of one of these signs is associated with a high risk of stroke (72%); if all three are present, the risk is as high as 85%. (Refer to Table 17-3 for an additional assessment tool for stroke.)

## What to Do

Call 9-1-1 and do the following while waiting for EMS:

1. Monitor breathing. If the person is not breathing, begin CPR.
2. Position the person on his or her back with head and shoulders slightly raised.
3. Loosen tight or constricting clothing.
4. Be prepared to turn the person onto his or her side to allow drool or vomit to drain.
5. If the person is unresponsive but breathing, place on his or her side.

### CAUTION

**DO NOT** give a person having a stroke anything to drink or eat. The throat can be paralyzed, which restricts swallowing.

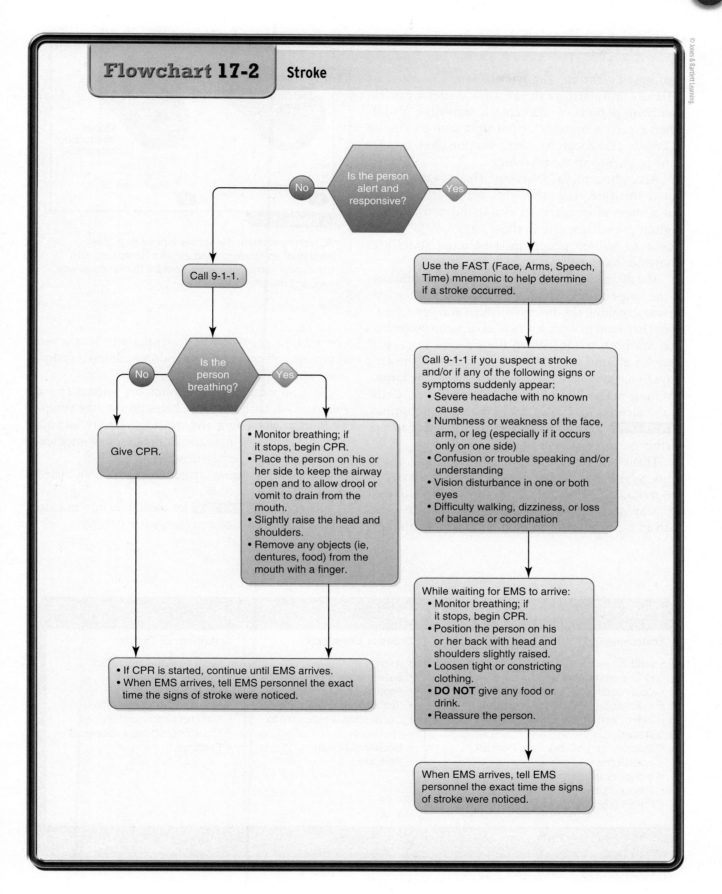

**Flowchart 17-2**   Stroke

Is the person alert and responsive?

**No** → Call 9-1-1.

Is the person breathing?

**No** → Give CPR.

**Yes** →
- Monitor breathing; if it stops, begin CPR.
- Place the person on his or her side to keep the airway open and to allow drool or vomit to drain from the mouth.
- Slightly raise the head and shoulders.
- Remove any objects (ie, dentures, food) from the mouth with a finger.

- If CPR is started, continue until EMS arrives.
- When EMS arrives, tell EMS personnel the exact time the signs of stroke were noticed.

**Yes** → Use the FAST (Face, Arms, Speech, Time) mnemonic to help determine if a stroke occurred.

Call 9-1-1 if you suspect a stroke and/or if any of the following signs or symptoms suddenly appear:
- Severe headache with no known cause
- Numbness or weakness of the face, arm, or leg (especially if it occurs only on one side)
- Confusion or trouble speaking and/or understanding
- Vision disturbance in one or both eyes
- Difficulty walking, dizziness, or loss of balance or coordination

While waiting for EMS to arrive:
- Monitor breathing; if it stops, begin CPR.
- Position the person on his or her back with head and shoulders slightly raised.
- Loosen tight or constricting clothing.
- **DO NOT** give any food or drink.
- Reassure the person.

When EMS arrives, tell EMS personnel the exact time the signs of stroke were noticed.

# ▶ Asthma

Asthma is a chronic (long-term) lung disease that inflames and narrows the airways. Asthma causes recurring periods of wheezing (a whistling sound when a person breathes), chest tightness, shortness of breath, and coughing. The coughing often occurs at night or early in the morning.

According to the National Heart, Lung, and Blood Institute, asthma affects people of all ages, but it most often starts in childhood and has the highest prevalence rate in those ages 5 to 17 years. About 23 million people in the United States are known to have asthma.

The airways are tubes that carry air into and out of the lungs. People who have asthma have inflamed airways, making the airways swollen and very sensitive. They tend to react strongly to certain substances that are breathed in. When the airways react, the muscles around them tighten. This causes the airways to narrow, allowing less air to flow to the lungs. Swelling makes the airways even narrower. Cells in the airways may make more mucus than normal **Figure 17-7**. Mucus is a sticky, thick liquid that can further narrow a person's airways.

This chain reaction can result in asthma symptoms. Symptoms can happen each time the airways are irritated. Sometimes symptoms are mild and go away on their own or after minimal treatment with an asthma medicine. At other times, symptoms

**Figure 17-7**

**A.** A cross-section of a normal airway. **B.** A cross-section of an airway during asthma symptoms, with the airway narrowed and inflamed, a thickened airway wall, and mucus.

continue to get worse. An asthma attack is when symptoms get more intense and/or additional symptoms appear.

It is important to treat symptoms when they are first noticed. Early response helps prevent the symptoms from worsening and causing a severe asthma attack. Severe asthma attacks may require medical care, and they can cause death.

Some of the known triggers of asthma are listed in **Table 17-4**.

Refer to **Flowchart 17-3** for additional information regarding the care of a person with asthma.

## Table 17-4 Common Asthma Triggers

| Environmental | Drugs or Chemicals | Conditions or Events |
|---|---|---|
| • Cold air | • Aspirin | • Gastroesophageal reflux |
| • House dust mites | • Beta-blocker medicine | • Allergic rhinitis |
| • Cockroaches | • Food or drug preservatives | • Panic attacks |
| • Animals (eg, cats, dogs, rodents) | • Seafood, shellfish | • Menstruation, pregnancy |
| • Indoor irritants (eg, wood-burning stoves) | • Occupational exposure to chemicals | • Viral respiratory infections |
| • Outdoor air pollution (eg, vehicle emissions) | • Household cleaning agents | • Emotional stress, excitement |
| • Indoor or outdoor molds and fungi | • Perfumes | • Exercise |
| • Tobacco smoke | | |
| • Pollen (eg, grass, trees) | | |

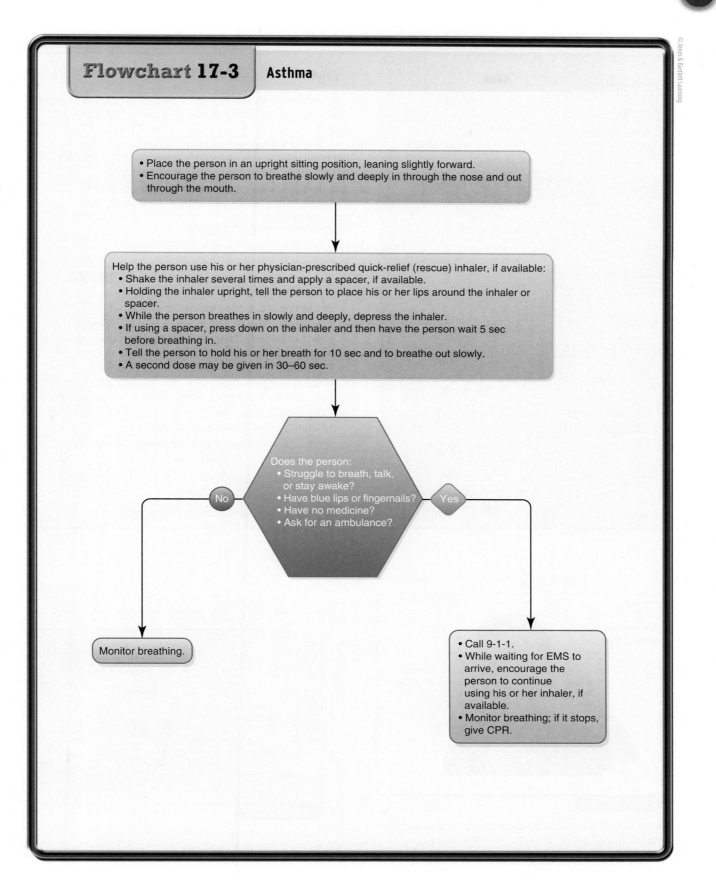

**Flowchart 17-3**   | Asthma

- Place the person in an upright sitting position, leaning slightly forward.
- Encourage the person to breathe slowly and deeply in through the nose and out through the mouth.

Help the person use his or her physician-prescribed quick-relief (rescue) inhaler, if available:
- Shake the inhaler several times and apply a spacer, if available.
- Holding the inhaler upright, tell the person to place his or her lips around the inhaler or spacer.
- While the person breathes in slowly and deeply, depress the inhaler.
- If using a spacer, press down on the inhaler and then have the person wait 5 sec before breathing in.
- Tell the person to hold his or her breath for 10 sec and to breathe out slowly.
- A second dose may be given in 30–60 sec.

Does the person:
- Struggle to breath, talk, or stay awake?
- Have blue lips or fingernails?
- Have no medicine?
- Ask for an ambulance?

No

Yes

Monitor breathing.

- Call 9-1-1.
- While waiting for EMS to arrive, encourage the person to continue using his or her inhaler, if available.
- Monitor breathing; if it stops, give CPR.

## What to Look For

- Frequent coughing
- Wheezing (high-pitched whistling sound or squeaky sound during breathing)
- Chest tightness
- Shortness of breath
- Sitting in tripod position (leaning forward with hands on knees or other support, trying to breathe)
- Inability to speak in complete sentences without stopping to breathe
- Nostrils flaring with each breath
- Fast breath and heart rates
- Blue lips or fingernails

## What to Do

1. Place the person in an upright sitting position, leaning slightly forward.
2. Encourage the person to sit quietly and to breathe slowly and deeply in through the nose and out through the mouth.
3. Call 9-1-1 immediately if the person is struggling to breathe, talk, or stay awake; has blue lips or fingernails; has no medicine; or asks for an ambulance.
4. Ask the person about any asthma medication he or she uses. Most people with asthma have a physician-prescribed quick-relief (rescue) inhaler with a spacer or holding chamber **Figure 17-8**.
5. Help the person use the quick-relief inhaler:
   - Shake the inhaler vigorously several times, remove the cap, and apply the spacer if available **Figure 17-9**.
   - Holding the inhaler upright, tell the person to place his or her lips around the inhaler or spacer.
   - For greater benefit, the person can take a breath and then exhale fully. Then, while the person breathes in slowly and deeply, depress the inhaler to release the medication.
   - If using a spacer, press down on the inhaler and then have the person wait 5 seconds before breathing in.
   - Tell the person to hold his or her breath for at least 10 seconds and to breathe out slowly.
   - A second dose may be given in 30 to 60 seconds.
6. Call 9-1-1 if:
   - There is no improvement after using the medication.
   - Repeated attacks occur.
   - A severe and prolonged attack occurs.

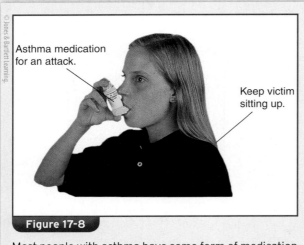

Asthma medication for an attack.

Keep victim sitting up.

**Figure 17-8**

Most people with asthma have some form of medication that may assist them during an asthma attack.

**Figure 17-9**

Spacer for inhaler.

**FYI**

**Using a Physician-Prescribed Quick-Relief Inhaler (Metered-Dose Inhaler)**

1. Check the inhaler's expiration date.
2. The inhaler should be at room temperature.
3. If there is a spacer/holding chamber, attach the inhaler to it.
4. Shake the inhaler several times.
5. The person should blow out the air in his or her lungs.
6. The person's lips should be placed around the inhaler, and the person should begin to inhale deeply.
7. The person depresses the handheld inhaler to release the medicine as he or she breathes in slowly until the lungs are full.
8. If using a spacer/holding chamber, the person should press down on the inhaler and then wait 5 seconds before breathing in.
9. The person should hold his or her breath for at least 10 seconds, allowing the medication to be absorbed into the lungs.
10. The person should wait for several breaths before taking a second dose.

**Q&A**

**Who gets asthma?**

Asthma is very common, affecting about 23 million people in the United States, including more than 6 million children. No one knows for sure why some people have asthma and others do not. People who have family members with allergies or asthma are more likely to have asthma.

In young children, boys are nearly twice as likely as girls to develop asthma, but this sex difference tends to disappear in older age groups. Obesity is a newly identified risk factor for asthma.

**What causes asthma?**

People generally think of asthma in terms of episodes or attacks. Actually, the asthmatic condition is always present, but symptoms may be dormant until triggered by an allergen, respiratory infection, or bad or cold weather. Other triggers may include some medicines, environmental irritants, physical exertion, and some foods and food additives.

*Source:* Centers for Disease Control and Prevention. "Asthma." http://www.cdc.gov/asthma

## ▶ Hyperventilation

Excessively fast breathing that occurs during emotional distress is called <u>hyperventilation</u>. The result is an abnormal decrease in the blood carbon dioxide level, which causes the symptoms of tingling and lightheadedness. It is important to rule out other causes of rapid breathing, such as untreated diabetes, severe shock, certain poisons, and brain swelling due to injury or high altitude.

**FYI**

**Breathing Into a Paper Bag**

A popular remedy for anxiety-related hyperventilation is to breathe into a paper bag. **DO NOT** do this. Tests on healthy people show that bag rebreathing rarely restores blood-gas balance but often causes dangerous stress to the heart and respiratory system, especially in people with a chronic respiratory disease.

*Source:* Callaham M. Hypoxic hazards of traditional paper bag rebreathing in hyperventilating patients. *Ann Emerg Med* 1989;18(6):622–628.

**What to Look For**

**What to Do**

| | |
|---|---|
| • Shortness of breath<br>• Fast breathing (more than 40 breaths per minute)<br>• Tingling or numbness of the hands, feet, and around the mouth<br>• Dizziness or light-headedness | 1. Calm and reassure the person.<br>2. Take the person to a quiet place or ask bystanders to leave. Have the person sit down.<br>3. Encourage the person to breathe slowly, using the abdominal muscles: inhale through the nose, hold the full inhalation for 1 to 2 seconds, then exhale slowly through pursed lips. |

## ▶ Chronic Obstructive Pulmonary Disease

Chronic obstructive pulmonary disease (COPD) is a broad term applied to emphysema, chronic bronchitis, and related lung diseases. COPD describes a disease that makes it hard for a person to breathe because the normal flow of air into and out of the person's lungs is partially obstructed.

The incidence of COPD is very high in North America, and the most common causative factor is cigarette smoking. Because COPD takes many years to develop before a person notices difficulty breathing, it is usually considered a disease of older adults and is most commonly diagnosed in people older than 60 years.

Chronic bronchitis is caused by chronic infection, which can be brought on by irritations such as tobacco smoke. The bronchi become thick, unable to stretch, and partially blocked. Early symptoms include a cigarette cough or a cough due to a cold. Later, more severe symptoms include difficulty breathing, increased sputum, and severe coughing.

Emphysema often occurs with chronic bronchitis. The alveoli of the lungs are partially destroyed, and the lungs have lost their elasticity, making it difficult for the person to exhale. Common symptoms include coughing, wheezing, and shortness of breath. Breathing is extremely difficult for people with emphysema.

**What to Look For**

**What to Do**

| | |
|---|---|
| The signs and symptoms of COPD are similar to those of asthma:<br>• Wheezing<br>• Prominent coughing and shortness of breath<br>• Person may depend on a constant low level of artificially supplied oxygen to maintain breathing | 1. People with COPD usually will have their own physician-prescribed medications. Assist the person to take any prescribed medications.<br>2. Place the person in the sitting position that provides the greatest comfort.<br>3. Encourage the person to cough up any secretions.<br>4. For acute breathing distress, obtain immediate medical assistance. The person might need oxygen, which is available from EMS and at hospital emergency departments. |

## ▶ Fainting

A sudden, brief loss of responsiveness not associated with a head injury is known as syncope (fainting) or psychogenic shock.

Simple fainting is common and benign and can have physical or emotional causes. Fainting can happen suddenly when blood flow to the brain is interrupted. The nervous system dilates blood vessels to three to four times their normal size and allows blood to pool in the legs and lower body.

Syncope, or simple fainting, can be precipitated by unpleasant emotional stimuli such as the sight of blood or strong fear. It usually occurs when the person is in the upright position.

Most fainting episodes are associated with decreased blood flow causing deficient oxygen or glucose in the brain. The decreased blood flow can be caused by a slow heart rate (vagal reaction, in which the vagus nerve, which slows the heart rate, is overstimulated by fright, anxiety, drugs, or fatigue), heart-rhythm disturbances, dehydration, heat exhaustion, anemia (low hemoglobin), or bleeding. Decreased glucose (**hypoglycemia**) can be caused by infections or medications used to treat diabetes.

Sitting or standing for a long time without moving, especially in a hot environment, can cause blood to pool in dilated vessels, which results in a loss of effective circulating blood volume, causing the blood pressure to drop. As the blood flow to the brain decreases, the person has a loss of consciousness and collapses.

Refer to **Flowchart 17-4** for additional information regarding the care of a person who has fainted.

## CAUTION

**DO NOT** use ammonia inhalants or smelling salts.

**DO NOT** give the person anything to drink or eat until he or she has fully recovered and can swallow.

**DO NOT** splash or pour water on the person's face.

**DO NOT** slap the person's face in an attempt to revive him or her.

| What to Look For | What to Do |
|---|---|
| • A person that has suddenly collapsed<br>• Pale skin, lips, and nail beds<br>• Clammy, sweaty skin | 1. Check breathing.<br>2. If breathing has stopped, call 9-1-1 and give CPR.<br>3. If the person is breathing:<br>  • Keep the person flat on his or her back. Feet can be raised 6 to 12 inches (15 to 30 cm) if doing so does not cause pain.<br>  • Monitor breathing; if it stops, give CPR.<br>  • Loosen tight clothing.<br>  • If the person fell, check and treat any injuries.<br>  • Wipe the person's forehead with a cool, wet cloth.<br>  • If vomiting occurs, roll the person onto his or her side.<br>4. Seek medical care if:<br>  • There are repeated episodes.<br>  • The person fainted for no apparent reason.<br>  • The person does not regain responsiveness quickly.<br>  • The person has diabetes, has seizures, is pregnant, has a loss of bowel or bladder control, or is older than 50 years. |
| A person who is about to faint, indicated by:<br>• Pale skin and lips<br>• Clammy, sweaty skin<br>• A person that complains about dizziness, nausea, and feeling unwell | 1. Prevent a hard fall if possible.<br>2. If the person collapses, take the steps discussed earlier. |

## Flowchart 17-4    Fainting

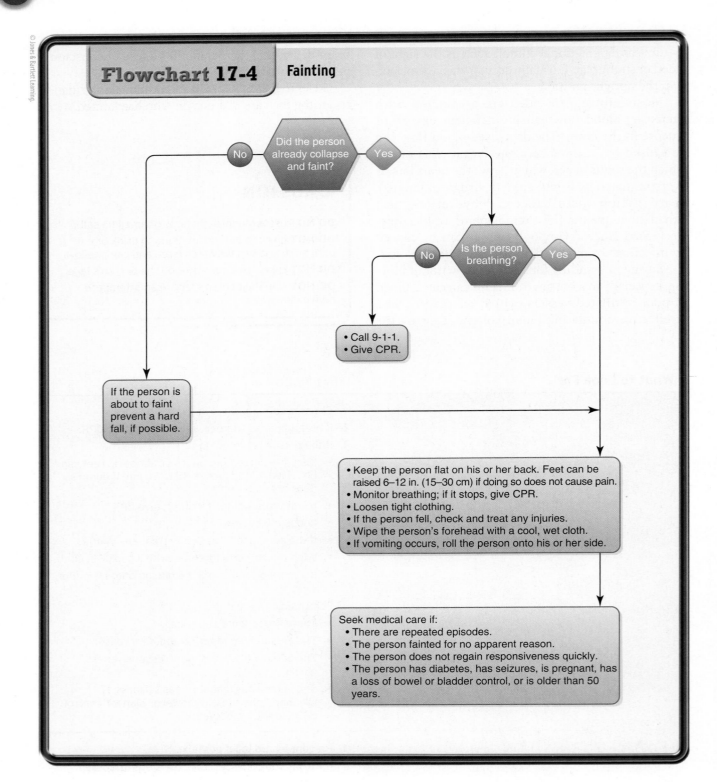

**Did the person already collapse and faint?**

- No
- Yes

**Is the person breathing?**

- No
- Yes

- Call 9-1-1.
- Give CPR.

If the person is about to faint prevent a hard fall, if possible.

- Keep the person flat on his or her back. Feet can be raised 6–12 in. (15–30 cm) if doing so does not cause pain.
- Monitor breathing; if it stops, give CPR.
- Loosen tight clothing.
- If the person fell, check and treat any injuries.
- Wipe the person's forehead with a cool, wet cloth.
- If vomiting occurs, roll the person onto his or her side.

Seek medical care if:
- There are repeated episodes.
- The person fainted for no apparent reason.
- The person does not regain responsiveness quickly.
- The person has diabetes, has seizures, is pregnant, has a loss of bowel or bladder control, or is older than 50 years.

# ▶ Seizure

A <u>seizure</u> is an abnormal firing of brain cells, usually resulting in jerking movements followed by an unresponsive period. Many different types of seizures exist. People may experience just one type or more than one. The type of seizure a person has depends on which part and how much of the brain is affected by the electrical disturbance that produces seizures.

The type of seizure that most first aid providers encounter is a generalized, tonic-clonic seizure (formerly and still commonly called grand mal) **Figure 17-10** . The person suddenly becomes completely stiff or tense (sometimes emitting a vocal cry), with arms and legs extended (tonic phase). The person then begins to jerk rigorously, with arms and legs contracting and then relaxing in unison (clonic phase). These two phases make up the convulsion phase.

In a generalized seizure, the person always has a loss of responsiveness. The person may foam at the mouth (sputum may be pink- or red-tinged due to tongue biting), and he or she may be incontinent. The heart beats during the convulsion, even though breathing temporarily stops. CPR chest compressions should not be done while the person is still jerking or twitching. The person having a seizure often makes a series of gasping sounds. The gasping generally lasts for 20 to 30 seconds, with several seconds in between gasps, but it can last longer in some cases.

**Figure 17-10**

Tonic and clonic phases of a seizure.

© Jones & Bartlett Learning

Seeing a generalized seizure can be frightening. Fortunately, the convulsion phase is over in about 60 seconds, usually before a call to 9-1-1 can even be made. Even if the person turns blue, the seizure will typically end long before brain damage would begin. Check for breathing after any convulsive episode has stopped. After the convulsion phase, the person becomes postictal (a state of confusion, sleepiness, and occasionally combativeness).

There are other types of seizures. In an absence, or staring, seizure (formerly known as a petit mal seizure), the person momentarily becomes mentally absent and appears to be daydreaming.

Several medical conditions increase the instability or irritability of the brain and can lead to seizures, including the following:

- Lack of oxygen
- Heat stroke
- Poisoning
- Electric shock
- Hypoglycemia
- High fever in children
- Brain injury, tumor, or stroke
- Alcohol withdrawal, drug abuse, or overdose

Nearly all seizures resulting from fever occur in children between the ages of 6 months and 5 years (23 months average). They affect 3% to 5% of all children by the age of 5 years. Febrile seizures may occur in the same child on more than one occasion, but this does not constitute epilepsy. Febrile seizures are very frightening to the child's parents. While these seizures are not life threatening, they may be a symptom of meningitis, a life-threatening brain infection that requires medical care.

Another cause of seizure is cardiac arrest. The brain is quickly affected when it runs out of blood glucose and oxygen. A person may incur irreversible brain damage or even die if the condition is not immediately recognized and the person is not rapidly resuscitated.

Additional causes of seizures include trauma, brain tumors, meningitis, alcohol withdrawal, and drug abuse (especially cocaine and amphetamines).

People with diabetes may be prone to seizures when their blood glucose falls below normal levels and they become hypoglycemic due to too much insulin.

Severe head injuries can cause rapid swelling of or bleeding into the brain, causing a seizure. Rapid action by surgeons can relieve the condition and be lifesaving.

Epilepsy, in contrast to the aforementioned causes of seizures, is an underlying condition (or permanent brain injury) that affects the delicate systems that govern how electrical energy behaves in the brain, making it susceptible to recurring seizures. Most people with epilepsy have seizures due to an unknown cause. Epilepsy is not a mental illness, and it is not a sign of low intelligence. It also is not contagious. Between seizures, a person with epilepsy can function as normally as a person who does not have epilepsy. Medication can often help control seizure frequency in people with epilepsy.

Refer to  Flowchart 17-5 for additional information regarding the care of a person with a seizure.

---

**FYI**

**Knowledge of Epilepsy**

A survey found that about half of all people have witnessed an epileptic seizure either in person or on television; about one-third of all people know someone with epilepsy, but relatively few are familiar with epilepsy, how to respond to a seizure, or the Epilepsy Foundation.

*Source:* Kobau R, Price P. Knowledge of epilepsy and familiarity with this disorder in the US population. *Epilepsia* 2003;44(11):1449-1454.

---

| What to Look For | What to Do |
|---|---|
| Convulsive seizures (eg, tonic-clonic seizures) typically last for 1 to 2 minutes (but may last longer), and the person may experience the following signs and symptoms:<br>• Sudden falling to the floor or ground<br>• Stiffening of arm and leg muscles followed by jerky movement with arching of the back<br>• Foaming at the mouth<br>• Grinding of teeth<br>• Blue-gray face and lips<br>• Eyes rolling upward<br>• Loss of bladder and bowel control<br><br>Nonconvulsive seizures (eg, absence or staring seizures) last only a few seconds and are so brief that they often escape detection. The person may experience the following signs and symptoms:<br>• Staring, confusion, or inattentiveness<br>• Frequent eye blinking<br>• Involuntary movements (eg, lip smacking, picking at clothes, fumbling) | 1. Move nearby objects to avoid injury.<br>2. Place something soft under the head such as a rolled towel. **DO NOT** use a pillow.<br>3. Time the seizure from start to finish.<br>4. Most seizures do not require medical care and end in 1 to 2 minutes. Stay with the person until the seizure is over.<br>5. Keep bystanders away.<br>6. Call 9-1-1 for any of the following:<br> • Seizure lasting longer than 5 minutes<br> • Series of seizures following one another<br> • The person has breathing difficulties after the seizure<br> • The person has diabetes or is pregnant<br> • Seizure happened in water<br> • This is the person's first known seizure<br> • The seizure is injury-related<br> • Slow recovery<br>7. After the seizure:<br> • Keep the airway open by placing the person on his or her side and head on a rolled towel.<br> • Monitor breathing and if it stops, give CPR.<br> • Allow the person to sleep.<br> • Stay with the person until he or she has fully recovered. |

## Flowchart 17-5    Seizures

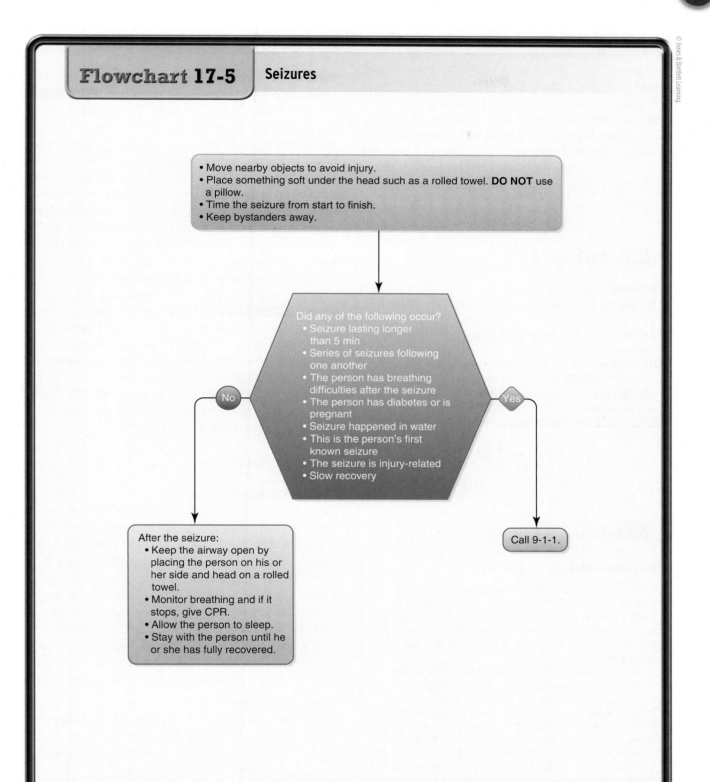

- Move nearby objects to avoid injury.
- Place something soft under the head such as a rolled towel. **DO NOT** use a pillow.
- Time the seizure from start to finish.
- Keep bystanders away.

Did any of the following occur?
- Seizure lasting longer than 5 min
- Series of seizures following one another
- The person has breathing difficulties after the seizure
- The person has diabetes or is pregnant
- Seizure happened in water
- This is the person's first known seizure
- The seizure is injury-related
- Slow recovery

No

Yes

After the seizure:
- Keep the airway open by placing the person on his or her side and head on a rolled towel.
- Monitor breathing and if it stops, give CPR.
- Allow the person to sleep.
- Stay with the person until he or she has fully recovered.

Call 9-1-1.

## Status Epilepticus

Most seizures end after a few seconds or a few minutes. However, in some cases, they are prolonged or occur in a series, a condition called **status epilepticus**. This is an emergency situation and requires immediate medical care. Repeated, uncontrolled seizures can lead to brain damage, fractures, severe dehydration, and aspiration. In adults, the most common cause of status epilepticus is failure to take prescribed medicines for epilepsy.

### CAUTION

**DO NOT** restrain the person.

**DO NOT** put anything between the person's teeth during the seizure.

**DO NOT** splash or pour water or any other liquid on the person's face.

**DO NOT** move the person to another place (unless it is the only way to protect the person from injury).

**DO NOT** leave a person until he or she is fully alert and recovered.

### FYI

**Seizures in Medical TV Dramas**

About half the time, the physicians and nurses on popular fictional TV medical shows give improper seizure first aid that, in reality, could lead to broken teeth, bruises, or dislocations, according to a study presented at the American Academy of Neurology's annual meeting.

In the study, around 280 hours of recent medical dramas were watched, and when a clip showing a seizure was found, it was reviewed and compared with the Epilepsy Foundation's first aid guidelines for seizures. Fifty-nine seizures were found, and 46% of the actions by the physician and nurse actors were considered inappropriate. They noted such poor medical actions as holding a patient down, attempting to stop involuntary movement, and putting something in a patient's mouth while a seizure was in progress. In about 29% of the cases, the action was medically correct. The remaining seizure incidents were on the screen too briefly to judge.

*Source:* Moeller A, Moeller JJ, Rahey SR, Sadler RM. Depiction of seizure first aid management in medical television dramas. *Can J Neurol Sci* 2011;38(5):723-727.

## ▶ Diabetic Emergencies

Insulin is a hormone produced by the pancreas that assists the body in using energy from food `Figure 17-11`. Insulin allows the transportation of glucose from the blood into the cells where it serves as a major source of fuel for the body. When excess glucose remains in the blood and is not transferred to the cells, the cells must rely on fat for fuel. When blood glucose cannot be used, it builds up in the blood. The glucose then overflows into the urine, passing through the body unused. When this occurs, a condition called **diabetes** develops `Table 17-5`. In diabetes, insulin is either ineffective or lacking in the body. This condition is not contagious and in most cases special diet and/or medication can control it.

The body is continuously balancing glucose and insulin `Figure 17-12`. Too much insulin and not enough glucose leads to low blood glucose and possibly an insulin reaction. An insulin reaction results from severe low blood glucose, causing unconsciousness and possibly death. Too much glucose and not enough insulin leads to high blood glucose, the production of ketones, and possibly **diabetic coma**. Ketones cause a sweet or fruity odor on the breath.

### Types of Diabetes

#### Type 1 Diabetes

Type 1 diabetes (formerly called juvenile-onset or insulin-dependent diabetes) is most commonly diagnosed in childhood, but it may present at any age in life. About 2 million of the individuals with diabetes have type 1 diabetes. This type of diabetes requires external insulin (not made by the body), which enables the glucose to enter the cells. External insulin is necessary because the body is unable to produce the insulin the cells require. When a person with type 1 diabetes is deprived of external insulin, he or she will become very ill. People with type 1 diabetes will usually be thin or not overweight.

#### Type 2 Diabetes

Type 2 diabetes used to be known as non-insulin-dependent or adult-onset diabetes. The incidence of type 2 diabetes is reaching epidemic proportions in the United States. According to the CDC, approximately 29 million people currently have type 2 diabetes. Excess body weight and a sedentary lifestyle are widely recognized risk factors, and this is especially because type 2 diabetes is being diagnosed in a growing number of children and adolescents. Other risk factors include a family history of type 2 diabetes and age older than 45 years. The age of onset is usually

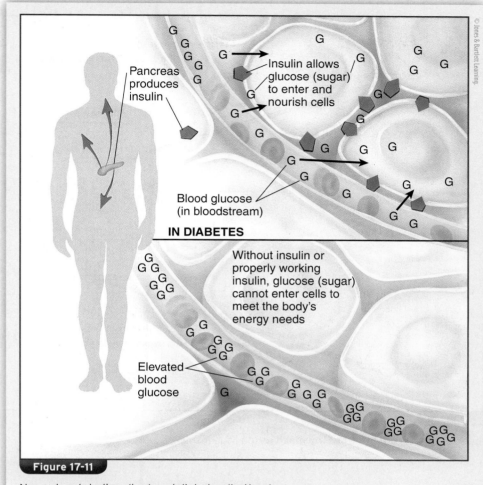

**Figure 17-11**

Normal metabolism (top) and diabetes (bottom).

## Table 17-5  Diabetic Emergencies

|  | Hyperglycemia (high blood glucose) | Hypoglycemia (low blood glucose) |
|---|---|---|
| Cause | Not enough insulin; too much glucose | Too much insulin; not enough glucose |
| Insulin level | Insufficient | Excessive |
| Onset of symptoms | Gradual | Sudden |
| Skin | Flushed, dry, warm | Pale, clammy |
| Breath | Fruity odor | Normal |
| Thirst | Severe | Normal |
| Urination | Frequent | Normal |
| Behavior | Normal to disorientation, drowsiness, and change in mood | Appearance of intoxication: combativeness, bad temper, anger, confusion, disorientation |
| Other symptoms | Drowsiness, vomiting, heavy breathing, eventual stupor or unconsciousness | Sudden hunger, eventual stupor, or unresponsiveness |
| First aid | • If in doubt, give sugar.<br>• Give fluids to fight dehydration.<br>• Take the person to the hospital. | • Give sugar.<br>• Seek medical care. |

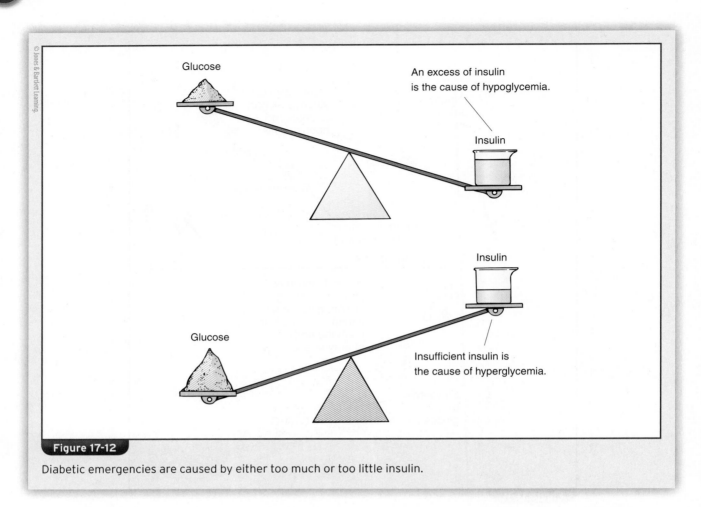

© Jones & Bartlett Learning

Glucose

An excess of insulin
is the cause of hypoglycemia.

Insulin

Insulin

Glucose

Insufficient insulin is
the cause of hyperglycemia.

**Figure 17-12**

Diabetic emergencies are caused by either too much or too little insulin.

over the age of 40 years, but it can occur at any age. This type of diabetes may require insulin replacement and other medication.

### Gestational Diabetes

Gestational diabetes occurs in some pregnancies. It usually ends after a baby is born, but when women who had gestational diabetes get older, type 2 diabetes can develop. Gestational diabetes results from the body's resistance to the action of insulin. This resistance is caused by hormones produced during pregnancy. Gestational diabetes is usually treated with diet, but some women need insulin.

### Low Blood Glucose (Hypoglycemia)

The condition of low blood glucose, called hypoglycemia, is sometimes referred to as an insulin reaction. This condition occurs in a person with diabetes for several reasons: too much insulin, too little or delayed food intake, exercise, alcohol, or any combination of these factors.

Hypoglycemia is not unusual for a person with diabetes who takes glucose-lowering medications, such as

insulin. The person must balance injecting the right amount of insulin, eating the right amounts of certain foods, and exercising. The wrong amount of any element can result in too much insulin in the blood, using up available glucose too rapidly. Because the brain's most usable fuel is sugar, it is the first organ at risk. Behaviors related to hypoglycemia often mimic those of people who have consumed too much alcohol; the person may stagger, may slur his or her speech, and may not follow simple commands. Unfortunately, some people with diabetes have been detained for intoxication by law enforcement personnel only to be found dead a few hours later.

Some people with diabetes are not dependent on insulin. Their bodies still make some insulin but not enough; with careful attention to diet and/or oral medication, the condition is more easily controlled. These people rarely become dangerously hypoglycemic.

People experiencing hypoglycemia may drool excessively. Profuse drooling can have the same effect as vomiting. Follow the same instructions as those for managing vomiting: quickly turn the person on his or her side.

| What to Look For | What to Do |
|---|---|
| • Responsive, alert, and can swallow<br>• Medical identification tag<br>• Sudden onset of symptoms (minutes to an hour) because no glucose is reaching the brain<br>• Staggering, poor coordination, clumsiness<br>• Anger, bad temper<br>• Cold, pale, moist, or clammy skin<br>• Confusion, disorientation<br>• Sudden hunger<br>• Excessive sweating<br>• Trembling, shakiness | The person may be able to tell you what to do.<br>1. If the person has a blood glucose monitor, allow him or her to check his or her blood glucose.<br>2. Use the Rule of 15 when:<br>  • Testing is not possible,<br>  • Testing shows a low blood glucose level, or<br>  • Profuse sweating or shaking occurs in a person with diabetes.<br>The Rule of 15 works as follows:<br>  • Have the person eat 15 grams of sugar (ie, 3 to 5 glucose tablets **Figure 17-13**, 3 to 5 teaspoons [15 mL to 25 mL] of table sugar, or 4 ounces [118 mL] of orange juice or regular soft drink [not diet]) **Table 17-6**.<br>  • Wait 15 minutes for the sugar to get into the blood.<br>  • Recheck the blood glucose level. If it is still low or no testing is available, give the person 15 more grams of sugar to consume **Figure 17-14**.<br>3. For some people who are prone to severe low hypoglycemia, a physician may write a prescription for a glucagon kit. Glucagon is a hormone that raises blood glucose and can be injected by trained friends, family, or coworkers in an emergency. |
| • Unresponsive<br>• Inability to follow simple instructions<br>• Seizure occurrence<br>• Inability to swallow | 1. Monitor breathing.<br>2. Look for a medical identification tag.<br>3. **DO NOT** give any food or drink.<br>4. Place the person on his or her side to keep the airway open and to drain fluids or vomit from the mouth.<br>5. If the person does not improve, call 9-1-1. |

**Figure 17-13**

Glucose tablets.

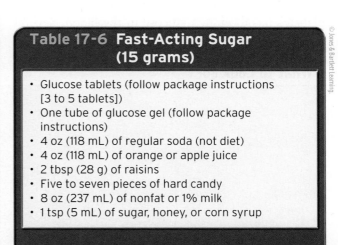

### Table 17-6 Fast-Acting Sugar (15 grams)

- Glucose tablets (follow package instructions [3 to 5 tablets])
- One tube of glucose gel (follow package instructions)
- 4 oz (118 mL) of regular soda (not diet)
- 4 oz (118 mL) of orange or apple juice
- 2 tbsp (28 g) of raisins
- Five to seven pieces of hard candy
- 8 oz (237 mL) of nonfat or 1% milk
- 1 tsp (5 mL) of sugar, honey, or corn syrup

**Figure 17-14**

Blood glucose meter with lancing device.

---

## FYI

### Summary of the Rule of 15 for Low Blood Glucose

The person with diabetes should check his or her blood glucose level. If it is not within the appropriate range, he or she should eat 15 grams of sugar, wait 15 minutes, check the blood glucose again, and, if low, eat 15 more grams of sugar, wait 15 minutes, and check the blood glucose again. If still low, seek immediate medical care.

## High Blood Glucose (Diabetic Coma, Hyperglycemia)

The opposite reaction of hypoglycemia is **hyperglycemia**. This condition occurs when a person with diabetes has too much glucose in the blood. Several scenarios can cause this medical condition, including insufficient insulin, overeating, illness, inactivity, stress, or a combination of these factors.

If the lack of insulin goes uncorrected for too long, the person's alertness slowly deteriorates to a state of unresponsiveness from which the person cannot be aroused. This serious condition is called diabetic coma; there is little that first aid providers or even EMS personnel can do to correct it. It requires careful rebalancing of insulin, fluids, and electrolytes in a medical facility, a process that can take days. Because diabetic coma has a generally slow onset and usually occurs in people with previously known diabetes, the person is most often brought to medical care long before unresponsiveness occurs.

Refer to Flowchart 17-6 for additional information regarding the care of a diabetic emergency.

## Q&A

### How can you tell the difference between hypoglycemia and hyperglycemia?

It is difficult to determine whether a person has hypoglycemia or hyperglycemia. Sugar helps the person with hypoglycemia, but not the person with hyperglycemia. However, do not debate whether to give sugar; sugar will cause no harm in either condition.

Ask the person with diabetes two questions: "Have you eaten today?" and "Have you taken your insulin today?" If the person with diabetes has taken his or her insulin but has not eaten, suspect hypoglycemia. If the person with diabetes has eaten but has not taken insulin, suspect hyperglycemia. If you are unsure which condition exists, give sugar.

---

## What to Look For

- Medical identification tag
- Gradual onset (hours to days) because some glucose is still reaching the brain
- Drowsiness
- Extreme thirst
- Very frequent urination
- Warm, red, dry skin
- Vomiting
- Fruity breath odor (has also been described to smell like nail polish remover)
- Heavy breathing
- Eventual unresponsiveness

## What to Do

1. Give frequent, small sips of water if the person with diabetes can swallow.
2. If uncertain whether the person with diabetes has a high or low blood glucose level, and if he or she is responsive and able to swallow, use the Rule of 15 for giving sugar, as previously described. The extra sugar will not cause significant harm in a person experiencing hyperglycemia.
3. **DO NOT** give insulin unless the person with diabetes can self-administer it.
4. Call 9-1-1 as soon as possible.

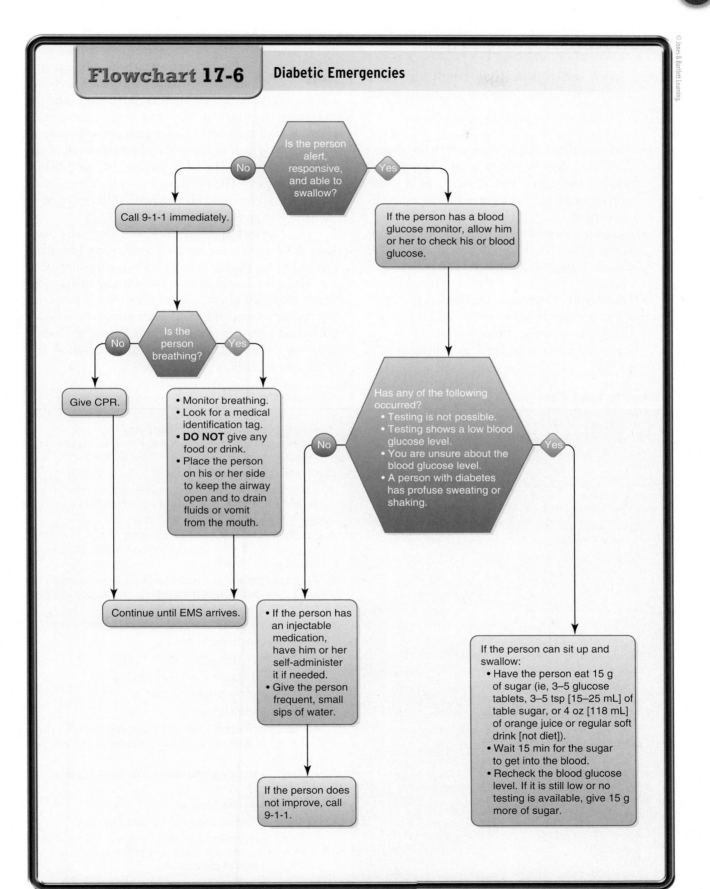

## Flowchart 17-6   Diabetic Emergencies

**Is the person alert, responsive, and able to swallow?**

**No** → Call 9-1-1 immediately.

→ **Is the person breathing?**
- **No** → Give CPR. → Continue until EMS arrives.
- **Yes** →
  - Monitor breathing.
  - Look for a medical identification tag.
  - **DO NOT** give any food or drink.
  - Place the person on his or her side to keep the airway open and to drain fluids or vomit from the mouth.

**Yes** → If the person has a blood glucose monitor, allow him or her to check his or blood glucose.

→ **Has any of the following occurred?**
- Testing is not possible.
- Testing shows a low blood glucose level.
- You are unsure about the blood glucose level.
- A person with diabetes has profuse sweating or shaking.

**No** →
- If the person has an injectable medication, have him or her self-administer it if needed.
- Give the person frequent, small sips of water.

→ If the person does not improve, call 9-1-1.

**Yes** → If the person can sit up and swallow:
- Have the person eat 15 g of sugar (ie, 3–5 glucose tablets, 3–5 tsp [15–25 mL] of table sugar, or 4 oz [118 mL] of orange juice or regular soft drink [not diet]).
- Wait 15 min for the sugar to get into the blood.
- Recheck the blood glucose level. If it is still low or no testing is available, give 15 g more of sugar.

# ▶ Abdominal Complaints

People with gastrointestinal conditions usually complain about one or more of the following symptoms:

- *Abdominal pain that is aching, cramping, sharp, or dull.* It might be constant, or it can come and go. The pain could indicate a mild condition or an acute condition requiring immediate surgery.
- *Nausea and vomiting.* Vomiting is the ejection of the stomach's contents through the mouth. Nausea is a feeling of the need to vomit.
- *Diarrhea or constipation.* Diarrhea is the frequent passage of loose, watery stools. Constipation is the opposite of diarrhea; stools are infrequent, hard, and difficult to pass.

## Abdominal Pain

The abdomen is the area between the diaphragm and the groin. Abdominal organs are either hollow or solid. Hollow organs are tubes, such as the stomach and the intestines, through which material passes, conducting food through the body. Solid organs are solid masses of tissue in which much of the chemical work of the body takes place. The liver, spleen, and gallbladder are solid organs. The peritoneum is a thin membrane lining the entire abdominal cavity. Inflammation of the peritoneum is called peritonitis.

There are many possible causes of abdominal pain—some not so serious and some life threatening. They often can be serious enough to require emergency surgery.

Abdominal conditions are so difficult to diagnose that even skilled physicians can have trouble pinpointing an exact cause. It is neither feasible nor useful for a first aid provider to distinguish among the many causes of abdominal pain because first aid usually will be similar regardless of the cause.

## What to Look For

A first aid provider should ask the following questions:
- When did the pain start? Where is it located?
- Is the pain constant, or does it come and go? Constant pain can be more serious than a cramping pain. Constant abdominal pain suggests inflammation of an organ; cramping suggests obstruction of a hollow organ.
- Does belching or passing gas relieve the pain? If so, the intestine might be affected.
- Does the person feel nauseated, or does he or she have a good appetite?
- Is there diarrhea or vomiting?
- Does the person feel warm (feverish)?
- Does anyone near the person have similar symptoms?
- For a woman is there any chance of pregnancy? Any pain with pregnancy should be treated as an emergency.
- Is the abdomen rigid to the touch? A rigid abdomen can be a sign of an emergency condition.

## What to Do

1. Give the person only clear fluids (anything you can see through, except alcohol and caffeinated beverages). Have the person slowly sip the fluids.
2. Give the person an antacid.
3. If practical, place a hot-water bottle against the person's abdomen or have the person soak in a warm bath.
4. Recognize the possibility of vomiting and be prepared for it. Keep the person on the left side to help prevent vomiting.
5. Keep the person in a comfortable position, usually lying down with knees bent (unless the person is nauseated).
6. Seek medical care if any of the following applies:
   - Pain is constant and severe.
   - The person is unable to drink fluids.
   - The person is or might be pregnant.
   - The abdomen is rigid and painful.
   - The abdomen is swollen.
   - More pain occurs after you press your fingers on the person's abdomen and suddenly release them.
   - There is bloody, blood-stained, or black stool or vomit.
   - The person has a fever.
   - There is light-headedness or fainting.
   - Pain began around the belly button and later moved to the lower right part of the abdomen. This is a sign of appendicitis.

> **CAUTION**
>
> **DO NOT** give enemas and laxatives, which can worsen the condition or cause complications such as ruptured bowel.
> **DO NOT** give fluids other than clear fluids as long as the pain continues.
> **DO NOT** give solid foods.
> **DO NOT** give milk products.

## Nausea and Vomiting

Nausea (upset stomach) and vomiting (throwing up) often occur with conditions such as altitude sickness, motion sickness, brain injury, intestinal viruses, eating or drinking too much, and being emotionally upset. In minor illnesses, nausea and vomiting should clear up in a day. Persistent nausea and vomiting can signal more serious illnesses such as appendicitis, food poisoning, or bowel obstruction. In general, if the condition lasts longer than 1 or 2 days, or if the person vomits multiple times in a short period, the person could become dehydrated (have a loss of too much fluid). Young children and older people can be more seriously affected.

| What to Look For | What to Do |
|---|---|
| **Nausea and vomiting**<br>• Is there abdominal pain?<br>• Is there blood or brown, grainy material in the vomit?<br>• Is there diarrhea? Vomiting and diarrhea together usually indicate a self-limited viral infection.<br>• Are there signs of dehydration (eg, the person is dizzy when standing; has dry, cracked lips; is very thirsty)?<br>• Does anyone else near the person have similar symptoms?<br>• Has the person had a recent head injury? | 1. Give the person small amounts of clear fluids (eg, sports drinks, clear soups, flat, decaffeinated soda, apple or cranberry juice), except alcohol and caffeinated beverages.<br>2. If the person is able to keep fluids down, offer carbohydrates (eg, bread, cereal, pasta) first; they are easier to digest. Avoid milk products and meats for 48 hours.<br>3. Have the person rest and avoid exertion until he or she is able to eat solid foods easily.<br>4. Prevent inhalation of vomit by positioning the person on his or her side to allow drainage. Inhaled vomit can result in severe pneumonia.<br>5. Seek medical care if:<br>  • Blood or brown, grainy material appears in the vomit.<br>  • There is constant abdominal pain.<br>  • The person faints when standing.<br>  • The person is unable to keep fluids down for more than 24 hours.<br>  • The person has severe, projectile vomiting (vomit shoots out in large quantities).<br>  • The vomiting follows a recent head injury. |
| **Motion sickness, indicated by:**<br>• Nausea<br>• Pale skin<br>• Cold sweats<br>• Vomiting<br>• Dizziness<br>• Headache<br>• Fatigue | 1. If the person is prone to motion sickness, he or she should sit near the midsection of a plane, boat, bus, train, or car. People susceptible to motion sickness should not read; should look far ahead to the horizon, not to the sides; and should avoid overeating.<br>2. A person prone to motion sickness should try taking dimenhydrinate (Dramamine) or a physician-prescribed scopolamine patch 1 hour before traveling (follow label directions). |

## Diarrhea

Diarrhea is the passage of loose, watery, or unformed stools (usually more than four times a day). Diarrhea can be a symptom of intestinal infection (bacterial, viral, or parasitic), food poisoning, or food sensitivity or allergy, among other ailments. Dehydration can occur if the body loses too much fluid through the stool and the person cannot drink enough fluid to keep up with the fluid losses from the diarrhea. Older people and very young people are especially prone to dehydration, which can result in dangerous chemical imbalances. Replacing fluids and electrolytes such as sodium and potassium is of primary importance for any person with diarrhea. Diarrhea flushes bacteria and parasites out of the body. Letting diarrhea run its course is best because then bacteria or parasites are not trapped in the intestines.

### What to Look For

Determine the answers to the following questions:
- Was the person recently exposed to untreated, possibly contaminated water or food?
- Is blood or mucus present in the stool? Their presence can signal more serious conditions.
- Are signs of dehydration present (eg, the person is dizzy when standing; has dry, cracked lips; is very thirsty)?
- Does the person have cramping abdominal pain?
- Has the person been incontinent?
- Is the person feverish?
- Does anyone else near the person have similar symptoms?

### What to Do

1. Have the person drink a lot of clear fluids (8 to 10 eight-oz [240-mL] glasses daily). This is the single most important treatment.

2. When the person can tolerate clear fluids, give mild foods such as soup and gelatin. Later, the BRAT diet—bananas, rice, applesauce, toast—is recommended.

3. Bismuth can help in most cases (follow label directions). Be aware that bismuth can turn the stool and the tongue black. People sensitive to aspirin should not use bismuth. If the person cannot let the diarrhea run its course, over-the-counter medications will calm the bowel, reducing movement through the intestines.

4. Seek medical care if:
   - The person has bloody stools, which might appear black or tarry. (Keep in mind that bismuth preparations can cause black stools.)
   - Symptoms do not improve after 24 hours.
   - The person has a fever.
   - The person has severe, constant abdominal pain.
   - The person is severely dehydrated.

## CAUTION

**DO NOT** give milk products and meats for 48 hours after diarrhea stops.

**DO NOT** give caffeine, which stimulates the intestine and causes urination, furthering dehydration.

**DO NOT** give soda or fruit juice; these contain high levels of sugar, which can worsen the condition, and do not provide electrolytes, which are essential for rehydration. Sports drinks, however, contain the right ratio of sugar and electrolytes to rehydrate without worsening the condition.

## Constipation

Constipation is the passage of hard, dry stools. Most physicians define constipation as two or fewer bowel movements a week, of which 25% require straining. Constipation is rarely more than a passing discomfort in otherwise healthy people. Normal bowel movements can occur three times a day or once every 3 days. Minor changes in diet, fluid intake, activity, or emotional state can cause bowel movement changes. Rectifying any of those changes will also relieve constipation in most cases. Bowel stimulants or laxatives are rarely needed.

| What to Look For | What to Do |
|---|---|
| • Bloating sensation of abdomen. A very painful or visibly swollen abdomen is a more serious condition than simple constipation.<br>• Hard, dry stools. Small strings of blood are not unusual if the stool was painful to evacuate. | 1. Have the person eat more fiber (fresh or dried fruits, vegetables, bran). Fiber causes the colon to contract. Over-the-counter fiber products can be used, but the label directions should be followed.<br>2. Make sure the person drinks plenty of fluids (8 to 10 eight-oz [240-mL] glasses daily). Excessively hard stools often are the result of dehydration.<br>3. Encourage the person to remain active. Activity such as walking stimulates colon contractions.<br>4. If symptoms do not improve, try one of the following:<br>  • A stool softener (docusate sodium)<br>  • Caffeine, which stimulates colon contractions<br>5. Seek medical care if the person experiences any of the following:<br>  • Severe abdominal pain<br>  • Visibly swollen or very painful abdomen<br>  • Fever<br>  • Vomiting |

### CAUTION

**DO NOT** give laxatives such as Epsom salt to people with severe abdominal pain or vomiting.
**DO NOT** give alcohol.
**DO NOT** give binding foods, such as bananas, cheese, and applesauce.

# prep kit

## ▶ Ready for Review

- A heart attack occurs when the heart muscle tissue dies because its blood supply is stopped.
- Angina pectoris results when blood flow to the heart muscle is restricted, but not completely blocked.
- A stroke occurs when part of the blood flow to the brain is suddenly cut off.
- Asthma is chronic, inflammatory lung disease characterized by repeated breathing conditions. Hyperventilation is fast, deep breathing and is common during emotional stress.
- Chronic obstructive pulmonary disease (COPD) is a broad term applied to emphysema, chronic bronchitis, and related lung diseases.
- Fainting is a sudden brief loss of responsiveness not associated with head injury.
- A seizure results from an abnormal stimulation of the brain' cells causing uncontrollable muscle movements.
- Diabetes is a condition in which insulin is lacking or ineffective.
- Hypoglycemia is very low blood glucose and can be caused by too much insulin, too little or delayed food intake, exercise, alcohol, or a combination of these factors.
- Hyperglycemia occurs when the body has too much glucose in the blood and can be caused by insufficient insulin, overeating, inactivity, illness, stress, or a combination of these factors.
- People with gastrointestinal conditions usually report pain, nausea, vomiting, diarrhea, or constipation.
- Nausea (upset stomach) and vomiting (throwing up) often occur with conditions such as altitude sickness, motion sickness, brain injury, intestinal viruses, eating or drinking too much, and being emotionally upset.
- Diarrhea is the frequent passage of loose, watery, or unformed stools and can be a symptom of intestinal infection, food poisoning, food allergy, or other ailments.
- Constipation is the passage of hard, dry stools and is rarely more than a passing discomfort in otherwise healthy people.

## ▶ Vital Vocabulary

**angina pectoris** A spasmodic pain in the chest, characterized by a sensation of severe constriction or pressure on the anterior chest; associated with insufficient blood supply to the heart, aggravated by exercise or tension, and relieved by rest or medication.

**asthma** A condition marked by recurrent attacks of breathing difficulty, often with wheezing, due to spasmodic constriction of the air passages, often as a response to allergens or to mucus plugs in the bronchioles.

**chronic obstructive pulmonary disease (COPD)** A disease that makes it hard for a person to breathe because the normal flow of air into and out of the person's lungs is partially obstructed.

**diabetes** A condition that develops when glucose builds up in the blood, overflows into the urine, and passes through the body unused.

**diabetic coma** A state of unresponsiveness caused by a lack of insulin that goes uncorrected for too long.

**heart attack** A lay term for a condition resulting from blockage of a coronary artery and subsequent death of part of the heart muscle; a myocardial infarction; sometimes called simply a coronary.

**hyperglycemia** An abnormally increased concentration of glucose in the blood.

**hyperventilation** Excessively fast breathing that occurs during emotional distress.

**hypoglycemia** An abnormally diminished concentration of glucose in the blood.

**psychogenic shock** A shock-like state due to severe emotional distress; may result in a fainting spell resulting from a transient decrease in blood flow to the brain.

**seizure** Generalized, uncoordinated muscular activity associated with a loss of responsiveness; a convulsion; an attack of epilepsy.

status epilepticus The occurrence of two or more seizures without a period of complete consciousness
between them.

stroke A brain injury due to bleeding in the brain tissue
or to a blockage of blood flow, causing permanent
damage.

syncope Fainting; a brief period of unresponsiveness.

transient ischemic attack A form of stroke that occurs
when a part of the brain is deprived of oxygen-rich
blood long enough to cause symptoms but not long
enough to cause permanent damage.

## ▶ Assessment in Action

You are on a 5-day backpack trip in the mountains
with your friends. On day 3, and after several tough
miles of hiking, your friend seems to be disoriented
and is stumbling over rocks and tree roots on the trail.
He falls to the ground and is responsive. You know
that this friend has type 1 diabetes and did take his
insulin in the morning.

*Directions:* Circle Yes if you agree with the statement;
circle No if you disagree.

Yes　　No　　**1.** This person is very likely suffering from
hyperglycemia.

Yes　　No　　**2.** Low blood glucose levels can be
caused by too much insulin, too little
or delayed food intake, exercise, and
alcohol.

Yes　　No　　**3.** To give sugar in this scenario, the person must be known to have diabetes,
have an altered mental status, and be
awake enough to swallow.

Yes　　No　　**4.** You should follow the Rule of 15
when giving sugar to the person in this
scenario.

## ▶ Check Your Knowledge

*Directions:* Circle Yes if you agree with the statement;
circle No if you disagree.

Yes　　No　　**1.** People having a heart attack can experience chest pain.

Yes　　No　　**2.** You can help the person with chest
pain take his or her nitroglycerin.

Yes　　No　　**3.** A responsive person having a stroke
should lie down with his or her head
slightly raised.

Yes　　No　　**4.** People with asthma may have a prescribed inhaler.

Yes　　No　　**5.** A person who is breathing fast (hyperventilation) should be encouraged to breathe
slowly by holding inhaled air for several
seconds and then exhaling slowly.

Yes　　No　　**6.** Immobilize the spine of a person having a seizure.

Yes　　No　　**7.** Some people having a seizure display
a rigid arching of the back.

Yes　　No　　**8.** A person having seizures always
requires medical attention.

Yes　　No　　**9.** If in doubt about the type of diabetic
emergency a person is experiencing,
give sugar to a responsive person who
can swallow.

Yes　　No　　**10.** Nitroglycerin can relieve chest pain
associated with angina.

# Poisoning

**18**

## Poison

### ▶ What Is a Poison?

The American Association of Poison Control Centers (AAPCC) defines a <u>poison</u> as anything that can harm someone if it is (1) used in the wrong way, (2) used by the wrong person, or (3) used in the wrong amount. A <u>toxin</u> is a poisonous substance produced by bacteria, animals, or plants that acts by changing the normal metabolism of cells or by destroying them.

Poisons can be classified by how they enter the body:

- Ingested (swallowed)—through the mouth
- Inhaled (breathed)—through the lungs
- Injected—through needlelike device (eg, snake's fangs, bee's stinger)
- Absorbed (direct contact)—through the skin or eyes

Poisons come in four forms: solids (eg, medicine pills and tablets, batteries, certain plants), liquids (eg, household cleaning products, antifreeze, paint), sprays (eg, spray cleaning products, bug spray), and gases (eg, carbon monoxide, formaldehyde).

Consumer products are typically safe to use as directed by their label; however, if label directions are not followed or are improperly followed, some of these products can be poisonous. The most common poisons are not necessarily the most dangerous ones. Some of the more dangerous poisons that could be found in a home include the following:

- Antifreeze and windshield washer products
- Some medicines
- Corrosive cleaners such as drain openers, oven cleaners, toilet bowl cleaners, and rust removers
- Fuels such as kerosene, lamp oil, gasoline
- Pesticides

## Q&A

**Are some poisons absorbed through the skin?**

Chemical substances, including some medicines and poisons, are absorbed through the skin. Heavy metals such as mercury and lead pass through the skin and can result in chronic poisoning. Chlordane, malathion, and other pesticides cross the skin barrier and can cause acute and chronic conditions. Cyanide readily absorbs through the skin and can be very deadly.

## ▶ Ingested (Swallowed) Poisons

Ingested poisoning occurs when the person swallows a toxic substance. Fortunately, most poisons have little toxic effect or are ingested in such small amounts that severe poisoning rarely occurs. However, the potential for severe or fatal poisoning is always present. According to the AAPCC, more than 80% of all poisonings happen by ingesting a toxic substance.

Swallowing nonfood substances is so common among children that it is unusual for a child to reach the age of 5 years without ingesting a nonfood substance at least once. Although many nonfood substances such as dirt and paper are not harmful, others present definite health threats. Some have the potential to block the airway. Others are poisonous. Hundreds of thousands of poisonings occur in the United States each year, but only a small percentage progress to severe or life-threatening conditions. The AAPCC reports that approximately 50% of all poison cases occur in children younger than 6 years.

Older people who are prescribed many medications may have difficulty keeping them straight and may inadvertently take an excessive dose if they forget having already taken a medication.

Analgesics (pain medications) account for the largest category of poisoning exposures. Basically, any substance that is accessible to a child is a potential

**Figure 18-1**

Sources of poisons.

poison. Analgesic products that contain acetaminophen, for example, are involved in poisoning incidents more often than other analgesics are, not because acetaminophen is more toxic but because products that contain acetaminophen outsell products that contain other analgesics **Figure 18-1**.

It is important not to confuse poisoning frequency with poisoning severity. Most plant and mushroom ingestions are minor, with harmless effects. In contrast, gun-blueing products (agents containing selenious acid that are used to maintain the blue color of gun barrels) account for fewer episodes of exposure, but the potential for harm is much greater. Fortunately, most poison ingestions involve products with minor toxic effects or amounts so small that severe poisoning rarely occurs **Table 18-1**.

## Table 18-1 Substances Most Frequently Involved in Human Exposures

| Substance Category | All Substances | Percentage of Total Exposures* |
|---|---|---|
| Analgesics | 291,062 | 11.29 |
| Cosmetics/personal care products | 199,291 | 7.73 |
| Cleaning substances (household) | 198,018 | 7.68 |
| Sedative/hypnotics/antipsychotics | 150,715 | 5.85 |
| Antidepressants | 112,412 | 4.36 |
| Antihistamines | 103,327 | 4.01 |
| Cardiovascular drugs | 102,170 | 3.96 |
| Foreign bodies/toys/miscellaneous | 99,835 | 3.87 |
| Pesticides | 83,005 | 3.22 |
| Topical preparations | 82,819 | 3.21 |
| Alcohols | 68,648 | 2.66 |
| Vitamins | 66,058 | 2.56 |
| Cold and cough preparations | 61,288 | 2.38 |
| Stimulants and street drugs | 59,869 | 2.32 |
| Anticonvulsants | 56,832 | 2.20 |
| Hormones and hormone antagonists | 56,775 | 2.20 |
| Antimicrobials | 56,726 | 2.20 |
| Bites and envenomations | 55,017 | 2.13 |
| Gastrointestinal preparations | 48,501 | 1.88 |
| Plants | 44,731 | 1.74 |
| Dietary supplements/herbals/homeopathic | 42,535 | 1.65 |
| Chemicals | 38.975 | 1.51 |
| Fumes/gases/vapors | 33,944 | 1.32 |
| Other/unknown nondrug substances | 32,001 | 1.24 |
| Hydrocarbons | 31,903 | 1.24 |

*Percentages are based on the total number of substances reported in all exposures (N-2,577,557).

Source: Mowry JB, Spyker DA, Brooks DE, McMillan N, Schauben JL. 2014 Annual Report of the American Association of Poison Control Centers' National Poison Data System (NPDS): 32nd annual report. Clin Toxicol 53(10):962-1147.

## What to Look For

- Abdominal pain and cramping
- Nausea or vomiting
- Diarrhea
- Burns, odor, or stains around and in the mouth
- Drowsiness or unconsciousness
- Seizure
- Poison container nearby

## What to Do

1. Try to determine:
   - Person's age and weight
   - Person's condition
   - What poison was swallowed
   - When the poison was taken
   - How much was taken
2. Call the **Poison Help** hotline, operated by the National Poison Control Center, at 1-800-222-1222 even if no signs of poisoning are present **Figure 18-2**. Follow their directions.
3. Place the person on his or her left side to delay poison moving into the intestines and prevent inhalation of vomit if it occurs **Figure 18-3**.
4. Monitor breathing; if it stops, give cardiopulmonary resuscitation (CPR).

**Figure 18-2**

Poison Help logo.

*Courtesy of the American Association of Poison Control Centers. To locate your local poison center call 1-(800) 222-1222 or visit aapcc.org.*

**Figure 18-3**

The left-side position delays the advance of the poison into the small intestine.

*© American Academy of Orthopaedic Surgeons.*

Refer to  Flowchart 18-1 for additional information regarding the care of a person who has ingested poison.

## CAUTION

**DO NOT** give water or milk to dilute poisons other than caustic or corrosive substances (acids and alkalis) unless told to do so by staff at a poison center. Fluids can dissolve a dry poison such as tablets or capsules more rapidly and fill up the stomach, forcing the stomach contents (the poison) into the small intestine, where it will be absorbed faster. Vomiting and aspiration could occur.

## FYI

**Poisoning: Where Can You Call for Help?**

If someone swallows poison, do not call the hospital emergency department unless the person is unconscious or has trouble breathing. Call the poison center. Researchers who made 156 test calls to 52 hospital emergency departments in Illinois found that the advice given was correct only 64% of the time. Calls to the same emergency department on different days for the same condition did not consistently produce the same advice. In contrast, poison centers gave correct advice in 17 of 18 (94%) test calls.

*Source:* Wigder HN, Erickson T, Morse T, Saporta V. Emergency department poison advice telephone calls. *Ann Emerg Med* 1995;25:349-352.

## CAUTION

**DO NOT** gag or tickle the back of the person's throat with a finger or a spoon handle. This method is usually ineffective in causing vomiting, and any vomiting produced is not very forceful.

**DO NOT** give dish soap, raw eggs, or mustard powder. They are not effective.

**DO NOT** use syrup of ipecac.

**DO NOT** follow the first aid procedures or recommendations on a container label without first getting confirmation from a medical source. Many labels are incorrect or out of date.

**DO NOT** try to neutralize a poison. Giving weak acids, such as lemon juice or vinegar, is not safe, contrary to the advice given on many drain cleaner and lye product labels. Chemical neutralization releases large quantities of heat that can burn sensitive tissues.

**DO NOT** think that a specific antidote exists for most poisons. An antidote is a substance that counteracts a poison's effects. Few poisons have specific antidotes that will effectively block their toxic effects.

**DO NOT** think that there is a universal antidote. No product is effective in treating most or all poisons.

## FYI

### About Poison Control Centers

- Fifty-five accredited poison control centers exist in the United States.
- They provide free assistance by phone to anyone in the 50 states, Puerto Rico, The Federated States of Micronesia, American Samoa, the US Virgin Islands, the US Virgin Islands, and Guam.
- All centers can be reached by calling the same telephone number: 1-800-222-1222.
- Centers are staffed by pharmacists, physicians, nurses, and other poison experts who are toxicology specialists.
- All calls to a center are answered by a trained medical professional.
- More than 70% of all the calls to a center about a potential poisoning are managed onsite and outside of a health care facility. This saves costly emergency department visits. About 20% of the calls are from a health care facility requesting advice.
- All calls are kept confidential and can be translated into 161 languages.
- Calls are free and can be made 24 hours a day, 7 days a week, 365 days a year.
- They also provide educational outreach poison prevention programs.

*Source:* American Association of Poison Control Centers.

## FYI

### Poison Center History

According to the US Department of Health and Human Services, the idea for a poison center came from a part-time secretary at the American Academy of Pediatrics during the early 1950s. She called hospitals in Chicago to find out why children were in the emergency department with certain conditions. What had they eaten? What did they drink?

At the time, companies did not have to tell people much about the ingredients in their products. The secretary asked companies what ingredients in their products might be making children sick. She then asked a group of medical professionals to set treatment guidelines. When physicians had questions, they would call her, and she would read medical advice to them off note cards.

Soon after, the US Surgeon General ordered copies of her 1,000 index cards to be sent to health departments across the country. From this, the first poison center was founded, and the idea spread throughout the nation.

*Source:* US Department of Health and Human Services. http://www.poisonhelp.hrsa.gov/poison-centers/about-poison-centers/index.html.

## FYI

### Highly Toxic and Potentially Fatal Plants

**Castor Beans and Jequirity Beans**

Symptoms: severe vomiting and diarrhea (often bloody), seizures, unresponsiveness, death

**Oleander and Foxglove**

Symptoms: vomiting and diarrhea, confusion, irregular heart beat

**Hemlock**

Symptoms: dry mouth, rapid heart rate, tremors, sweating, seizures, muscle weakness, coma

*Source:* O'Malley GF, O'Malley R. Chemical food poisoning. Merck Manual, Consumer Version. https://www.merck-manuals.com/home/injuries-and-poisoning/poisoning/chemical-food-poisoning.

## FYI

### Preventing Poisoning

**Follow these precautions to reduce the risk of poisoning:**

1. Keep household products and medicines out of reach and out of sight of children, preferably in a locked cabinet or closet. When an adult who is using household products or taking medicine leaves the room, even briefly, he or she should move the containers to a safe place.
2. Store medicines separately from other household products and keep them in their original containers—never in cups or soft-drink bottles.
3. Properly label all products, and read the label before use.
4. Turn on a light when giving or taking medicine.
5. Because children tend to imitate adults, avoid taking medications in their presence.
6. Refer to medicines by their correct names. Do not tell children that medicines are candy; they are not.
7. Use household substances in child-resistant packaging. Prescription medicines should be kept in safety packaging.

**To avoid poisonings among older people:**

1. Always read the label and follow instructions when taking medicine.
2. Turn on a light at night when taking medicine.
3. Never mix medicines and alcohol, and never take more than the prescribed amount of medicine.
4. Do not borrow a friend's medicine or take old medicines.
5. Inform the physician what other medicines are being taken to avoid the risk of **adverse drug interactions**.

*Source:* US Consumer Product Safety Commission.

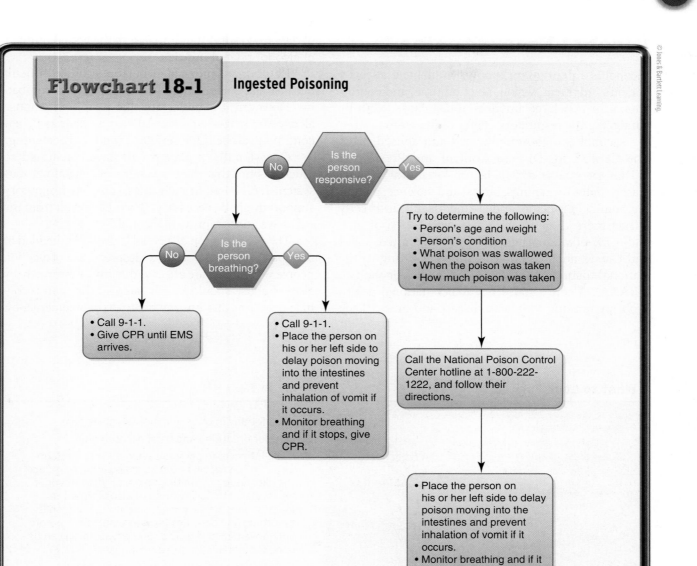

**Flowchart 18-1**　Ingested Poisoning

Is the person responsive?

- No → Is the person breathing?
  - No:
    - Call 9-1-1.
    - Give CPR until EMS arrives.
  - Yes:
    - Call 9-1-1.
    - Place the person on his or her left side to delay poison moving into the intestines and prevent inhalation of vomit if it occurs.
    - Monitor breathing and if it stops, give CPR.
- Yes:
  - Try to determine the following:
    - Person's age and weight
    - Person's condition
    - What poison was swallowed
    - When the poison was taken
    - How much poison was taken
  - Call the National Poison Control Center hotline at 1-800-222-1222, and follow their directions.
  - Place the person on his or her left side to delay poison moving into the intestines and prevent inhalation of vomit if it occurs.
  - Monitor breathing and if it stops, give CPR.

## Q&A

**Why place a person who has ingested poison on his or her left side?**

Placing the person on his or her left side (recovery position) positions the end of the stomach, where it enters the small intestine, straight up. Gravity will delay (up to 2 hours) the poison from moving into the small intestine, where absorption into the person's circulatory system is faster. The side position also helps prevent inhalation into the lungs if vomiting begins.

## Q&A

**Why call a Poison Control Center?**

A poison expert will decide whether the person is in danger. The poison expert will give you the advice you need and may stay on the phone with you while you get help or call you later to follow up. Most calls (more than 70%) can be handled outside of a hospital. If you need a physician or an ambulance, the poison expert will tell you right away.

# Alcohol Emergencies

Alcohol is a **depressant**, not a stimulant. It affects a person's judgment, vision, reaction time, and coordination. In very large amounts, it can cause death by paralyzing the respiratory center of the brain.

Alcohol is a commonly used and abused drug. The Centers for Disease Control and Prevention (CDC) cites it as a risk factor for motor vehicle crashes, falls, drownings, burns, and violence, including homicide, suicide, and sexual assault. It directly affects more than 16 million people (9.4% of men and 4.7% of women) annually in the United States and causes about 88,000 deaths, according to the National Institute on Alcohol Abuse and Alcoholism (NIAAA). Alcohol abuse is a major national health problem, ranking with heart disease and cancer. Lack of data makes it difficult to assess the actual number of alcohol-related injuries.

Helping an intoxicated person is often difficult because the person could be belligerent and combative. However, it is important that people who abuse alcohol be helped and not labeled as drunks. Their condition can be quite serious, even life threatening.

Occasionally, a person will have consumed so much alcohol that there are signs of central nervous system depression. In such cases, complete respiratory support might be necessary. Death can result from the excessive consumption of alcohol.

The consumption of alcohol is deeply embedded in our society. Because of the widespread use of alcohol, people whose lives are affected directly or indirectly by alcohol abuse should be educated so they can recognize problems and know what to do in an emergency.

## What to Look For

Although the following signs indicate alcohol intoxication, some might also mean illness or injury other than alcohol abuse, such as diabetes or heat injury:

- The odor of alcohol on a person's breath or clothing
- Unsteady, staggering walking
- Slurred speech and the inability to carry on a conversation
- Nausea and vomiting
- Flushed face
- Seizures (Any seizures related to alcohol require medical evaluation. Hyperglycemia can mimic alcohol intoxication, as can poisoning and neurologic conditions. [For additional information, see Chapter 17, *Sudden Illnesses*.])

## What to Do

1. Look for any injuries. Alcohol can mask pain.
2. Monitor breathing and treat accordingly.
3. If the intoxicated person is lying down, place him or her in the recovery (left-side) position to reduce the likelihood of vomiting and aspiration of vomit and to delay the absorption of alcohol into the bloodstream. Be sure to check that the person is breathing and does not have a spinal injury before you move him or her. The recovery position can be used for responsive and unresponsive people.
4. Call the poison center for advice or the local emergency number for help. It might be best to let emergency medical services (EMS) personnel decide whether the police should be alerted.
5. If the person becomes violent, leave the scene and find a safe place until police arrive.
6. Provide emotional support.
7. Assume that an injured or unresponsive person has a spinal injury and needs to be stabilized against movement. Because of decreased pain perception, a person who is intoxicated cannot be assessed reliably. If you suspect a spinal injury, wait for EMS personnel to arrive. They have the proper equipment and training to stabilize and move a person.
8. Because many intoxicated people have been exposed to the cold, suspect hypothermia (dangerously low body temperature) and move the person to a warm place whenever possible. Remove wet clothing and cover the person with warm blankets. Handle a person with hypothermia gently because rough handling could induce a deadly heart rhythm.

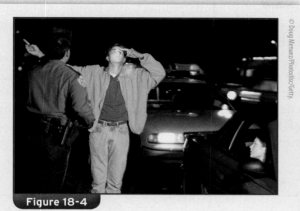

**Figure 18-4**

Field sobriety test.

**Figure 18-5**

Cocaine.

**Figure 18-6**

Marijuana.

## CAUTION

**DO NOT** let an intoxicated person sleep on his or her back.

**DO NOT** leave an intoxicated person alone unless he or she becomes violent.

**DO NOT** try to handle a hostile, intoxicated person by yourself. Find a safe place, and then call the police for help.

# Drug Emergencies

Drugs are classified according to their effects on the user:

- *Uppers* are stimulants of the central nervous system. They include amphetamines, cocaine, and caffeine **Figure 18-5** .
- *Downers* are depressants of the central nervous system. They include **barbiturates**, **tranquilizers**, marijuana, and **narcotics** **Figure 18-6** .
- *Hallucinogens* alter and often enhance the sensory and emotional information in the brain centers. They include lysergic acid diethylamide (LSD), mescaline, peyote, and phencyclidine hydrochloride (PCP). Marijuana also has some hallucinogenic properties.
- *Inhalants* usually are inhaled and can cause serious damage to many body organs. They include plastic model glue and cement, paint solvent, gasoline, spray paint, and nail polish remover **Figure 18-7** .

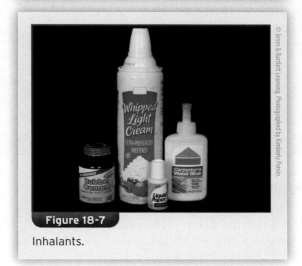

**Figure 18-7**

Inhalants.

## ▶ Sympathomimetics

Sympathomimetics are stimulants. A **stimulant** is any agent that produces an excited state. Amphetamine and methamphetamine are commonly taken by mouth. They are also injected in many cases. They typically are taken to make the user feel good, improve task performance, suppress appetite, or prevent sleepiness. Sympathomimetic drugs are frequently called uppers.

Methamphetamine production is dangerous because it is often produced illegally in makeshift labs using hazardous materials and techniques.

Cocaine can be taken in a number of different ways—through the nose, by injection, and by smoking. Crack is pure cocaine and is smoked. Smoked crack produces the most potent effect. Cocaine is one of the most addictive substances known. It can induce strokes, seizures, and heart attacks.

| What to Look For | What to Do |
|---|---|
| • Disorganized behavior, hyperactivity, restlessness, and sometimes anxiety or great fear<br>• Paranoia (which can put the user and others in danger) and delusions | 1. Check breathing.<br>2. Call the poison center for advice or 9-1-1 for help.<br>3. Check for injuries.<br>4. Keep the person on the left side to reduce the likelihood of vomiting and aspiration of vomitus and to delay absorption of drugs.<br>5. Provide reassurance and emotional support.<br>6. If the person becomes violent, seek safety until the police arrive. Let law enforcement officers handle dangerous situations.<br>7. Call 9-1-1. |

## ▶ Hallucinogens

**Hallucinogens** produce changes in mood and sensory awareness; a person using these drugs might hear colors and see sounds. They can cause hallucinations and bizarre behavior that might make users dangerous to themselves and others. Acute intoxication requires medical attention. Users should be protected from hurting themselves. The classic hallucinogen is LSD. Abuse of another hallucinogen, PCP, often called angel dust, is dangerous because it causes severe behavioral changes.

| What to Look For | What to Do |
|---|---|
| The user reports:<br>• Visual hallucinations<br>• Increased intensity of vision and hearing | 1. Check breathing.<br>2. Call the poison center for advice or 9-1-1 for help.<br>3. Check for injuries.<br>4. Keep the person on the left side to reduce the likelihood of vomiting and aspiration of vomit and to delay absorption of drugs.<br>5. Provide reassurance and emotional support.<br>6. If the person becomes violent, seek safety until the police arrive. Let law enforcement officers handle dangerous situations.<br>7. Call 9-1-1. |

## ▶ Marijuana

The flowering hemp plant called marijuana is used throughout the world. It has been estimated that as many as 20 million people use marijuana daily in the United States.

| What to Look For | What to Do |
|---|---|
| • Euphoria, relaxation, and drowsiness<br>• Impaired short-term memory and capacity to do complex thinking and work<br>• Altered perception of time<br>• Anxiety and panic<br>• Hallucinations (produced by very high doses) | 1. Check breathing.<br>2. Call the poison center for advice or 9-1-1 for help.<br>3. Check for injuries.<br>4. Keep the person on the left side to reduce the likelihood of vomiting and aspiration of vomit.<br>5. Provide reassurance and emotional support.<br>6. If the person becomes violent, seek safety until the police arrive. Let law enforcement officers handle dangerous situations.<br>7. Call 9-1-1. |

## ▶ Depressants

Depressants are often prescribed as a part of legitimate medical treatment. They are easy to obtain, and people intent on misusing them sometimes solicit prescriptions from several physicians. This class of drug includes **opiates** (narcotics) and **sedative-hypnotics** (barbiturates and tranquilizers).

## Sedative-Hypnotics

Sedative-hypnotics are prescribed as anesthetics, sedatives, and anti-anxiety treatments. The effects of sedative-hypnotic drug overdose are similar to those of alcohol.

| What to Look For | What to Do |
|---|---|
| • Drowsiness and sleepiness<br>• Slurred speech<br>• Slow breathing rate | 1. Check breathing.<br>2. Call the poison center for advice or 9-1-1 for help.<br>3. Check for injuries.<br>4. Keep the person on the left side to reduce the likelihood of vomiting and aspiration of vomit and to delay absorption of drugs.<br>5. Provide reassurance and emotional support.<br>6. If the person becomes violent, seek safety until the police arrive. Let law enforcement officers handle dangerous situations.<br>7. Call 9-1-1. |

## Opiates

The pain relievers called opiates are named for the opium in poppy seeds, the origin of heroin, codeine, and morphine. On the list of frequently abused drugs, they have been joined by a number of synthetic opiates, called **opioids**, that originated in a laboratory, with most of them having legitimate medical uses. With the exception of heroin, which is illegal in the United States, many addicts started using an opiate drug with an appropriate medical prescription.

| What to Look For | What to Do |
|---|---|
| • Reduced breathing rate<br>• Pinpoint pupils<br>• Sedated condition and unresponsiveness | 1. Check breathing.<br>2. Call the poison center for advice or 9-1-1 for help.<br>3. Check for injuries.<br>4. Keep the person on the left side to reduce the likelihood of vomiting and aspiration of vomit and to delay absorption of drugs.<br>5. Provide reassurance and emotional support.<br>6. If the person becomes violent, seek safety until the police arrive. Let law enforcement officers handle dangerous situations.<br>7. Call 9-1-1. |

## ▶ Abused Inhalants

Inhaling glue or other solvents (gasoline, lighter fluid, nail polish remover) produces effects similar to those from ingesting alcohol. People who sniff these substances can die of suffocation. In addition, some inhalants can cause death by changing the rhythm of the heartbeat and can cause permanent brain damage.

| What to Look For | What to Do |
| --- | --- |
| • Mild drowsiness to unresponsiveness<br>• Slurred speech and clumsiness<br>• Seizures<br>• Slow breathing rate<br>• Smell of solvents | 1. Check breathing.<br>2. Call the poison center for advice or 9-1-1 for help.<br>3. Check for injuries.<br>4. Keep the person on the left side to reduce the likelihood of vomiting and aspiration of vomit.<br>5. Provide reassurance and emotional support.<br>6. If the person becomes violent, seek safety until the police arrive. Let law enforcement officers handle dangerous situations.<br>7. Call 9-1-1. |

# Carbon Monoxide Poisoning

<u>Carbon monoxide</u>, because of its common presence in our environment, along with its insidious nature, is a leading cause of poisoning death in the United States each year. Carbon monoxide is an odorless, colorless, nonirritating gas produced by the incomplete combustion of carbon-based fuels. According to a report from the CDC, each year more than 400 Americans die of unintentional carbon monoxide poisoning. Carbon monoxide poisoning sends more than 20,000 to the hospital annually.

People who ride long distances in older, poorly maintained cars are at increased risk of carbon monoxide poisoning. Rust can damage an automobile's exhaust system and create holes in the car's body, through which carbon monoxide can enter. A common source of carbon monoxide poisoning is motor vehicle exhaust. Some people will attempt suicide by running the engine inside a closed garage and inhaling the fumes. Many unintentional deaths involve people sleeping inside a running car, often after consuming alcohol.

People in a closed room where there is cigarette smoking experience mild increases in the level of carbon monoxide in their blood. Less familiar and, therefore, more dangerous sources of carbon monoxide are faulty furnaces, water heaters, and kerosene heaters. Recreational fires, whether open-flame, charcoal, or hibachi grills, also give off carbon monoxide.

People with carbon monoxide poisoning are often unaware of its presence. The gas is invisible, tasteless, odorless, and nonirritating. It is produced by the incomplete burning of organic material such as gasoline, wood, paper, charcoal, coal, and natural gas.

Carbon monoxide causes hypoxia, or lack of oxygen, in two ways. First, the hemoglobin in red blood cells is about 200 times more likely to bind to carbon monoxide than to oxygen if both are present in the blood; thus, even a small amount of carbon monoxide can greatly reduce the amount of oxygen carried in the bloodstream. Second, carbon monoxide does not allow the cells to use what little oxygen is delivered. In short, carbon monoxide restricts oxygen to the body parts that need oxygen the most—the heart and the brain.

Refer to **Flowchart 18-2** for additional information regarding the care of an inhaled poison emergency.

---

### FYI

**Carbon Monoxide After Hurricane Katrina**

Hurricane Katrina made landfall on August 29, 2005, on the Gulf Coast of the United States, causing loss of life, widespread property damage, and power outages. After the hurricane, some residents used portable generators and other gasoline-powered appliances for electrical power and cleanup. These devices produce carbon monoxide, and improper use can cause carbon monoxide poisoning. From August 29 through September 24, a total of 51 cases of carbon monoxide poisoning were reported by hyperbaric oxygen facilities (facilities that house large chambers in which oxygen levels are higher than normal to treat carbon monoxide poisoning) in Alabama, Louisiana, and Mississippi. Carbon monoxide poisoning can be prevented by reducing exposure to carbon monoxide through appropriate placement and ventilation of gasoline-powered engines.

*Source:* Centers for Disease Control and Prevention. Carbon monoxide poisoning after Hurricane Katrina–Alabama, Louisiana, and Mississippi. *Morb Mortal Wkly Rep* 2005;54(39):996-998.

---

### What to Look For

It is difficult to determine if a person is poisoned by carbon monoxide. Sometimes, a complaint of having flulike symptoms is actually a sign of carbon monoxide poisoning:

- Headache
- Ringing in the ears (tinnitus)
- Chest pain (angina)
- Muscle weakness
- Nausea and vomiting
- Dizziness and visual changes (blurred or double vision)
- Unresponsiveness
- Respiratory and cardiac arrest

The traditionally cited sign of carbon monoxide poisoning is cherry-red skin and lips. This sign is uncommon, however, and occurs only at death; therefore, it is a poor initial indicator of carbon monoxide poisoning.

The following are earmarks of possible carbon monoxide poisoning:

- The symptoms come and go.
- The symptoms worsen or improve in certain places or at certain times of the day.
- People around the person have similar symptoms.
- Pets seem ill.

### What to Do

1. Get the person out of the toxic environment and into fresh air *immediately.*
2. Call 9-1-1, who will send EMS personnel who will be able to give the person 100% oxygen, improving oxygenation and disassociating the linkage between the carbon monoxide and the hemoglobin. For a responsive person, it takes 4 to 5 hours with ordinary air (21% oxygen) or 30 to 40 minutes with 100% oxygen to reverse the effects of carbon monoxide poisoning.
3. Monitor breathing.
4. Place an unresponsive breathing person in the recovery position.
5. Seek medical care. All people with suspected carbon monoxide poisoning should obtain a blood test to determine the level of carbon monoxide.

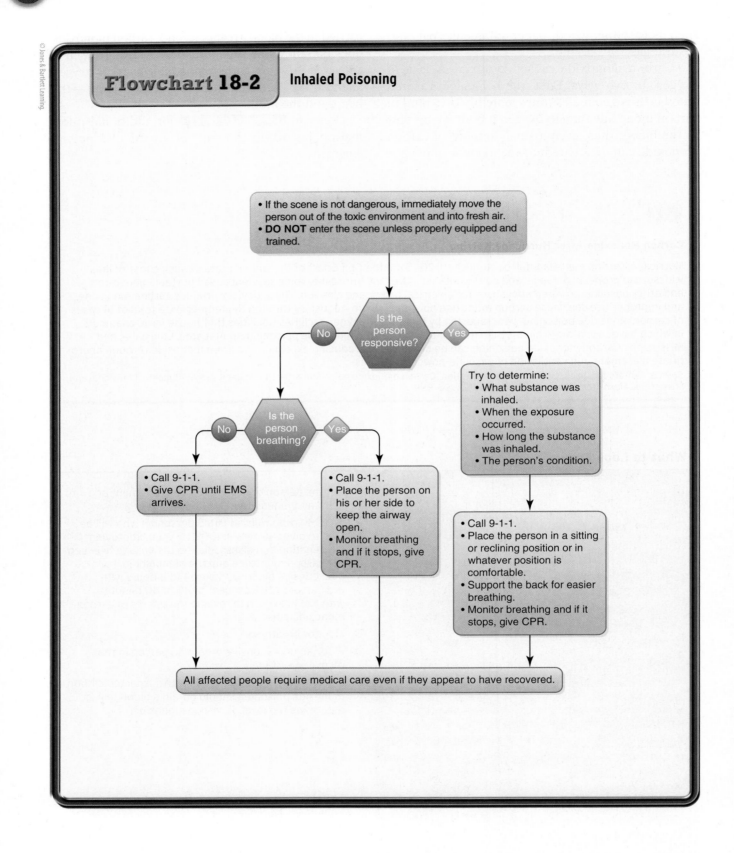

**Flowchart 18-2**    Inhaled Poisoning

- If the scene is not dangerous, immediately move the person out of the toxic environment and into fresh air.
- **DO NOT** enter the scene unless properly equipped and trained.

Is the person responsive?

**No** / **Yes**

Try to determine:
- What substance was inhaled.
- When the exposure occurred.
- How long the substance was inhaled.
- The person's condition.

Is the person breathing?

**No** / **Yes**

- Call 9-1-1.
- Give CPR until EMS arrives.

- Call 9-1-1.
- Place the person on his or her side to keep the airway open.
- Monitor breathing and if it stops, give CPR.

- Call 9-1-1.
- Place the person in a sitting or reclining position or in whatever position is comfortable.
- Support the back for easier breathing.
- Monitor breathing and if it stops, give CPR.

All affected people require medical care even if they appear to have recovered.

**Carbon Monoxide Poisoning Deaths Associated With Camping**

Exposure to carbon monoxide is responsible for more fatal, unintentional poisonings in the United States than any other agent, with the highest incidence occurring during the cold-weather months. Although most of these deaths occur in residences or motor vehicles, two incidents among campers in Georgia illustrate the danger of carbon monoxide in outdoor settings.

**Case 1**

A 51-year-old man, his 10-year-old son, a 9-year-old boy, and a 7-year-old girl were found dead inside a zipped-up, 10 x 14-inch (3 x 4-m), two-room tent at their campsite in southeast Georgia (a pet dog also died). A propane gas stove, still burning, was found inside the tent; the stove apparently had been brought inside to provide warmth.

**Case 2**

A 34-year-old man and his 7-year-old son were found dead inside their zipped-up tent at a group camping site in central Georgia. They were discovered by other campers. A charcoal grill was found inside the tent; the grill apparently had been brought inside to provide warmth after it had been used outside for cooking.

During 1990 to 1994, in the United States, portable fuel-burning camp stoves and lanterns were involved in 10 to 17 carbon monoxide poisoning deaths each year, and charcoal grills were involved in 15 to 27 deaths each year. During this same time, an annual average of 30 fatal carbon monoxide poisonings occurred inside tents or campers.

*Source:* Centers for Disease Control and Prevention. Carbon monoxide poisoning deaths associated with camping–Georgia, March 1999. *Morb Mortal Wkly Rep* 1999;48(32):705-706.

**Carbon Monoxide Detectors Can Save Lives**

The US Consumer Product Safety Commission recommends that consumers purchase and install carbon monoxide detectors with labels showing they meet the requirements of the Underwriters Laboratories (UL) voluntary standard (UL 2034). The standard requires detectors to sound an alarm when the carbon monoxide concentration reaches a potentially hazardous level.

Properly working carbon monoxide detectors can provide an early warning before the deadly gas builds up to a dangerous level. Exposure to a low concentration during several hours can be as dangerous as exposure to a high carbon monoxide level for a few minutes. The detectors react to both conditions. Each home should have at least one carbon monoxide detector in the area outside individual bedrooms. Carbon monoxide detectors are as important as smoke detectors to home safety.

*Source:* US Consumer Product Safety Commission. Carbon monoxide detectors can save lives. October 5, 2004. http://www.energy.wsu.edu/Documents/carbon_mono.pdf.

# Plant-Induced Dermatitis

## ▶ Poison Ivy, Poison Oak, and Poison Sumac

The American Skin Association reports about 85% of the population is sensitive to poison ivy, poison oak, and poison sumac. With more people venturing into the outdoors, episodes of dermatitis caused by exposure to poison ivy **Figure 18-8**, poison oak **Figure 18-9**, and poison sumac **Figure 18-10** are increasing. (Actually, more than 60 plants can cause allergic reactions, but these three are by far the most common offenders.) Of those who do react, 10% to 15% will have incapacitating swelling and blistering eruptions that require medical care **Figure 18-11**, according to the American Skin Association. There is no routine test to determine a person's degree of sensitivity; a history of dermatitis is the most reliable indicator.

The resin (urushiol) of these plants is a colorless or slightly yellow oil. It runs in resin canals just under the surface, from the roots through the

**Figure 18-8**

Poison ivy, found in all 48 contiguous states in the United States.

**Figure 18-9**

Poison oak.

**Figure 18-10**

Poison sumac.

**Figure 18-11**

Poison ivy dermatitis.

stems, into the leaves and flowers, and just under the surface of the fruit. It is not present in the nectar. The leaves of the plants are fragile and easily ruptured by strong winds or by humans or animals brushing against them. The oil immediately oozes onto the surface.

The light-colored oil generally is not visible on human skin. If present on the sole of a shoe, on the palm of a hand or glove, or on the surface of an animal's fur, it can be spread by direct contact. On some objects, the oil can stay in an active form for months or years. Urushiol can be on the handle of a rake for years and still bond to human skin within 5 or 10 minutes. Poison ivy leaves have been kept for up to 5

years with no loss of potency. Contaminated clothing has caused rashes even after more than 1 year. Smoke from burning plants can produce severe dermatitis. People downwind from these burning leaves can be affected by airborne oil, which can be inhaled and cause airway irritation.

Most people cannot identify these irritating plants. Poison ivy and poison oak are low bushes or climbing vines with waxy, broad, green leaves in the summer that change to brown to red in the fall. The leaflets of poison ivy and poison oak grow in groups of three (three leaves radiating from a single attachment point), giving rise to the warning, "leaves of three, let them be." Poison ivy flourishes throughout most of the United States, except in Alaska and Hawaii; poison oak is found on the West and East Coasts and some South Central areas of the United States. Poison sumac is found chiefly in damp, swampy areas in the eastern United States. These plants tend not to grow at elevations higher than 5,000 feet (1,500 m) or in hot, dry deserts. A helpful method of identifying these plants is the black spot test. When the sap is exposed to the air, it turns brown in a matter of minutes and black by the next day.

People can come in contact with the urushiol of these plants from their clothes or shoes, pet fur, or the smoke from burning plants. Contrary to popular belief, no one can develop a rash by touching the fluid from the blisters (their own or others') because the fluid in the blister does not contain the oily resin. Any apparent spreading is actually a delayed reaction to contact with the resin.

Refer to **Flowchart 18-3** for additional information regarding the care of plant-induced dermatitis from poison ivy, poison oak, and poison sumac.

**Conducting a Black Spot Test**

Most people with poison ivy dermatitis do not recognize the plant. Poison ivy and poison oak leaves have three leaflets; poison sumac has 7 to 13 leaflets per leaf. The mature fruit is an off-white berry. These botanical characteristics explain the axioms, "leaves of three, let them be" and "berries white, poisonous sight!"

The black spot test is another means of identifying these plants. To check a suspicious plant, grasp a leaf and its stem where it attaches to the branch with a folded sheet of white paper (do not touch the leaf). Crush the end of the leaf stalk in the folded sheet of white paper with a rock. The paper needs to be wet with the sap of the leaf stem. The clear sap of poison ivy, poison oak, and poison sumac on the paper will turn dark brown within 10 minutes and black within 24 hours. This test is not conclusive but can strongly suggest that the plant is one of the three plants.

*Source:* Schram SE, Willey A, Lee PK, Bohjanen KA, Warshaw EM. Black-spot poison ivy. *Dermatitis* 2008;19(1):48-51.

**Preventing Poisonous-Plant Dermatitis**

To reduce the likelihood of poisonous-plant dermatitis developing, follow these suggestions:

- Avoid the plants.
- Wear protective clothing and use appropriate commercial barrier preparations.
- Replenish the barrier protection every 4 to 6 hours, if practical.
- Decontaminate after known exposure with liberal amounts of soap and water, and then reapply the barrier preparation.
- Decontaminate at the end of the day with isopropyl alcohol and a water rinse.
- Dispose of all contaminated clothing and equipment.

| What to Look For | What to Do |
|---|---|
| Known contact within 5 minutes for people with sensitive skin and up to 1 hour for people with moderately sensitive skin | If within 1 hour of an exposure:<br>1. Gently wipe skin with rubbing alcohol. **DO NOT** rub it in. **DO NOT** use packaged alcohol wipes.<br>2. Next, or if rubbing alcohol is not available, wash the skin with lots of cold running water. Soap is not necessary, but if used, rinse with lots of cold running water. **DO NOT** scrub skin.<br>3. **DO NOT** use gasoline. |
| Mild dermatitis: itching | 1. Apply any of the following:<br>  • Colloidal oatmeal bath (Aveeno Soothing Bath Treatments)<br>  • Baking soda paste (1 teaspoon [5 mL] water mixed with 3 teaspoons [15 mL] baking soda)<br>  • Calamine lotion<br>  • Aluminum acetate solution (Burow's solution)<br>  • Physician-prescribed medication<br>2. If none of the above are available, the application of over-the-counter hydrocortisone may be beneficial in mild cases. |
| Moderate dermatitis: itching and swelling | 1. Treat the same as for mild signs and symptoms.<br>2. Apply a physician-prescribed steroid ointment. |
| Severe dermatitis: itching, swelling, and blisters | 1. Treat the same as for mild and moderate symptoms.<br>2. Apply a physician-prescribed topical or oral steroid.<br>3. Seek medical care if the person inhales smoke from a burning plant or if the reaction involves the face, eyes, genitals, or large areas of the body. |

## Flowchart 18-3 Plant-Induced Dermatitis

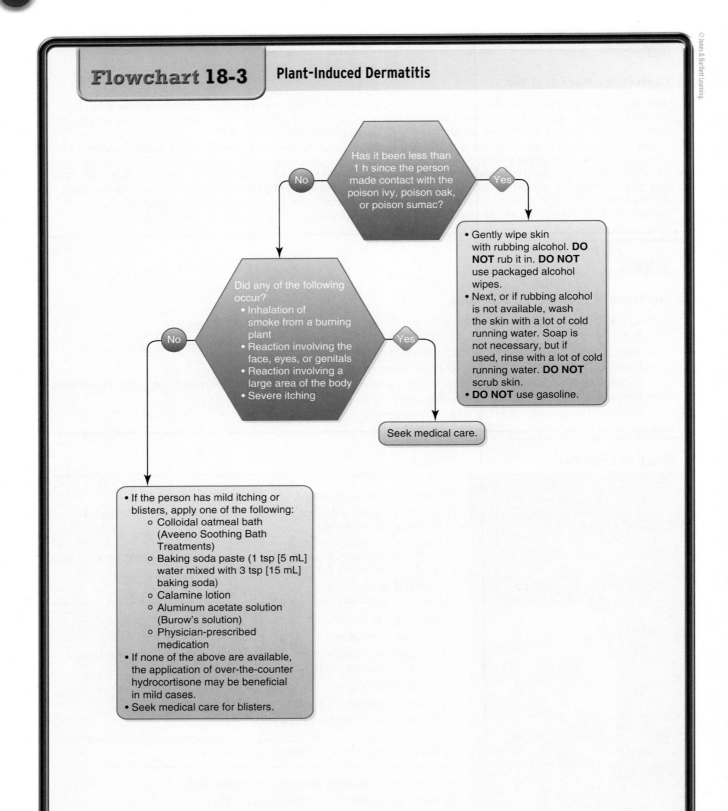

**Has it been less than 1 h since the person made contact with the poison ivy, poison oak, or poison sumac?**

**No** / **Yes**

**Yes:**
- Gently wipe skin with rubbing alcohol. **DO NOT** rub it in. **DO NOT** use packaged alcohol wipes.
- Next, or if rubbing alcohol is not available, wash the skin with a lot of cold running water. Soap is not necessary, but if used, rinse with a lot of cold running water. **DO NOT** scrub skin.
- **DO NOT** use gasoline.

**Did any of the following occur?**
- Inhalation of smoke from a burning plant
- Reaction involving the face, eyes, or genitals
- Reaction involving a large area of the body
- Severe itching

**No** / **Yes**

**Yes:** Seek medical care.

**No:**
- If the person has mild itching or blisters, apply one of the following:
  - Colloidal oatmeal bath (Aveeno Soothing Bath Treatments)
  - Baking soda paste (1 tsp [5 mL] water mixed with 3 tsp [15 mL] baking soda)
  - Calamine lotion
  - Aluminum acetate solution (Burow's solution)
  - Physician-prescribed medication
- If none of the above are available, the application of over-the-counter hydrocortisone may be beneficial in mild cases.
- Seek medical care for blisters.

## CAUTION

**DO NOT** use over-the-counter anti-itch lotions that also have antihistamines because they can cause further skin irritation. Oral antihistamines often are used in conjunction with prescription creams to help decrease itching.

**DO NOT** let the person rub or scratch the rash or itching skin.

# ▶ Stinging Nettle

The stinging nettle plant has stinging hairs on its stem and leaves. The stinging hair is a fine, hollow tube with a bladder at its base that contains a chemical irritant. When the stinging hair is touched, a fine needlepoint that penetrates the skin and injects an irritating chemical is formed.

Stinging nettle affects almost all people. Its effects are not an allergic response, as with poison ivy, but rather result from the direct irritant effect of the plant's sap.

## What to Look For

- Immediate, intense redness, burning, and itching to the exposed area, lasting for an hour or more, depending on the area of the body exposed to the plant
- The thicker skin on the soles and the palms retards the stinging hairs better than areas of thinner skin, such as the backs of the hands and the arms.
- Usually, no systemic (whole-body) effects are noted.

## What to Do

1. Wash the exposed area with soap and water to remove irritant chemicals.
2. Apply a cold, wet pack to help soothe the painful itching. Other treatments might include a paste of colloidal oatmeal, an over-the-counter hydrocortisone cream (1%), or calamine lotion.
3. Take an over-the-counter antihistamine, if desired. Be sure to follow package directions, and be aware that antihistamines cause drowsiness.
4. The duration of the stinging nettle reaction is measured in hours, rather than days, so little therapy is needed.

# prep kit

## ▶ Ready for Review

- A poison is any substance that impairs health or causes death by its chemical action when it enters the body or comes in contact with the skin.
- Poisons are classified by how they enter the body. They can be ingested, inhaled, absorbed, and injected.
- Ingested poisoning occurs when the person swallows a toxic substance.
- Alcohol is a depressant that affects a person's judgment, vision, reaction time, and coordination.
- Drugs are classified according to their effects on the user:
  - Uppers (stimulants)
  - Downers (depressants)
  - Hallucinogens
  - Inhalants
- Carbon monoxide is a leading cause of poisoning death in the United States each year.
- About 85% of the population is sensitive to poison ivy, poison oak, and poison sumac.

## ▶ Vital Vocabulary

**adverse drug interactions** An unintended or harmful response to two or more drugs being taken concurrently.

**barbiturates** A group of drugs in the class of drugs known as sedative-hypnotics.

**carbon monoxide** A colorless, odorless, poisonous gas formed by incomplete combustion, such as in fire.

**depressant** An agent that produces a depressed or reduced level of stimulation.

**hallucinogens** An agent that produces false perceptions in any one of the five senses.

**ingested poisoning** Poisoning caused by swallowing a toxic substance.

**naloxone** A medication used to counter the effects of opioids.

**narcotics** A drug that produces sleep or altered mental status.

**opiates** A drug containing or derived from opium.

**opioids** A synthetically produced narcotic not derived from opium.

**poison** Any substance that impairs health or causes death by its chemical action when it enters the body or comes in contact with the skin.

**Poison Help** A medical facility operated by the National Poison Control Center that provides immediate, free, expert advice any time; can be reached by calling 1-800-222-1222.

**sedative-hypnotics** A class of drugs that act as a central nervous system depressant.

**stimulant** An agent that produces an excited state.

**toxin** A poisonous substance produced by bacteria, animals, or plants that acts by changing the normal metabolism of cells or by destroying them.

**tranquilizers** A group of drugs in the class of drugs known as sedative-hypnotics.

## ▶ Assessment in Action

You have been helping your sister paint three rooms in her home. While taking a break, your 2-year-old niece enters the room with a small cup of paint used for touch up. There is paint around and inside her mouth.

*Directions:* Circle Yes if you agree with the statement; circle No if you disagree.

Yes   No   1. Immediately give your niece water or milk to dilute the ingested paint.

Yes   No   2. Use syrup of ipecac to induce vomiting.

Yes   No   3. Determine how much of the paint was swallowed, when it was swallowed, and the age and size of your niece.

Yes   No   4. Call the National Poison Control Center for advice (1-800-222-1222).

## ▶ Check Your Knowledge

*Directions:* Circle Yes if you agree with the statement; circle No if you disagree.

Yes   No   1. Swallowing a poison can produce nausea.

Yes   No   2. Milk should be given to all people who ingest poison.

Yes   No   **3.** A person with alcohol intoxication does not require medical care.

Yes   No   **4.** Carbon monoxide has a unique smell.

Yes   No   **5.** Everyone who touches a poison ivy, poison oak, or poison sumac plant will have some type of skin reaction.

Yes   No   **6.** Causing a person who is poisoned to vomit is a recommended first aid practice.

Yes   No   **7.** Some cases of poison ivy, poison oak, or poison sumac require medical care.

Yes   No   **8.** Calamine lotion can help relieve itching caused by poison ivy, poison oak, or poison sumac.

Yes   No   **9.** If a person who is intoxicated or drugged becomes violent, leave the area.

Yes   No   **10.** Move a person with carbon monoxide poisoning to fresh air.

# Bites and Stings

## 19

## ▶ Animal Bites

Animal bites represent a major, largely unrecognized public health issue. Two concerns result from an animal bite: immediate tissue damage and later infection from microorganisms.

Dogs are responsible for the majority of all animal bite injuries Figure 19-1. According to the American Veterinary Medical Association (AVMA), about 30 to 40 bite-related deaths occur in the United States each year Table 19-1. However, 80% of the nearly 5 million dog bites that occur yearly are trivial or minor, and medical care is not required or sought, which demonstrates the importance of knowing first aid.

A dog's mouth can carry more than 60 species of bacteria, some of which are dangerous to humans Table 19-2. Two examples of infection—tetanus and rabies—have been almost eradicated by medical advances, but they still pose a potential issue.

Although cat bites are less mutilating than dog bites, cat bites have a much higher rate of infection than dog bites. Cats have very sharp teeth, which can create deep puncture wounds and involve muscle, tendon, and bone.

Another pet especially likely to bite children is the ferret. These animals are often unpredictable. Ferrets are prone to unprovoked attacks, rapidly and repeatedly biting and slashing their target; they can cause severe facial injury to infants.

Besides children, older adults and people unable to help themselves are especially prone to animal bites because they are sometimes unable to detect or prevent a dangerous situation. Many animal-related deaths occur when the person is left alone with the offending pet. Contrary to popular belief, wild or stray dogs seldom are involved in fatal attacks.

Damage mostly occurs on the hands, arms, legs, and face. A damaged face presents several issues because the proximity of blood vessels to the skin surface makes the face susceptible to copious bleeding. Facial disfigurement and scarring can result in emotional trauma. Complete or partial loss of an eye also is possible.

Wild animal attacks occur most often in rural or wilderness locations (see Chapter 24, *Wilderness First Aid*, for more information). Not all injuries are bites. Severe injuries result from people being thrown in the air, gored by an antler, butted, or trampled on the ground.

## Rabies

Rabies is one of the most ancient and feared of diseases Figure 19-2 . Although human rabies rarely occurs in the United States or in other industrialized nations, it remains a scourge in developing countries. A virus found in warm-blooded animals causes rabies, which

© E.M. Singletary, M.D. Used with permission.

**Figure 19-1**

Dog bite.

## Table 19-1 Animal-Related Human Deaths in the United States (1999-2007)

| | Number of deaths | Percent of deaths (from total) | Average number of fatalities per year |
|---|---|---|---|
| **VENOMOUS ANIMALS** | | 39.6 | 79.5 |
| Hornets, wasps, and bees | 509 | 28.3 | 56.6 |
| Venomous spiders | 70 | 3.9 | 7.8 |
| Other venomous arthropods | 63 | 3.5 | 7.1 |
| Venomous snakes and lizards | 59 | 3.3 | 6.6 |
| Scorpions | 5 | 0.3 | 0.6 |
| Unspecified venomous animal or plant | 4 | 0.2 | 0.4 |
| Centipedes and venomous millipedes | 2 | 0.1 | 0.2 |
| Venomous marine animals and plants | 1 | 0.1 | 0.2 |
| **NONVENOMOUS ANIMALS** | | 60.4 | 121.3 |
| Other mammal | 655 | 36.4 | 72.9 |
| Dog | 250 | 13.9 | 27.8 |
| Other nonvenomous insect or other nonvertebrate | 85 | 4.7 | 9.4 |
| Other reptiles | 77 | 4.3 | 8.6 |
| Marine animal | 10 | 0.6 | 1.2 |
| Crocodile or alligator | 9 | 0.5 | 1.0 |
| Rat | 3 | 0.2 | 0.4 |
| **TOTAL** | 1802 | | 200.8 |

*Reproduced from:* Wilderness and Environmental Medicine, 23:2, Forrester, J.A., et.al., Fatalities from venomous and nonvenomous animals in the United States, 146-152, Copyright (2012), with permission from Elsevier.

## Table 19-2 Facts About Dog Bites

- Carefully choose your pet dog. Evaluate your environment and lifestyle, and speak with a professional to determine the appropriate type of pet.
- Dogs should be neutered to reduce aggressive tendencies.
- Never leave infants or young children alone with a dog. Be sensitive to cues that a child is fearful or apprehensive about a dog.
- Teach children basic safety around dogs, and review regularly.
- Dogs with histories of aggression are inappropriate for families with children.
- **DO NOT** play aggressive games, such as wrestling, with your dog.
- Never approach an unfamiliar dog. Immediately report stray dogs or dogs displaying unusual behavior.
- Remain motionless when approached by an unfamiliar dog—never run or scream.
- **DO NOT** disturb a dog that is sleeping, eating, or caring for puppies.
- If knocked down by a dog, lie still and remain in a ball.
- If bitten by a dog, immediately report the bite.

*Data from:* Centers for Disease Control and Prevention: Nonfatal dog bite-related injuries treated in hospital emergency departments–United States 2001. *MMWR Weekly*,;52(26):605–610. Retrieved December 23, 2015 from www.cdc.gov/mmwr/preview/mmwrhtml/mm5226a1.htm.

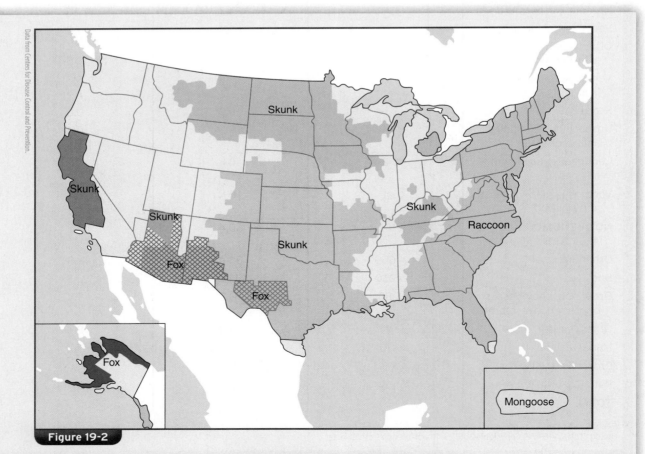

**Figure 19-2**

Distribution of rabies virus among wild animals in the United States, 2009-2013.

spreads from one animal to another in the saliva, usually through a bite or by licking. Bites from cold-blooded animals such as reptiles do not carry the danger of rabies.

A bite or a scratch is considered a significant rabies exposure if it penetrates the skin. Unprovoked attacks are more likely to have been inflicted by a rabid animal than are provoked attacks. Nonbite exposure consists of contamination of wounds, including scratches, abrasions, and weeping skin rashes.

Consider an animal as possibly rabid if any of the following applies:

- The animal made an unprovoked attack.
- The animal acted strangely, that is, out of character (for example, a usually friendly dog is aggressive, or a wild fox seems docile and friendly).
- The animal was a high-risk species (skunk, raccoon, or bat).

Report animal bites to the police or animal control officers; they should be the ones to capture the animal for observation. If a healthy domestic dog or cat up to date with its rabies vaccination bit the person, the animal should be confined and observed for 10 days for any illness. If a wild animal bit the person, it should be considered a possible rabies exposure and medical care should be sought immediately. According to the Centers for Disease Control and Prevention (CDC), wild animals account for 92% of reported rabies cases **Figure 19-3**. Raccoons are the most frequently reported rabid wildlife species followed by bats, skunks, and foxes.

For bites from a pet animal, notify the animal's owner, or, if you are the owner, notify the family of the person who was bitten. When doing so, use good judgment, because encounters may become very emotional and lead to violence. If the bite came from a wild animal, notify the proper authorities.

Refer to **Flowchart 19-1** for additional information regarding the care of animal bites.

## Human Bites

After dogs and cats, the animal most likely to bite humans is another human. Human bites can cause severe injury, often more so than other animal bites. The human mouth contains a wide range of bacteria

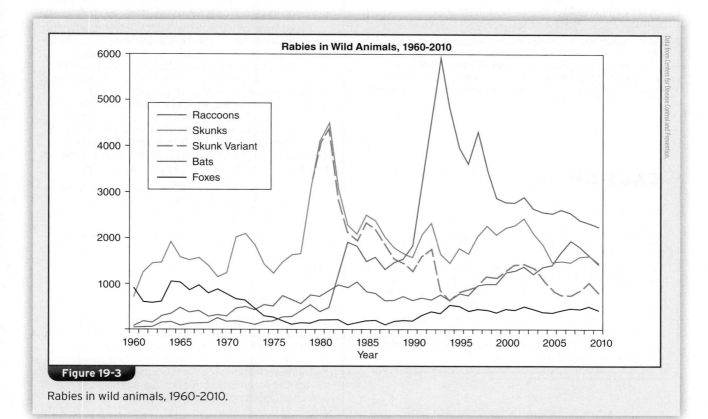

**Figure 19-3**

Rabies in wild animals, 1960–2010.

Data from Centers for Disease Control and Prevention.

| What to Look For | What to Do |
|---|---|
| **Bite that has broken the skin**<br>• Puncture wound from the animal's sharp, pointed teeth<br>• Crushed tissue and skin<br>• Open wound on fingers, knuckles, and/or hand | 1. Stop the bleeding by applying direct pressure over the wound.<br>2. For a shallow wound:<br>  • Wash inside and around it with soap and running water.<br>  • Flush the inside of the wound with clean running water.<br>  • Cover the wound with a thin layer of an over-the-counter antibiotic ointment and a sterile dressing.<br>3. Severe bites should be cleaned at a medical facility. For all bites that break the skin, seek medical care to:<br>  • Clean the wound.<br>  • Close wide and gaping open wounds.<br>  • Receive a tetanus booster, if necessary. |
| **Bite that did not break the skin** | Apply an ice pack to the skin for up to 20 minutes. |
| **Wild animal bite** | 1. **DO NOT** try to capture the animal.<br>2. **DO NOT** kill the animal. If you must kill it, **DO NOT** hit or shoot its head (brain). Though often impossible, the animal's brain can be tested for the rabies virus.<br>3. Contact the local health department. |

---

**Dog Bites: Which Breeds Are Most Dangerous?**

The AVMA reviewed a range of studies listing the dog breeds most frequently reported in biting incidents; at the top of the list were German Shepherds, Pit Bulls, Rottweilers, and Jack Russell Terriers. However, the AVMA noted breed is a poor sole predictor of dog bites. More predictive factors include the dog's training, sex, and neutering status.

*Source:* American Veterinary Medical Association. Dog bite risk and prevention: The role of breed. https://www.avma.org/KB/Resources/LiteratureReviews/Pages/The-Role-of-Breed-in-Dog-Bite-Risk-and-Prevention.aspx. March 12, 2015.

---

**Dog Bites**

The *Journal of American Veterinary Medical Association* published a study of fatalities related to dog bites. The researchers found 256 fatalities during a 10-year period. Nearly half of the fatalities were children under 5 years of age (45%) and the majority were men. Most cases (84%) involved a dog who had not been neutered or spayed.

Breed was not a predictive factor determined in the study. Instead, the researchers found the co-ocurrence of a number of owner-related factors to be more predictive of dog bites. These factors include lack of positive human contact; mismanagement by owner(s); abuse or neglect by owner(s); owner(s) lack of supervision of the dog with a child or vulnerable adult who may be unfamiliar with the dog; and an isolated living environment. The researchers suggested breed-specific legislation be reviewed in light of the findings of the study and stressed the need for animal services programs that focus on responsible ownership.

*Source:* Patronek GJ, Sacks JJ, Delise KM, Cleary DV, Marder AR. Co-occurrence of potentially preventable factors in 256 dog bit-related fatalities in the United States (2000-2009). *J Am Vet Med Assoc* 2013;243(12):1726-1736.

---

**CAUTION**

**DO NOT** try to capture the animal yourself.

**DO NOT** go near the animal.

**DO NOT** kill the animal unless absolutely necessary. If it must be killed, protect the head and brain from damage so they can be examined for rabies. Transport a dead animal intact to limit exposure to potentially infected tissues or saliva. The animal's remains should be refrigerated to prevent decomposition.

**DO NOT** handle the animal without taking appropriate precautions. Infected saliva might be on the animal's fur, so wear heavy gloves or use a shovel if you have to move a dead animal.

---

**Human Rabies**

The number of human deaths in the United States attributed to rabies has declined from 100 or more each year to an average of 1 or 3 each year. Two programs have been responsible for this decline. First, animal control and vaccination programs, which were begun in the 1940s; and second, effective human rabies vaccines and immunoglobulins have been developed.

*Sources:* Centers for Disease Control and Prevention; United States Rabies Surveillance Data.

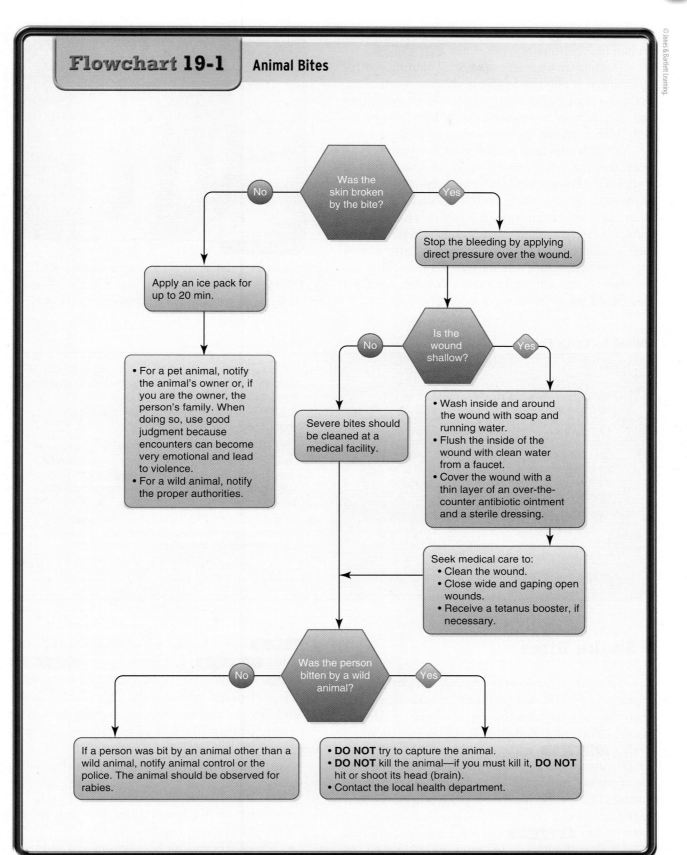

**Flowchart 19-1**   **Animal Bites**

Was the skin broken by the bite?

**No** → Apply an ice pack for up to 20 min.

→ • For a pet animal, notify the animal's owner or, if you are the owner, the person's family. When doing so, use good judgment because encounters can become very emotional and lead to violence.
• For a wild animal, notify the proper authorities.

**Yes** → Stop the bleeding by applying direct pressure over the wound.

Is the wound shallow?

**No** → Severe bites should be cleaned at a medical facility.

**Yes** → • Wash inside and around the wound with soap and running water.
• Flush the inside of the wound with clean water from a faucet.
• Cover the wound with a thin layer of an over-the-counter antibiotic ointment and a sterile dressing.

→ Seek medical care to:
• Clean the wound.
• Close wide and gaping open wounds.
• Receive a tetanus booster, if necessary.

Was the person bitten by a wild animal?

**No** → If a person was bit by an animal other than a wild animal, notify animal control or the police. The animal should be observed for rabies.

**Yes** → • **DO NOT** try to capture the animal.
• **DO NOT** kill the animal—if you must kill it, **DO NOT** hit or shoot its head (brain).
• Contact the local health department.

and viruses, so the chance of infection is great from a human bite, especially on the hand .

Most human bites are inflicted by fighting youths, by children at play, by people in mental institutions, or during sexual assaults. Embarrassment sometimes causes a person not to seek medical care immediately, which greatly increases the risk of infection.

Although most human bites occur during acts of violence, they may also be unintentional or sports-related, sustained by hospital workers trying to restrain children or patients having a seizure, or self-inflicted during nail chewing or thumb sucking. A study published in the *Journal of Emergencies, Trauma, and Shock* reported that men are more often bit than women, mostly during aggressive altercations, with the peak age being 28 years. The most common injury location is the hand, sustained on a closed fist as the result of a punch.

**Figure 19-4**

Human bites can result in serious, spreading infection.

| What to Look For | What to Do |
|---|---|
| There are two types of human bites:<br>• True bite<br>  • Part of the body's flesh is caught between teeth, usually deliberately<br>  • Occurs during fights and in cases of abuse (Mandatory reporting laws apply if spousal or child abuse is involved. A schoolyard bite, with one child biting another, generally is not reportable.)<br>• Clenched-fist injury<br>  • Results from cutting a fist on teeth, usually during a fight (although unintentional injury can happen during sports and play)<br>  • Associated with a high likelihood of infection<br>  • Injury is usually a laceration over the knuckles | 1. If the wound is not bleeding heavily, wash it with soap and water for 5 to 10 minutes. Avoid scrubbing, which can bruise tissues.<br>2. Flush the wound thoroughly with running water under pressure from a faucet.<br>3. Control bleeding with direct pressure.<br>4. Cover the wound with a sterile dressing. **DO NOT** close the wound with tape or butterfly bandages. Closing the wound traps bacteria in the wound, increasing the chance of infection.<br>5. Seek medical care for possible further wound cleaning, a possible tetanus shot, and sutures to close the wound, if needed. |

## ▶ Snake Bites

According to the World Health Organization, approximately 100,000 people die of snake bites each year. The CDC reports that each year in the United States, 7,000 to 8,000 people are bitten by venomous snakes **Figure 19-5**. Amazingly, fewer than a dozen Americans die each year of snake bites. People who die of snake bites in the United States usually do so during the first 48 hours after the bite. Only four snake species in the United States are venomous: rattlesnakes **Figure 19-6** (which account for about 65% of all venomous snake bites and nearly all the snake bite deaths in the United States), copperheads

**Figure 19-7**, water moccasins (also known as cottonmouths) **Figure 19-8**, and coral snakes **Figure 19-9**. Although uncommon, snake bites can be painful, costly, and potentially deadly. Other than death, disabilities such as partial or complete loss of an extremity or finger or loss of movement in a joint can occur. Most people fully recover.

The first three species of venomous snakes are pit vipers, which have three characteristics in common:

- Triangular, flat heads wider than their necks
- Elliptical pupils (cat-like eyes)
- A heat-sensitive pit between the eye and the nostril on each side of the head

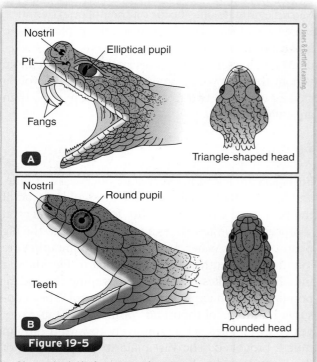

Nostril

Pit

Elliptical pupil

Fangs

Triangle-shaped head

**A**

Nostril

Round pupil

Teeth

Rounded head

**B**

**Figure 19-5**

Characteristic features of venomous snakes (pit vipers) **(A)** and of harmless snakes **(B)**.

**Figure 19-7**

Copperhead snake.

**Figure 19-8**

Water moccasin (cottonmouth).

**Figure 19-6**

Rattlesnake.

**Figure 19-9**

Coral snake; the United States' most venomous snake.

The coral snake is small and colorful, with a series of bright red, yellow, and black bands around its body (every other band is yellow). Coral snakes are found in Arizona, the southeastern United States, and Texas.

At least one species of venomous snake is found in every state except Alaska, Hawaii, and Maine **Figure 19-10**. Exotic snakes, whether imported legally or smuggled into the United States, can be found in zoos, schools, snake farms, and amateur and professional collections, and account for at least 15 bites a year. Some of the exotic snakes can be venomous.

A legitimate snake bite is one in which the person was bitten before the encounter with a snake was recognized or while trying to move away from the snake. They most often involve the lower extremities and are accidental (Table 19-3).

An illegitimate snake bite is one in which, before being bitten, the person recognized the encounter with a snake but did not attempt to move away from the snake.

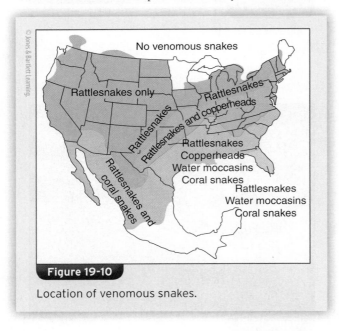

**Figure 19-10**
Location of venomous snakes.

Most illegitimate bites occur on the upper extremities. Most bites of this type occur when the person tries to kill, capture, play with, or move a snake. Adult snakes deliver more serious bites because they inject more venom than do young snakes, even though a young snake's venom is two to three times more toxic than an adult's.

## Pit Vipers

Pit vipers are found in every state but Alaska, Maine, and Hawaii. Rattlesnakes are the most widespread of the pit vipers. Copperheads are found in the central southeastern United States and westward into the Big Bend of Texas. Water moccasins (cottonmouths) are found in the southeast from Virginia to Florida and into Texas. Snakes benefit us by keeping the rodent population from exploding out of control. They consume hundreds of thousands of mice and rats every year. Few snakes act aggressively toward a human unless provoked. The vast majority of bites are not deadly and can be effectively treated.

According to the Wilderness Medical Society, most people are bit on the extremities. Alcohol intoxication of the person is a factor in many bites. The majority of bites in the United States occur in the southwestern part of the country, partly due to the near-extinction of pit vipers in the eastern United States. Deaths occur most often in children, in older people, and in people to whom **antivenom** is not given or is inappropriately given.

## Table 19-3  How to Avoid a Snake Bite

- **DO NOT** handle venomous snakes—keep away. They usually do not have to be killed for identification purposes.
- Avoid hiking and camping in snake-infested areas; avoid caves, rock crevices, dens, stonewalls, and wood piles.
- Watch where you sit and step; **DO NOT** sit on or step over logs until closely checked. **DO NOT** reach into holes or hidden ledges.
- Wear protective gear such as boots, gloves, long pants, and long-sleeved shirts when in snake habitats.
- **DO NOT** handle a dead venomous snake. The reflex action of the jaws can still inflict a bite up to 90 minutes after the snake has been killed, even if decapitated.
- **DO NOT** surprise or corner a snake. Use a walking stick to prod in front of you while walking, and make noise so that a snake can sense you coming.
- **DO NOT** keep venomous snakes as pets.
- When unintentionally encountering a snake, remain silent and motionless. If the snake has not fled, step away slowly and cautiously.

## FYI

**Blue Jeans and Snake Bites**

Researchers studied whether ordinary clothing (denim material from blue jeans) reduces the amount of venom injected by a rattlesnake.

The investigators used saline solution-filled gloves to simulate human limbs and elicited bites from small and large southern Pacific rattlesnakes. Each snake was videotaped biting a bare glove and a denim-covered glove. The results were that the snakes injected significantly less venom into the denim-covered gloves than into the bare gloves—up to 60% reduction for the small snakes and 66% reduction for the large snakes. The investigators felt that denim interfered with venom delivery and induced a high proportion of dry bites (no venom released), as well as harmless spillage of venom from the fangs of the snakes onto the surface of the denim cover. It was interesting to note that larger rattlesnakes struck more readily, maintained longer fang contact during their bites, and delivered 26 to 41 times more venom into the gloves than did the small snakes. This adds to the body of evidence that indicates large venomous snakes are much more dangerous to humans than small ones.

Wearing long denim pants can be an inexpensive and effective way to reduce the severity of snake bites. Other forms of clothing (eg, high leather boots or other types of long pants) may be equally or more effective at deflecting a bite and preventing a snakebite.

*Source:* Herbert SS, Hayes WK. Denim clothing reduces venom expenditure by rattlesnakes striking defensively at model human limbs. *Ann Emerg Med* 2009; 54(6):830-836.

In about 25% of venomous snake bites, venom is not injected—only fang and tooth wounds (known as a dry bite) occur. Never assume, however, that the bite is a dry bite. Take the following steps if you see fang marks and positively identify a pit viper:

- Get the person and bystanders away from the snake because of the risk of a second bite. A dead snake can still bite even if decapitated.
- Encourage the person to rest, stay calm, and be still.
- **DO NOT** try to capture or kill the snake. These actions could lead to a second person being bitten. Try to remember the snake's color and the shape of its head. Taking a good photograph from a safe distance (more than the length of the snake) can help with identifying the snake.
- Remove any rings, jewelry, or tight clothing from the bitten body part to avoid constriction from swelling.
- Gently wash the bite with soap and running water and apply a sterile dressing over the fang marks.
- Call 9-1-1 or transport the person to a medical facility as soon as possible.

## What to Look For

Snake characteristics:
- Triangular, flat head, wider than the neck
- Vertical, elliptical pupils (cat's eye)
- Heat-sensitive pit located between the eye and nostril

Following a bite, the following signs and symptoms may be present:
- Severe, burning pain at the bite site
- Two small puncture wounds (the person may have only one) **Figure 19-11**
- Swelling within 10 to 15 minutes; can involve entire extremity
- Discoloration and blood-filled blisters possible in 6 to 10 hours
- Nausea, vomiting, sweating, and weakness (in severe cases)

## What to Do

1. Call 9-1-1. You do not need to capture or kill the snake.
2. When possible, carry the person. If alone and capable, walk slowly.
3. **DO NOT** apply a pressure bandage for a pit viper snakebite; this action has not been proven to be beneficial. According to a number of toxicology associations and the Wilderness Medical Society's Practice Guidelines, the application of pressure bandages for pit viper snakebites is not recommended.

**Figure 19-11**

Rattlesnake bite on the foot **(A)** and thumb **(B)**.

## CAUTION

**DO NOT** apply cold or ice to a snake bite. It does not inactivate the venom and poses a danger of frostbite.

**DO NOT** use the cut-and-suck procedure—you could damage underlying structures (for example, blood vessels, nerves, or tendons). Cutting the skin may cause infection and poor wound healing.

**DO NOT** apply mouth suction. Your mouth is filled with bacteria, increasing the likelihood of wound infection.

**DO NOT** use any form of suction.

**DO NOT** apply electric shock. No medical studies support this method.

**DO NOT** apply a constriction band—their use remains controversial. They may increase tissue damage. If applied too tightly or if swelling occurs, they can act as a tourniquet.

**DO NOT** apply a pressure bandage. A number of toxicology associations and the Wilderness Medical Society's Practice Guidelines do not recommend pressure bandages for pit viper snakebites.

## Coral Snake Bites

The coral snake is America's most venomous snake, but it rarely bites people. The coral snake has short fangs and tends to hang on and chew its venom into the person rather than to strike and release, like a pit viper. Coral snake venom is a neurotoxin, and symptoms can begin 1 to 5 hours after the bite.

### What to Look For

Snake characteristics:
- Small and very colorful, with a series of bright red, yellow, and black bands going all the way around its body
- Every alternate band is yellow.
- Black snout

Following a bite, the following signs and symptoms may be present:
- Few immediate signs (absence of immediate symptoms is not evidence of a harmless bite)
- Several hours may pass before the onset of:
  - Nausea
  - Vomiting
  - Sweating
  - Tremors
  - Drowsiness
  - Slurred speech
  - Blurred vision
  - Swallowing difficulty
  - Breathing difficulty

### What to Do

1. Call 9-1-1. You do not need to capture or kill the snake.
2. Apply a wide elastic bandage using overlapping turns.
3. Start wrapping at the end of the bitten arm or leg and wrap upward, covering its entire length.
4. Use similar tightness as when wrapping a sprained ankle. You should be able to slip a finger under the wrapping.
5. Stabilize the bitten arm or leg as you would for a broken bone and keep it below heart level.
6. **DO NOT** cut skin or use suction.

## Nonvenomous Snake Bites

Nonvenomous snakes inflict the most snake bites. If you are not positive about a snake, assume it was venomous. Some so-called nonvenomous North American snakes such as the hognose and garter snakes have venom that can cause painful local reactions but no systemic (whole-body) symptoms.

Refer to **Flowchart 19-2** for additional information regarding the care of snake bites.

| What to Look For | What to Do |
|---|---|
| • Horseshoe shape of tooth marks on skin<br>• Bleeding<br>• Possible swelling, mild itching, and tenderness | 1. Gently clean the bite site with soap and water.<br>2. Treat the bite the same as you would a shallow wound. (Refer to Chapter 8, *Bleeding*, and Chapter 9, *Wounds*.)<br>3. Consult with a physician. |

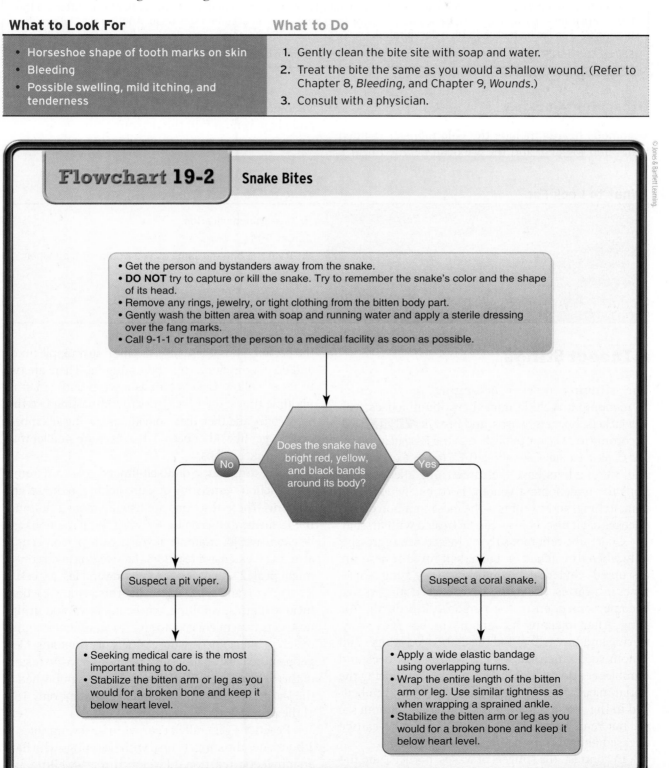

### Flowchart 19-2    Snake Bites

• Get the person and bystanders away from the snake.
• **DO NOT** try to capture or kill the snake. Try to remember the snake's color and the shape of its head.
• Remove any rings, jewelry, or tight clothing from the bitten body part.
• Gently wash the bitten area with soap and running water and apply a sterile dressing over the fang marks.
• Call 9-1-1 or transport the person to a medical facility as soon as possible.

Does the snake have bright red, yellow, and black bands around its body?

No → Suspect a pit viper.

• Seeking medical care is the most important thing to do.
• Stabilize the bitten arm or leg as you would for a broken bone and keep it below heart level.

Yes → Suspect a coral snake.

• Apply a wide elastic bandage using overlapping turns.
• Wrap the entire length of the bitten arm or leg. Use similar tightness as when wrapping a sprained ankle.
• Stabilize the bitten arm or leg as you would for a broken bone and keep it below heart level.

---

## FYI

**Dead Snakes Can Still Bite**

Data collected at the Good Samaritan Regional Medical Center in Phoenix show that fatal injuries do not prevent rattlesnakes from biting humans. Of the 34 patients admitted to the Phoenix Center for Rattlesnake Bites in an 11-month period, 5 were bitten by snakes that had been fatally injured and were presumed dead. One patient was bitten on the index finger after picking up a snake he had bludgeoned in the head and assumed was dead. Another was bitten after picking up a snake he had shot, then decapitated.

*Source:* Suchard JR, LoVecchio F. Envenomations by rattlesnakes thought to be dead. *N Engl J Med* 1999; 340(24):1930.

---

### Other Reptile Bites

Venomous lizards include the Gila monster (United States and Mexico) and the Mexican bearded lizard. Venomous lizards may firmly hang on during the bite and chew venom into the person's skin.

| What to Look For | What to Do |
|---|---|
| • Puncture wounds—teeth may break off<br>• Swelling and pain, often severe and burning<br>• Sweating<br>• Vomiting<br>• Increased heart rate<br>• Shortness of breath | 1. Give pain medication.<br>2. Call 9-1-1.<br>3. Treat the bite the same as you would for a pit viper bite. |

---

## ▶ Insect Stings

The stinging insects belonging to the order Hymenoptera include honeybees, bumblebees, yellow jackets, hornets, wasps, and fire ants **Figure 19-12**. According to a review published in the *Journal of Allergy and Clinical Immunology*, about 0.4% to 0.8% of children and 3% of adults have life-threatening allergic reactions to Hymenoptera venom. Fortunately, localized pain, itching, and swelling—the most common consequences of an insect bite—can be treated with first aid.

Generally, venomous flying insects are aggressive only when threatened or when their hives or nests are disrupted. Under such conditions, they sting, sometimes in swarms. Honeybees have barbed stingers that become embedded in the person's skin during the sting. After injecting its venom, the bee flies away, tearing and leaving behind the embedded stinger and venom sac, which causes it to die. Honeybees and bumblebees do not release all their venom during the initial injection; some remains in the stinger embedded in the person's skin. If the stinger and venom sac are not removed properly, additional venom can be released and worsen the person's reaction.

In contrast, the stingers of wasps, hornets, and fire ants are not barbed and do not become embedded in the person. Thus, these insects can sting multiple times, and do not die as a result of the stinging. There are two types of yellow jackets: one is a wasp and can sting multiple times; the other is a ground-nesting bee that stings once and then dies, sometimes leaving an embedded stinger like other bees. These bees are smaller than yellow jacket wasps.

Most stings cause only self-limited, local inflammatory reactions consisting of pain, itching, redness, and swelling. These reactions are usually more a nuisance than a medical emergency. However, local reactions can be extensive; for example, involving the person's entire arm. In an extensive reaction, the swelling and redness might peak 2 to 3 days after the sting and last a week or longer. Signs and symptoms of life-threatening reactions include nausea, vomiting, wheezing, fever, and drippy nose. A person might go into **anaphylaxis** almost immediately or after experiencing a variety of symptoms. Most people who have anaphylactic reactions have no history of them. In a study of 400 fatal bee stings published in the *Journal of Allergy and Clinical Immunology*, only 15% of the people had a known sensitivity.

Reactions generally occur within a few minutes to 1 hour after the sting. People with bee stings who have anaphylactic reactions develop throat swelling and bronchospasm, which are manifested by difficulty

**Figure 19-12**

Bees. **A.** Honeybee. **B.** Yellow jacket. **C.** Hornet. **D.** Wasp.

speaking, tightness in the throat or chest, wheezing, shortness of breath, and chest pain. Respiratory tract obstruction accounts for the majority of deaths among people with flying insect stings.

For the severely allergic person, a single sting could be fatal within minutes. Although there are accounts of people who have survived some 2,000 stings at one time, 500 stings will usually kill even people who are not allergic to stinging insects.

Massive numbers of stings are rare. They might occur if a person stumbled into a hive or if a truck carrying a load of honeybee hives crashed. With the slow migration of Africanized bees (so-called killer bees) from South and Central America into the United States, the number of cases involving multiple stings is likely to increase. The venom of the Africanized bee is no more potent than that of the European type; it is just that the African type is extremely aggressive and, thus, more likely to be involved in multiple stings. A number of child deaths have resulted from the multiple stings of fire ants, which are common in the southeastern United States.

A rule of thumb is that the sooner symptoms develop after a sting, the more serious the reaction will be.

- Usual reactions are instant pain, redness around the sting site, and itching.
- Worrisome reactions include hives, swelling of lips or tongue, a tickle in the throat, and wheezing.
- Life-threatening reactions are blue or gray skin color, seizures, unresponsiveness, and an inability to breathe because of swelling and spasm of the airway.

About 60% to 80% of anaphylactic deaths are caused by the person being unable to breathe because swollen airway passages obstruct airflow to the lungs. The second most common cause of death is shock, caused by collapse of blood circulation through the body.

One of the difficulties in dealing with stings is the lack of uniformity in people's responses. One sting is not necessarily equivalent to another, even within the same species, because the amount of venom injected varies from sting to sting. A person who experiences anaphylactic shock after being stung by a hornet might respond to a bee sting with only a small amount of swelling. One person might have a local reaction involving an entire limb, although the more typical response is a small circle of redness and swelling that disappears without incident in a few days. In beekeepers, for whom stings are an accepted occupational hazard, the response is likely to be even less than in most other people, because they have become tolerant to the toxins in the venom from having been stung many times on different occasions. There seems to be no easy way to predict how a person will react. Most people who are stung, however, have local reactions: redness, swelling, and pain.

Stings to the mouth or eye tend to be more dangerous than stings to other body areas. Also, people tend to react more severely to multiple stings, especially 10 or more. The most dangerous single stings in nonallergic individuals are those inside the throat, which can result from swallowing an insect that has dropped into a soft drink can or from inhaling one that flies into the person's open mouth. A sting in the mouth or throat can cause swelling that obstructs the airway even in a person who is not allergic to insect stings. If the sting is not life threatening, have the person suck on ice or flush his or her mouth with cold water. For a bee sting, dissolve a teaspoon (5 mL) of baking soda in a glass of water. Have the person rinse his or

## FYI

### Fire Ants

Fire ants are aggressive, will defensively attack anything that disturbs them, and can sting repeatedly **Figure 19-13**. The fire ant bites by securing itself to the skin of a person with its mandibles, causing pain; then, using its head as a pivot, the ant swings its abdomen in an arc, repeatedly stinging the person with an abdominal stinger. According to a study published in the *Journal of Allergy and Clinical Immunology*, up to 60% of the people who live in infested urban areas are stung each year, and more than 80 deaths have been attributed to these insect bites.

The fire ant sting usually produces immediate pain and a red, swollen area, which disappears within 45 minutes **Figure 19-14**. A blister then forms, rupturing in 30 to 70 hours, and the area often becomes infected. In some cases, a red, swollen, itchy patch develops instead of a blister. Although the stings are not usually life threatening, they are easily infected and can leave permanent scars.

Some people become sensitive to fire ant stings and should seek the advice of an allergist. Anaphylaxis (a life-threatening allergic reaction) occurs in about 1% to 2% of people stung by fire ants. Therefore, if a sting leads to shortness of breath, tightness and swelling in the throat, tightness in the chest, increased pulse rate, swelling of the tongue and mouth, dizziness, or nausea, the person should be taken to a hospital emergency department immediately. Some people lapse into a coma from even one sting.

First aid for fire ant stings includes placing an ice cube over the sting to reduce the pain and to slow absorption of the venom. A topical corticosteroid cream can help combat local swelling and itching. An antihistamine can prevent some local symptoms if given early, but it works too slowly to counteract a life-threatening allergic reaction. People who are allergic to stings should always carry a kit with antihistamine tablets and a preloaded syringe of epinephrine.

| What to Look For | What to Do |
|---|---|
| • Usual reactions:<br>  • Instant pain, redness, itching<br>• Worrisome reactions:<br>  • Hives<br>  • Swollen lips/tongue<br>  • Tickle in throat<br>  • Wheezing<br>• Life-threatening reactions:<br>  • Blue/gray skin color | 1. Look for a stinger; if found, immediately scrape the stinger and venom sac off the skin with a fingernail or plastic card (eg, credit card), or brush it off with your hand. Only bees leave their stinger embedded. **DO NOT** use tweezers. **DO NOT** squeeze the venom sac, which may or may not be attached to the stinger.<br>2. Wash the area with soap and water.<br>3. Apply an ice pack to the area for up to 20 minutes, placing a paper towel or thin damp cloth between the skin and ice pack. Baking soda paste may also help, except for wasp stings. |

*(Continues)*

## What to Look For

- Seizures
- Unresponsiveness
- Inability to breathe because of swollen vocal cords (cause of about 60% to 80% of anaphylactic deaths)

## What to Do

4. Give pain medication.
5. Apply hydrocortisone cream (1%) and give antihistamine (Benadryl) to relieve itching and swelling.
6. For a severe allergic reaction, help the person self-administer epinephrine. (See Chapter 7, *Shock*.) A person with a known allergy to insect stings should have a physician-prescribed epinephrine auto-injector to take wherever stinging insects are known to exist. When a person with anaphylaxis does not respond to the first dose, and arrival of EMS will exceed 5 to 10 minutes, consider administering a second dose.
7. Monitor breathing; if it stops, give cardiopulmonary resuscitation (CPR).
8. A sting in the throat or mouth can cause swelling even in a person without an allergy; have the person suck on ice.

**Figure 19-13**

Fire ants.

**Figure 19-14**

Fire ant stings.

her mouth and then hold the water in the mouth for several minutes.

Refer to Flowchart 19-3 for additional information regarding the care of insect stings.

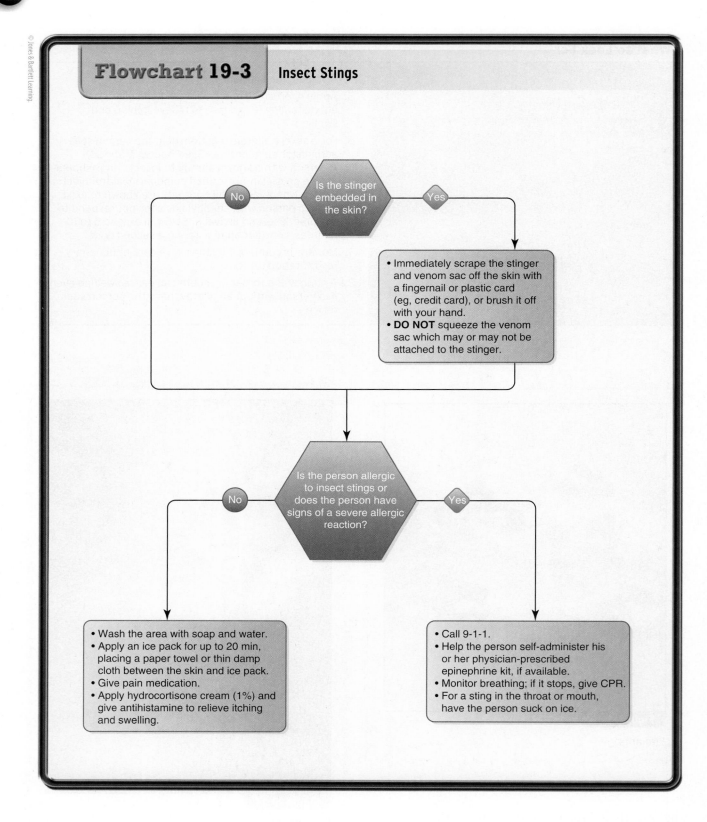

**Flowchart 19-3** | **Insect Stings**

Is the stinger embedded in the skin?

**No** →

**Yes** →

- Immediately scrape the stinger and venom sac off the skin with a fingernail or plastic card (eg, credit card), or brush it off with your hand.
- **DO NOT** squeeze the venom sac which may or may not be attached to the stinger.

Is the person allergic to insect stings or does the person have signs of a severe allergic reaction?

**No** →

**Yes** →

- Wash the area with soap and water.
- Apply an ice pack for up to 20 min, placing a paper towel or thin damp cloth between the skin and ice pack.
- Give pain medication.
- Apply hydrocortisone cream (1%) and give antihistamine to relieve itching and swelling.

- Call 9-1-1.
- Help the person self-administer his or her physician-prescribed epinephrine kit, if available.
- Monitor breathing; if it stops, give CPR.
- For a sting in the throat or mouth, have the person suck on ice.

## FYI

**Preventing Insect Stings**

People who know they are allergic to insect stings need to exercise extra care to avoid being stung. They should carry a bee sting kit and follow these guidelines:

- Wear long pants and long-sleeved shirts.
- Because insects are attracted to bright colors and floral patterns, wear white, green, tan, and khaki—the colors least attractive to insects.
- Wear shoes outdoors.
- Avoid yard work and other activities in which insect contact is frequent.
- Keep garbage cans away from the house.
- Remove insect-attracting plants from inside as well as the immediate proximity of the house.
- **DO NOT** use scented soaps, lotions, or perfumes.
- Keep car windows closed.
- If an insect confronts you, avoid quick movements and **DO NOT** provoke it. Turn away, lower your face, and walk away slowly. **DO NOT** run about wildly or move erratically when bees are nearby.
- **DO NOT** eat when bees are nearby.
- Have insect nests around the house removed by professional exterminators.

## ▶ Spider and Insect Bites

Most spiders are venomous, which is how they paralyze and kill their prey. However, most spiders lack an effective delivery system—long fangs and strong jaws—to bite a human. About 60 species of spiders in North America are capable of biting humans, although only a few species have produced significant poisonings **Figure 19-15**.

Most bites are by female spiders. Male spiders are almost always smaller than females and have fangs that are too short and fragile to bite humans. Death rarely occurs and only from bites by brown recluse and black widow spiders.

The number of deaths from spider bites is not accurately known. A spider bite is difficult to diagnose, because most people never see the spider and the bites typically cause little immediate pain.

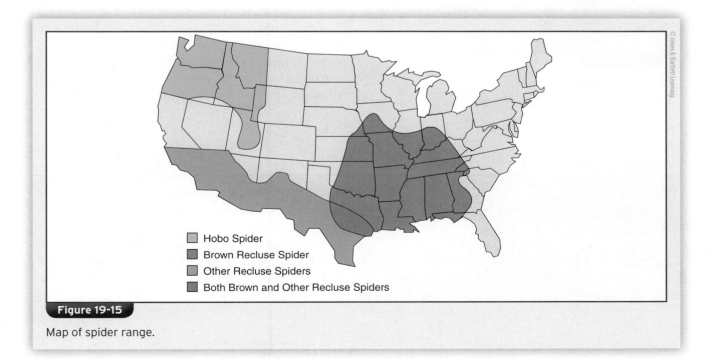

☐ Hobo Spider
☐ Brown Recluse Spider
☐ Other Recluse Spiders
☐ Both Brown and Other Recluse Spiders

**Figure 19-15**

Map of spider range.

An article in *American Family Physician* cites a study of 600 suspected spider bites, of which 80% were caused by other arthropods (eg, kissing bugs, ticks, fleas, mites, and bedbugs) and disease states (eg, poison ivy, diabetic ulcer, bedsore, Lyme disease, and gonococcus). Spiders rarely bite more than once, and they do not always release venom.

## Black Widow Spiders

Black widow spiders are also commonly known as brown widow spiders and red-legged spiders, depending on the species **Figure 19-16**. The term *black* widow is actually inaccurate, because only three of the five species of widow spider are actually black; the others are brown and gray. Newly hatched spiders are almost entirely red. Males have white stripes along the outside of the abdomen.

The female black widow spider is one of the largest spiders, with a body that ranges up to 0.5 inch (1 cm) in length and a leg span of up to 2 inches

**Figure 19-16**

Black widow spider.

(5 cm). It is her large size that allows the female black widow's fangs to be large and strong enough to penetrate human skin. The female black widow can live as long as 3 years. Black widow spiders have round abdomens that vary from gray to brown to black, depending on the species. In the female black widow, the abdomen is shiny black with a red or yellow spot (often in the shape of an hourglass) or white spots or bands.

The male is only one-third of the size of the female. Contrary to popular myth, the male usually mates safely with the female. Because he is small, his fangs are incapable of penetrating human skin, so bites are from the female. Black widow spiders produce one of the most potent venoms known in terms of volume. The venom is chiefly a neurotoxin in humans, with symptoms most often manifested as severe muscle pain and cramping.

Black widow spiders are found throughout the world. In the Western Hemisphere, they are found from southern Canada, throughout every state in the continental United States and in Hawaii, to the tip of South America.

The web of the black widow spider is an extensive, irregular, shaggy trap for the insects she normally eats. The black widow rarely leaves the web and stays close to her egg mass. She aggressively defends the egg mass and bites if it is disturbed. When she is not guarding eggs, the spider often attempts to escape rather than bite.

Frequent cleaning to remove spiders and their webs from buildings, outbuildings, and outdoor living areas decreases the chance of accidental contact with black widow spiders. Insecticides could decrease the population of the food for the black widows but do not usually affect the spiders themselves.

| What to Look For | What to Do |
|---|---|
| • Sharp pinprick sensation followed by dull, numbing pain<br>• Two small fang marks seen as tiny red spots<br>• Severe abdominal pain (bites on an arm can produce severe chest pain, thus mimicking a heart attack)<br>• Headache, chills, fever, heavy sweating, nausea, and vomiting | 1. Clean with soap and water.<br>2. Apply an ice pack to the area.<br>3. Give pain medication.<br>4. Seek medical care as soon as possible.<br>5. If facial swelling or anaphylaxis occurs, call 9-1-1 and treat appropriately. |

## Brown Recluse Spiders

Brown recluse spiders are also known in North America as fiddle-back and violin spiders **Figure 19-17**. They have a violin-shaped figure on their backs (several other spider species have a similar configuration on their backs). Color varies from fawn to dark brown, with darker legs. Male and female spiders are venomous. Brown recluse spiders are found primarily in the southern and midwestern states, with other less toxic but related spiders found throughout the rest of the country. They are absent from the Pacific Northwest.

If you suspect a brown recluse spider bite, remember the following:

- The brown recluse spider bites only when it is trapped against the skin.
- A local reaction usually occurs within 2 to 8 hours with mild to severe pain at the bite site and the development of redness, swelling, and local itching.
- In 48 to 72 hours, a blister develops at the bite site, becomes red, and bursts. During the early stages, the affected area often takes on a bull's-eye appearance, with a central white area surrounded by a reddened area, ringed by a whitish or blue border. A small, red crater remains, over which a scab forms. When the scab falls away in a few days, a larger crater

**Figure 19-17**
Brown recluse spider.

remains. That too scabs over and falls off, leaving a larger crater. The craters are known as volcano lesions. This process of slow tissue destruction can continue for weeks or months. The ulcer sometimes requires skin grafting.
- Fever, weakness, vomiting, joint pain, and a rash could occur.
- Stomach cramps, nausea, and vomiting might occur. Death is rare.

**What to Look For**

- Mild to severe pain that occurs within 2 to 8 hours
- Blister that develops within 48 to 72 hours; becomes red and bursts; takes on a bull's-eye appearance
- Nausea, vomiting, headache, and fever

**What to Do**

1. Treat the bite the same as you would a black widow spider bite.
2. If the wound becomes infected, apply antibiotic ointment under a sterile dressing.
3. Seek medical care.

## Tarantulas

Tarantulas bite only when vigorously provoked or roughly handled **Figure 19-18**. The bite varies from almost painless to a deep throbbing pain lasting up to 1 hour. The tarantula, when upset, will roughly scratch the lower surface of its abdomen with its legs and flick hairs onto a person's skin.

**What to Look For**

Varies from mild to severe throbbing pain that lasts up to 1 hour

**What to Do**

1. Treat the bite the same as you would a black widow spider bite.
2. For hairs in the skin, remove with sticky tape, wash with soap and water, and apply hydrocortisone cream (1%).
3. Give an antihistamine and pain medication.

© Nick Simon/Shutterstock

**Figure 19-18**

Tarantula.

## Common Aggressive House Spider (Hobo Spider)

Another biter is the common aggressive house spider, or hobo spider. It arrived in the Pacific Northwest in 1936 and slowly made its way across Washington State and into surrounding states. In those areas, the hobo spider is the most common large spider.

Refer to **Flowchart 19-4** for additional information regarding the care of spider bites.

| What to Look For | What to Do |
|---|---|
| Same as for brown recluse spiders | Treat the bite the same as you would a brown recluse spider bite. |

## Scorpions

Scorpions look like miniature lobsters, with lobster-like pincers and a long, up-curved tail-like appendage with a venomous stinger **Figure 19-19**. Several species of scorpions inhabit the southwestern United States, but only the bark scorpion poses a threat to humans. Severe reactions, which usually appear only in children, could include paralysis, spasms, or breathing difficulties. Death due to scorpion stings in the United States is rare.

The bark scorpion is found primarily in Arizona. Rare stings have been reported in other parts of the United States, after the scorpions traveled from Arizona as stowaways in luggage or in car trunks. The bark scorpion is pale tan and is 0.75 to 1.25 inches (2 to 3 cm) long, not including the so-called tail.

Stings to adults usually are not life threatening. Stings to small children, however, are often dangerous. When a child is stung, every effort should be made to get the child to medical care as quickly as possible. Pay close attention to make sure the person's airway is open and that he or she is breathing.

Recently, bark scorpion antivenom production has been discontinued. Its use was controversial. The US Food and Drug Administration has given approval for clinical trials to evaluate a Mexican antivenom for use in the United States.

| What to Look For | What to Do |
|---|---|
| • The following symptoms begin from within minutes to half an hour, reach their height within the first few hours, and usually last from 6 to 24 hours: <br>   • Local, immediate pain and burning around the sting site (Tapping a finger over the sting site [the tap test] could serve to indicate a scorpion sting.) <br>   • Numbness or tingling that occurs later <br> • Severely affected people will experience: <br>   • Pain along the stung arm or leg, even paralysis <br>   • Uncontrolled jerking movements of the legs or arms and facial twitching <br>   • A fast heart rate <br>   • Salivation <br>   • Breathing distress | 1. Monitor breathing. <br> 2. Gently wash the sting site with soap and water. <br> 3. Apply an ice pack to the sting site to reduce pain and venom absorption. <br> 4. Give pain medication. <br> 5. Apply dressing. <br> 6. Seek medical care for severe reactions. |

## Flowchart 19-4 | Spider Bites

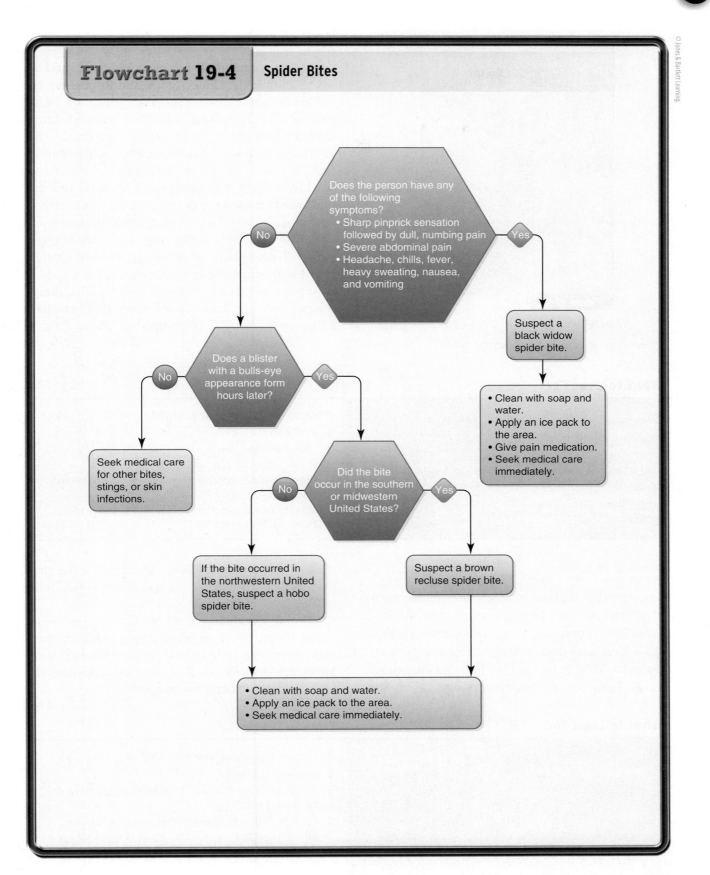

Does the person have any of the following symptoms?
- Sharp pinprick sensation followed by dull, numbing pain
- Severe abdominal pain
- Headache, chills, fever, heavy sweating, nausea, and vomiting

No → Does a blister with a bulls-eye appearance form hours later?

Yes → Suspect a black widow spider bite.

- Clean with soap and water.
- Apply an ice pack to the area.
- Give pain medication.
- Seek medical care immediately.

No → Seek medical care for other bites, stings, or skin infections.

Yes → Did the bite occur in the southern or midwestern United States?

No → If the bite occurred in the northwestern United States, suspect a hobo spider bite.

Yes → Suspect a brown recluse spider bite.

- Clean with soap and water.
- Apply an ice pack to the area.
- Seek medical care immediately.

**Figure 19-19**

Bark scorpion.

## Centipedes

Centipedes come in various sizes and colors and are found all over the United States and throughout the world. The giant desert centipede, which can be up to 8 inches (20 cm) long, is the only centipede in the United States that is dangerous to humans. Do not confuse centipedes with millipedes, which cannot inject venom but can irritate the skin.

Like spiders, any centipede with fangs that can penetrate human skin can inject venom. These arthropods inject toxic substances into the skin from a pair of hollow jaws that act like fangs. Contrary to popular belief, centipedes do not inject venom with their feet. Exaggerated stories about the deadly effects of their bites and reports that the tip of each leg carries a venomous spur have caused many people to have an unreasonable fear of centipedes. Their venom is relatively weak.

| What to Look For | What to Do |
|---|---|
| • Burning pain<br>• Local inflammation of the wound<br>• Mild swelling of lymph nodes<br>• The bite of the giant desert centipede causes inflammation, swelling, and redness that last 4 to 12 hours. | 1. Clean the wound with soap and water.<br>2. Apply an ice pack.<br>3. Give pain medication.<br>4. If symptoms persist, give an antihistamine (Benadryl) or apply hydrocortisone cream (1%) on the bite site.<br>5. Most bites will get better even without treatment; however, for severe reactions, seek medical care. |

## Mosquitoes

Mosquitoes bite millions of people. Mosquitoes are not only a nuisance, but they also carry many diseases. In developing countries, mosquitoes transmit malaria, yellow fever, and dengue fever; in the United States, they carry West Nile, Zika, and equine encephalitis viruses. There is no evidence that mosquitoes transmit the human immunodeficiency virus (HIV), the virus that causes acquired immunodeficiency syndrome (AIDS).

Female mosquitoes need blood to lay their eggs. Because they breed in water, mosquitoes are most often found in marshes, wetlands, and wooded areas. Mosquitoes usually can be separated into daytime and nighttime biters, but most bite at twilight.

| What to Look For | What to Do |
|---|---|
| • Itching<br>• Mild swelling | 1. Wash the affected area with soap and water.<br>2. Apply an ice pack.<br>3. Apply calamine lotion or hydrocortisone cream (1%) to decrease itching.<br>4. For a person with numerous stings or a delayed allergic reaction, an antihistamine (Benadryl) every 6 hours or a physician-prescribed cortisone might be helpful. |

## FYI

**Preventing Mosquito Bites**

To minimize being bitten by mosquitoes, follow these guidelines:

- Wear protective clothing: pants, long-sleeved shirt, and full-brimmed hat. Mosquito netting draped over a hat will protect the face and neck. Mosquito bed nets should be used when sleeping in unscreened rooms.
- Use insect repellents on exposed skin. DEET (diethyltoluamide)-containing repellents are most effective against mosquitoes and, to a lesser extent, helpful in repelling ticks and black flies.
- DEET is considered to have low toxicity. However, it is absorbed through the skin, and hives, skin rashes, and blisters can result when it is used for prolonged periods or in excessive amounts. The long-acting 35% solution has a polymer that prevents evaporation and skin absorption.
- Products that contain 100% DEET are available but unnecessary, especially for children. Long-acting formulations of 35% DEET seem equally effective in protecting against mosquitoes and have far less potential for toxic effects.
- DEET products can be applied over other creams such as sunscreens and moisturizers. Use DEET only on exposed skin, and avoid the hands of young children because they often put their hands in their mouths. Keep DEET out of the reach of small children because ingestion could be fatal. Children younger than 5 years should not be exposed to concentrations greater than 10%, according to the American Academy of Pediatrics. Children younger than 2 months of age should not have DEET applied to their skin. For children ages 5 or older, the DEET concentration should not exceed 30%.
- Other nontoxic insect repellents seem to be less effective than DEET. They might be only 25% as effective as DEET and might need to be reapplied every half hour. Mixed opinions exist about whether 100 mg of vitamin $B_1$ (thiamine) taken daily for 1 week before being exposed is an effective preventive agent. Some experts believe that a diet high in garlic will make a person undesirable to a mosquito.
- Permethrin is a pesticide, not a repellent. It should be applied to clothing and not the skin.

## FYI

**Mosquito Bites**

In tropical climates, mosquitoes are important carriers of infectious diseases such as malaria and yellow fever. Mosquito bites can also provoke unpleasant skin lesions. In many areas of the world, massive and disturbing mosquito infestations occur. For example, in Alaska it is possible to be bitten by mosquitoes as many as 1,000 times in one hour. Under such conditions, complete avoidance of bites is impossible without use of effective repellents and protective clothing. Topical treatment with over-the-counter sticks, creams, and lotions containing antihistamines, hydrocortisone, or other antipruritic agents is common. However, only a few studies have been made on the effectiveness of these products.

*Source:* Reunala T, et al. Treatment of mosquito bites with cetirizine. *Clin Exp Allergy* 1993; 23(1):72-75.

## Ticks

Ticks are not insects but are close relatives of mites and spiders. They have eight legs and are classified as hard ticks and soft ticks. Hard ticks are more familiar because of their wide distribution and common occurrence on domestic animals. Soft ticks are found mainly in western states. In the United States, seven kinds of hard ticks and five kinds of soft ticks carry diseases (for example, Lyme disease), are a nuisance (causing itching and swelling), or cause paralysis (toxin injected). Ticks hatch from eggs and grow through three distinct stages: nymph (too small to see), larva (just visible), and adult (ready to lay eggs) **Figure 19-20**.

The adult is most likely to be seen. Ticks at any stage of development can use humans for food; at each stage, they need a blood meal before they can grow to the next stage. Ticks are limited in their ability to find their meals. They cannot fly, they crawl very slowly, and, without some help, they cannot travel more than a few yards from where they were hatched. When they are ready for their next meal, they might wait months, years, or even decades for the right host to come along. Bites are nearly painless, so the tick attachment is not noticed until later.

The front part of a tick consists of the head area and the mouthparts. The mouthparts have a central structure, the hypostome, which is shaped like a blunt harpoon. A tick makes a hole in the person's skin with the sharp teeth (barbs) on the front of the hypostome and inserts its hypostome **Figure 19-21**. The barbs anchor the tick to the skin and make it difficult to pull the tick out. Some ticks produce a substance that helps cement them to the host. As they feed, some ticks increase in size 20 to 50 times.

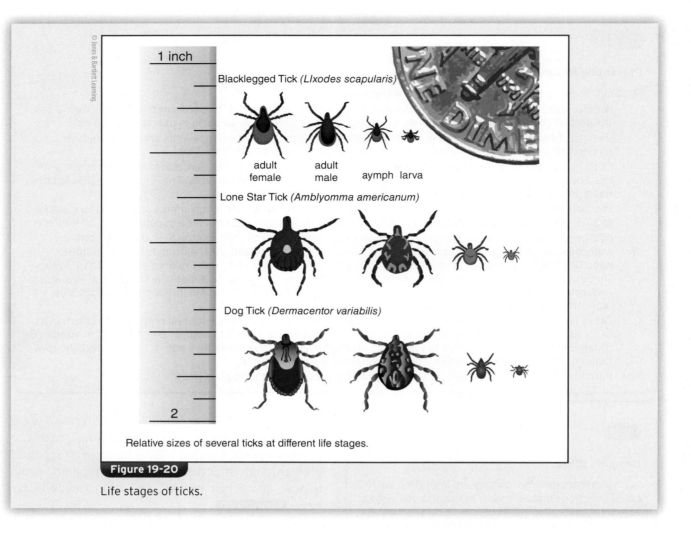

1 inch

Blacklegged Tick (*LIxodes scapularis*)

adult
female

adult
male

aymph   larva

Lone Star Tick (*Amblyomma americanum*)

Dog Tick (*Dermacentor variabilis*)

2

Relative sizes of several ticks at different life stages.

**Figure 19-20**

Life stages of ticks.

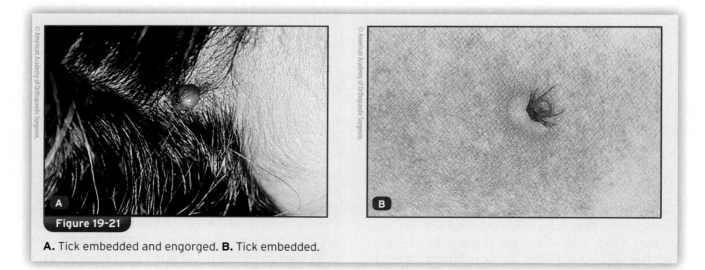

**A.** Tick embedded and engorged. **B.** Tick embedded.

**Figure 19-21**

Most ticks are harmless, but they can carry diseases (ie, Lyme disease, Rocky Mountain spotted fever, Colorado tick fever, tularemia, etc). The longer the tick stays embedded or the more engorged it is with blood, the greater the chance a disease will be transmitted.

---

## FYI

**Preventing Tick Bites**

- Wear light-colored clothing so you can see any ticks on your clothes.
- Wear a long-sleeved shirt that fits tightly at the wrists and neck and tuck the shirt into your pants.
- Wear long pants and tuck the pant legs into your boots or socks, or use masking tape to tape the pant legs tightly to your socks, shoes, or boots.
- Check your clothes while you are outdoors and before entering a house. Wash your clothes as soon as possible.
- Inspect your pets for ticks before they come inside.
- After coming indoors, shower or bathe and check your body for ticks, especially in areas that have hair or where clothing was tight. Another person could do the checking.
- Treat your body and clothing with a repellent. The most common, Environmental Protection Agency-approved, and effective tick repellent is DEET.
- You can buy DEET and apply it directly to your skin. Ticks crawling on the treated area are irritated by the repellent and drop off. DEET is most effective against ticks when applied to clothing from a spray can.
- There have been a few reports of adverse toxic reactions to DEET, such as seizures, allergic responses, and skin irritation. To minimize reactions, do the following:
  - Apply DEET sparingly to your skin.
  - Avoid applying high-concentration products (more than 35% DEET) to the skin.
  - **DO NOT** inhale or ingest DEET-containing products or get them in your eyes.
  - **DO NOT** apply DEET to wounds or irritated skin.
  - Wash your skin after coming indoors.
  - **DO NOT** use products with more than 10% DEET on infants and small children (younger than 5 years).
- You can also use 0.5% preparations of permethrin (a pesticide). Permethrin should be applied only to clothing (especially shirt sleeves, pants legs, and collars), never directly on the skin.

---

| What to Look For | What to Do |
|---|---|
| • No initial pain; the tick may go unnoticed for days<br>• Red area around tick, indicating the tick has punctured the skin and is feeding on the person's blood<br>• Rash, fever, and chills **Figure 19-22**<br>• The bite varies from a small bump to extensive swelling and ulcer. | Ticks are difficult to remove. Partial removal may lead to infection.<br>To remove the tick:<br>1. Use tweezers or one of the specialized tick-removal tools to grasp the tick as close to the skin as possible **Figure 19-23**.<br>2. Pull upward with steady, even pressure.<br>3. Lift the tick to tent the skin surface. Hold in this position until the tick lets go (about 1 minute).<br>4. Pull the tick away from the skin. Try not to pull hard enough to break the tick apart, which leaves parts of the mouth embedded. |
| Completely removed tick | 1. Wash your hands and the area with soap and water. Apply rubbing alcohol to further disinfect the area.<br>2. Apply an ice pack to reduce pain.<br>3. Apply calamine lotion or hydrocortisone cream to relieve itching.<br>4. Place the tick in a plastic bag and bring it to a physician within 72 hours for identification and possible antibiotic treatment in order to prevent serious illness such as Lyme disease.<br>5. If a rash, fever, or flulike symptoms (headache, body aches, and/or nausea) occur in 3 to 30 days after the tick's removal, seek medical care—with or without the tick. |
| Tick's mouth parts broke off and remain in the skin | 1. If unable to remove the parts, leave them in place and treat with warm soaks and antibiotic ointment. The retained parts will usually expel and the skin will heal.<br>2. If infection develops, seek medical care. |

Refer to [Flowchart 19-5] for additional information regarding the care of tick bites.

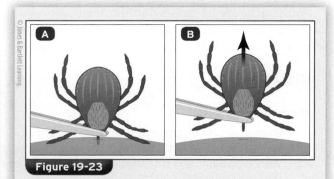

**Figure 19-23**

Removing a tick with tweezers. **A.** Grasp the tick as close to the skin as possible. **B.** Pull upward with steady, even pressure.

**Figure 19-22**

A bull's-eye rash is a distinctive finding in Lyme disease, but is not always present in people.

## FYI

**The Knot Method of Tick Removal**

An embedded tick should be removed as soon as possible. The longer an infected tick stays embedded, the more likely it is to transmit a disease. An alternative to using tweezers and special commercial tick removal devices, especially when they are not available, is the knot method. Use cotton thread or dental floss and tie an overhand knot (similar to a shoelace knot without the bows). The open overhand knot is placed over the tick as close as possible to the skin surface and then gently closed to form a loop around the tick. Lift the tick's body over its head in a somersault-type fashion to remove the tick. This method removes the entire tick and is simple and effective.

*Source:* Celensa A. The knot method of tick removal. *Wilderness Environ Med* 2002; 13(2):181.

## CAUTION

**DO NOT** use any of the following ineffective methods to remove a tick:
- Petroleum jelly
- Fingernail polish
- Rubbing alcohol
- Touching with a blown-out hot match, needle, or paper clip
- Gasoline

**DO NOT** grab a tick at the rear of its body. The tick's internal organs could rupture, resulting in their contents being squeezed into the person, causing infection.

**DO NOT** twist or jerk the tick, which could result in incomplete removal.

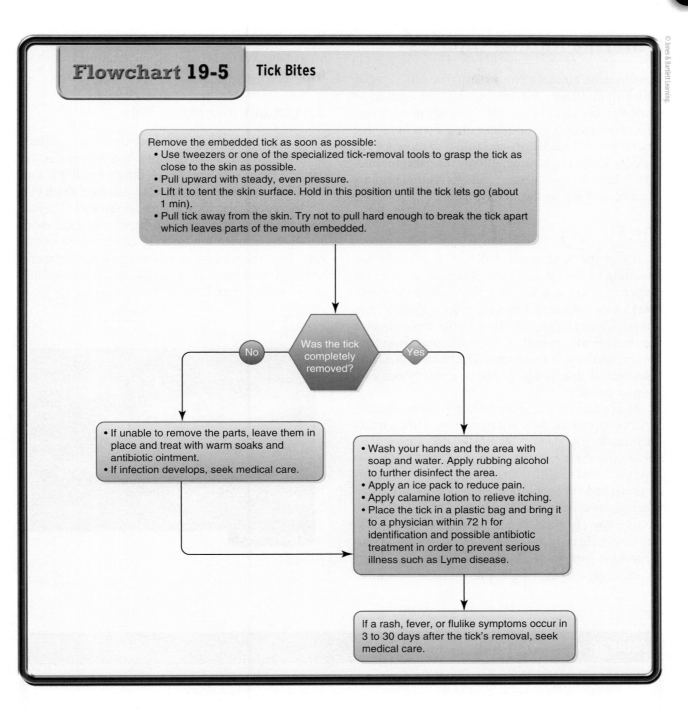

**Flowchart 19-5** | **Tick Bites**

Remove the embedded tick as soon as possible:
- Use tweezers or one of the specialized tick-removal tools to grasp the tick as close to the skin as possible.
- Pull upward with steady, even pressure.
- Lift it to tent the skin surface. Hold in this position until the tick lets go (about 1 min).
- Pull tick away from the skin. Try not to pull hard enough to break the tick apart which leaves parts of the mouth embedded.

Was the tick completely removed?

No

Yes

- If unable to remove the parts, leave them in place and treat with warm soaks and antibiotic ointment.
- If infection develops, seek medical care.

- Wash your hands and the area with soap and water. Apply rubbing alcohol to further disinfect the area.
- Apply an ice pack to reduce pain.
- Apply calamine lotion to relieve itching.
- Place the tick in a plastic bag and bring it to a physician within 72 h for identification and possible antibiotic treatment in order to prevent serious illness such as Lyme disease.

If a rash, fever, or flulike symptoms occur in 3 to 30 days after the tick's removal, seek medical care.

© Jones & Bartlett Learning.

## FYI

### Lyme Disease

Lyme disease has been reported in every state in the United States, with the Northeast, upper Midwest, and mid-Atlantic regions accounting for a vast majority of cases. It is caused by a bacterium, *Borrelia burgdorferi*, transmitted by the bite of the deer tick. Nearly 30,000 confirmed cases were reported in 2008, easily making Lyme disease the most common insect-borne infection in the United States.

The disease has two distinct phases—early and late. The best-known early symptom, a bull's-eye rash, affects up to 80% of affected people. Other early symptoms include headache, chills and fever, acute arthritis, and heart and spinal nerve root conditions. Lyme disease can include chronic arthritis, peripheral nerve injury, and brain and spinal cord symptoms.

*Source:* Lipman MM. Lyme disease: Beyond the rash. *Consumer Rep Health* 2010; 22(8):11.

## ▶ Marine Animal Injuries

Most marine animals bite or sting in self-defense, rather than attack. Marine venoms are similar to many venoms found in reptiles and arthropods and can cause anaphylaxis or other types of reactions. The general first aid guidelines are similar to those for any disorder involving trauma, allergy, or cardiopulmonary failure. Serious allergic reactions require primary attention to keeping the airway open.

### Sharks

Sharks are the most feared of all marine animals, but, according to the International Shark Attack File, the chance of being attacked by a shark along the North American coastline is 1 in 11.5 million Table 19-4. Although exact figures are unavailable, it is estimated that, worldwide, more than 50 attacks and fewer than a dozen deaths occur each year. The number of unprovoked shark attacks has grown at a steady rate over the past century.

Most attacks occur within 100 feet (30 m) of shore, and most people are attacked by a single shark without warning. In the majority of attacks, the person does not see the shark before the attack Figure 19-24. The leg is the most frequently bitten part. Sharks are clearly more attracted to people on the surface than to underwater scuba divers. The greatest attraction for sharks seems to be chemicals found in fish blood—sharks can detect them in quantities as small as one part per million parts of water. Shark bite wounds, among the most devastating of all animal bites, are similar to injuries caused by boat propellers and chainsaws. Immediate control of bleeding and treatment for shock are essential.

### Barracudas and Moray Eels

Barracudas have a fearsome appearance, but they have an undeserved reputation as attackers of humans. The risk of a barracuda bite is exceedingly small. First aid for a barracuda bite is identical to that for a shark bite.

Moray eels also have a fierce appearance. They are frequent biters of divers who handle or tease them, usually in competition for food or in pursuit of lobsters. The multiple puncture wounds created by moray eel bites have a high infection risk. Treat these wounds as you would shark bites.

**Figure 19-24**

Shark.

### Table 19-4 Preventing Shark Attacks

- Avoid swimming in areas frequented by sharks or where shark attacks have occurred. (In the United States, the greatest concentration of great white shark attacks is off the northern California coast.)
- **DO NOT** swim or dive alone.
- **DO NOT** swim far offshore, in murky water, or along deep drop-offs.
- People with open wounds and menstruating women should avoid swimming in areas where there is risk of a shark attack.
- Avoid swimming in the vicinity of seal or sea lion colonies or turtle habitats.
- **DO NOT** spear fish for an extended period in the same area, and **DO NOT** attach fish to your body.
- Avoid swimming at dawn, dusk, or night in potentially dangerous waters.

## Marine Animals That Sting

Stings from marine animals lead the list of adverse marine animal encounters. It is important to identify the offending animal, because in many cases, first aid is quite specific. Reactions to being stung vary from mild dermatitis to severe reactions. Most people recover without medical attention.

Jellyfish and Portuguese man-of-wars have long tentacles equipped with stinging devices called **nematocysts**. When cast ashore or onto rocks, detached nematocysts retain their ability to sting for a long time, usually until they are completely dried out.

The Portuguese man-of-war sting is usually in the form of well-defined linear welts or scattered patches of welts with redness, which usually disappear within 24 hours **Figure 19-25**. The jellyfish sting produces severe muscle cramping with multiple, thin lines of welts crossing the skin in a zigzag pattern **Figure 19-26**. Pain usually is a burning type that lasts 10 to 30 minutes. The welts on the skin usually disappear within an hour.

Anemones are beautiful but potentially dangerous **Figure 19-27**. Many anemone stings result from the improper handling of aquarium animals.

**Figure 19-26**
Jellyfish.

**Figure 19-25**
Portuguese man-of-war.

**Figure 19-27**
Anemones.

**Treatment for Envenomation by Jellyfish**

Nineteen reputable medical articles on various treatments for jellyfish stings found vinegar increases pain and nematocyst discharge in most jellyfish species in North America. (Vinegar may be beneficial for stings caused by the Portuguese man-of-war or the Hawaiian box jellyfish.) Instead of using vinegar to treat a jellyfish sting, consider washing the injury with ocean water. Although hot water and topical lidocaine were found to be more beneficial in treating jellyfish stings, they are often unavailable at locations where these injuries occur, such as at the beach or a diving site.

*Source:* Ward NT, et al. Evidence-based treatment of jellyfish stings in North America and Hawaii. *Ann Emerg Med* 2012; 60(4): 399-414.

**CAUTION**

**DO NOT** try to rub the tentacles off of the person's skin—rubbing activates the stinging cells.

**DO NOT** use fresh water for rinsing because it will cause the nematocysts to fire.

**DO NOT** apply cold packs—they also will cause the nematocysts to fire.

**DO NOT** touch the tentacles with your bare hands.

## Stingrays

Stingrays, commonly found in tropical and subtropical waters, are peaceful, reclusive bottom feeders that generally lie buried in the sand or mud **Figure 19-28**. Most wounds inflicted by stingrays are produced on the ankle or foot when the person steps on a ray. The ray reacts by thrusting its barbed tail upward and forward into the person's leg or foot. According to the American College of Emergency Physicians, approximately 2,000 stingray injuries occur each year in coastal US waters. The stingray's venomous tail barb easily penetrates human skin. The sting usually is more like a laceration because the large tail barb can do significant damage. The venom causes intense burning pain at the site.

**Figure 19-28**

Stingray.

Refer to **Flowchart 19-6** for additional information regarding the care of marine animal injuries.

| Injury Type | Marine Animal | What to Do |
|---|---|---|
| Bite, rip, or puncture | • Sharks<br>• Barracudas<br>• Eels<br>• Seals | 1. Monitor breathing.<br>2. Control bleeding.<br>3. Wash wound with soap and water.<br>4. Flush the area with water under pressure.<br>5. Treat for shock. |

*(Continues)*

| Injury Type | Marine Animal | What to Do |
|---|---|---|
| Sting | • Jellyfish<br>• Portuguese man-of-war<br>• Sea anemone<br>• Fire coral | **For North American species:**<br>1. Wash tentacles off with ocean water. **DO NOT** use fresh water.<br>2. Controversy exists about the use of vinegar for jellyfish stings; what works for one species may make another worse. For only Hawaiian box jellyfish and Portuguese man-of-wars, soak the area in vinegar for 30 seconds.<br>3. Remove clinging tentacles quickly with tweezers or by scraping with a credit card, razor blade, or clean stick.<br>4. For all jellyfish stings in North America and Hawaii, soak the area in non-scalding hot water for 20 minutes. Xylocaine (Lidocaine), an over-the-counter medication, can be applied on the affected skin.<br>5. **DO NOT** use the following remedies: human urine, meat tenderizer, alcohol, and pressure bandages. These remedies are either not supported by research or have been shown to be ineffective. |
| Venomous bite | • Sea snake<br>• Octopus<br>• Cone snail | 1. Monitor breathing.<br>2. Control bleeding.<br>3. Apply pressure bandage on entire arm or leg. |
| Puncture (by spine) | • Stingray<br>• Scorpion fish<br>• Stonefish<br>• Starfish<br>• Catfish | 1. Soak the area in hot water for 30 to 90 minutes or until pain subsides. **DO NOT** use water that is hot enough to burn.<br>2. Remove pieces of debris with tweezers.<br>3. Wash the area with soap and water.<br>4. Flush the area with water under pressure.<br>5. Treat the wound. |

## Flowchart 19-6 Marine Animal Injuries

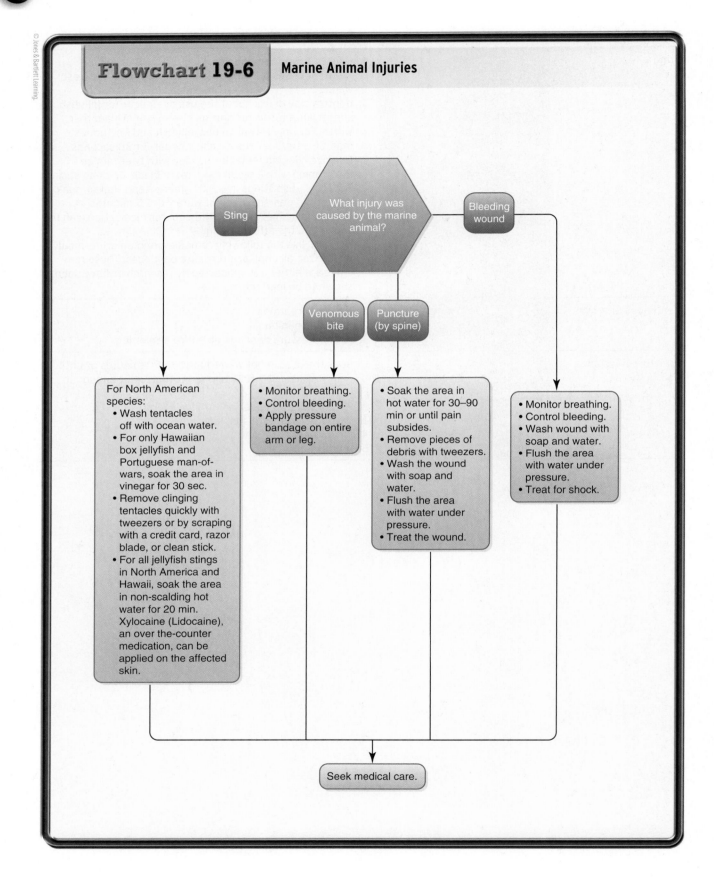

**What injury was caused by the marine animal?**

**Sting**

**Bleeding wound**

**Venomous bite**

**Puncture (by spine)**

For North American species:
- Wash tentacles off with ocean water.
- For only Hawaiian box jellyfish and Portuguese man-of-wars, soak the area in vinegar for 30 sec.
- Remove clinging tentacles quickly with tweezers or by scraping with a credit card, razor blade, or clean stick.
- For all jellyfish stings in North America and Hawaii, soak the area in non-scalding hot water for 20 min. Xylocaine (Lidocaine), an over the-counter medication, can be applied on the affected skin.

- Monitor breathing.
- Control bleeding.
- Apply pressure bandage on entire arm or leg.

- Soak the area in hot water for 30–90 min or until pain subsides.
- Remove pieces of debris with tweezers.
- Wash the wound with soap and water.
- Flush the area with water under pressure.
- Treat the wound.

- Monitor breathing.
- Control bleeding.
- Wash wound with soap and water.
- Flush the area with water under pressure.
- Treat for shock.

**Seek medical care.**

## ▶ Ready for Review

- Almost half of all Americans will suffer a bite from either an animal or human.
- Throughout the world, about 100,000 people die each year of snake bites.
- The stinging insects belonging to the order Hymenoptera include honeybees, bumblebees, yellow jackets, hornets, wasps, and fire ants.
- Most spiders are venomous, which is how they paralyze and kill their prey. However, most spiders lack an effective delivery system—long fangs and strong jaws—to bite a human.
- Most marine animals bite or sting in self-defense, rather than attack.

## ▶ Vital Vocabulary

anaphylaxis A life-threatening allergic reaction.

antivenom An antiserum containing antibodies against reptile or insect venom.

nematocysts Stinging cells found on certain marine animals.

rabies An acute viral infection of the central nervous system transmitted by the bite of an infected animal.

## ▶ Assessment in Action

You are enjoying an overnight campout with your family in the springtime. As you get ready for bed, you notice a small lump on your belly and are startled to find an embedded tick.

*Directions:* Circle Yes if you agree with the statement; circle No if you disagree.

Yes No 1. You should leave the tick alone because it will cause no harm to humans.

Yes No 2. Covering the tick with petroleum jelly is very effective for removing the embedded tick.

Yes No 3. You should touch a hot, blown-out match to the tick.

Yes No 4. Grabbing the tick as close to the skin as possible with tweezers and pulling upward is usually effective.

Yes No 5. After removing the tick, clean the wound and use an ice pack to reduce pain.

## ▶ Check Your Knowledge

*Directions:* Circle Yes if you agree with the statement; circle No if you disagree.

Yes No 1. Severe abdominal pain is a sign of a black widow spider bite.

Yes No 2. Apply an ice or cold pack over a snake bite.

Yes No 3. Use the cut and suck method for a snake bite.

Yes No 4. Remove a bee's stinger by using tweezers to pull it out.

Yes No 5. Apply an ice or cold pack over an insect sting or a suspected spider bite.

Yes No 6. A baking soda paste can help reduce the itching and swelling from an insect sting.

Yes No 7. A person's prescribed epinephrine auto-injector might have to be used if the person has a life-threatening reaction to an insect sting.

Yes No 8. Care for stings from marine animals (for example, jellyfish) by pouring hydrogen peroxide on the affected area.

Yes No 9. Covering an embedded tick with petroleum jelly causes the tick to back out because of the lack of oxygen.

Yes No 10. Ticks can transmit disease.

# Cold-Related Emergencies

**20**

## Chapter
### at a glance

## Cold-Related Emergencies

Heat flows from an area with a higher temperature to an area with a lower temperature. When a person is surrounded by air or water cooler than body temperature, the body experiences heat loss. If heat escapes faster than the body produces heat, the body's temperature falls. Normal body temperature is 98.6°F (37°C), and if body temperature falls much below that, cold injuries can result.

### ▶ How Cold Affects the Body

Humans protect themselves from cold primarily by avoiding or reducing cold exposure through the use of clothing and shelter. When that protection proves inadequate, the body has biologic defense mechanisms to help maintain correct body temperature. The internal mechanisms to maintain body temperature during cold exposure include vasoconstriction and shivering. Triggering of these responses is a signal that clothing and shelter are inadequate.

**Vasoconstriction** is the tightening of blood vessels. During cold exposure, vasoconstriction occurs in the exposed skin. The reduced blood flow in the skin conserves body heat but can lead to discomfort, numbness, loss of dexterity in the hands and fingers, and, eventually, cold injuries.

Cold triggers shivering, which increases internal heat production and helps offset the heat loss. Shivering is the body's main involuntary defense against the cold. Shivering produces body heat by forcing muscles to contract and relax rapidly. About 80% of the muscle energy used in shivering is turned into body heat. When the core temperature rises, shivering is no longer needed and is shut down by the brain. When the core temperature falls to about 86°F to 90°F (30°C to 32.3°C), the shivering reflex stops. Likewise, when there is no further fuel for the body, shivering stops. Several drugs suppress the shivering response, including barbiturates, narcotics, beta-blocking agents, and alcohol.

Internal heat production is also increased by physical activity; the more vigorous the activity, the greater the heat production. In fact, heat production during intense exercise or strenuous work usually is sufficient to compensate completely for heat loss, even when it is extremely cold. However, high-intensity exercise and hard physical work are fatiguing and cannot be sustained indefinitely. If clothes become wet with sweat, heat loss is markedly increased after exertion.

Susceptibility to cold injuries can be minimized by maintaining proper hydration and nutrition; avoiding alcohol, caffeine, and nicotine; and limiting periods of inactivity in cold conditions. Humans do not acclimatize to cold weather nearly as well as they acclimatize to hot weather.

The colder the surrounding temperature, the greater the potential for body heat to escape. When the skin is exposed to cold, the brain signals the blood vessels in the skin to tighten, and blood flow to the skin decreases. This is the body's attempt to prevent heat inside the body from being carried to the skin, where heat loss will occur. However, because of reduced blood flow to the skin, the skin temperature falls.

When cold exposure lasts more than an hour, cooling of the skin and reduced blood flow to the hands will blunt sensation, touch, and pain, and will cause a loss of dexterity and agility. These changes can impair a person's ability to perform manual tasks and, because symptoms could go unnoticed, can lead to more severe cold injuries.

## Heat Loss From the Body

Normal body temperature is maintained by a balance of heat production and heat loss. Heat is produced by food metabolism and muscle activity, and shivering can increase heat production up to 500%. Shivering causes a large increase in heat production, but it rapidly consumes calories stored in the liver and muscles as glycogen. Lack of food limits the body's ability to produce heat; when glycogen stores are depleted, heat output decreases.

Heat loss occurs primarily through the skin. Blood flow to the skin varies in different parts of the body, and some areas allow more heat loss than others. Heat loss measurements demonstrate high losses from the head and neck (up to 50%), axillary area (armpits), and groin area. The constriction of blood vessels caused by cold conserves heat.

Body heat loss can occur via four mechanisms:

- Conduction, or direct contact with a colder object (for example, lying on the snow), normally accounts for only a small fraction of heat loss. The exception is immersion in cold water, in which heat loss can be 25 to 30 times greater than in air and even more in moving water.
- Convection is the loss of heat from the body by air blowing over the skin or through porous clothing. Windchill is the combined effect of the ambient temperature and wind speed.
- Evaporation, or conversion of liquid on the skin to a vapor, normally accounts for about 20% of heat loss (two-thirds through sweating and one-third through breathing).
- Radiation is the primary method of heat loss, accounting for about 65% of the body's heat loss. A warm object gives off (radiates) heat to cooler air. It has been demonstrated that up to 50% of the body's total heat production can be lost by radiation through a person's unprotected head **Figure 20-1** .

## Q&A

### How is shivering related to the muscular system?

Shivering is the body's natural way of keeping warm and can actually serve as a lifesaver in extreme cold. Shivering produces heat by forcing skeletal muscles to contract and relax rapidly. About 80% of the muscle energy used in this process is turned into body heat. Studies have shown that applying hot water bottles or hot objects can actually be harmful in some cases of hypothermia because the shivering reflex is shut down.

## How Cold Is It?

In addition to cold, two other factors account for body heat loss: moisture and wind. Moisture—whether from rain, snow, or perspiration—speeds the conduction of heat away from the body.

Wind causes sizable amounts of body heat loss. If the thermometer reads 20°F (minus 6.7°C) and the wind speed is 20 mph (32 kmph), the exposure is comparable to 4°F (minus 15.6°C). This is called the windchill factor. Use the following rough measures of wind speed: if you feel the wind on your face, wind speed is at least 10 mph (16 kmph); if small branches move or if dust or snow is raised, it is 20 mph (32 kmph); if large branches are moving, it is 30 mph (48 kmph); and if a whole tree bends, it is about 40 mph (65 kmph).

To determine the windchill factor:

1. Estimate the wind speed by checking for the aforementioned signs.
2. Look at an outdoor thermometer reading (in degrees Fahrenheit).
3. Match the estimated wind speed with the actual thermometer reading in the following table.

# Wind Chill Chart

*Effective 11/01/01*

| Calm | 40 | 35 | 30 | 25 | 20 | 15 | 10 | 5 | 0 | -5 | -10 | -15 | -20 | -25 | -30 | -35 | -40 | -45 |
|---|---|---|---|---|---|---|---|---|---|---|---|---|---|---|---|---|---|---|
| 5 | 36 | 31 | 25 | 19 | 13 | 7 | 1 | -5 | -11 | -16 | -22 | -28 | -34 | -40 | -46 | -52 | -57 | -63 |
| 10 | 34 | 27 | 21 | 15 | 9 | 3 | -4 | -10 | -16 | -22 | -28 | -35 | -41 | -47 | -53 | -59 | -66 | -72 |
| 15 | 32 | 25 | 19 | 13 | 6 | 0 | -7 | -13 | -19 | -26 | -32 | -39 | -45 | -51 | -58 | -64 | -71 | -77 |
| 20 | 30 | 24 | 17 | 11 | 4 | -2 | -9 | -15 | -22 | -29 | -35 | -42 | -48 | -55 | -61 | -68 | -74 | -81 |
| 25 | 29 | 23 | 16 | 9 | 3 | -4 | -11 | -17 | -24 | -31 | -37 | -44 | -51 | -58 | -64 | -71 | -78 | -84 |
| 30 | 28 | 22 | 15 | 8 | 1 | -5 | -12 | -19 | -26 | -33 | -39 | -46 | -53 | -60 | -67 | -73 | -80 | -87 |
| 35 | 28 | 21 | 14 | 7 | 0 | -7 | -14 | -21 | -27 | -34 | -41 | -48 | -55 | -62 | -69 | -76 | -82 | -89 |
| 40 | 27 | 20 | 13 | 6 | -1 | -8 | -15 | -22 | -29 | -36 | -43 | -50 | -57 | -64 | -71 | -78 | -84 | -91 |
| 45 | 26 | 19 | 12 | 5 | -2 | -9 | -16 | -23 | -30 | -37 | -44 | -51 | -58 | -65 | -72 | -79 | -86 | -93 |
| 50 | 26 | 19 | 12 | 4 | -3 | -10 | -17 | -24 | -31 | -38 | -45 | -52 | -60 | -67 | -74 | -81 | -88 | -95 |
| 55 | 25 | 18 | 11 | 4 | -3 | -11 | -18 | -25 | -32 | -39 | -46 | -54 | -61 | -68 | -75 | -82 | -89 | -97 |
| 60 | 25 | 17 | 10 | 3 | -4 | -11 | -19 | -26 | -33 | -40 | -48 | -55 | -62 | -69 | -76 | -84 | -91 | -98 |

Wind (mph) *(vertical axis label)*

Frostbite Times: ■ 30 minutes ■ 10 minutes ■ 5 minutes

$$\text{Wind Chill (°F)} = 35.74 + 0.6215T - 35.75 (V^{0.16}) + 0.4275T (V^{0.16})$$

Where, T=Air Temperature (°F) V=Wind Speed (mph)

*Source:* Courtesy of the National Weather Service/NOAA.

Courtesy of the National Weather Service/NOAA.

## Susceptibility to Cold Injury

A person's susceptibility to cold injury is affected by many factors. People who are physically unfit are more susceptible to cold injury. They tire more quickly and are unable to stay active to keep warm as long as people who are physically fit.

Dehydration reduces blood flow in the skin, which increases susceptibility to cold injury. Fat functions as an insulator against heat loss because it has less blood flow than muscle and loses less heat. Therefore, a very lean person may be susceptible to the effects of cold if clothing is inadequate or wet or if the person is relatively inactive. Older people are less tolerant of the cold than younger people because of a decline in physical fitness, poor circulation, other illnesses, and medications that affect thermoregulation.

Alcohol and, to a lesser extent, caffeine cause the blood vessels in the skin to open, which can accelerate body heat loss. Also, alcohol and caffeine both increase urine formation, leading to dehydration, which can further degrade the body's defenses against cold. Most important, alcohol blunts the senses and impairs judgment, so a person may not feel the signs and symptoms of developing cold injury.

Because nicotine decreases blood flow to the skin, smoking and chewing tobacco can increase susceptibility to frostbite. Inadequate nutrition,

**Figure 20-1**

Sources of heat loss.

Labels on figure: Evaporation, Radiation, Convection, Conduction

© Jones & Bartlett Learning.

illness, and injury compromise the body's responses to cold and a person's ability to recognize and react appropriately to the symptoms of developing cold injury. People who have experienced a cold injury are at greater risk of experiencing another cold injury.

## Effects of Altitude

Assessing weather conditions in mountainous regions must include altitude considerations, especially if the assessment is based on weather measurements obtained at lower elevations. Temperatures, windchill, and the risk of cold injury at high altitudes can differ considerably from those at lower elevations.

In general, it can be assumed that air temperature drops 3.6°F every 1,000 feet (305 m) above the original measurement site. Winds usually are more severe at high altitudes, and there is less cover above the tree line. People are more susceptible to frostbite and other cold injuries at altitudes above 8,000 feet (2400 m) than at sea level because of lower temperatures, higher winds, and less oxygen.

## Effects of Water

Water can conduct heat away from the body much faster than air of the same temperature. When clothing becomes wet because of snow, rain, splashing water, or accumulated sweat, the body's loss of heat is accelerated up to 25 times faster. Swimmers and people working or wading in water can have a great deal of body heat loss, even when the water temperature is only mildly cool. People entering very cold water should be closely watched because sudden plunging into cold water can produce an irregular heartbeat, gasping, and hyperventilation, which can cause inhalation of water, heart failure, and drowning.

## Effects of Wind

For any given air temperature, the potential for body heat loss, skin cooling, and decreased internal temperature is increased by wind. Wind increases heat loss from skin exposed to cold air, in effect lowering the temperature. The windchill index integrates wind speed and air temperature to provide an estimate of the cooling power of the environment and the associated risk of cold injury.

Windchill temperatures obtained from weather reports do not take into account artificial wind, which worsens the windchill effect of natural wind. For example, riding in an open vehicle can subject the passengers to dangerous windchill, even when natural winds are low.

## Effects of Metals and Liquid Fuels

Metal objects and liquid fuels that have been left outdoors in the cold pose a serious hazard. Both can conduct heat away from the skin rapidly. Fuels and solvents remain liquid at very low temperatures. Skin contact with fuel or metal at below-freezing temperatures can result in nearly instantaneous freezing. Fuel handlers must use great care and not allow exposed skin to come into contact with spilled fuels or metals.

## Minimizing Effects of Cold on the Body

When adequately protected, humans can tolerate temperatures as low as minus 72°F (minus 57.8°C). Adequate clothing maintains the microclimate surrounding the body. Air is an excellent insulator, and the basis for most clothing is to trap a layer of air around the body. Layering, which has been used for centuries, allows the removal or opening of a garment to vent excess heat during times of greater activity or changes in environment, and it accommodates individual needs and preferences. Wearing layered clothing is especially important for people who frequently change environments by going in and out of buildings or who periodically undertake vigorous physical activity **Figure 20-2**.

Three important layers are recommended for most outdoor activities. The first layer (undergarments) removes perspiration from the skin, the middle layers insulate, and the outer layer or outer shell protects against wind and water. By understanding this principle, people can vary their clothing for protection and comfort.

For the first layer, use underwear that wicks away perspiration; that is, it stays dry by drawing moisture away from the skin to the next layer of clothing. Wet clothing transfers heat away from the body. Cotton holds moisture next to the skin, so the person feels cold and clammy. Silk feels warm and soft, but it also retains moisture. Fabrics such as polypropylene or one of the new types of polyesters such as Capilene or Thermax should be considered.

The middle layer can be a synthetic pile or fleece jacket that is warm and dries quickly or a wool or synthetic sweater. Synthetic insulating materials, unlike down or wool, provide warmth without bulk or heavy weight. Insulation should be effective even when wet. In that respect, synthetics are clearly superior to natural fibers and natural products. Duck or goose down, for example, is virtually useless when wet, and it dries slowly. One exception, however, is the insulating ability of wool, even when wet.

People who are physically active can sweat even in extremely cold weather. Therefore, the best choice for an outside layer is a jacket that is waterproof, wind resistant, and breathable. Materials such as Gore-Tex allow perspiration to evaporate. A zipper is preferable, so the clothing can be opened easily to increase ventilation. Nylon and vinyl are poor choices because they produce a sauna effect by holding in perspiration. Because more body heat loss occurs through the head than any other part (up to 50%), heed the admonition, "If the feet are cold, cover the head." A wool or synthetic cap serves well.

Figure 20-2
Wearing layered clothing can help your body adapt to changing conditions.

## ▶ Nonfreezing Cold Injuries

Nonfreezing cold injuries can occur when conditions are cold and wet (air temperatures between 32°F and 55°F [0°C and 12.8°C]) and the hands and feet cannot be kept warm and dry. The most prominent nonfreezing cold injuries are chilblain and trench foot.

### Chilblain

Chilblain is a nonfreezing cold injury that, while painful, causes little or no permanent damage. Chilblain can develop in 3 to 6 hours in skin exposed to cold and moisture.

## What to Look For

- Swollen skin
- Skin that is tender, hot to the touch, and possibly itchy
- Blisters
- Condition can worsen to an aching, prickly (pins and needles) sensation and then numbness.

## What to Do

1. Get the person out of the cold.

## Trench Foot/Immersion Foot

<u>Trench foot</u> (also called immersion foot) is a serious, nonfreezing cold injury that develops when the skin on the feet is exposed to moisture and cold for prolonged periods (12 hours or longer). Wearing wet boots or shoes and socks causes trench foot; prolonged immersion of the feet in cold water causes immersion foot.

The combination of cold and moisture softens the skin, causing tissue loss and, often, infection. The risk of this potentially crippling injury is high during wet weather. People who wear rubberized or tight-fitting boots in cold weather are at risk for trench foot regardless of weather conditions because sweat accumulates inside the boots and keeps the feet wet.

## What to Look For

- Itching, numbness, or tingling pain
- Swollen feet and pale skin that feels cold when touched
- Red or blue blotches on the skin, sometimes with open weeping or bleeding

## What to Do

1. Dry the skin.
2. Rewarm the foot gradually.
3. Care for open weeping areas by cleansing with mild soap and water and applying breathable dressings.

## Q&A

**What is the origin of the term *trench* or *immersion foot*?**

The term *immersion foot* was coined during World War I to describe an injury that occurred to people who were shipwrecked and isolated in a lifeboat for a prolonged period of time. Similarly, the term *trench foot* was coined during World War I to describe an injury that occurred to soldiers who were stuck for a prolonged period of time in trenches filled with cold mud and water.

  Both conditions occur after prolonged exposure to a wet and cold environment. Temperatures range from just above freezing to about 50°F (10°C). The duration of exposure usually exceeds 10 to 12 hours.
*Source:* Stewart C. Local cold injuries in children: Diagnosis, management, and prevention. *Pediatr EM Rep* 1991;4:1.

# ▶ Freezing Cold Injuries

Freezing cold injuries can occur whenever the air temperature is below freezing (32°F [0°C]). Freezing limited to the skin surface is <u>frostnip</u>. Freezing that extends deeper through the skin and into the flesh is <u>frostbite</u>.

Frostbite is prevalent during military campaigns and is a known hazard for outdoor workers, the homeless, mountain climbers, and explorers. As more people pursue cross-country skiing, snowmobiling, and other outdoor winter sports, the number of frostbite cases probably will increase. However, it is still thought to be rare in nonmilitary situations.

## Frostnip

Frostnip is caused when water on the skin surface freezes. Frostnip should be taken seriously because it could be the first sign of impending frostbite. It may be difficult to tell the difference between frostnip and frostbite.

| What to Look For | What to Do |
|---|---|
| • Yellow to gray skin color<br>• Frost (ice crystals) on the skin<br>• Initial tingling or numbness that may become painful | • Get the person out of the cold and to a warm place.<br>• Gently warm the affected area by placing it against a warm body part (eg, have the person put bare hands under the armpits) or by applying a warm chemical heat pack covered by a cloth. For the nose, breathe with cupped hands over the nose.<br>• **DO NOT** rub the area. |

## Frostbite

Frostbite happens only in below-freezing temperatures. Tissue is not composed of water alone, so it will not freeze until it has been cooled to about 28°F (minus 2.2°C). Tissue is damaged in two ways: (1) actual tissue freezing, which results in the formation of ice crystals within the tissue (the ice crystals expand as they freeze, damaging cells), and (2) the obstruction of the blood supply to the tissue, which causes sludged blood clots and further prevents blood from flowing to the tissues. The second type of tissue damage is more extensive than the first. In severely cold temperatures, flesh can freeze in less than a minute **Figure 20-3**.

Frostbite affects mainly the feet, hands, ears, and nose. These areas do not contain large heat-producing muscles and are some distance from the body's heat-generation sources. The severity and extent of frostbite are difficult to judge until hours after thawing. The most severe consequences of frostbite occur when tissue dies (<u>gangrene</u>), and the affected part might have to be amputated.

Courtesy of Neil Malcom Winkelmann.

**Figure 20-3**

Frostbitten fingers 6 hours after rewarming in 108°F (42.2°C) water.

The longer the tissue stays frozen, the worse the injury. Check for hypothermia in any person with frostbite.

Refer to **Flowchart 20-1** for additional information regarding the care of frostbite.

**What to Look For**

**What to Do**

Before thawing, frostbite can be classified as superficial or deep:

- Superficial frostbite
  - White, waxy, or gray-yellow skin
  - The affected part feels very cold and numb. There might be tingling, stinging, or an aching sensation.
  - The skin surface feels stiff or crusty and the underlying tissue feels soft when depressed gently and firmly.
- Deep frostbite
  - The affected part feels cold, hard, and solid and cannot be depressed; it feels like a piece of wood or frozen meat.
  - Skin in the affected body part is pale and waxy.
  - A painfully cold part stops hurting.

1. Get the person out of the cold and to a warm place. If possible, **DO NOT** use a frozen extremity until medical care is reached.
2. Remove any wet clothing and constricting items, such as rings, that could impair blood circulation.
3. **DO NOT** attempt to thaw the part if: (a) medical care is less than 2 hours away; (b) the affected area has thawed; (c) shelter, warm water, and a container are not available; or (d) a risk of refreezing exists.
4. Use the wet, rapid rewarming method if (a) medical care is more than 2 hours away; (b) there is no possibility of refreezing the affected area, or (c) shelter, warm water, and a container are available. If the wet, rapid rewarming method is not possible, slow rewarming can be done by moving into a warm location and warming the part with the body heat of the person or another person (eg, armpit or abdomen).
5. *Wet, rapid, rewarming method:* Place the frostbitten part in warm (100 to 104°F [38 to 40°C]) water. **DO NOT** use other heat sources (eg, fire, space heater, oven). If you do not have a thermometer, you can put your hand into the water for 30 seconds to test that it is warm but not hot enough to burn. Maintain water temperature by adding warm water as needed. Rewarming usually takes 20 to 40 minutes or until the part becomes soft and pliable to touch and takes on a red/purple appearance. Air dry the area; **DO NOT** rub. To help control the severe pain during rewarming, give the person ibuprofen. For ear or facial injuries, it is best to apply warm, moist cloths, changing them frequently.

After thawing, frostbite can be categorized by degrees, similar to the classification of burns:

- First-degree frostbite
  - The affected part is warm, swollen, and tender.
- Second-degree frostbite
  - Blisters form minutes to hours after thawing and enlarge over several days **Figure 20-4**.
- Third-degree frostbite
  - Blisters are small and contain red-blue or purple fluid. The surrounding skin may be red or blue and might not blanch when pressure is applied.

After thawing:
1. If the feet are affected, **DO NOT** allow the person to walk. The feet will be impossible to use after they are rewarmed unless only the toes are affected.
2. Protect the affected area from contact with clothing and bedding.
3. Place bulky, dry, clean gauze on the affected part and between the toes and the fingers to absorb moisture and keep them from sticking together.
4. Slightly elevate the affected part above heart level to reduce pain and swelling.
5. Apply aloe vera gel to promote skin healing.
6. Give ibuprofen to limit pain and inflammation.
7. Give fluids if the person is alert and can swallow.
8. Seek medical care as soon as possible.

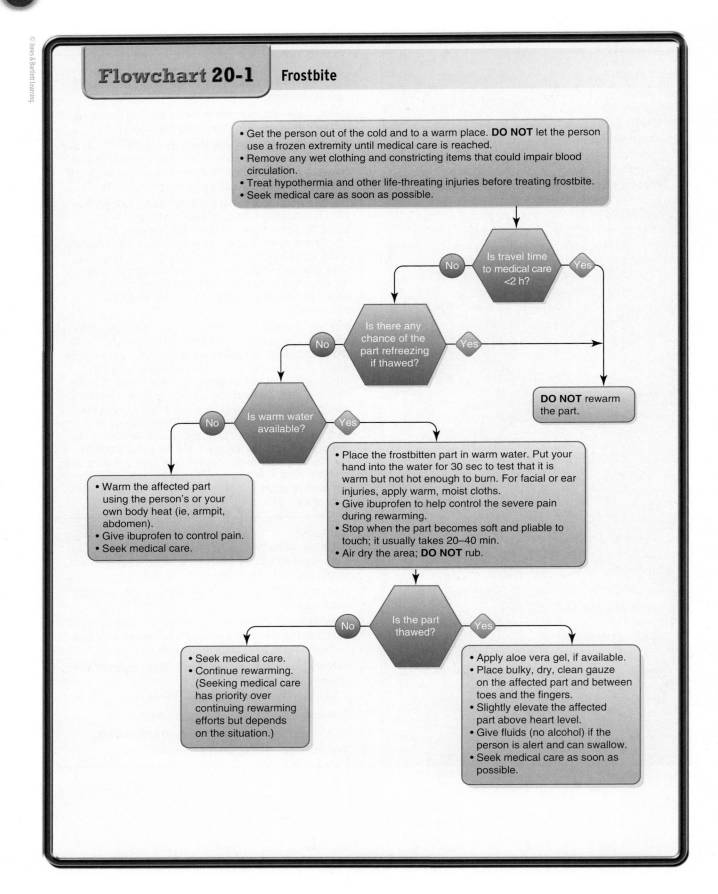

**Flowchart 20-1**  Frostbite

- Get the person out of the cold and to a warm place. **DO NOT** let the person use a frozen extremity until medical care is reached.
- Remove any wet clothing and constricting items that could impair blood circulation.
- Treat hypothermia and other life-threating injuries before treating frostbite.
- Seek medical care as soon as possible.

Is travel time to medical care <2 h?

No — Yes

Is there any chance of the part refreezing if thawed?

No — Yes →

**DO NOT** rewarm the part.

Is warm water available?

No — Yes

- Warm the affected part using the person's or your own body heat (ie, armpit, abdomen).
- Give ibuprofen to control pain.
- Seek medical care.

- Place the frostbitten part in warm water. Put your hand into the water for 30 sec to test that it is warm but not hot enough to burn. For facial or ear injuries, apply warm, moist cloths.
- Give ibuprofen to help control the severe pain during rewarming.
- Stop when the part becomes soft and pliable to touch; it usually takes 20–40 min.
- Air dry the area; **DO NOT** rub.

Is the part thawed?

No — Yes

- Seek medical care.
- Continue rewarming. (Seeking medical care has priority over continuing rewarming efforts but depends on the situation.)

- Apply aloe vera gel, if available.
- Place bulky, dry, clean gauze on the affected part and between toes and the fingers.
- Slightly elevate the affected part above heart level.
- Give fluids (no alcohol) if the person is alert and can swallow.
- Seek medical care as soon as possible.

## CAUTION

**DO NOT** use water hotter than 104°F (40°C)–burns can result.

**DO NOT** use water cooler than 100°F (37.8°C)–it will not thaw frostbite rapidly enough.

**DO NOT** break any blisters.

**DO NOT** rub or massage the affected part–ice crystals can be pushed into body cells, rupturing them.

**DO NOT** rub the affected part with ice or snow.

**DO NOT** rewarm the part with a heating pad, hot-water bottle, stove, sunlamp, radiator, exhaust pipe, or over a fire. Excessive temperatures cannot be controlled, and burns can result.

**DO NOT** allow the person to drink alcoholic beverages. Alcohol dilates blood vessels and causes loss of body heat.

**DO NOT** allow the person to smoke. Smoking constricts blood vessels, thus impairing circulation.

**DO NOT** rewarm if there is any possibility of refreezing.

**DO NOT** allow the thawed part to refreeze because the ice crystals formed will be larger and more damaging. If refreezing is likely or even possible, it is better to leave the affected part frozen.

**DO NOT** use the dry rewarming technique (putting the person's hands in your armpits) because that takes three to four times longer than the wet, rapid method to thaw frozen tissue. Slow rewarming results in greater tissue damage than rapid rewarming.

**DO NOT** rewarm if close to a medical facility.

**Figure 20-4**

Second-degree frostbite of the toes **(A)** and ear **(B)**.

## ▶ Hypothermia

Body temperature falls when the body cannot produce heat as fast as it is lost. **Hypothermia** is a life-threatening condition in which the body's core temperature falls below 95°F (35°C). Generally, the core temperature will not fall until after many hours of continuous exposure to cold air if the person is healthy, physically active, and reasonably dressed. However, because wet skin and wind accelerate body heat loss and the body produces less heat during inactive periods, the core body temperature can fall even when the air temperature is above freezing if conditions are windy, clothing is wet, or the person is inactive.

Hypothermia can occur year round. Most people think of hypothermia as related only to cold outdoor exposure. It can happen indoors, in the southern states, and even on a summer day. It does not require subfreezing temperatures.

Hypothermia happens when heat loss occurs faster than heat production. Most people will die if the body temperature falls to 80°F (26.7°C). Hypothermia can occur in indoor or outdoor situations. Hypothermia occurs rapidly during cold-water immersion (1 hour or less when the water temperature is less than 45°F [7.2°C]). Because water has a tremendous capacity to drain heat from the body, prolonged immersion (several hours) in even slightly cool water (less than 70°F [21.1°C]) can cause hypothermia. Hypothermia is a medical emergency. Untreated, it can result in death.

Even though people with hypothermia might have no heartbeat, breathing, or response to touch or pain, they may not be dead. Sometimes, the heartbeat and breathing of a person with hypothermia will be so faint or slow that they are not detected. If the person has no signs of life, begin CPR immediately. If hypothermia has resulted from submersion in cold water, CPR should be started without delay. People with hypothermia should be treated as gently as possible because rough handling can cause life-threatening disruptions in heart rhythm. All people with hypothermia, even those who do not seem to be alive, must be evaluated by a physician.

In the past, the people believed most vulnerable to hypothermia were hunters, hikers, backpackers, careless drinkers, and people who had been in an accident. However, disadvantaged urban dwellers exposed to the elements and older people with impaired thermoregulatory mechanisms also are susceptible. Lightly clad people almost anywhere can quickly become chilled outdoors when it is raining, even though the temperatures are only cool, and people immersed for some time in cool or cold water can have rapid heat loss. Even well-conditioned athletes such as long-distance runners can experience hypothermia. Hypothermia should be considered whenever the person's behavior and history and the weather conditions indicate abnormal heat loss. Hypothermia is an underreported cause of death in the United States. In most cases, death is attributed to other factors, with hypothermia considered a secondary cause.

The person's history may be sufficient to determine hypothermia has occurred. Hypothermia is likely if a person is reported by companions to be acting strangely and is shivering after exposure to cold or moisture or if he or she has been immersed in cold water. Hypothermia is not likely if the person is shivering but able to function well and to care for himself or herself. If there is any doubt, assume that the person has hypothermia.

Predisposing factors are important: drinking alcoholic beverages is commonly associated with hypothermia. A typical scenario involves one or more people in lightweight garments who drink too much, fall asleep outdoors or in a poorly heated shelter, become chilled by cold air or moisture, and remain exposed for many hours. Certain medications predispose people to hypothermia because they interfere with the hypothalamus, which acts as the brain's thermostat in regulating body heat.

Especially vulnerable to hypothermia are very old and very young people. Infants and children have a small muscle mass, so the shivering response is poor in children and nonexistent in infants. They also have less body fat. Younger children need help to protect themselves against the cold because they cannot put on or take off clothes. People who are less fit are also more likely to become hypothermic.

## Types of Exposure

There are three classifications of cold exposure:

- Acute exposure (also known as immersion) occurs when body heat loss occurs very rapidly, usually in water. Acute exposure is considered to be 6 hours or less.
- Subacute exposure (also known as mountain or exhaustion exposure) occurs when exposure is 6 to 24 hours and can be land- or water-based.
- Chronic exposure (also known as urban exposure) involves long-term cooling. It generally occurs on land and exceeds 24 hours.

## Recognizing Hypothermia

Consider hypothermia in all people who have been exposed to cold and who have an altered mental status. Suspect hypothermia in any person who has a body temperature of less than 95°F (35°C). (Keep in mind that some thermometers do not measure below 95°F [35°C].) Shivering is a good clue, but it could be suppressed when energy stores (glycogen) are depleted. Suspect hypothermia in people with frostbite and those injured in a cold environment.

Some people die of hypothermia because they or those around them do not recognize the symptoms, which are difficult to recognize in the early stages. Here are some signs to watch for:

- *Change in mental status.* This is one of the first symptoms of developing hypothermia. Examples are disorientation, apathy, and changes in personality, such as unusual aggressiveness.
- *Shivering.* Shivering is the first, and most important, body defense against a falling body temperature. Shivering starts when the body temperature drops 1°F and can produce more heat than many rewarming methods. As the core temperature continues to fall, shivering decreases and usually stops at about 86°F (30°C). Shivering also stops as body temperature rises. If shivering stops as responsiveness

decreases, assume that the core temperature is falling. If, on the other hand, shivering stops while the person is becoming more coordinated and feeling better, assume that the core temperature is rising.

- *Cool abdomen.* Place the back of your hand between the clothing and the person's abdomen to assess the person's temperature. When the person's abdominal skin under clothing is cooler than your hand, consider the person to have hypothermia until proven otherwise.
- *Low core body temperature.* The best indicator of hypothermia is a thermometer reading of the core body temperature. The ability to reliably measure core temperature depends on the availability of an appropriate thermometer and access to the person's rectum. Normal thermometers do not register below 94°F (34.4°C) and so do not indicate whether the hypothermia is mild or severe. Because first aid for mild hypothermia is different from that for severe hypothermia, it is helpful to have a rectal thermometer that registers below 90°F (32.2°C). Oral and axillary (armpit) temperatures are influenced by too many external factors to make them reliable.

Measuring rectal temperatures in wilderness or remote locations is seldom done, mainly because low-reading rectal thermometers usually are not readily available. Also, taking a rectal temperature can be difficult, inconvenient, and embarrassing to the person and first aid provider. If done outdoors, such a procedure can further expose the already cold person.

## Types of Hypothermia

The difference between mild and severe hypothermia is based on the core body temperature, but taking a rectal temperature often is not possible. The second most significant difference is that with severe hypothermia, the person becomes so cold that shivering stops, which means the person's body cannot rewarm itself internally and requires external heat for recovery.

The National Association of Emergency Medical Services Physicians recommends that CPR not be started on a person with severe hypothermia if one of the following applies:

- The person's core body temperature is less than 60°F (15.6°C).

- The person's chest is frozen (cannot be compressed).
- The person was submerged in water for more than 60 minutes.
- The person has a lethal injury.
- Transport for controlled rewarming will be delayed.
- Rescuers are endangered.

For CPR to be effective, heart activity must be restored within a short time, which requires defibrillation, oxygen, and medications. **DO NOT** start CPR until you have checked the person's circulation for one minute. A person with hypothermia will have an extremely slow pulse rate. CPR can cause cardiac arrest in an already beating heart. If there is no detectible pulse after one minute, start CPR. If it is not safe to perform continuous CPR, CPR can be delayed or can be given intermittently during evacuation for people with severe hypothermia. CPR can be given for several hours, if necessary. (See Chapter 5, *CPR*, for additional information.)

Do the following to care for all people with hypothermia:

1. Stop further heat loss.
   - Get the person out of the cold.
   - Handle the person gently.
   - Replace wet clothing with dry clothing.
   - Add insulation (eg, blankets, towels, pillows, sleeping bags) beneath and around the person. Cover the person's head (50% to 80% of the body's heat loss is through the head).
   - Cover the person with a vapor barrier (eg, tarp, plastic, trash bags). **DO NOT** cover the mouth and/or nose. If you are unable to remove wet clothing, place a vapor barrier between clothing and insulation. For a dry person, the vapor barrier can be placed outside of the insulation.
2. Keep the person in a horizontal (flat) position.
   - **DO NOT** raise the legs. **DO NOT** let the person walk or exercise. **DO NOT** massage the person's body. These activities could drive cold blood from the extremities to the torso and produce what is known as temperature after-drop.

Refer to Flowchart 20-2 for additional information regarding the care of hypothermia.

**What to Look For**

**What to Do**

Mild hypothermia, as indicated by:

- Vigorous, uncontrollable shivering. Shivering is desirable because it generates heat that will rewarm the person with mild hypothermia.
- The "umbles":
  - Grumbles—decreased mental skills
  - Mumbles—slurred speech
  - Fumbles—difficulty using fingers or hands
  - Stumbles—staggers while walking
  - Tumbles—collapses or falls down
- Cool or cold skin on abdomen, chest, or back

1. Follow the previously stated steps for treating a person with hypothermia.
2. Apply heat to the chest, armpits, and back (in that order). Use large electric pads, electric blankets, or warm water bottles. Place insulation between the skin and heat source to prevent burning the skin.
3. Warming the arms and legs up to the elbows and knees in 107°F to 113°F (42°C to 45°C) water is effective in people who are alert and have mild hypothermia. **DO NOT** use a warm shower or bath for rewarming even if a person appears to have only mild hypothermia; doing so may cause cardiovascular collapse.
4. Give warm, sugary drinks, which can provide energy (calories) and a psychologic boost. These drinks will not provide enough warmth to rewarm the person.
5. If the person is adequately rewarmed and has a normal mental status, you will usually not need to evacuate him or her to medical care.

## Q&A

**What is the coldest body temperature?**

The lowest recorded body temperature with a full recovery was 56.6°F (13.7°C). This was the temperature of Anna Bagenholm, age 29, who was trapped under ice for 80 minutes in May 2000, while skiing with friends near Narvik, Norway.

*Source:* Martin DS. 2009. From an icy slope, a medical miracle emerges. CNN. http://edition.cnn.com/2009/HEALTH/10/12/cheating.death.bagenholm/index.html

## CAUTION

**DO NOT** give the person alcohol to drink; it dilates blood vessels, allowing more heat loss.
**DO NOT** allow the person to use tobacco.

**What to Look For**

**What to Do**

Severe hypothermia, as indicated by:

- Rigid and stiff muscles
- No shivering
- Skin feels ice cold and appears blue
- Altered mental status
- Slow heart rate
- Slow breathing rate
- The person may appear to be dead

1. Follow the previously stated steps for treating a person with hypothermia.
2. Cut off the person's wet clothing.
3. Monitor the person's breathing, and give CPR if necessary. **DO NOT** start CPR if:
   - The person has been submerged in cold water for more than 1 hour.
   - The person has obvious fatal injuries.
   - The person is frozen (eg, ice in airway).
   - The person has a chest that is stiff or that cannot be compressed.
   - Rescuers are exhausted or in danger.
4. Call 9-1-1.
5. Check the person's heart rate for 1 minute before starting CPR.
6. Provide rewarming if possible by applying heat to the person's chest, armpits, and back (in that order). Use large electric pads or electric blankets, large chemical heat pads, or warm water bottles. (Small chemical heat packs [ie, those used for hand and foot warming] do not provide sufficient heat to affect body core temperature.) Place insulation between the skin and heat source to prevent burning the skin.

## CAUTION

**DO NOT** allow the person to exert himself or herself (no walking, no climbing).

**DO NOT** use small chemical heat packs for rewarming; they have a risk of burning and do not provide sufficient heat to affect body temperature.

**DO NOT** use warm showers or baths for rewarming. It may cause cardiovascular collapse.

**DO NOT** give the person alcohol. Alcohol interferes with shivering and accelerates heat loss by dilating the blood vessels in the skin. The person might feel warmer temporarily, but there is a greater risk of hypothermia.

**DO NOT** give the person a caffeinated drink. Caffeine has a diuretic effect, and the person probably is already dehydrated.

**DO NOT** rub or massage the person's arms or legs. Rubbing the skin suppresses shivering, dilates the blood vessels in the skin (resulting in more heat loss), and produces temperature after-drop.

**DO NOT** raise the person's legs, which allows cold blood from the legs to flow into the body core and adversely affect the heart. Keep the person in a flat position.

### Adding Heat

Adding heat to a person is extremely difficult. The longer the person has been exposed to the cold, the longer it will take to raise the core temperature to normal. Trying to rewarm a person with hypothermia could cause cardiac arrest.

Although surface rewarming suppresses shivering, it might be the only option when the person is far from medical care. In that case, the person must be warmed by any available external heat source.

According to the Wilderness Medical Society, there are issues with the commonly recommended rewarming methods:

Warm water immersion requires a lot of warm water (no hotter than 106°F [41.1°C]) and a bathtub—both rarely found in remote locations. Hot baths can produce rapid changes in the blood that can produce cardiac arrest.

Recent studies show that body-to-body contact in an insulated sleeping bag is no better than shivering for rewarming. Reasons include the following:

- All the heat produced by the rescuer's body is not enough to rewarm a person. For example, heat loss of adults cooled to 91°F (32.8°C) exceeds 300 kcal (kilocalories); heat production of a rescuer is only 100 kcal per hour.
- There usually is only a small amount (less than 50%) of direct skin contact, which is essential for effective heat transfer, between the person and the rescuer.
- The person's peripheral blood vessel constriction can impair heat transfer to the body's core.
- Skin warming can slow the person's shivering response.

Because skin rewarming suppresses shivering, which slows the rate of core rewarming, only use body-to-body rewarming when there will be a long delay in getting the person to medical care and when more appropriate methods of adding heat are unavailable. Several types of chemical heating pads are available. Although they might be effective for warming hands and feet, there is no evidence that they are capable of rewarming a person with hypothermia. For example, one type of heating pad is 70 × 90 inches (178 × 229 cm) and provides 14.5 kcal of total heat, with a maximum temperature of about 125°F (51.7°C). A minimum of 20 pads would be needed to provide enough heat to rewarm a person with a temperature of 91°F (32.8°C), even if heat transfer were 100% efficient. This method can stop the desirable effects of shivering, leaving the person with hypothermia.

## ▶ Dehydration

**Dehydration** occurs because of unperceived fluid loss combined with inadequate fluid intake. In very cold weather, the humidity approaches zero, and large quantities of fluid loss occurs through exhaled breath.

People in a cold environment must drink even when they are not thirsty. Inactive people in comfortable climates need two quarts (about 2 L) of water a day to prevent dehydration.

A person's hydration status can be monitored by noting the color and the volume of the urine. The lighter the color, the better hydrated; dark yellow urine is a definite indication that fluid consumption should be increased.

Unmelted snow and ice should not be consumed for water. Eating snow and ice irritates the mouth, wastes body heat, and, if enough is consumed, lowers body temperature. When snow and ice are the only available sources of water, they should be melted before being consumed. Melted snow or ice should not be considered drinkable until it has been appropriately disinfected (by boiling, filtering, or using chemicals).

## Flowchart 20-2 | Hypothermia

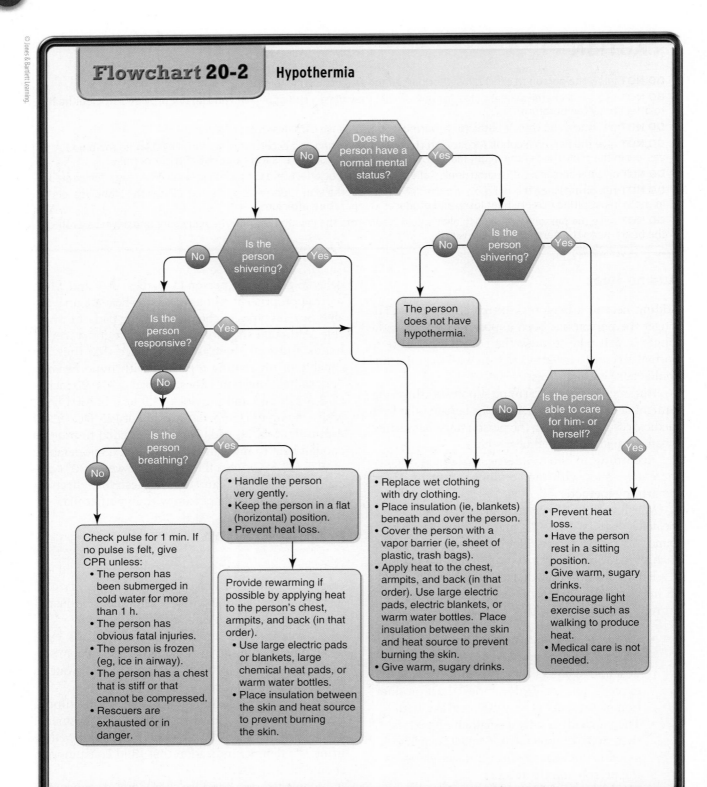

**Does the person have a normal mental status?**

**No** →

**Is the person shivering?** — **No / Yes**

**Is the person responsive?** — **Yes** →

**No**

**Is the person breathing?** — **No / Yes**

Check pulse for 1 min. If no pulse is felt, give CPR unless:
- The person has been submerged in cold water for more than 1 h.
- The person has obvious fatal injuries.
- The person is frozen (eg, ice in airway).
- The person has a chest that is stiff or that cannot be compressed.
- Rescuers are exhausted or in danger.

- Handle the person very gently.
- Keep the person in a flat (horizontal) position.
- Prevent heat loss.

Provide rewarming if possible by applying heat to the person's chest, armpits, and back (in that order).
- Use large electric pads or blankets, large chemical heat pads, or warm water bottles.
- Place insulation between the skin and heat source to prevent burning the skin.

**Yes** →

**Is the person shivering?** — **No / Yes**

The person does not have hypothermia.

**Is the person able to care for him- or herself?** — **No / Yes**

- Replace wet clothing with dry clothing.
- Place insulation (ie, blankets) beneath and over the person.
- Cover the person with a vapor barrier (ie, sheet of plastic, trash bags).
- Apply heat to the chest, armpits, and back (in that order). Use large electric pads, electric blankets, or warm water bottles. Place insulation between the skin and heat source to prevent burning the skin.
- Give warm, sugary drinks.

- Prevent heat loss.
- Have the person rest in a sitting position.
- Give warm, sugary drinks.
- Encourage light exercise such as walking to produce heat.
- Medical care is not needed.

## ▶ Ready for Review

- When a person is surrounded by air or water cooler than body temperature, body heat loss occurs.
- Humans protect themselves from cold primarily by avoiding or reducing cold exposure through the use of clothing and shelter.
- Nonfreezing cold injuries can occur when conditions are cold and wet and the hands and feet cannot be kept warm and dry.
- Freezing cold injuries can occur whenever the air temperature is below freezing.
- Hypothermia is a life-threatening condition in which the body's core temperature falls below 95°F (35°C).
- Dehydration occurs because of unperceived fluid loss combined with inadequate fluid intake.

## ▶ Vital Vocabulary

<u>chilblain</u>  A nonfreezing cold injury that, while painful, causes little or no permanent damage.

<u>dehydration</u>  Loss of water from the tissues of the body.

<u>frostbite</u>  The damage to tissues as a result of prolonged exposure to extreme cold.

<u>frostnip</u>  The superficial local tissue destruction caused by freezing; it is limited in scope and does not destroy the full thickness of skin.

<u>gangrene</u>  Permanent damage or death of tissue.

<u>glycogen</u>  Main form in which carbohydrate is stored in the liver and then broken down into glucose (sugar) for energy.

<u>hypothermia</u>  Decreased body temperature; severe hypothermia is life threatening.

<u>trench foot</u>  A serious nonfreezing cold injury that develops when the skin on the feet is exposed to moisture and cold for prolonged periods (12 hours or longer); also called immersion foot.

<u>vasoconstriction</u>  The narrowing of the diameter of a blood vessel.

<u>windchill</u>  The relationship of wind velocity and temperature in determining the effect of cold on living organisms.

## ▶ Assessment in Action

You are on a winter hike with five friends high in the mountains. The snowshoeing has been great, but it is very cold. At the trailhead, the temperature was 15°F (minus 9°C), and it has not warmed up much during your hike. One of your friends wore only tennis shoes but has not been complaining. When you return to the trailhead and begin to warm up in your car, your friend begins to complain of tingling and aching in his toes.

*Directions:* Circle Yes if you agree with the statement; circle No if you disagree.

| Yes | No | **1.** It is difficult to determine if your friend has frostnip or frostbite. |
| --- | --- | --- |
| Yes | No | **2.** Frostbite requires freezing temperatures (below 32°F [0°C]). |
| Yes | No | **3.** The skin and underlying tissue affected by superficial frostbite feel hard and solid. |
| Yes | No | **4.** As long as there is no danger of refreezing, you could begin warming his toes in warm water. |
| Yes | No | **5.** If you do not have warm water, you could rub his toes to increase circulation. |

## ▶ Check Your Knowledge

*Directions:* Circle Yes if you agree with the statement; circle No if you disagree.

| Yes | No | **1.** Shivering is a signal that clothing and shelter are inadequate to protect the body from the cold. |
| --- | --- | --- |
| Yes | No | **2.** Up to 100% of the body's total heat production can be lost by radiation through a person's unprotected head. |
| Yes | No | **3.** Physically unfit people are more susceptible to cold injury. |
| Yes | No | **4.** Frostnip is caused when water on the skin surface freezes. |
| Yes | No | **5.** Shivering produces body heat. |
| Yes | No | **6.** Rub a frostbitten part to rewarm it. |
| Yes | No | **7.** Rewarm a person with hypothermia quickly in a hot shower or with small chemical heat packs. |
| Yes | No | **8.** Replace any wet clothing with dry clothing for a person with hypothermia. |
| Yes | No | **9.** Seek medical care for a person with severe hypothermia. |
| Yes | No | **10.** Below-freezing temperatures are required for hypothermia to occur. |

# Heat-Related Emergencies

## Heat-Related Emergencies

When the temperature goes up, a multitude of issues can—and do—arise. Given the right (or wrong) conditions, anyone can develop a heat illness. Some people will develop __heat cramps__, while others may be sickened by __heat exhaustion__ or even die from __heat stroke__.

## ▶ How the Body Stays Cool

The human body is constantly engaged in a life-and-death struggle to disperse the heat that it produces. If allowed to accumulate, the heat would quickly increase your body temperature beyond its comfortable 98.6°F (37°C). That does not normally happen, because your body has enough heat loss to maintain a steady temperature. Usually, you are aware of this struggle only during hard labor or exercise in a hot environment, when your body produces heat faster than it can lose it. In certain circumstances, your body can build up too much heat, your temperature might rise to life-threatening levels, and you can become delirious or have a loss of consciousness. This condition is called heat stroke and is a serious medical emergency. If you do not rid your body of excess heat fast enough, damage to the brain and other vital organs will result. Heat stroke is often fatal. Before your temperature reaches heat-stroke level, however, you might experience heat exhaustion with its flulike symptoms. By treating the symptoms of heat exhaustion, you avoid heat stroke.

How does the body dispose of excess heat? Humans experience heat loss largely through their skin, much like heat loss occurs in a car through its radiator. Exercising muscles warms the blood, just as the car's hot engine warms its radiator fluid. Warm blood travels through the skin's dilated blood vessels, losing heat by evaporating sweat to the surrounding air, just as the car loses engine heat through the radiator.

When blood delivers heat to the skin, the body loses heat primarily in two ways: **radiation** and **evaporation**. When the air temperature is 70°F (21.1°C) or less, the body releases heat into its surroundings by radiation. As the environmental temperature approaches the body's temperature, however, heat loss through radiation is greatly reduced. In fact, people working or exercising on a hot summer day actually gain heat through radiation from the sun, leaving evaporation as the only way to control body temperature effectively.

---

### FYI

**World Record: Highest Body Temperature**

The person with the highest recorded body temperature who lived to tell about it is Willie Jones. On July 10, 1980, a day when the temperature reached 90°F (32.2°C) with 44% humidity, Mr. Jones was admitted to Grady Memorial Hospital, Atlanta, Georgia, with heat stroke. His temperature was 115.7°F (46.5°C). The record temperature was taken after he had been immersed for 25 minutes in cold water. The attending physician said that his body temperature may have exceeded 120°F (48.9°C) when he first arrived at the hospital. After 24 days in the hospital, he was discharged. A body temperature of 109°F (42.8°C) can be fatal.

*Source: Guinness World Records 2008, p. 112. New York, 2008, Bantam Books.*

---

## Water Loss

Water makes up about 50% to 60% of an adult's body weight. You lose about 2 quarts (about 2 L) every day through breathing, urinating, bowel movements, and sweat. The fluid loss must be replaced. Although the amount of water used each day varies from person to person, an adult requires about 2 quarts (about 2 L) a day from water, other beverages, and food (about 70% of most food is water). A working adult can produce 2 to 3 quarts (about 2 to 3 L) of sweat an hour for short periods and up to 10 to 15 quarts (about 10 to 15 L) a day. When the body's water absorption rate of 1.5 quarts (about 1.5 L) per hour is pitted against a sweat loss of 2 quarts (about 2 L) per hour, dehydration results—drinking water cannot keep up with sweat losses.

When you are thirsty, you are already dehydrated. Thirst is not a good guide for when to drink water. In fact, in hot and humid conditions, people could be so dehydrated by the time they become thirsty that they have trouble catching up with their fluid losses. One guideline regarding water intake is to monitor urine output. You are getting enough water if you are producing clear urine at least five times a day. Cloudy or dark urine or urinating fewer than five times a day probably means you should drink more.

If possible while working, especially in hot weather, drink 1 cup (8 ounces) of water every 20 minutes. Usually, 1 pint (16 ounces) is the most a person can comfortably drink at once. It takes time for water to pass from the stomach into the blood, so you cannot catch up by drinking extra water later; about 1 quart (about 1 L) of water per hour can pass out of the stomach.

Cool water (50°F [10°C]) is easier for the stomach to absorb than warm water, and a little flavoring can make the water more tasty. The best fluids are those that leave the stomach fast and contain little sodium and less than 8% sugar. Coffee and tea should be avoided because they contain caffeine, a diuretic that increases water loss through urination. Alcoholic beverages also dehydrate by increasing urination. Soda pop contains about 10% sugar and, therefore, is not absorbed as well as water or commercial sports drinks (which contain about 5% to 8% sugar). Fruit juices range from 11% to 18% sugar and have an even longer absorption time.

## Electrolyte Loss

Sweat and urine contain potassium and sodium, essential electrolytes that control the movement of water into and out of the cells. These electrolytes can be found in many everyday foods. Bananas and nuts are rich in potassium, and most American diets have up to 10 times as much sodium as their bodies need. Acclimatizing to heat (heat exposure 1 to 2 hours a day for 10 to 14 days) can reduce sodium loss tenfold. Getting enough salt (sodium chloride) is rarely an issue in the typical American diet. In fact, most Americans consume an excessive amount of sodium, averaging 5 to 10 grams of sodium per day, although humans probably require only 1 to 3 grams. Sodium loss, therefore, is seldom an issue, unless a person is sweating profusely for long periods and drinking large amounts of water (more than 1 quart [about 1 L] an hour).

Most people require only water most of the time. Commercial sports drinks can be useful for participants in vigorous physical activity lasting for longer than 1 hour. The human body needs water more than it needs salt. Whenever extra sodium is added to a diet, more water should be consumed. Otherwise, excessive sodium can draw water out of the cells, accelerating dehydration.

Drinking large amounts of water (more than 1 quart [about 1 L] an hour) and profuse sweating for long periods can lead to a condition called water intoxication, in which electrolytes are flushed from the body. Symptoms of water intoxication include frequent urination and behavior changes (irrationality, combativeness, seizures, and coma). These symptoms are the result of inadequate sodium in the body, a condition known as **hyponatremia**.

**Water Intoxication in Recreational Hikers**

Water intoxication, often seen in endurance athletes, has been reported in recreational hikers. Water intoxication results when people replace sweat loss with plain water instead of an enhanced product that more nearly resembles sweat. Differentiating water intoxication from heat exhaustion is difficult. Recreational wilderness hikers performing sustained exercise in the heat might require electrolyte replacement similar to endurance athletes.

*Source:* Backer H, et al. 1993. Hyponatremia in recreational hikers in Grand Canyon National Park. *J Wilderness Med* 4(4):391-406.

## Effects of Humidity

Sweat can cool the body only if it evaporates. In dry air, you will not notice sweat evaporating. The higher the humidity, the less sweat can evaporate. It drips off the skin without cooling the body. At about 75% humidity, sweating is ineffective in cooling the body.

Because humidity can significantly reduce evaporative cooling, a very humid but mildly warm day can be more stressful than a very hot, dry day. The higher the humidity, the lower the temperature at which heat risk begins, especially for people generating heat with vigorous work.

**FYI**

**Heat-Related Deaths in Cars**

**Case 1**

Hawaii, March 2007: A 3-year-old girl from Honolulu died from hyperthermia. The child's father told police that he left her in a child seat in the back seat of the car for an hour and a half late that morning while he visited friends in a Makiki apartment building. The outside temperature was only 81°F (27.2°C).

**Case 2**

South Carolina, April 2006: A mother left her 15-month-old son locked in a car. He was left in the car for 9 hours while his mother went to work. She is currently serving a 20-year prison sentence.

**Case 3**

Colorado, August 2008: Two children who died in an overheated car may have been on their own for more than 3 hours as their mother slept after working a night shift. The children died in a closed but unlocked car; investigators believe the temperature where the children were found may have reached 123°F (50.6°C).

**Case 4**

Mississippi, July 2001: A man died of heat stroke after falling asleep in his car with the windows up in a supermarket parking lot.

**Case 5**

North Carolina, April 2014: A mother intentionally left her infant alone in the car while she worked as a cook at a restaurant. The outside temperature was 80°F (26.6°C). The mother was charged with involuntary manslaughter.

*Source:* Null J. Heatstroke deaths of children in vehicles. Department of Meteorology & Climate Science San Jose State University. Updated February 21, 2016. http://noheatstroke.org/hyperthermia2014.htm.

## Who Is at Risk?

Everyone is susceptible to heat illness if environmental conditions overwhelm the body's temperature-regulating mechanisms. Heat waves can set the stage for multiple cases of heat stroke. For example, in the 1995 Chicago heat wave, the death toll reached 591 in 5 days. Several groups are at particular risk, including people with obesity, people with a chronic illness, and people with alcoholism.

Older people are at higher risk because of impaired cardiac output and decreased ability to sweat. Infants and young children are also susceptible to heat stroke. Children (and pets) are especially vulnerable when they are left in automobiles. The temperature in a parked car can soar to 150°F (65.6°C), even when a window is open. The fluid loss and dehydration resulting from physical activity put outdoor laborers and athletes at particular risk.

## FYI

**Heat-Related Deaths of Young Children in Parked Cars**

Each year, many young children in the United States die of heat stroke caused by being enclosed in parked motor vehicles. Researchers located and analyzed 171 heat-related deaths in children under age 5 years:

- 39% involved a child forgotten by a caregiver.
- 27% involved a child playing in an unattended vehicle.
- 20% involved a child intentionally left in a vehicle by an adult.
- 14% involved unclear circumstances.

*Source:* Guard A, Gallagher SS. Heat-related deaths to young children in parked cars: An analysis of 171 fatalities in the United States. *Inj Prev* 2005;11(1):33-37.

Certain medications predispose to heat stroke. They include drugs that alter sweat production (for example, antihistamines, antipsychotics, and antidepressants) and those that interfere with **thermoregulation**.

## ▶ Heat Illnesses

Heat illnesses include a range of disorders. Some of them are common, but only heat stroke is life threatening. People with untreated heat stroke always die.

### Heat Cramps

Heat cramps are painful muscle spasms that occur suddenly during or after vigorous exercise or activity. They usually involve the muscles in the back of the leg

## FYI

**Hot Weather Precautions**

These simple preventive measures can reduce heat stress:

1. Keep cool indoors.
   - Stay in air conditioned areas, if available.
   - Take cool baths or showers.
   - Use your stove and oven less.
2. Wear lightweight, loose-fitting clothing.
3. If you must go outdoors, put on sunscreen of SPF 15 or higher 30 minutes prior to going out.
4. Limit your outdoor activity to the morning and evening, and make sure to rest often in shady areas.
5. Increase intake of fluids, regardless of your activity level.
   - Thirst is not always a good indicator of adequate fluid intake.
   - People who engage in strenuous activities, such as sports, should drink 2 to 4 glasses of cool fluids each hour in hot weather.
   - People for whom fluid is restricted or who are taking water pills should consult their physicians for instructions on appropriate fluid intake.
   - **DO NOT** drink liquids that contain alcohol or large amounts of sugar.
   - Monitor your urine color. Urine color that is pale yellow or light yellow indicates a person is hydrated; dark yellow urine may be a sign of dehydration
6. Stay in contact with other people and monitor those who are at greater risk of suffering from heat-related illnesses, such as infants, young children, older adults, and people who are overweight, ill, or taking certain medications.
7. Listen or watch local news and weather stations for weather updates and recommended procedures and precautions.
8. **DO NOT** leave infants, children, or pets unattended in a parked car.

*Source:* Extreme heat prevention guide. Centers for Disease Control and Prevention. http://emergency.cdc.gov/disasters/extreme-heat/heat_guide.asp. Published May 31, 2012. Updated September 22, 2015.

## Q&A

**What is the difference between fever and hyperthermia?**

Fever and hyperthermia have different causes. Body temperature is regulated by a natural thermostat in the part of the brain called the hypothalamus. If the "set point" is increased by illness or certain drugs, a fever results. In other words, in a fever, the body is trying to raise the temperature above normal to fight a disease (eg, a virus).

Hyperthermia is related to environmental heat exposure. It occurs when the body absorbs more heat than it can handle. It is caused by an inability to cool the body. Hyperthermia can rapidly progress to heat stroke if not corrected.

| What to Look For | What to Do |
|---|---|
| Painful muscle spasms affecting the muscle in the back of the leg or abdomen that happen suddenly during or after physical exertion | Relief may take several hours.<br>1. Have the person rest in a cool area.<br>2. Give lightly salted cool water (dissolve 1/4 teaspoon [1.25 mL] of salt in 1 quart [about 1 L] of water) or a commercial sports drink. **DO NOT** give salt tablets.<br>3. Stretch any cramped muscle.<br>4. For a lower leg calf muscle cramp, try the acupressure method of pinching the upper lip, just below the nose. |

(calf and hamstring muscles) or the abdominal muscles. Some experts state they are caused by water and electrolyte losses during times of excessive sweating. People who experience heat cramps might be drinking fluids without adequate salt content. However, other experts disagree, because the typical American diet is heavy with salt.

## Heat Exhaustion

Heat exhaustion is characterized by heavy perspiration with a normal or slightly above-normal body temperature. Heavy sweating causes water and electrolyte losses. Some experts believe that a better term would be *severe dehydration*. Heat exhaustion affects workers and athletes who do not drink enough fluids while working or exercising in hot environments. Symptoms include severe thirst, heavy sweating, fatigue, headache, nausea, vomiting, and sometimes diarrhea. The affected person often mistakenly believes he or she has the flu.

Uncontrolled heat exhaustion can evolve into heat stroke. The difference between heat exhaustion and heat stroke is that the person with heat exhaustion has (1) no altered mental status and (2) skin that is clammy, but not hot.

| What to Look For | What to Do |
|---|---|
| • Sweating<br>• Thirst<br>• Fatigue<br>• Flulike symptoms (headache, body aches, and nausea)<br>• Shortness of breath<br>• Rapid heart rate | 1. Move the person out of the heat to a cool place.<br>2. Remove excess clothing.<br>3. Spray or douse cold water on the person's skin and vigorously fan.<br>4. If the person is able to swallow, give a commercial sports drink, fruit juice, or lightly salted water; if none of these options are available, give cold water. **DO NOT** give salt tablets.<br>5. Call 9-1-1 if improvement does not occur within 30 minutes. Heat exhaustion can turn into heat stroke. |

## Heat Stroke

Two types of heat stroke exist: classic and exertional Table 21-1 . Classic heat stroke, also known as the slow cooker, can take days to develop. It is often seen during summer heat waves and typically affects people who are poor, older, chronically ill, and those with alcoholism and obesity. Because older people, who often have medical conditions, are frequently afflicted, this type of heat stroke has a 50% death rate, even with medical care. It results from a combination of a hot environment and dehydration. Under normal conditions, temperature and humidity are the most important elements influencing body comfort. The heat index compiled by the National Weather Service lists apparent temperatures (how hot it feels) at various combinations of temperature and humidity Table 21-2 .

Exertional heat stroke is also more common in the summer. It is frequently seen in athletes, laborers, and military personnel, all of whom often sweat profusely. This type of heat stroke is known as the fast cooker. It affects healthy, active people who are strenuously working or playing in a warm environment. Because its rapid onset does not allow enough time for severe dehydration to occur, 50% of people with exertional heat stroke usually are sweating. (People with classic heat stroke are not sweating.)

## Table 21-1 Classic or Exertional Heat Stroke?

| Characteristics | Classic | Exertional |
|---|---|---|
| Age group usually affected | Older people | Men, 15-45 years |
| Claims many people at the same time | During heat waves | During athletic competition |
| Health status of people | Chronically ill | Healthy and physically fit |
| Activity at the time of incident | Sedentary | Strenuous exercise |
| Medication use | Common | Usually none |
| Sweating | Absent | Often present (50% of people) |

## Table 21-2 Heat Index

**Temperature (°F)**

| Relative Humidity (%) | 80 | 82 | 84 | 86 | 88 | 90 | 92 | 94 | 96 | 98 | 100 | 102 | 104 | 106 | 108 | 110 |
|---|---|---|---|---|---|---|---|---|---|---|---|---|---|---|---|---|
| 40 | 80 | 81 | 83 | 85 | 88 | 91 | 94 | 97 | 101 | 105 | 109 | 114 | 119 | 124 | 130 | 136 |
| 45 | 80 | 82 | 84 | 87 | 89 | 93 | 96 | 100 | 104 | 109 | 114 | 119 | 124 | 130 | 137 | |
| 50 | 81 | 83 | 85 | 88 | 91 | 95 | 99 | 103 | 108 | 113 | 118 | 124 | 131 | 137 | | |
| 55 | 81 | 84 | 86 | 89 | 93 | 97 | 101 | 106 | 112 | 117 | 124 | 130 | 137 | | | |
| 60 | 82 | 84 | 88 | 91 | 95 | 100 | 105 | 110 | 116 | 123 | 129 | 137 | | | | |
| 65 | 82 | 85 | 89 | 93 | 98 | 103 | 108 | 114 | 121 | 128 | 136 | | | | | |
| 70 | 83 | 86 | 90 | 95 | 100 | 105 | 112 | 119 | 126 | 134 | | | | | | |
| 75 | 84 | 88 | 92 | 97 | 103 | 109 | 116 | 124 | 132 | | | | | | | |
| 80 | 84 | 89 | 94 | 100 | 106 | 113 | 121 | 129 | | | | | | | | |
| 85 | 85 | 90 | 96 | 102 | 110 | 117 | 126 | 135 | | | | | | | | |
| 90 | 86 | 91 | 98 | 105 | 113 | 122 | 131 | | | | | | | | | |
| 95 | 86 | 93 | 100 | 108 | 117 | 127 | | | | | | | | | | |
| 100 | 87 | 95 | 103 | 112 | 121 | 132 | | | | | | | | | | |

**Likelihood of Heat Disorders with Prolonged Exposure or Strenuous Activity**

■ Caution  ■ Extreme Caution  ■ Danger  ■ Extreme Danger

There are several ways to tell the difference between heat exhaustion and heat stroke.

- If the person's body feels extremely hot when touched, suspect heat stroke.

- Altered mental status (behavior) occurs with heat stroke, ranging from slight confusion and disorientation to coma. Between those extreme conditions, people usually become

**Heat Illness Among High School Athletes**

Heat illness during practice or competition is a leading cause of death and disability among high school athletes in the United States. The 100 schools sampled by the CDC reported a total of 118 heat illnesses among high school athletes resulting in at least 1 day of time lost from athletic activity (ie, time-loss heat illness). The highest rate of time-loss heat illness was among football players at a rate 10 times higher than the average rate for the eight other sports surveyed. Time-loss heat illnesses occurred most frequently during August and while practicing or playing football.

Consistent with guidelines from the National Athletic Trainers' Association (NATA), to reduce the risk for heat illness, high school athletic programs should implement heat-acclimatization guidelines (eg, set limits on summer practice duration and intensity). All athletes, coaches, athletic trainers, and parents/guardians should be aware of the risk factors for heat illness, follow recommended strategies, and be prepared to respond quickly to symptoms of illness. Coaches should also continue to stress to their athletes the importance of maintaining proper hydration before, during, and after sports activities.

*Source:* Centers for Disease Control and Prevention. Heat illness among high school athletes—United States, 2005-2009. *MMWR Morb Mortal Wkly Rep* 2011;59(32):1009-1013.

irrational, agitated, or even aggressive, and they might have seizures.

- In severe heat stroke, a coma can occur in less than an hour. The longer a coma lasts, the lower the chance for survival.
- Rectal temperature can also distinguish heat stroke from heat exhaustion, although obtaining a rectal temperature is usually not practical. A responsive person with heat stroke might not cooperate, taking a rectal temperature can be embarrassing to the person and the first aid provider, and rectal thermometers are seldom available.

## What to Look For

- Extremely hot skin when touched; skin is usually dry, but may be wet from sweating related to strenuous work or exercise
- Altered mental status ranging from slight confusion, agitation, and disorientation to unresponsiveness

## What to Do

1. Move the person from the hot environment to a cool, shaded area.
2. Remove clothing, down to the person's underwear.
3. Cool the person quickly by any means possible. In some remote locations, this might be difficult. **DO NOT** delay cooling the person if any of the following methods (given in the order of effectiveness) are possible:
   - Whole-body cold water immersion: Place the person in cold water, up to the neck. **DO NOT** leave the person alone.
   - Evaporative cooling: Spray or douse cold water on the skin and vigorously fan Figure 21-1.
   - Place ice packs against the person's armpits, groin, and sides of the neck.
4. Stop cooling when the person's mental status improves.
5. Monitor the person frequently, as temperatures can rise again after cooling.
6. Call 9-1-1 as soon as possible.

Keep the sheet wet by continually sprinkling it with water.

Vigorously fan the victim to keep the person cool.

© Jones & Bartlett Learning

**Figure 21-1**

Spraying with water and fanning are effective in low humidity conditions.

## CAUTION

**DO NOT** delay initiating cooling while waiting for an ambulance. The longer the delay, the greater the risk of tissue damage and prolonged hospitalization.

**DO NOT** continue cooling after the person's mental status has improved. Unnecessary cooling could lead to hypothermia.

**DO NOT** use rubbing alcohol to cool the skin. It can be absorbed into the blood and cause alcohol poisoning. Also, the vapors are a potential fire hazard.

**DO NOT** give the person aspirin or acetaminophen. The brain's temperature control center is not elevated, as it is with fever caused by diseases, so these products are not effective for lowering body temperature.

### Other Heat Illnesses

Less serious heat illnesses include heat syncope, heat edema, heat rash, and hyponatremia.

Refer to **Flowchart 21-1** for additional information regarding care for heat-related emergencies.

| Heat Illness | What to Look For | What to Do |
|---|---|---|
| Heat syncope | • Dizziness or fainting that occurs immediately after strenuous physical activity in a hot environment | 1. If the person is unresponsive, check his or her breathing. A person with heat syncope will usually recover quickly.<br>2. If the person fell, check for injuries.<br>3. Have the person rest and lie down in a cool area.<br>4. Wet the skin with a cool, damp cloth or a spray bottle.<br>5. If the person is not nauseated and is fully alert and able to swallow, give lightly salted cool water (dissolve 1/4 teaspoon [1.25 mL] of salt in 1 quart [about 1 L] of water) or a commercial sports drink. **DO NOT** give salt tablets. |
| Heat edema | • Swollen ankles and feet that occur during the first few days in a hot environment | 1. Have the person wear support stockings.<br>2. Elevate the person's legs. |
| Heat rash (prickly heat) | • Itchy rash on skin that is wet from sweating; this condition is seen in humid regions after prolonged sweating. | 1. Dry and cool the person's skin.<br>2. Limit heat exposure. |
| Hyponatremia (water intoxication) | • The person drank too much water (>1 quart [about 1 L] per hour)<br>• Frequent urination; urine is clear<br>• Profuse sweating for long periods<br>• Dizziness, weakness, nausea, vomiting, headache<br>• Altered mental status<br>• Severe sodium loss may result in seizures or unresponsiveness and can be fatal. | 1. Move the person to a cool location.<br>2. **DO NOT** give more fluids.<br>3. Give salty foods. **DO NOT** give salt tablets because they can irritate the stomach and cause nausea and vomiting.<br>4. For a person with altered mental status, call 9-1-1 as soon as possible. |

## Flowchart 21-1 Heat-Related Emergencies

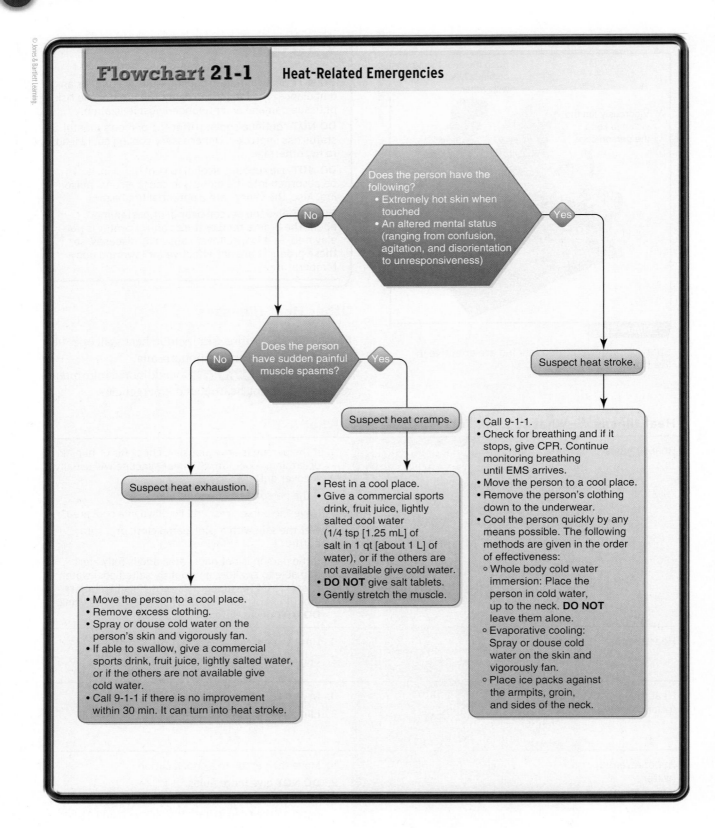

**Does the person have the following?**
- Extremely hot skin when touched
- An altered mental status (ranging from confusion, agitation, and disorientation to unresponsiveness)

No → **Does the person have sudden painful muscle spasms?**

Yes → **Suspect heat stroke.**

**Does the person have sudden painful muscle spasms?**

No → **Suspect heat exhaustion.**

Yes → **Suspect heat cramps.**

**Suspect heat exhaustion.**
- Move the person to a cool place.
- Remove excess clothing.
- Spray or douse cold water on the person's skin and vigorously fan.
- If able to swallow, give a commercial sports drink, fruit juice, lightly salted water, or if the others are not available give cold water.
- Call 9-1-1 if there is no improvement within 30 min. It can turn into heat stroke.

**Suspect heat cramps.**
- Rest in a cool place.
- Give a commercial sports drink, fruit juice, lightly salted cool water (1/4 tsp [1.25 mL] of salt in 1 qt [about 1 L] of water), or if the others are not available give cold water.
- **DO NOT** give salt tablets.
- Gently stretch the muscle.

**Suspect heat stroke.**
- Call 9-1-1.
- Check for breathing and if it stops, give CPR. Continue monitoring breathing until EMS arrives.
- Move the person to a cool place.
- Remove the person's clothing down to the underwear.
- Cool the person quickly by any means possible. The following methods are given in the order of effectiveness:
  - Whole body cold water immersion: Place the person in cold water, up to the neck. **DO NOT** leave them alone.
  - Evaporative cooling: Spray or douse cold water on the skin and vigorously fan.
  - Place ice packs against the armpits, groin, and sides of the neck.

## ▶ Ready for Review

- Given the right conditions, anyone can develop a heat illness.
- The human body is constantly dispersing the heat that it produces.
- Heat illnesses include a range of disorders from heat cramps to heat stroke. Heat stroke is life threatening.

## ▶ Vital Vocabulary

**evaporation** Conversion of water or another fluid from a liquid to a gas.

**heat cramps** A painful muscle cramp resulting from excessive loss of salt and water through sweating.

**heat exhaustion** A prostration caused by excessive loss of water and salt through sweating; characterized by clammy skin and a weak, rapid pulse.

**heat stroke** A life-threatening condition of severe hyperthermia caused by exposure to excessive natural or artificial heat.

**hyponatremia** A condition that occurs when the level of sodium in the body is inadequate.

**radiation** The transfer of heat to colder objects in the environment by radiant energy.

**thermoregulation** The body's ability to maintain a normal body temperature despite environmental conditions of heat or cold.

## ▶ Assessment in Action

You decide to watch your local high school football team practice before its first game in late August. The coach has the defense running sprints for the last 30 minutes without rest breaks. At the end of the sprints, all but one player walk over to the water station. That player falls to the ground and you are the first to respond. The person is responsive and his skin is moist and clammy.

*Directions:* Circle Yes if you agree with the statement; circle No if you disagree.

Yes    No    **1.** The person is most likely suffering from heat stroke.

Yes    No    **2.** The first thing you should do is to help the coach and athletic trainer move the person out of the heat and to a cool place.

Yes    No    **3.** The person should drink cool water or a sports drink.

Yes    No    **4.** Giving several salt tablets, if available, should always be considered.

Yes    No    **5.** Removing the player's jersey, shoulder pads, and helmet and sponging him with cool water is recommended.

Yes    No    **6.** The coach and/or athletic trainer should seek medical care if there is no improvement within 30 minutes.

## ▶ Check Your Knowledge

*Directions:* Circle Yes if you agree with the statement; circle No if you disagree.

Yes    No    **1.** For heat cramps in the legs, stretch the cramped muscle.

Yes    No    **2.** Commercial sports drinks can be given to people experiencing heat-related emergencies.

Yes    No    **3.** Move a person with a heat-related illness to a cool place.

Yes    No    **4.** People with heat stroke need immediate medical care—it is a life-threatening condition.

Yes    No    **5.** Rapidly cool a person with heat stroke, including the use of ice packs applied to the neck, armpits, and groin.

Yes    No    **6.** Fruit juices are digested quickly and rehydrate the body most rapidly.

Yes    No    **7.** You can drink too much water and cause water intoxication.

Yes    No    **8.** Humidity cannot significantly reduce evaporative cooling.

Yes    No    **9.** Certain medications may predispose people to heat stroke.

Yes    No    **10.** Heat exhaustion can feel like the flu.

# Childbirth and Gynecologic Emergencies

## 22

## Childbirth and Gynecologic Emergencies

Handling childbirth and gynecologic situations of pregnancy requires that a first aid provider be familiar with the terminology used to describe female reproductive anatomy and physiology.

- The <u>birth canal</u> includes the vagina and the lower part of the uterus.
- The <u>cervix</u> is the small opening at the lower end of the uterus through which the baby passes.
- The <u>placenta</u> (afterbirth) is the organ through which the mother and the fetus exchange nourishment and waste products during pregnancy. It is expelled after the baby's birth.
- The <u>umbilical cord</u> is the extension of the placenta through which the <u>fetus</u> receives nourishment while in the uterus.
- The <u>amniotic sac</u> (bag of waters) surrounds the fetus inside the uterus. Amniotic fluid in the sac cushions the fetus and helps protect it from injury.
- <u>Crowning</u> occurs when the fetus's head presses against the vaginal opening and begins to bulge out.

- <u>Bloody show</u> is the mucus and blood that might be discharged from the vagina as labor begins.
- <u>Labor</u> is the process of childbirth (defined in three stages), from the first regular uterine muscle contractions until delivery of the placenta.
- A <u>miscarriage</u> (medical term is *spontaneous abortion*) is the delivery of a fetus before it can live independent of the mother.

# Predelivery Emergencies

## ▶ Miscarriage

Miscarriages usually occur during the first 3 months (first trimester) of pregnancy. Most occur because the fetus was not developing properly and was unable to survive. The woman will be emotionally upset. She might be hesitant about confiding in a stranger, especially a man; obtaining help from a woman, if possible, might be wise.

### What to Look For

| What to Look For | What to Do |
| --- | --- |
| <ul><li>Cramping pain in lower abdomen resembling menstrual cramps</li><li>Aching in the lower back</li><li>Vaginal bleeding, which could be sudden and heavy</li><li>Passage of tissue from the vagina</li></ul> | 1. Reassure the woman.<br>2. Help her into a comfortable position with legs bent.<br>3. Have the woman place a sanitary pad over the outside of the vagina. **DO NOT** place pads in the vagina. Replace blood-soaked pads or dressings.<br>4. Any tissue that passes through the vagina should be transported with the woman to the hospital. **DO NOT** try to pull tissue out of the vagina; instead, cover it with a sterile pad.<br>5. Seek medical care.<br>6. Call 9-1-1 if bleeding is heavy or signs of shock are present. |

# Vaginal Bleeding

## ▶ Vaginal Bleeding During Pregnancy

A woman experiencing vaginal bleeding late in her pregnancy (third trimester, or last 3 months) usually constitutes an emergency. Find out how long she has been bleeding and how many sanitary pads she has used so that you can report the information to medical personnel. An increase in pulse rate of more than 20 beats per minute when the woman goes from a lying-down to a sitting position suggests blood loss of more than 1 pint (473 mL). The woman might feel embarrassed. She might be hesitant about confiding in a stranger, especially a man; therefore, obtaining help from a woman might be wise.

### What to Look For

| What to Look For | What to Do |
| --- | --- |
| <ul><li>Bleeding may be mild spotting but can indicate a severe condition.</li><li>Bleeding may be heavy.</li><li>Signs of shock may be present.</li></ul> | To care for someone with vaginal bleeding during late pregnancy, do the following:<br>1. Place the woman on her left side to relieve pressure from the fetus on the inferior vena cava (large vein between the spine and the abdominal organs).<br>2. Have the woman place a sanitary pad over the outside of the vagina.<br>3. Call 9-1-1 immediately.<br>4. Treat for shock (eg, maintain body temperature, avoid giving fluids). |

## ▶ Vaginal Bleeding Caused by Injury

It is difficult to determine the source of the bleeding. Vaginal bleeding can be difficult to care for because of the woman's modesty and pain.

### What to Look For

- Injuries of the external female genitalia, including all types of soft-tissue injuries (such as wounds or contusions)
- Severe pain
- Blood in the vaginal area
- Massive vaginal bleeding

### What to Do

1. Use direct pressure over a bulky dressing or sanitary pad to control external bleeding from a laceration or other injury.
2. Apply an ice pack to reduce swelling and pain.
3. Never place or pack dressings into the vagina. It is useless and dangerous to introduce packs blindly into the vagina in an attempt to control bleeding.
4. Place the woman on her left side to help prevent vomiting, to prevent aspiration of vomitus, and, if the woman is pregnant, to relieve pressure on the **vena cava** from the fetus.
5. In the case of a sexual assault, sympathetically explain that evidence needs to be preserved and that the person should not change clothes, wash, urinate, defecate, or douche.
6. Seek medical care.

### Q&A

**Are pregnant women more susceptible to injury?**

More injuries are seen in pregnant women because many of them are active and often work and travel throughout all stages of pregnancy. In addition, there is a significant incidence of violence toward pregnant women.

Factors predisposing a woman to injury in early pregnancy are fainting episodes, hyperventilation, and becoming easily fatigued. In the last trimester, an enlarged abdomen changes the woman's center of gravity, making her more susceptible to falls, and pelvic pressure causing leg pain.

Motor vehicle crashes in which the seat belt is not used or is used in an improper position are also a common cause of injury.

## ▶ Non–Injury-Related Vaginal Bleeding

Bleeding from the vagina in women of childbearing age who are not pregnant is most likely to be menstrual bleeding. However, such bleeding can indicate more serious conditions (such as miscarriage, childbirth, infection).

### What to Look For

- Abdominal cramps
- Blood in the vaginal area

### What to Do

1. Reassure the woman.
2. Help her into a comfortable position with legs bent.
3. Have the woman place a sanitary pad over the outside of the vagina.
4. Seek medical care.

# Emergency Childbirth

Emergency childbirth occurs when a baby is born at an unplanned time or at an unplanned place. Most babies in the United States are delivered in a hospital. Occasionally, the birth process moves along faster than expected. Because emergency childbirth is encountered infrequently, taking care of an anxious mother and her newborn infant is a stressful event for a first aid provider. On the other hand, assisting in the birth of a baby is one of the few situations in which first aid providers have the opportunity to participate in a happy event rather than an unpleasant one.

## ▶ Imminent Delivery

Consider transporting the woman to a hospital only if she does not have the urge to push or the baby is not crowning and this is her first pregnancy. Making a hasty decision to transport the woman means that the delivery could take place under the worst possible circumstances. When there is enough time to transport the woman to a hospital, the woman should wear a seat belt. Neither the lap belt nor the shoulder harness should be worn alone—both should be worn at the same time to avoid rupturing the uterus if a crash occurs. If she needs to lie down, place her on her left side. This position prevents a possible drop in blood pressure caused by pressure of the fetus on the inferior vena cava, which reduces venous blood returning to the heart.

If the woman has the urge to push or the baby is crowning, the woman has had previous pregnancies, and there is not enough time to get to the hospital, you must prepare to assist in the delivery. First, call (or have a bystander call) 9-1-1. Then, if the woman is in a crowded or public place, try to find a private, clean area. The mother might find it reassuring to have a companion, such as her husband, a friend, or a relative, present. Follow these guidelines:

- Wear exam gloves. If available, wear a mask, a gown, and eye protection.
- **DO NOT** touch the vaginal area except during delivery and, if possible, with a witness present.
- **DO NOT** let the mother use the toilet.
- **DO NOT** hold the mother's legs together.

If the baby's head is not the presenting part (the first part to come out of the birth canal), the delivery will be complicated. Tell the mother not to push and attempt to calm and reassure her. Call 9-1-1 if you have not already done so.

> **CAUTION**
>
> **DO NOT** allow the mother to go to the toilet if delivery seems imminent.
>
> **DO NOT** attempt to delay or restrain delivery in any way (for example, holding the mother's legs together).

## Stages of Labor

Labor is a three-stage process that begins with the first regular uterine contractions, includes delivery of the baby, and ends with delivery of the placenta. The first stage usually lasts several hours (possibly 12 hours or more for a first baby), from the first contraction until the cervix is fully open (dilated). The cervix gradually stretches until it is large enough to let the baby pass through. (Outside a hospital setting, first aid providers cannot safely check for dilation of the cervix.) The contractions usually begin as acutely aching sensations in the small of the back; in a short time, they turn into cramplike pains recurring regularly in the lower abdomen. At first, the contractions are 10 to 15 minutes apart, are not very severe, and last less than 1 minute. Gradually, the intervals between contractions grow shorter, and the contractions increase in intensity. A slight, watery, bloodstained discharge (bloody show) from the vagina might accompany contractions or might occur before labor begins.

At the end of the first stage of labor, the amniotic sac breaks, and 1 pint (473 mL) or more of watery fluid, the amniotic fluid, discharges. Sometimes the amniotic sac breaks during the first stage of labor, but this is no cause for concern because it usually does not affect labor. If the amniotic sac breaks prematurely and labor does not begin within 12 hours, the risk of infection to mother and baby is great, and medical care should be sought.

The second stage usually lasts from 30 minutes to 2 hours. It begins when the neck of the cervix is fully open and ends with the actual birth of the baby. The baby is normally head down; once the head gets through the pelvis, the rest of the body should follow easily. During the third stage, which lasts about 15 minutes or more, the afterbirth (placenta) is expelled **Figure 22-1** .

**Figure 22-1**

Normal stages of childbirth. **A.** End of the first stage of labor. **B.** Head delivers facedown. **C.** Support the head. **D.** Placenta is expelled in 5 to 20 minutes.

## Recognizing Signs of Imminent Delivery

At the scene of a woman in labor, you will need to determine whether delivery is imminent or whether there is time to transport the woman to the hospital. To make that decision, answer the questions in the following table. Only if the answers to these questions seem to indicate an imminent birth should you examine the mother for crowning. Look to see if there is bulging at the vaginal opening or if part of the baby is visible. Crowning indicates that the baby is about to be born and that there is no time to get to a hospital before delivery. Because this step might be embarrassing to the mother, the father, bystanders, or even you, it is important that you explain fully what you are doing and why. Make every effort to protect the woman from embarrassment during such an examination by removing only enough clothing to expose the vaginal area. Use something to shield the woman from prying eyes—for example, a blanket used to make a tent, or even a human shield, with people standing with their backs toward her.

### FYI

**Supplies for Delivery**

Ideally, you should have the following supplies for delivery:

- Clean sheets, towels, and blankets to cover the mother and baby
- A plastic bag or towel to wrap the placenta for delivery to the hospital
- Clean, unused exam gloves to reduce the likelihood of infection
- Sanitary pads
- Newspapers, plastic, or a cloth sheet to place under the woman to provide a clean delivery area
- Rubber bulb syringe for suctioning the baby's mouth and nostrils
- Sterile gauze pads for wiping blood and mucus from the baby's mouth and nose
- Strips of gauze, new or clean shoelaces, or similar materials to tie the cord. (**DO NOT** use thread, wire, or string because they might cut through the cord.) Gauze bandages or pads opened into strips can be used.

## What to Look For

To determine whether delivery is imminent or whether there is time to transport the woman to the hospital, answer the following questions:

- *Has the woman had a baby before?* Labor during a first pregnancy is usually longer than in subsequent pregnancies. If this is her first pregnancy, there might be more time for transport to a hospital.

- *How frequent are the contractions?* Contractions more than 5 minutes apart are a good indication that there will be enough time to get the mother to a nearby hospital. Contractions less than 2 minutes apart that last 45 to 60 seconds, especially in a woman who has had more than one pregnancy, signal imminent delivery.

- *Has the amniotic sac ruptured? If so, when?* Labor usually proceeds more rapidly after rupture. If the sac ruptures more than 18 hours before birth occurs, the likelihood of fetal infection increases, and the hospital staff should be alerted. Delivery might be more difficult when the amniotic sac ruptures prematurely because amniotic fluid serves as a lubricant.

- *Does the mother feel as though she has to move her bowels?* That sensation is caused by the fetal head in the vagina pressing against the rectum and indicates that delivery is imminent.

## What to Do

If you are faced with an imminent delivery, follow the steps in **Skill Sheet 22-1**:

1. Take standard precautions by washing your hands thoroughly and wearing exam gloves. If possible, wear a mask, a gown, and eye protection.
2. Have the mother lie on her back with her head slightly elevated, knees drawn up, and legs spread apart. The mother might want to be in a different position. Other safe positions for childbirth include the following:
   - Sitting up or squatting, with someone behind supporting her. These two positions place less tension on the vaginal tissues, reducing the likelihood of a tear, and allow the force of gravity to help.
   - Lying on her left side, which improves blood return to her heart and prevents aspiration should she vomit. Have someone hold the woman's right leg up out of the way.
   - Kneeling in a knee-chest position, which is used in many countries and in cases of breech presentations.
3. Remind the woman to take short, quick breaths during each contraction. Between contractions, she should rest and breathe deeply through her mouth.
4. Place absorbent, clean materials (such as sheets or towels) under the mother's buttocks.
5. Elevate her buttocks with blankets or a pillow.
6. When the baby's head appears, place the palm of your hand on top of the head and exert very gentle pressure to prevent an explosive delivery. Have the woman stop pushing. **DO NOT** push on the **fontanelles** (soft spots on the top and back of the infant's head).
7. If the amniotic sac does not break or has not broken, tear it with your fingers and push it away from the baby's head and mouth as they appear. The baby could suffocate if the sac is not removed.
8. As the baby's head emerges from the vagina, determine whether the umbilical cord is wrapped around the baby's neck. If it is, gently slip the cord over the baby's head. If you cannot do that, attempt to alleviate pressure on the cord.
9. Support the baby's head as it emerges.
10. Suction the baby's mouth and then the nostrils two or three times with the bulb syringe. Use caution to avoid contact with the back of the baby's mouth. If a bulb syringe is not available, wipe the baby's mouth and then the nose with gauze.
11. As the torso and full body emerge, support the baby with both hands— he or she will be slippery.
12. **DO NOT** pull on the baby, which could cause cervical spine damage. **DO NOT** put your fingers in the baby's armpits; pressure on the nerve centers there could cause paralysis.
13. Keep the baby level with the vagina, slightly head down, to improve drainage from the mouth and nose.
14. Wipe blood and mucus from the baby's mouth and nose with sterile gauze; suction the mouth, and then suction the nose again.
15. Dry the infant to reduce heat loss and help stimulate breathing. Rub the baby's back or flick the soles of its feet to stimulate breathing. The baby should breathe within 30 seconds, especially after the cord stops pulsating. (**DO NOT** hold the baby up by the feet and slap its buttocks, which could cause an increase in intracranial pressure.) If breathing does not start within 30 seconds, begin cardiopulmonary resuscitation (CPR).

*(Continues)*

| What to Look For | What to Do |
|---|---|
| | **16.** Wrap the infant in a warm blanket and place on his or her side, head slightly lower than the trunk. Keep the infant level with the mother's vagina until the cord is cut. Raising the baby above the mother's abdomen (location of the placenta) while the umbilical cord is intact will allow the baby's blood to drain out and might result in shock in the baby. Holding the baby below the mother's abdomen allows her blood to flow into the baby, and the extra blood cells can cause serious conditions such as jaundice. |
| | **17.** When the umbilical cord stops pulsating, tie it with gauze (or similar material) or a clean shoelace between the mother and the infant. |
| | **18.** If the mother is going to the hospital soon after the birth, and it was a normal delivery, there is no need to cut the cord. Keep the infant warm and wait for EMS personnel, who will have the proper equipment to clamp and cut the cord. If you are in a remote location, you might have to cut the cord yourself. In such a situation and after cord pulsations stop, tie the cord about 4 inches (10 cm) away from the baby and make a second tie 2 inches (5 cm) from the first tie. Cut the cord between the two ties. |
| | **19.** Watch for delivery of the placenta, which usually takes a few minutes, but could take as long as 30 minutes. **DO NOT** pull on the end of the umbilical cord to speed the delivery of the placenta. |
| | **20.** When the placenta is delivered, wrap it in a towel with three quarters of the umbilical cord and place the towel in a plastic bag. Keep the bag at the level of the infant. Take the placenta to the hospital, where it will be examined for completeness. This procedure is necessary because pieces of placenta retained in the uterus can cause persistent bleeding or infection. |
| | **21.** Place a sterile pad over the vaginal opening, lower the mother's legs, and help her hold them together. |
| | **22.** Gently massage the woman's abdomen, just below the navel, to help control bleeding. |

## Skill Sheet

### 22-1    Childbirth

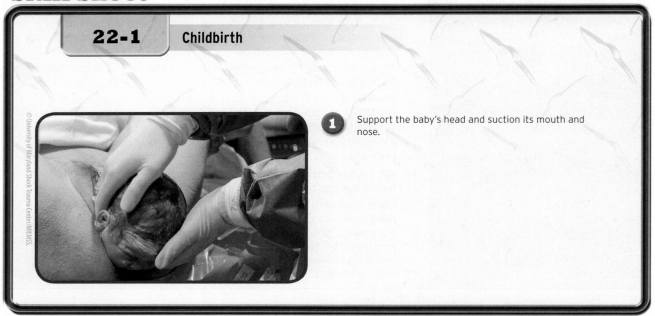

© University of Maryland Shock Trauma Center/MIEMSS

**1** Support the baby's head and suction its mouth and nose.

# Skill Sheet Continued

**22-1**    Childbirth

**2** Once the head delivers, the upper shoulder will be visible.

**3** Support the baby's head and body as the shoulders deliver.

**4** Clean and dry the infant to reduce heat loss and stimulate breathing.

**5** Allow the placenta to deliver. **DO NOT** pull on the umbilical cord.

© University of Maryland Shock Trauma Center/MIEMSS.

## Delivery Aftercare

After delivery, monitor the mother's breathing and pulse. Replace any blood-soaked sheets and blankets while awaiting transport. A woman can expect from 1 to 2 cups (300 to 500 mL) of blood loss after delivery. You should be aware of this amount of blood loss so it does not cause undue psychological stress to the new mother or to you. If blood loss continues, massage the uterus. Uterine massage stimulates the uterus to contract, thus constricting blood vessels within its walls and decreasing bleeding.

1. Use your hand with your fingers fully extended.
2. Place the palm of your hand on the lower abdomen, where you should be able to feel a grapefruit-sized mass.
3. Gently massage over the area with a firm, circular motion.
4. If bleeding continues, check your massage technique.
5. The mother can also breastfeed the baby following delivery of the placenta to stimulate uterine contractions and thus help control bleeding.

## Initial Care of the Newborn

Normal findings in a newborn are a pulse rate of more than 100 beats per minute (feel the brachial artery, which runs between the shoulder and elbow) and a respiratory rate of more than 40 breaths per minute. The baby often will be crying. The most important care is positioning, drying, keeping warm, and stimulating the newborn to breathe. Wrap the newborn in a blanket, making sure the head is covered. Newborns are at risk for hypothermia; premature and low-weight newborns are at greater risk. Repeat suctioning if necessary, and continue to stimulate the newborn if he or she is not breathing (flick the soles of the feet and rub the infant's back).

If the newborn is motionless, tap the infant on the bottom of a foot or a shoulder for a response. If the infant does not respond and is not breathing, or is only gasping, begin CPR starting with 30 chest compressions followed by two breaths. Initially, give a total of five sets of 30 chest compressions and two breaths before calling 9-1-1 unless a bystander has already called. Continue sets of 30 chest compressions and two breaths until EMS personnel take over. (See Chapter 5, *CPR*.)

## ▶ Abnormal Deliveries

Most childbirths are normal and natural. Sometimes, however, complications arise. It is essential that you be calm, deliberate, and gentle in a situation that becomes even more stressful because of complications. Call 9-1-1 for all of these situations.

### FYI

**Emergencies During Pregnancy**

**What Medical Specialties Take Care of Women?**

A gynecologist specializes in treating conditions related to the female reproductive tract. An obstetrician specializes in treating pregnant women. A pediatrician specializes in treating newborn babies, toddlers, and teens.

**How Is Emergency Care for a Pregnant Woman Different?**

There are two people involved—the mother and fetus. Even minor trauma to the mother's abdomen can result in life-threatening consequences. All pregnant women with trauma to the abdomen need a medical examination in a hospital emergency department and often need fetal monitoring. Fetal viability is determined by maternal viability. Position the mother on her left side to help venous blood return to the heart. Care for the pregnant woman the same way you would treat a nonpregnant woman.

**What Are Some Indications of Pregnancy Emergencies?**

- The three key warning signs of a serious condition are bleeding, abdominal cramps, and weakness.
- Morning sickness, swollen ankles, and urinary tract infections are not usually dangerous, but call the physician anyway.
- If a pregnant woman is spotting (small amount of vaginal bleeding), have her lie down immediately. Call for medical attention. Spotting can signal the onset of a miscarriage.

### Prolapsed Cord

A **prolapsed cord** is a condition in which the umbilical cord comes through the birth canal before delivery of the head. The cord is squeezed between the baby's head and the mother's body (vaginal wall), and oxygen supply to the baby could be stopped. This puts the baby in danger of suffocation **Figure 22-2**. This situation is rare and very dangerous.

| What to Look For | What to Do |
|---|---|
| The umbilical cord can be seen before the baby's head. | 1. Position the woman with her head down or buttocks raised to use gravity to lessen pressure in the birth canal.<br><br>2. Insert fingers of your gloved hand into the vagina, placing fingers on either side of the cord to hold pressure from the presenting part (most often the head) of the fetus away from the pulsating cord. Continue until EMS arrives. **DO NOT** push the cord back into the vagina. This is one of only two circumstances for putting your fingers into the vagina.<br><br>3. Call 9-1-1 immediately. |

## CAUTION

**DO NOT** attempt to push the cord back into the vagina.

## Breech Birth Presentation

A breech presentation occurs when the baby's buttocks or lower extremities emerge before the head or shoulders. Breech presentation is the most common type of abnormal delivery and occurs in 3% to 4% of all deliveries. Place the mother in a kneeling, head-down position, with her pelvis elevated, and seek medical care immediately Figure 22-3.

In a breech presentation, if the baby's head is not delivered within 3 minutes of the body, you must act to prevent suffocation of the baby. Suffocation can occur when the baby's face is pressed against the vaginal wall or when the umbilical cord is compressed by the baby's head in the vagina.

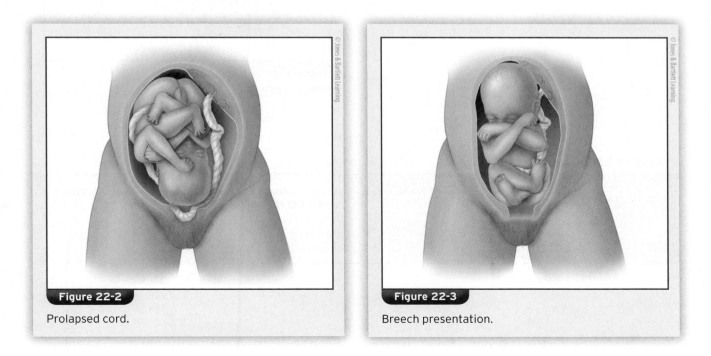

**Figure 22-2**
Prolapsed cord.

**Figure 22-3**
Breech presentation.

**What to Look For**

**What to Do**

| The baby's buttocks come out first. | 1. To establish an airway, do the following:<br>  • Place one hand in the vagina, positioning the palm toward the baby's face. This is one of only two circumstances for putting your fingers into the vagina.<br>  • Form a V with your fingers on either side of the baby's nose.<br>  • Push the vaginal wall away from the baby's face until the head is delivered.<br>2. Have someone call 9-1-1 immediately.<br>3. Have the woman continue to push with contractions and attempt to deliver the baby. |

**CAUTION**

**DO NOT** pull out the baby's head during a breech delivery.

## Limb Presentation

Limb presentation occurs when an arm, leg, or foot of the infant protrudes from the birth canal. A foot more commonly presents when the infant is in a breech presentation **Figure 22-4** .

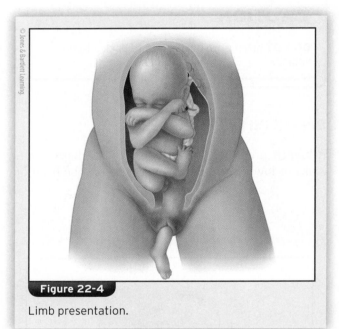

**Figure 22-4**

Limb presentation.

**What to Look For**

**What to Do**

| An arm, leg, or foot appears first. | 1. Place the mother in a head-down position with the pelvis elevated. **DO NOT** pull on the baby or attempt to push the limb back into the vagina.<br>2. Call 9-1-1 immediately. The baby cannot be delivered in this position by a first aid provider. |

## Meconium

<u>Meconium</u> is the baby's first feces (bowel movement) and can be present in the amniotic fluid. Its presence is associated with fetal distress during labor and a greater risk for infant death. The danger to the baby is the possibility of breathing the meconium into the lungs, where it can cause severe respiratory conditions.

| What to Look For | What to Do |
|---|---|
| Amniotic fluid that is:<br>• Green or brown-yellow<br>• Tarry<br>• Almost odorless | 1. Keep the infant in a moderately head-down position to aid with drainage.<br>2. Suction the mouth and nostrils thoroughly, or the baby will inhale meconium with its first breath into the lungs. Clear amniotic fluid, however, is harmlessly absorbed through the baby's lungs. Try not to stimulate the infant to breathe before suctioning.<br>3. Maintain the baby's open airway.<br>4. Call 9-1-1 immediately. |

## Premature Birth

Any baby born prior to 37 completed weeks of pregnancy is defined as premature and will require special care. Premature babies develop conditions because they are smaller and less developed than full-term infants. For example, their cardiovascular and respiratory systems are often immature.

Refer to **Flowchart 22-1** for additional information regarding emergency childbirth.

| What to Look For | What to Do |
|---|---|
| • A premature infant will be smaller and thinner than a full-term infant.<br>• A premature infant has a head proportionately larger in comparison with the rest of the body.<br>• The cheesy, white coating on the skin (*vernix caseosa*) of a full-term infant will be minimal or absent on the premature infant. | 1. Keep the baby warm. Premature babies are especially at risk for hypothermia.<br>2. Keep the mouth and nose clear of mucus.<br>3. Monitor breathing and perform CPR, if necessary. |

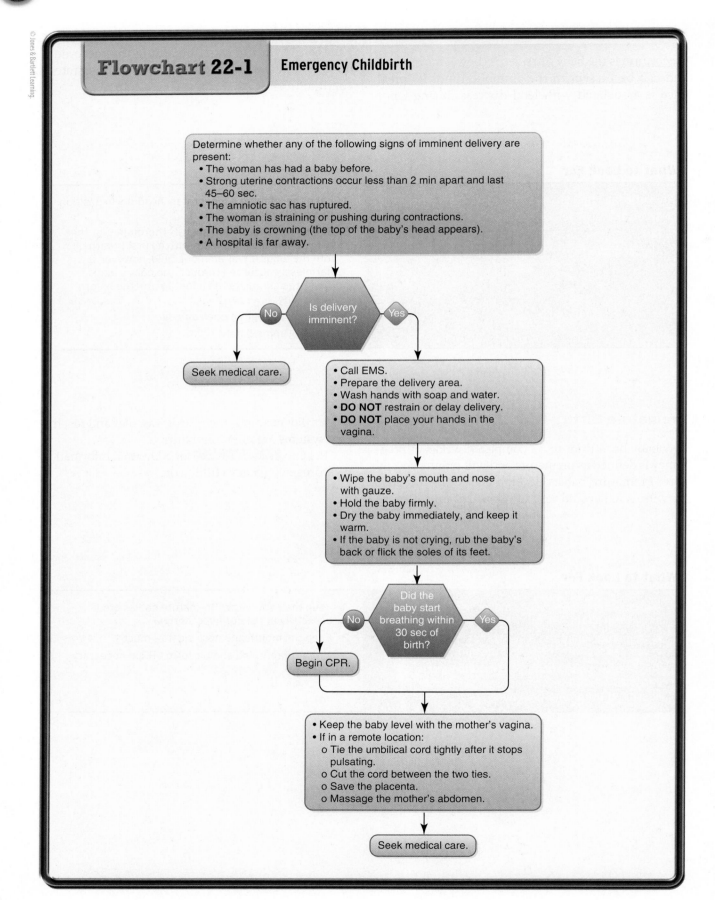

**Flowchart 22-1**    **Emergency Childbirth**

Determine whether any of the following signs of imminent delivery are present:
- The woman has had a baby before.
- Strong uterine contractions occur less than 2 min apart and last 45–60 sec.
- The amniotic sac has ruptured.
- The woman is straining or pushing during contractions.
- The baby is crowning (the top of the baby's head appears).
- A hospital is far away.

**Is delivery imminent?**

No → Seek medical care.

Yes →
- Call EMS.
- Prepare the delivery area.
- Wash hands with soap and water.
- **DO NOT** restrain or delay delivery.
- **DO NOT** place your hands in the vagina.

- Wipe the baby's mouth and nose with gauze.
- Hold the baby firmly.
- Dry the baby immediately, and keep it warm.
- If the baby is not crying, rub the baby's back or flick the soles of its feet.

**Did the baby start breathing within 30 sec of birth?**

No → Begin CPR.

Yes →

- Keep the baby level with the mother's vagina.
- If in a remote location:
  o Tie the umbilical cord tightly after it stops pulsating.
  o Cut the cord between the two ties.
  o Save the placenta.
  o Massage the mother's abdomen.

Seek medical care.

# Gynecologic Emergencies

Gynecologic emergencies are reproductive system conditions that occur in nonpregnant women.

## Q&A

**What is pelvic inflammatory disease (PID)?**

PID is caused by the spread of microorganisms from the vagina and cervix to reproductive organs. The organisms (the most common being *Chlamydia* and *Neisseria gonorrhoeae* are typically sexually transmitted. A person with PID can have more than one sexually transmitted disease (STD) at the same time. Other important conditions (eg, ectopic pregnancy, acute appendicitis) may cause confusion about the condition. The inflammatory response can range from mild to severe. No reliable signs or symptoms exist, but may involve vaginal discharge and abdominal tenderness. Because the consequences of unrecognized and untreated PID can be severe, medical care should be sought.

## Q&A

**What are the signs and symptoms of an ectopic pregnancy?**

A fertilized egg that implants in one of the <u>fallopian tubes</u> instead of in the uterus is called an <u>ectopic pregnancy</u>. The embryo is not viable and must be removed as soon as the condition is identified to avoid serious complications, such as rupture of the fallopian tube.

Pelvic pain and vaginal bleeding or spotting in a woman of childbearing age should be treated as an ectopic pregnancy until the condition is ruled out by a physician. Predisposing factors for ectopic pregnancy are previous ectopic pregnancies, surgeries, pelvic infections, and presence of an intrauterine device (IUD). Common signs and symptoms are vaginal bleeding and abdominal tenderness.

## Q&A

**What should be done about urinary tract infections?**

- Women, especially during pregnancy, are very susceptible to urinary tract infections. Often, when one infection clears, another replaces it.
- Seek advice from a physician. Self-care measures to help relieve the burning pain include taking shallow, lukewarm sitz baths sprinkled with baking soda; urinating while standing in the shower; and practicing good personal hygiene. Wiping from front to back after going to the bathroom helps keep bacteria, including *Escherichia coli*, away from the urinary tract. Drinking more fluids helps prevent and treat urinary tract infections. Some experts report that drinking cranberry juice (tablets are also available with fewer calories) might help inhibit urinary tract infections.
- A urinary tract (bladder) infection can lead to the more serious kidney infection. Signs of a kidney infection include pain in the lower back or flank, fever, and nausea or vomiting.

## ▶ Sexual Assault and Rape

Perhaps one of the most difficult emergency situations that a first aid provider might have to deal with is sexual assault. According to the Rape, Abuse & Incest National Network (RAINN), 68% of sexual assault cases are not reported to authorities. In most cases, the sexual assault survivor is a woman. The Centers for Disease Control and Prevention (CDC) reports 1 in 5 women in the United States have been raped at some point in their life. It should be noted, however, that men, heterosexual and homosexual, also can be raped.

There are many definitions of rape, but in general, rape involves the criminal act of forcing another person to submit to sexual intercourse. Related physical injury is common, but the psychological trauma may be more damaging. It is essential that you be calm and sympathetic when dealing with a person who has experienced sexual assault. (For more information, see Chapter 23, *Behavioral Emergencies*.)

## What to Look For

## What to Do

A person who has been sexually assaulted might display:

- Headaches
- Sleeplessness, nightmares
- Nausea and/or muscle spasms
- Confusion
- Depression
- Anxiety, jumpiness

1. **DO NOT** ask a lot of questions. Confine your questions to an assessment of the person's injuries, not a detailed description of the events. Ask questions based on the SAMPLE history (see Chapter 4, *Finding Out What Is Wrong*).

2. **DO NOT** blame the survivor in any way or talk about what might have been done or what you would have done. Be supportive. Remind him or her that he or she is safe now.

3. Determine which injuries require immediate care. Whenever it is necessary that a woman disrobe, try to have another woman present.

4. **DO NOT** expose the genitalia unless an injury in that area requires immediate care (for example, severe bleeding). Examining genitalia, except when childbirth is imminent, has serious legal implications and therefore usually should be avoided.

5. Try, if possible, to preserve evidence but leave the actual investigation to the police. To preserve evidence, encourage the person not to change clothes, wash, urinate, defecate, or douche. Explain to the person in a sympathetic way that it would be best not to clean up. Keep in mind that a person who has been raped, like any other person, has the right to refuse first aid and transport to a hospital.

6. Even if the person refuses aid, **DO NOT** leave him or her alone. Try to have a trusted friend or relative stay with the person. Protect the privacy of the person. Emotional support is vital. Most large communities have rape crisis centers; furnishing the person with the name and number of the nearest center (look in the telephone directory) is probably as important as treating any physical injuries. Trained volunteers can talk to the person and give you and the person information about what to do next.

7. Get the person medical care. The person could be in shock and unaware of the severity of her or his injuries. Strongly encourage a person who has been raped to receive medical care, even if the person does not show any signs of injury and does not want medical care. However, be aware that the medical exam following a rape is intrusive and, for women, includes a full gynecologic exam. The person will need information about what is going to happen before receiving medical care.

## ▶ Ready for Review

- Miscarriages usually occur during the first trimester of pregnancy.
- If a woman experiences vaginal bleeding late in her pregnancy, it usually constitutes an emergency.
- Emergency childbirth occurs when a baby is born at an unplanned time or at an unplanned place.
- In most cases, childbirth is normal and natural. Sometimes complications can arise.
- Perhaps one of the most difficult emergency situations that a first aid provider might have to deal with is sexual assault.

## ▶ Vital Vocabulary

amniotic sac A thick, transparent sac that holds the fetus suspended in the amniotic fluid.

birth canal The vagina and the lower part of the uterus.

bloody show The bloody mucus plug that is discharged from the vagina when labor begins.

cervix The small opening at the lower end of the uterus through which the baby passes.

crowning The stage of birth when the presenting part of the baby is visible at the vaginal orifice.

ectopic pregnancy A pregnancy that develops outside the uterus, typically in a fallopian tube.

fallopian tubes The tubes that connect each ovary with the uterus.

fetus The developing, unborn infant inside the uterus.

fontanelles Areas where the infant's skull has not fused together; usually disappear at approximately 18 months of age.

labor The process or period of childbirth; especially, the muscular contraction of the uterus designed to expel the fetus from the mother.

meconium A dark green material in the amniotic fluid that can indicate fetal distress; the infant's first bowel movement.

miscarriage Delivery of the fetus before it is mature enough to survive outside the womb (about 20 weeks), from either natural (spontaneous abortion) or induced causes.

placenta The vascular organ attached to the uterine wall that supplies oxygen and nutrients to the fetus; also called afterbirth.

prolapsed cord A condition in which the umbilical cord comes out of the vagina before the infant.

umbilical cord The flexible structure that connects the fetus to the placenta.

vena cava Large vein between the spine and the abdominal organs.

## ▶ Assessment in Action

You are visiting a local museum when you respond to calls for help in the exhibit hall. A young woman has gone into labor. When you arrive on scene, she tells you this is her third child and that her due date is next week. She says she thought she would have time to get to the hospital when the contractions started. However, the contractions intensified and got closer together very quickly. Contractions are now less than 2 minutes apart and last up to 60 seconds. A hospital is 10 minutes away.

*Directions:* Circle Yes if you agree with the statement; circle No if you disagree.

Yes   No   **1.** Labor during a third pregnancy is usually longer than in previous pregnancies.

Yes   No   **2.** Allow the woman to use the toilet.

Yes   No   **3.** With contractions less than 2 minutes apart, you should have time to get her to the hospital.

Yes   No   **4.** Call 9-1-1 and immediately prepare a delivery area.

Yes   No   **5.** If the baby is crowning, you should not restrain or delay delivery.

## ▶ Check Your Knowledge

*Directions:* Circle Yes if you agree with the statement; circle No if you disagree.

Yes  No  **1.** An aching in the lower back is a sign of a miscarriage.

Yes  No  **2.** It is normal for a woman to experience vaginal bleeding in her last trimester.

Yes  No  **3.** Most babies in the United States are delivered at home.

Yes  No  **4.** Place a pregnant woman on her left side when transporting her to the hospital.

Yes  No  **5.** Labor is a four-stage process.

Yes  No  **6.** The second stage of labor lasts from 30 minutes to 2 hours.

Yes  No  **7.** New or clean shoelaces can be used to tie the umbilical cord.

Yes  No  **8.** A prolapsed umbilical cord is a normal occurrence.

Yes  No  **9.** The placenta is also called the after-birth.

Yes  No  **10.** Whether or not the woman has given birth before will usually affect the length of the labor.

© Antonio Guillem/Shutterstock

# Behavioral Emergencies

## Behavioral Emergencies

Behavior is how a person acts. Although each person acts or behaves differently, sometimes a person exhibits unacceptable or intolerable behavior. The abnormal behavior may be due to a psychological condition (such as a mental illness) or a physical condition. For example, a person with diabetes who has an uncorrected low blood glucose level can display aggressiveness, restlessness, or anxiety. Because the brain lacks energy in the form of blood glucose, altered mental status results. Likewise, lack of oxygen and inadequate blood flow to the brain also cause altered mental status, resulting in similar behavior. Behavior that leads to violence or other inappropriate activities is known as a **behavioral emergency**.

Several factors can change a person's behavior, including situational stresses, medical illnesses, psychiatric conditions, alcohol, and drugs. The following are common reasons for behavioral changes:

- Low blood glucose level in a person with diabetes
- Lack of oxygen (known as hypoxia)
- Inadequate blood flow to the brain
- Head trauma
- Excessive cold
- Excessive heat
- Mind-altering substances, such as alcohol, depressants, stimulants, hallucinogens, and narcotics
- Psychogenic or psychiatric illness that leads to psychotic thinking, depression, or panic

## ▶ Depression

Depression is more than the sad feeling that everyone experiences at times. Depression is one of the most common and treatable of all mental illnesses. There are several types of depression: reactive depression (following tragic events), major or clinical depression (with no apparent cause, lasts more than 2 weeks, and prevents functioning in top form at work or in social situations), and bipolar depression, a type that includes episodes of euphoria. Depression is believed to be due to a chemical imbalance in the brain, which causes the nerves in the brain not to work properly. This is why it is often treated using medications that act on the brain. Depression can lead to suicide; in fact, untreated depression is the main cause of suicide.

### What to Look For

Not everyone who is depressed experiences every symptom. Severity of symptoms varies with people and also varies over time.

- Persistent sad, anxious, or empty moods
- Feelings of hopelessness, pessimism
- Feelings of guilt, worthlessness, helplessness
- Loss of interest or pleasure in hobbies and activities that were once enjoyed, including sex
- Decreased energy, fatigue, feeling slowed down
- Difficulty concentrating, remembering, making decisions
- Insomnia, early-morning awakening, or oversleeping
- Appetite and/or weight loss or overeating and weight gain
- Thoughts of death or suicide; suicide attempts
- Restlessness, irritability
- Persistent physical symptoms that do not respond to treatment such as headaches, digestive disorders, and chronic pain

### What to Do

1. Some depressed people do not feel like talking. In such cases, saying, "You look very sad," often allows the person to talk about the depressed feelings. The person might burst into tears. **DO NOT** discourage the crying. Maintain a sympathetic silence and let the person "cry it out."
2. Provide empathetic attention and reassurance. Let the person know you are concerned.
3. Attempt to interview the person in private because the presence of several people may make the person uncomfortable. Ask open-ended questions such as, "Tell me how you feel."
4. Tell the person that many people have periods of unhappiness, but they can be helped to feel better. Mention community resources where such help can be found.

## ▶ Suicide

Suicide is defined as any willful act that ends one's own life. Each year, over 40,000 Americans commit suicide; it is the 10th reported leading cause of death in the United States, according to the National Center for Injury Prevention and Control. Many experts, however, believe that suicide is vastly underreported. Suicide in the United States is increasingly an issue for adolescents, college-age students, and older adults.

The Centers for Disease Control and Prevention (CDC) reports the rate for suicide in men is four times that for women. It is most common in men who are single, widowed, or divorced. Slightly more than half of all people who commit suicides—both men and women—use firearms. The next most common method is hanging. Poisoning by solids or liquids is the most common method used by people who attempt but do not complete suicide. Jumping from high places, carbon monoxide poisoning by auto exhaust, drowning, and self-inflicted (non-firearm) wounds are less common methods.

The number of suicides peaks during spring months and is lowest in the winter. Suicide rates are lowest in the Northeast and highest in the mountain states.

Suicide attempts are eight times more common than completed suicides. In addition, although men complete suicide four times more often than women, women are reported to attempt suicide three times more often, according to the American Foundation for Suicide Prevention (AFSP). It is not known if men are more reluctant to seek help and, thus, less likely to report their attempts. It also is not known if the lower rate of suicide among women results from their choice of less-lethal methods.

Suicide is often attempted by people who are depressed or have alcoholism. The AFSP reports about 60% of all people who commit suicide previously attempted suicide, and about 75% gave clear warning that they intended to kill themselves. Typically, a suicide attempt occurs when a person's close emotional attachments are in danger or when a significant family member or friend dies. People who are contemplating suicide often feel unable to manage their lives. Frequently, they lack self-esteem.

Many people who are planning to commit suicide make last-minute attempts to communicate their intentions. When a person phones to threaten suicide, try to keep the person on the line until EMS reaches the scene.

If you encounter a person who is attempting or threatening suicide, discreetly remove any dangerous articles. Talk quietly with the person and encourage the person to discuss the situation. Ask the following: "Have you attempted suicide before? Have you made any concrete plans for a method of suicide? Has any family member committed suicide?" People who have made a previous suicide attempt, who have detailed suicide plans, or who have a close relative who committed suicide are more likely to try to kill themselves Table 23-1. They must be reassured and taken to medical help, usually at a medical facility. **DO NOT** leave them alone under any circumstances.

When a person attempts suicide, first aid care has priority. Drug overdoses must be managed. Bleeding from slashed wrists must be controlled. As you give first aid, try to encourage the person to talk about the situation. If a drug overdose is involved, collect any medication containers, pills, or other drugs found on the scene and take the items to the hospital emergency department with the person. In all cases, law enforcement authorities should be contacted.

## Table 23-1 Suicide Risk Factors

The SAD PERSONS scale is a mnemonic list of known suicide high-risk characteristics. A score of nine or greater indicates the probable need for psychiatric consultation.

| Mnemonic | Characteristics | Score |
| --- | --- | --- |
| **S** Sex | Male | 1 |
| **A** Age | Younger than 19 years or older than 45 years | 1 |
| **D** Depression or hopelessness | Admits to depression or decreased concentration, appetite, sleep, libido | 2 |
| **P** Previous attempts or psychiatric care | Previous inpatient or outpatient psychiatric care | 1 |
| **E** Excessive alcohol or drug use | Chronic addiction or recent frequent drug use | 1 |
| **R** Rational thinking loss | Brain dysfunction (unknown or nonspecific cause) or psychosis | 2 |
| **S** Separated, widowed, or divorced | | 1 |
| **O** Organized or serious attempt | Well-thought-out plan or life-threatening display | 2 |
| **N** No social support | No close family, friends, job, or active religious affiliation | 1 |
| **S** Stated future intent | Determined to repeat attempt | 2 |

Determining whether high-risk factors are involved will help first aid providers maintain objectivity. It is important to maintain a nonjudgmental approach. Using the SAD PERSONS mnemonic acknowledges the seriousness of the situation and reminds first aid providers that ridiculing, making demeaning comments, or ignoring the person is not helpful or proper.

Take precautions by keeping the person under close observation, removing any potentially dangerous items (for example, glass, razors, and medicines) from the immediate area, and not allowing the person to go anywhere, even to the bathroom, unaccompanied.

*Source:* Data from Hockberger RS, Rothstein RJ. Assessment of suicide potential by non-psychiatrists using the SAD PERSONS score. *J Emerg Med* 6(2):99–107.

### What to Look For

A person who is:

- Getting his or her affairs in order (paying off debts, making or changing a will)
- Giving away articles of either personal or monetary value
- Exhibiting signs of planning a suicide such as obtaining a weapon or writing a suicide note

### What to Do

1. If someone tells you he or she is thinking about suicide, take the distress seriously Table 23-2.
2. Ways to be helpful to someone who is threatening suicide include the following:
   - Be direct. Talk openly and matter-of-factly about suicide.
   - Be willing to listen. Allow expressions of feelings. Accept the feelings.

*(Continues)*

| What to Look For | What to Do |
|---|---|
| A person who says:<br>• "Life is not worth living."<br>• "My family would be better off without me. "<br>• "Next time I will take enough pills to do the job right."<br>• "Take my (prized collection, valuables); I do not need this stuff anymore."<br>• "I will not be around to deal with that."<br>• "You will be sorry when I am gone."<br>• "I will not be around much longer."<br>• "I just cannot deal with everything—life is too hard."<br>• "Nobody understands me; nobody feels the way I do."<br>• "There is nothing I can do to make it better."<br>• "I would be better off dead."<br>• "I feel like there is no way out." | • Be nonjudgmental. **DO NOT** debate whether suicide is right or wrong.<br>• Get involved. Become available. Show interest and support.<br>• **DO NOT** dare him or her to do it.<br>• **DO NOT** act shocked. This will put distance between the two of you.<br>• **DO NOT** be sworn to secrecy. Seek support.<br>• Offer hope that alternatives are available but **DO NOT** offer glib reassurance.<br>• Take action. Remove means of suicide, such as guns or stockpiled pills.<br>• Get help from people or agencies specializing in crisis intervention and suicide prevention. |

## CAUTION

**DO NOT** ignore a suicide threat. Every suicidal act or gesture should be taken seriously and the person referred to a professional counselor.

### Table 23-2 Common Myths About Suicide

| Myth | Fact |
|---|---|
| People who talk about suicide do not commit suicide. | Of every 10 people who kill themselves, 8 have given definite warnings of their suicidal intentions. Suicide threats and attempts must be taken seriously. |
| Suicide happens without warning. | Studies reveal that the person contemplating suicide gives many clues and warnings about suicidal intentions. Being alert to these cries for help may prevent suicidal behavior. |
| People who contemplate or attempt suicide are fully intent on dying. | Most people who contemplate suicide are undecided about living or dying, and they gamble with death, leaving it to others to save them. Almost no one commits suicide without letting others know how he or she is feeling. Often this cry for help is given in code. Decoding these distress signals can save lives. |
| Once a person attempts suicide, he or she is suicidal forever. | Fortunately, people who want to kill themselves are suicidal only for a limited time. If they are saved from self-destruction, they can lead useful lives. |
| Improvement following a suicidal crisis means that the suicidal risk is over. | Most suicides occur within 3 months after the beginning of improvement, when the person has the energy to put morbid thoughts and feelings into effect. Relatives and physicians should be especially vigilant during this period. |
| Suicide strikes more often among the rich—or, conversely, it occurs more frequently among the poor. | Suicide strikes all classes and is represented proportionately at all levels of society. |
| Suicide is inherited or runs in a family (that is, is genetically determined). | Suicide risk is not inherited. It is an individual decision and can be prevented. |
| All people who attempt or commit suicide have a mental illness. | Studies of hundreds of genuine suicide notes indicate that although a person who attempts or commits suicide is extremely unhappy, he or she does not necessarily have a mental illness. The overpowering unhappiness may result from a temporary emotional upset, a long and painful illness, or a complete loss of hope. |

*Source:* US Department of Health and Human Resources.

# ▶ Emotional Injury

First aid for an emotional injury means being supportive of people with emotional injuries, whether the injuries are from physical injury or excessive or unbearable strain on the person's emotions.

Emotional first aid often goes hand in hand with physical first aid because a physical injury and the circumstances surrounding it may actually cause emotional injury. On the other hand, emotional injury may occur when there is no physical injury. Emotional injuries usually are not as obvious as physical injuries, but both can be severe and require first aid.

Although most emotional reactions are temporary, lasting only minutes, hours, or, at the most, a few days, they are seriously disabling and may upset others. It is important to know that first aid can be applied to emotional as well as to physical injuries.

## Typical Reactions

With few exceptions, all people experience fear in the face of an emergency. Feeling shaky, perspiring profusely, and becoming nauseated are common. Such reactions are normal and no cause for concern. Most people are able to regain their composure reasonably quickly.

Extensive training is not needed to recognize severe, abnormal reactions. To determine whether a person needs help, find out whether he or she is doing something that makes sense and is able to take care of him- or herself. For the most part, emotional first aid measures are simple and easy to understand Table 23-3 .

However, improvisation is often needed, just as it is in splinting a fracture. Whatever the situation, you will have your own emotional reactions toward the person. These reactions are important; they can enhance or hinder your ability to help the person. Especially when you are tired or worried, you may easily become impatient with the person who seems to be "making a mountain out of a molehill." You may feel resentful toward the person for being a burden. Be on guard against becoming impatient, intolerant, or resentful. People who can see the first aid provider's calmness, confidence, and competence will be reassured.

On the other hand, do not be overly sympathetic or overly solicitous. Excessive sympathy for an incapacitated person can be as harmful as negative feelings. The person needs solid help but does not need to be overwhelmed with pity.

## Table 23-3 Psychological First Aid for Reactions to Emergency Situations

| Reaction | Symptoms | Do ... | Do Not ... |
|---|---|---|---|
| Normal | • Trembling<br>• Muscle tension<br>• Perspiration<br>• Nausea<br>• Mild diarrhea<br>• Urinary frequency<br>• Pounding heart<br>• Rapid breathing<br>• Anxiety | • Give reassurance.<br>• Encourage the person.<br>• Talk with the person.<br>• Observe to see that the person is gaining composure, not losing it. | • Show resentment.<br>• Overdo sympathy. |
| Individual panic (flight reaction) | • Unreasoning attempt to flee<br>• Loss of judgment<br>• Uncontrolled weeping<br>• Wildly running about | • Try kind firmness.<br>• Give the person something warm to eat or drink.<br>• Get help to isolate the person from others, if necessary.<br>• Be empathetic.<br>• Encourage the person to talk.<br>• Be aware of your own limitations. | • Use forceful physical restraint.<br>• Strike the person physically.<br>• Douse the person with water.<br>• Give sedatives. |

© Jones & Bartlett Learning

(Continues)

## Table 23-3 Psychological First Aid for Reactions to Emergency Situations, Continued

| Reaction | Symptoms | Do ... | Do Not ... |
|---|---|---|---|
| Depression (under-active reactions) | • Stands or sits without moving or talking<br>• Vacant expression<br>• Lack of emotional display | • Make contact gently.<br>• Secure a rapport.<br>• Get the person to tell you what happened.<br>• Be empathetic.<br>• Recognize feelings of resentment in the person and yourself.<br>• Give the person a simple, routine task to complete.<br>• Offer warm food or drink. | • Tell the person to "snap out of it."<br>• Overdo sympathy.<br>• Give sedatives.<br>• Argue with the person. |
| Overactive | • Argumentative<br>• Talks rapidly<br>• Jokes inappropriately<br>• Makes endless suggestions<br>• Jumps from one activity to another | • Let the person talk about the situation.<br>• Find the person a job that requires physical effort.<br>• Offer warm food or drink.<br>• Supervision is necessary.<br>• Be aware of your own feelings. | • Suggest that the person is acting abnormally.<br>• Give sedatives.<br>• Argue with the person. |
| Physical (conversion disorder [a mental disorder in which psychological conflict manifests itself as physical symptoms]) | • Severe nausea and vomiting<br>• Cannot use some part of the body | • Show interest in the person.<br>• Find a small job for the person to distract and occupy his or her thoughts.<br>• Make the person comfortable.<br>• Get medical care as soon as possible. | • Tell the person that there is nothing wrong with him or her.<br>• Place blame.<br>• Ridicule the person.<br>• Ignore the disability. |

*Source:* Modified from M51-400-603-1, Department of Nonresident Instruction, Medical Field Service School, Brooke Army Medical Center, Fort Sam Houston, Texas.

## What to Look For

- Aggressive, hostile, or violent behavior, which may be a response to illness or may be a way of coping with feelings of helplessness
- Person standing or sitting in a threatening position (eg, clenched fists)
- Presence of lethal object
- Yelling or verbal threats of harm to others

## What to Do

1. Size up the situation before you do anything. An angry, violent person is ready to fight with anyone who approaches and may be difficult to control. If the scene appears unsafe, **DO NOT** enter. If necessary, contact law enforcement officers.
2. Avoid responding with anger. Many angry or violent people can be calmed by someone who is trained and who appears confident that the person will behave well.
3. Encourage the person to speak directly about the cause of his or her anger. A statement like "I am not sure I understand why you are angry." often brings results. Reassure the person that you are there to help.

**What to Look For**

**What to Do**

4. Notify the police if you are unable to communicate with a person who is dangerous to him- or herself or to others.

5. Confronting a person who is experiencing a behavioral emergency can be a trying and frustrating experience. Use these guidelines if you must try to calm a person who is upset:

   - Acknowledge that the person seems upset, and reiterate that you are there to help.
   - Maintain a comfortable distance.
   - Encourage the person to state what is troubling him or her.
   - **DO NOT** make quick moves.
   - Respond honestly to the person's questions.
   - **DO NOT** threaten, challenge, or argue with a disturbed person.
   - Tell the truth—**DO NOT** lie.
   - **DO NOT** play along with any of a disturbed person's visual or auditory disturbances.
   - Involve trusted family members or friends.
   - Be prepared to stay with the person for an extended period of time.
   - Never leave the person alone.
   - Avoid unnecessary physical contact.
   - Maintain eye contact.

## ▶ Sexual Assault and Rape

The definitions of rape and sexual assault vary widely. *Rape* is generally defined as the criminal act of forcing another person to submit to sexual intercourse. Categories of rape include the following:

- *Acquaintance rape*, which involves people who knew each other before the rape; includes relatives, neighbors, or friends.
- *Date rape*, which takes place within a relationship but without the consent of one person and may involve harm or the threat of harm by the other person.
- *Marital rape*, which occurs when the person and the offender are married to each other.
- *Stranger rape*, which occurs when the person and the offender have no relation to each other.

The person may hesitate to report a rape for various reasons, such as shame, guilt, fear of retaliation, or reluctance to deal with law enforcement officials or the judicial system. The person may even begin to doubt whether a "real" rape occurred. Rape is a traumatic crisis that disrupts the physical, psychological, social, and sexual aspects of the person's life. The most common physical injuries are bruises, black eyes, and cuts.

As a first aid provider, you must be tactful and sensitive with the person. The person may find it extremely difficult to discuss what happened and may feel fear or hostility toward a first aid provider of the opposite sex. Every effort should be made to understand the person's feelings and to respond with kindness and reassurance. The emotional trauma of rape is usually more prolonged and severe than the physical trauma. The attitude shown toward the person during the initial care can have a substantial influence—for good or ill—on future psychological and physical recovery. Convince the person to seek counseling through community resources such as a rape crisis center and to report the crime to the police. Ask the person not to change clothes or to bathe because doing so can alter legal evidence. For the same reason, suggest that the person not urinate, douche, defecate, or wash before being examined by a physician. Care for any injuries incurred during the attack. For more information, see Chapter 22, *Childbirth and Gynecologic Emergencies*.

## ▶ Child Abuse and Neglect

Because <u>child abuse</u> and <u>neglect</u> usually occur in the privacy of the home, no one knows exactly how many children are affected. According to the Administration for Children and Families, approximately 3.6 million cases of child abuse and neglect are reported each year. Of these, 75% involve neglect, 17% involve physical abuse, and 8% involve sexual abuse; 7% of cases also involve other forms of maltreatment, such as emotional abuse, threats, exposure to drugs and alcohol, or lack of supervision. Child abuse and neglect can cause permanent damage to a child's physical, emotional, and mental development. The physical effects can include damage to the brain, vital organs, eyes, ears, arms, and legs, which, in turn, can result in mental retardation, blindness, deafness, or loss of a limb. At its most serious, abuse or neglect can result in a child's death.

Child abuse and neglect are usually divided into four major categories: physical abuse, neglect, sexual abuse, and emotional maltreatment. Each has recognizable characteristics, and all may be encountered by a first aid provider. Still, children who have been mistreated are often afraid to tell anyone because they think they will be blamed or that no one will believe them. Other parents or teachers also tend to overlook symptoms because they do not want to face the truth. The longer a child continues to be abused or is left to deal with the situation on his or her own, the less likely he or she is to make a full recovery.

The National Center on Child Abuse and Neglect has set forth physical and behavioral indicators of child abuse and neglect. The list is not intended to be exhaustive; many more indicators exist than can be included. The presence of a single indicator does not necessarily prove that child abuse or neglect has occurred Table 23-4.

However, the repeated occurrence of an indicator, the presence of several indicators in combination, or the appearance of serious injury should alert you to the possibility of child abuse Figure 23-1.

**Table 23-4 Physical and Behavioral Indicators of Child Abuse and Neglect**

| Type of Child Abuse or Neglect | Physical Indicators | Behavioral Indicators |
|---|---|---|
| Physical Abuse | • Unexplained bruises and welts on face, lips, mouth, torso, back, buttocks, and/or thighs in various stages of healing<br>• Clustered injuries on several different surface areas; formed by regular patterns reflecting the shape of the articles used to inflict the injury (electric cord, belt buckle)<br>• Regularly appearing injuries after an absence, weekend, or vacation, especially about the trunk and buttocks<br>• Old bruises in addition to fresh ones<br>• Unexplained burns (such as those from a cigar or cigarette) especially on soles, palms, back, or buttocks<br>• Immersion burns (socklike, glovelike, doughnut shaped on buttocks or genitalia)<br>• Pattern burns as from an electric burner or iron, for example<br>• Rope burns on arms, legs, neck, or torso<br>• Unexplained fractures (particularly if multiple) to skull, nose, and/or facial structures in various stages of healing | • Wary of adult contacts<br>• Apprehensive when other children cry<br>• Behavioral extremes: aggressiveness or withdrawal<br>• Frightened of parents<br>• Afraid to go home<br>• Reports injury by parents<br>• Acts apathetic and does not cry despite injuries<br>• Has been seen by emergency personnel for related complaints<br>• Was injured several days before medical attention was sought |

## Table 23-4  Physical and Behavioral Indicators of Child Abuse and Neglect, Continued

| Type of Child Abuse or Neglect | Physical Indicators | Behavioral Indicators |
|---|---|---|
| | • Multiple or spiral fractures<br>• Unexplained lacerations or abrasions to mouth, lips, gums, eyes, and/or external genitalia | |
| Physical Neglect | • Consistent hunger, poor hygiene, inappropriate dress<br>• Consistent lack of supervision, especially in dangerous activities or for extended periods of time<br>• Unattended physical conditions or medical needs<br>• Abandonment | • Begs, steals food<br>• Extended stays at school (early arrival and late departure)<br>• Constant fatigue, listlessness, or falling asleep in class<br>• Alcohol or drug abuse<br>• Delinquency (for example, thefts)<br>• States there is no caretaker |
| Sexual Abuse | • Difficulty walking or sitting<br>• Torn, stained, or bloody underclothing<br>• Pain or itching in genital area<br>• Bruises or bleeding in external genitalia or vaginal or anal areas<br>• Sexually transmitted disease, especially in preteens<br>• Pregnancy | • Unwillingness to change for gym or participate in physical education class<br>• Withdrawal, fantasizing, or infantile behavior<br>• Bizarre, sophisticated, or unusual sexual behavior or knowledge<br>• Poor peer relationships<br>• Delinquency or truancy<br>• Reports sexual assault by caretaker |
| Emotional Maltreatment | • Speech disorders<br>• Lags in physical development<br>• Failure to thrive | • Habit disorders (for example, sucking, biting, rocking)<br>• Conduct disorders (for example, antisocial, destructive)<br>• Neurotic traits (sleep disorders, inhibition of play)<br>• Psychoneurotic reactions (hysteria, obsession, compulsion, phobias, hypochondria)<br>• Behavior extremes: compliant, passive-aggressive, demanding<br>• Overly adaptive behavior: inappropriately adult or inappropriately infantile<br>• Developmental lags (mental, emotional)<br>• Attempted suicide |

*Source:* Data from National Center on Child Abuse and Neglect.

Courtesy of Ronald Dieckmann, MD.

Courtesy of Ronald Dieckmann, MD.

Courtesy of Ronald Dieckmann, MD.

**Figure 23-1**

**A.** The face is a common target for physical abuse. **B.** Stocking-glove burns of the hands and feet are almost always inflicted injuries. **C.** Rope or cord bruises are a commonly inflicted injury.

| What to Look For | What to Do |
|---|---|
| The best way to check for signs of abuse is to be alert to any unexplainable changes in a child's body or behavior.<br>• Physical abuse:<br>  • Any injury (bruise, burn, fracture, abdominal or head injury) that cannot be explained<br>• Sexual abuse:<br>  • Fearful behavior (nightmares, depression, unusual fears, attempts to run away)<br>  • Abdominal pain, bedwetting, urinary tract infection, genital pain or bleeding, sexually transmitted disease<br>  • Extreme sexual behavior that seems inappropriate for the child's age<br>• Emotional abuse:<br>  • Sudden change in self-confidence<br>  • Headaches or stomachaches with no medical cause<br>  • Abnormal fears, increased nightmares<br>  • Attempts to run away<br>• Emotional neglect:<br>  • Failure to gain weight (especially in infants)<br>  • Desperately affectionate behavior<br>  • Large appetite and stealing of food | 1. Care for the neglected infant or child. Give appropriate first aid for injuries.<br>2. **DO NOT** accuse parents or caregivers, especially at the scene.<br>3. Report any suspected abuse to the local welfare and social service agency responsible for investigating the issue. Report what you saw and heard, not what you think. |

## ▶ Domestic Violence

Domestic violence, also known as partner abuse, spouse abuse, or battering, occurs when one person inflicts injury—either emotional or physical—upon another person with whom they had or have a relationship. It occurs between spouses and partners, parents and children, children and grandparents, and brothers and sisters. Domestic violence may be the single most common source of serious injury to women.

---

### FYI

**Are You Being Abused?**

Just one "yes" answer to these questions means you are involved in an abusive relationship. If so, you are not alone and you have choices. No one deserves to be abused. Does your partner:
  • Threaten to hurt you or your children?
  • Say it is your fault if he or she hits you; then promise it will not happen again (but it does)?
  • Put you down in public?
  • Keep you from contacting family or friends?
  • Throw you down or push, hit, choke, kick, or slap you?
  • Force you to have sex when you do not want to?

*Source:* American College of Obstetricians and Gynecologists, www.acog.org.

### What to Look For

- Bruises or injuries on the head, neck, or chest
- Type or extent of an injury that is inconsistent with the person's explanation
- Substantial delay between when the injury occurred and when the person sought help
- Injuries during pregnancy
- Evidence of alcohol or drug abuse
- Needs medical care as a result of a suicide attempt or rape

### What to Do

1. If you are not aware of immediate danger, but you suspect abuse, check with welfare and social service agencies. Most cities and counties, according to state law, will investigate and protect vulnerable adults. The issue cannot be remedied until it is reported.
2. Call the police if a person is in imminent danger.
3. Treat any injuries.

## ▶ Elder Abuse

Elder abuse ranges from passive neglect to active assault and includes emotional abuse. Some physically abused older people report having had something thrown at them; some are pushed, grabbed, or shoved; others are slapped, bitten, or kicked. Elder abuse occurs most often in women older than 75 years. Signs of abuse may be quite obvious or subtle. Burns are a common form of elder abuse.

### What to Look For

- Physical injury:
  - Bruises, cuts, burn or rope marks, and broken bones that cannot be explained
  - Comments about being battered
  - The refusal of the caregiver to allow you to visit the older person alone
- Lack of physical care:
  - Dehydration, malnourishment, weight loss, and poor hygiene
  - Bed sores, soiled bedding
  - Unmet medical needs
  - Comments about being mistreated
- Unusual behaviors:
  - Agitation, withdrawal, fear or anxiety, apathy
  - Reports of being treated improperly

### What to Do

1. If you are not aware of immediate danger, but you suspect abuse, check with welfare and social service agencies. Most cities and counties, according to state law, will investigate and protect vulnerable adults. The issue cannot be remedied until it is reported.
2. If you suspect elder abuse in an institutional setting, such as a nursing home, report your concerns to your state long-term care ombudsman. Each state has a long-term care ombudsman to investigate and address nursing home complaints.
3. Call the police if a person is in imminent danger.
4. First aid includes calling 9-1-1 when needed and treating any injuries.

## ▶ Ready for Review

- Behavior that leads to violence or other inappropriate activities is known as a behavioral emergency.
- Depression is one of the most common and treatable of all mental illness.
- Suicide in the United States is increasingly an issue for adolescents, college-age students, and older people.
- First aid for an emotional injury means being supportive of people with emotional injuries, whether the injuries are a result of physical injury or excessive or unbearable strain on the person's emotions.
- Because child abuse and neglect usually occur in the privacy of the home, no one knows exactly how many children are affected.
- Domestic violence may be the single most common source of serious injury to women.
- The types of physical abuse of older people vary from passive neglect to active assault.

## ▶ Vital Vocabulary

**behavioral emergency** Situations in which a person exhibits abnormal behavior that is unacceptable or cannot be tolerated by the person themselves, or by family, friends, or the community.

**child abuse** A general term applying to all forms of child abuse and neglect.

**depression** A persistent mood of sadness, despair, and discouragement.

**domestic violence** Injury (emotional or physical) that a person inflicts upon another person with whom they had or have a relationship.

**elder abuse** Any action on the part of an older person's family member, caregiver, or other associated person that takes advantage of the older person, his or her property, or emotional state.

**neglect** Refusal or failure on the part of the caregiver to provide life necessities.

**suicide** Any willful act that ends one's own life.

## ▶ Assessment in Action

Your good friend has been married for about 3 years. He is normally a quiet, reserved person who cares deeply for others. Lately, you have seen him change; he has been argumentative, jokes inappropriately, and appears to have a hard time concentrating. He no longer engages in several of his hobbies and does little else when not at work. You then find out that he separated from his wife about 1 month ago.

*Directions:* Circle Yes if you agree with the statement; circle No if you disagree.

Yes   No   **1.** Your friend is exhibiting an overactive reaction to his situation.

Yes   No   **2.** You should avoid being too argumentative with your friend.

Yes   No   **3.** You should not give sedatives to calm him down.

Yes   No   **4.** Supervision and perhaps even some type of professional therapy may be helpful for your friend.

Yes   No   **5.** Letting him talk to you about his situation will make things worse.

## ▶ Check Your Knowledge

*Directions:* Circle Yes if you agree with the statement; circle No if you disagree.

Yes   No   **1.** Abnormal behavior may be due to a psychological condition or a physical condition.

Yes   No   **2.** Low blood glucose in a person with diabetes can affect behavior.

Yes   No   **3.** Depression cannot be treated.

Yes   No   **4.** The rate of suicide for men is higher than the rate for women.

Yes   No   **5.** Most people who talk about suicide are not serious.

Yes   No   **6.** The only way for you to react to an aggressive person is with anger.

Yes   No   **7.** A failure to gain weight may be a sign of emotional neglect in an infant.

Yes   No   **8.** Women are rarely subjected to domestic violence.

Yes   No   **9.** Burns are a common form of elder abuse.

Yes   No   **10.** Feeling shaky during an emergency is not normal.

# Wilderness First Aid

**24**

## Wilderness First Aid

At some time, anyone living, working, traveling, or recreating in remote locations will probably encounter dangers unfamiliar to most people. Regardless of precautions, injuries and illnesses happen.

The term *wilderness,* as defined by the Wilderness Medical Society (WMS), is a remote geographic location more than 1 hour from definitive medical care. According to that definition, wilderness could describe a variety of situations, including the following:

- Recreation (for example, fishing, camping, hiking, hunting)
- Occupations in remote areas (such as farming, forestry, fishing)
- Urban areas with overwhelmed emergency medical services (EMS) after a natural or manmade disaster
- Residences in remote communities (such as farms, ranches, vacation homes)
- Developing countries

The millions of people in these wildernesses should be as medically prepared as possible to manage a condition for others and for themselves. First aid with a wilderness focus seems indispensable in the following situations:

1. Occurrence of injuries and illnesses in the outdoors, where adverse environmental conditions such as heat, cold, altitude, rain, or snow may be a major concern

2. Delay of definitive medical care for hours or days because of location, bad weather, lack of transportation, or lack of communication

3. Occurrence of injuries and illnesses not commonly seen in urban or suburban areas (for example, altitude illness, frostbite, wild animal encounters)

4. The need for advanced medical care (for example, reduction of some dislocations, wound cleansing)

5. Limited first aid supplies and equipment

6. Need to make difficult decisions (cardiopulmonary resuscitation [CPR], evacuation) in a remote setting

Most first aid texts and training courses describe situations in which EMS response is expected within 10 to 20 minutes. In these cases, the first aid provider usually helps for only a few minutes before an ambulance arrives. When the person is transported to a medical facility, the first aid provider's job is finished.

Wilderness first aid is similar to that needed in urban situations, except that extra or extended skills are needed. Consideration must be given to time, distance, and availability of medical care. A first aid provider in the wilderness may have to remain many hours or days with a sick or injured person.

# ▶ Cardiac Arrest

Because heart activity must be restored within a short time (which requires defibrillation and medications) for a person with cardiac arrest to survive, CPR has limited use in a wilderness or remote setting, especially if severe trauma such as massive head or chest injury, severe blood loss, or a severed spinal cord accompanies the cardiac arrest. In addition, CPR is difficult to continue during a wilderness evacuation.

The WMS recommends *stopping* CPR if:

- The person revives.
- The rescuers are exhausted.
- The rescuers are in danger.
- The person is turned over to higher-level trained personnel.
- The person does not respond to prolonged (about 30 minutes) resuscitation efforts.

The State of Alaska Cold Injuries Guidelines, the WMS, and the National Association of EMS Physicians (NAEMSP) say that CPR should not be started if:

- The person has been submerged in cold water for more than 1 hour.
- The person has a core temperature of less than 60°F (15°C).
- The person has obvious signs of death or fatal injuries (eg, rigor mortis, decapitation, decomposition).
- The person is frozen (eg, ice formation in the airway).
- The person has a chest wall that is so stiff that compressions are impossible.
- Rescuers are exhausted or in danger.
- Definitive care is not available within 3 hours.

## CPR for People with Hypothermia

The person with severe hypothermia must be handled very gently. The cold heart is very prone to spontaneous ventricular fibrillation due to any movement. Even cautious movement of the person may induce ventricular fibrillation.

It is difficult to assess breathing in an unresponsive person with hypothermia. If the person is unresponsive and not breathing, you should begin CPR. **DO NOT** wait to check the person's temperature, and **DO NOT** wait until the person is rewarmed, to start CPR. Prevent further heat loss by removing the person's wet clothes; insulate and shield the person from wind and additional cold exposure. Avoid rough handling and activate the EMS system as soon as possible. Continue CPR until EMS arrives. In a person with severe hypothermia, CPR can be delayed ("scoop and run") and can be given intermittently during evacuation if it is not possible or safe to perform continuous CPR. CPR can be given for several hours, if necessary. Deliver chest compressions at 100 to 120 beats per minute.

## CPR for People in an Avalanche

Avalanche-related deaths are on the rise in North America due to winter recreational activities (eg, backcountry skiing and snowboarding, helicopter and snowcat skiing, snowmobiling, out-of-bounds skiing, ice climbing, mountaineering, and snowshoeing). The most common causes of avalanche-related death are suffocation (hypoxia), injury, hypothermia, or a combination of these three. If the person is unresponsive and is not breathing, begin CPR. Use an automated external defibrillator (AED) as soon as it becomes available. **DO NOT** attempt resuscitation in a person buried for 35 minutes or longer with an airway that is obstructed by snow or ice.

### CPR for Drowning

First aid providers should give CPR as soon as an unresponsive submersed person is removed from the water. If you are alone, give 5 sets (about 2 minutes) of CPR before leaving the person to activate the EMS system and get an AED. If you are not alone, send someone to activate the EMS system and get an AED while you continue giving CPR. An AED should be used as soon as it becomes available.

People with only respiratory arrest usually respond after a few rescue breaths. Rescue breathing can be started once the person is in shallow water; however, chest compressions are difficult to perform in water and may not be effective. There is no need to attempt to clear the airway of water because only a small amount of water is aspirated by most drowning people and is absorbed by the body. **DO NOT** try to remove water by performing abdominal thrusts.

If vomiting occurs during CPR, turn the person to the side and remove the vomitus using a finger or a cloth. If a spinal injury is suspected, the person should be turned as a unit with no twisting. A suggestion is to keep the person's nose and navel pointed in the same direction as they are turned.

### CPR for People Struck by Lightning

The National Weather Service estimates an average of 49 deaths occur from lightning strikes in the United States each year. The main cause of death in these people is cardiac arrest. When multiple people are struck at the same time by lightning, rescuers should give the highest priority to people who are unresponsive and not breathing by beginning CPR. An AED should be used as soon as it becomes available.

### ▶ Dislocations

In a wilderness situation, reducing (a technical term that means aligning) some dislocated joints is recommended. The WMS gives the following

reasons for reducing a joint dislocation quickly after it happens:

1. Reduction is easier immediately after the injury, before swelling develops.
2. It is easier to transport a person after reduction.
3. Reduction dramatically relieves pain.
4. The joint can be stabilized and better protected.
5. Reduction lessens the possibility of jeopardizing circulation in the extremity. (If the blood supply is cut off, gangrene could develop, which could result in amputation.)
6. Several simple dislocations can be reduced using simple and safe techniques.

A dislocation is considered simple if it involves the anterior (front) part of the shoulder, a finger, or the patella (the knee cap, not the knee itself). **DO NOT** attempt to reduce a dislocated elbow or hip. Elbow and hip dislocations resemble fractures; reduction techniques for those joints are painful and can cause further injury.

### Shoulder Dislocation

Anterior (frontal) shoulder joint dislocations account for more than 90% of shoulder dislocations Figure 24-1.

There are several methods for reducing a shoulder dislocation; two of the easiest methods are

Figure 24-1

The shoulder almost always dislocates anteriorly. Note the absence of the normal rounded appearance of the shoulder.

## What to Look For

- The person is in extreme pain.
- Because the problem often recurs, the person can identify the dislocation if it has happened before.
- The upper arm is held away from the body in various positions and cannot be brought next to the body into a sling-type position.
- The person is unable to touch the uninjured shoulder with the hand of the injured extremity.
- Compare the injured shoulder with the uninjured one. The shoulder joint will appear squared off or flattened and a prominence may be seen or felt in the front of the shoulder.

## What to Do

*Traction and external rotation method (easiest and most effective method)* **Figure 24-2** :

1. Gently but steadily pull the arm out to the side while another rescuer provides countertraction against the chest wall, just below the armpit, using straps, a sleeping bag, clothing, or a flotation vest. (If there is only one rescuer, countertraction can be applied by the rescuer's padded or bare feet against the person's chest [not armpits].)
2. Tell the person to relax. Massage may help.
3. As you pull, gently and steadily rotate the arm one-half to two-thirds of the way up to a baseball-throwing position (take 5 to 15 minutes). Keep the arm in that position; the muscles will fatigue within 15 minutes, allowing the joint to slip back into place.
4. After successful reduction, stabilize the arm with a sling and swathe (binder).

*Simple hanging traction method:*

1. Lay the person face down on a surface high enough so the injured arm can hang over the side. Place some cushioning (a folded towel or clothing) under the armpit, between the arm and the surface **Figure 24-3** .
2. Attach a 5- to 10-lb (2- to 5-kg) weight to the person's lower arm, between the elbow and the wrist. Cushion and strap the weight, being careful not to impede circulation. Keep the person's palm facing inward.
3. It may take up to 60 minutes to stretch and tire the muscles, allowing the joint to pop back in.
4. After successful reduction, stabilize the arm with a sling and swathe. Secure a sling and swathe (binder) using the method shown in Chapter 16, *Splinting Extremities*.

© Jones & Bartlett Learning

**A**   **B**

**Figure 24-2**

Applying traction **(A)** and external rotation **(B)** to an anterior shoulder dislocation.

**Figure 24-3**

Simple hanging traction to reduce an anterior shoulder dislocation.

discussed here. With either method, stop if pain increases or resistance is met. Do not try pulling on the person's arm with your foot in the person's armpit. Check the circulation, sensation, and movement of the hand before and after reducing.

## Finger Dislocation

The fingers are injured easily, and even a minor injury may cause a dislocation **Figure 24-4**.

Often, people with this injury can reduce the finger dislocation themselves. In a remote location, you should try to reduce a finger dislocation only once. **DO NOT** attempt to reduce a dislocation at the base of the index finger or at the base of the thumb—those areas may require surgery for reduction.

**Figure 24-4**

Dislocation of the finger joint. Do not be tempted to try to "pop" the joint back into place.

## What to Look For

- Deformity and inability to use or bend the finger
- Pain and swelling
- An abnormal position of the two adjoining bones; looks like a lump at the joint

## What to Do

To reduce a finger dislocation, use one of two methods.

*Method 1* **Figure 24-5** :

1. Hold the end of the finger with one hand and the rest of the finger in the other.
2. Gently hyperextend the dislocated joint (bend it backwards).
3. Pull gentle traction.
4. Push the dislocated bone into place.
5. Unbend the finger.
6. Buddy tape it to the next finger.
7. Splint the finger in the position of function (fingers and hand in a cupping shape, as though holding a baseball).

*Method 2:*

1. Hold the end of the finger with one hand and the rest of the finger in the other.
2. Pull the end of the finger first in the direction it is pointing, then, while maintaining traction, gently swing it back into the normal anatomic position.
3. Regardless of whether the reduction is successful, stabilize the joint in the position of function (fingers and hand in a cupping shape, as though holding a baseball) by the buddy-taping method—using adhesive tape to secure the injured finger to an adjacent uninjured finger.

© Jones & Bartlett Learning.

**Figure 24-5**

Reducing a finger dislocation.

## Knee Cap Dislocation

For most dislocated knee caps, you should only apply an ice pack and use a splint to stabilize the leg in place as you found it. For remote locations, however, always consider reducing a dislocated knee cap by using the method described in the following table. All dislocations, whether successfully reduced in the field or not, should be seen by a physician.

## What to Look For

- Some people have recurrent dislocations of the patella (knee cap) and can tell you what is wrong.
- The patella has moved to the outside of the knee joint (large bulge under the skin) with the leg bent **Figure 24-6** .
- The person is in pain.
- Compare the injured portion with the patella on the other leg.

## What to Do

1. Slowly straighten the knee as you gently push the knee cap back into its normal position. Straightening alone may replace the knee cap.
2. Stabilize the leg straight. The person usually can walk on the injured leg.
3. With the knee extended (straight) and stabilized, the person may be able to walk well enough for self-evacuation. Because of the heavy physical demands and usually higher altitudes in the backcountry, carrying a person can take 8 to 16 rescuers rotating the task. In the wilderness, a ski pole or a tree branch makes a good walking aid. Helicopter evacuation usually is not justified for a knee cap dislocation.
4. Seek follow-up care from a physician.

Figure 24-6

A dislocated patella typically will appear with the patella displaced lateral to the knee and with the knee moderately flexed.

## ▶ Spinal Injury

The necessity of stabilizing the spine after trauma is well known. A person with a cervical spinal injury who is moved without stabilization may become quadriplegic or die. In urban settings, first aid providers should have the person remain as still as possible and wait for EMS to arrive. **DO NOT** apply a cervical collar.

In the wilderness, spinal stabilization may not always be necessary—such a procedure can be difficult, impractical, impossible, or even dangerous during prolonged evacuation in severe environments. For example, an injured climber far above the timberline could wait for hours or days, depending on the distance someone has to go for help. The injured climber would have to wait in a hostile environment and risk death from avalanche, rockfall, or hypothermia. However, if the person were cleared of a spinal injury, he or she could self-evacuate.

Spinal fractures can be difficult to determine, even by physicians reading x-rays. Suspect a spinal injury when a significant cause of injury (ie, a vehicle crash involving ejection, a rollover, or high speed; a head injury causing unresponsiveness; penetrating wounds of the neck or trunk; diving into shallow water; fall from a height; collisions involving recreational vehicles or bicycles) has occurred.

To clear a spinal injury in the wilderness, determine if the person is reliable or unreliable. A reliable person meets the following criteria:

- Alert, knows name and where he or she is
- Not intoxicated by drugs or alcohol
- Calm, cooperative
- Has no painful, distracting injury

An unreliable person has one or more of the following criteria:

- Unresponsive; altered mental status
- Intoxicated by drugs or alcohol
- Combative, confused
- Has a painful, distracting injury

| What to Look For | What to Do |
|---|---|
| A reliable person with:<br>• Back pain and leg numbness and tingling<br>• Tenderness/pain when you run fingers all the way down the spine (if possible); press each bump of vertebrae and on the depressions produced on each side when you touch or push on the spinal bones. | When a spinal injury is suspected:<br>1. Send for medical help. **DO NOT** attempt to evacuate the person. Wait for trained rescuers with proper equipment.<br>2. Leave the person on the ground. Cover to prevent heat loss by log rolling the person, keeping the nose and navel pointing in the same direction, and place insulating materials under and over the person. |

| What to Look For | What to Do |
|---|---|
| A reliable person who fails the following tests for sensation and movement (test all four extremities):<br>• Upper body<br>  • Pinch several fingers with the person's eyes closed and ask, "Can you feel this? Where am I touching you?"<br>  • Ask, "Can you wiggle your fingers?"<br>  • Ask, "Can you squeeze my hands?"<br>• Lower body<br>  • Pinch several toes with the person's eyes closed or looking away and ask, "Can you feel this? Where am I touching you?"<br>  • Ask, "Can you wiggle your toes?<br>  • Ask, "Can you push and pull your feet simultaneously against my hands?" | 1. Stabilize the person against movement. Improvised cervical collars (ie, blanket, SAM Splint) alone are inadequate.<br>  • Place the person's head between your knees, as this is less tiring than kneeling and holding the person's head with your hands.<br>  • An alternative method is to improvise sandbags by placing dirt, sand, or rocks cushioned with clothing in stuffed sacks or plastic bags and securely place them on both sides of the person's head. |
| A reliable person who is injured and:<br>• Is alert, not intoxicated, and has no distracting injuries.<br>• Does not report neck pain or neurological symptoms (ie, tingling, numbness).<br>• Has no neck tenderness when felt, no loss of sensation when fingers and toes are pinched, can move the fingers and toes, and can squeeze your hands and push and pull their feet against your hands.<br>• Can rotate his or her neck 30° left and right when requested. | 1. Suspect no spinal injury.<br>2. Treat other injuries (ie, wounds, bruises, fractures). |
| An unreliable person who has a significant cause of injury | Assume that a spinal injury exists. Stabilize the person against movement. Have the person remain as still as possible |

# ▶ Splinting Femur Fractures

A person with a femur fracture can easily have 2 quarts (about 2 L) of blood loss in the thigh and develop massive swelling. Because EMS personnel have the training, experience, and equipment, it is best to let them apply traction splints, if possible. However, first aid providers can use the methods in Chapter 16, *Splinting Extremities*, to stabilize a femur fracture.

## Q&A

**Do improvised traction splints work?**

Although the advantages of stabilizing a broken femur by applying a traction splint are cited in various manuals, there are dissenting opinions about the effectiveness of improvised traction splints. For example, the Outward Bound organization says, "Improvised traction splints for field use employing ski poles, canoe paddles, and other pieces of equipment are usually more architecturally interesting than medically useful. The simplest, safest, and most universal splint is firm immobilization on a long board or litter without traction." The WMS suggests stabilizing the fractured extremity to the uninjured leg with adequate padding and placing padding behind the knee to create a slight bend, which is more comfortable than being straight.

## ▶ Avalanche Burial

Avalanches are falling masses of snow that may also contain rocks, soil, or ice. Since the early 1970s, the number of deaths caused by avalanches has increased rapidly as a result of the tremendous growth in backcountry winter mountain travel (eg, skiing, mountaineering, snowmobiling). According to the American Avalanche Association and Avalanche Canada, there are approximately 37 deaths annually in the United States and 13 in Canada.

Snow sets up solid after an avalanche. It is almost impossible for people to dig themselves out, even if they are buried under less than a foot of snow. The pressure of several feet of snow sometimes is so great that people are unable to expand their chests to breathe. A completely buried person has a poor chance of survival. During the first 15 minutes, more people are found alive than dead. Between 16 and 30 minutes after an avalanche, an equal number are found dead and alive (50% chance of survival). After 30 minutes, more are found dead than alive.

Most people buried by an avalanche die of suffocation; therefore, in the absence of fatal injuries, speed of extrication from the avalanche and existence of an air pocket are the main factors that determine survival of a buried person. There are no documented reports of anyone surviving a burial of 7 feet (2 m) or more.

---

### FYI

**Avalanche Rescue**

If you survive an avalanche, follow these steps to find other people:

1. With a piece of equipment, clothing, or tree branch, mark the spot where a person was last seen.
2. Search the area below the last-seen point for any clues of the person. Make probes into likely burial spots with a ski, ski pole, or tree limb.
3. If beacons were being used, all survivors must immediately switch their units to the receive mode and listen for a beeping sound from buried beacons.
4. If a second avalanche is possible, place one person in a safe location to shout a warning so rescuers can flee to safety.
5. Send a person to notify the ski patrol immediately if you are near a ski area and there are several rescuers. If you are the only rescuer, do a fast surface search for clues before leaving to notify the ski patrol. In remote backcountry, all survivors should remain and search until they cannot or should not continue.

Rescue transceivers or beacons are an efficient way of locating people. Organized probe lines have found more people than any other method, but because of the time involved, most of the people were dead. Trained search dogs can locate buried people quickly, but they often are brought to the scene only after long periods of burial. One trained dog can search more effectively than 30 searchers.

---

| What to Look For | What to Do |
|---|---|
| Avalanches kill and injure in two ways:<br>• The first is from the serious injury the person acquires while tumbling down an avalanche path. Trees, rocks, cliffs, and the wrenching action of snow are hazards. About one-third of all deaths are related to trauma, especially trauma to the head and neck.<br>• The second way is snow burial, which causes suffocation in the other two-thirds of avalanche deaths. Inhaled snow clogs the mouth and nose, and people can suffocate quickly if they are buried with the airway already blocked. | After you have first checked for further avalanche danger and then found a person, follow these steps:<br>1. Quickly free the person's head, chest, and stomach.<br>2. Send for help.<br>3. Clear the person's airway and check breathing.<br>4. If not breathing, begin CPR.<br>5. Check for severe bleeding.<br>6. Examine for and stabilize a spinal injury.<br>7. Treat for hypothermia. |

## ▶ Altitude Illness

If you live in or visit mountainous regions, you need to know about altitude illness. Altitude illness is not simply an exotic affliction of mountaineers but is a common environmental risk to which millions of people are exposed, often without adequate knowledge.

Altitude illnesses actually are a spectrum of a single problem, <u>hypoxia</u>. Hypoxia occurs when the body's tissues do not have enough oxygen. Altitude illnesses include acute mountain sickness (AMS), high-altitude pulmonary edema (HAPE), and high-altitude cerebral edema (HACE) `Table 24-1`.

The least serious altitude illness is AMS, which affects about one in four people from lower elevations who visit areas 6,000 to 12,000 feet (1,829 to 3,658 m) above sea level. Such elevations are common at ski resorts and on mountain hiking trails.

The actual incidence of altitude illness varies with rate of ascent and altitude attained. A study published in the *Annals of Emergency Medicine* cited about 67% of climbers on Mt. Rainier in Washington have at least mild AMS because of rapid ascent to a moderately higher altitude. The incidence of AMS in a study of Colorado skiers at lower altitudes (usually one day's ascent from Denver or lower) was only 15% to 40%.

Although anyone can get altitude illness, certain factors increase the risk. Under similar conditions, different people sometimes respond quite differently to altitude. For most people, at least four factors deter-mine whether they will be sick or well at a higher altitude: (1) the speed of ascent (the slower the climb, the fewer the symptoms); (2) the altitude reached (the higher one goes, the more likely one will become ill); (3) health at the time (malnutrition, dehydration, fatigue, and any of several illnesses increase the risk); and (4) individual differences and genetic influences.

Altitude illness occurs because oxygen levels decrease as elevation increases, and it takes a few days to adapt to the thinner air. At 11,500 feet (3,505 m), the amount of oxygen in the air is about 65% the amount at sea level, so the body struggles to maintain normal levels of oxygen. As the person breathes more deeply, he or she "blows off" more carbon dioxide than normal, creating a more alkaline (less acidic) condition in the body, which in turn causes altitude illnesses.

It is important to recognize the symptoms of altitude illness and take steps to treat it. In a small number of people, acute altitude illness can progress to HAPE, in which fluid builds up in the lungs, or HACE, in which fluid collects in the brain. HAPE and HACE occur when

## Table 24-1 Characteristics of Altitude Illnesses

| | AMS | HAPE | HACE |
|---|---|---|---|
| Elevation | Above 8,000 ft (2,438 m) | Usually above 10,000 ft (3,048 m) | Above 12,000 ft (3,658 m) |
| Time after ascent | 1 to 2 days | 3 to 4 days, possibly later | 4 to 7 days, possibly later |
| Cause and symptoms | Symptoms of hypoxia: headache, sleep disturbance, fatigue, shortness of breath, dizziness, loss of appetite, vomiting | Symptoms of fluid in the lungs: shortness of breath, dry cough, mild chest pain, weakness, insomnia, rapid pulse, cyanosis, rales (crackles) or gurgling sounds | Symptoms of increased fluid and pressure in the brain: severe headache (unrelieved), vomiting, Cheyne-Stokes breathing (irregular breathing pattern that includes periods of apnea [no breathing]), ataxia (irregular gait or lack of coordination), unconsciousness |
| First aid | • Stop ascending or return to a lower altitude.<br>• Drink fluids.<br>• Rest.<br>• Take aspirin or ibuprofen.<br>• Take acetazolamide.<br>• If you are trained, give high-flow supplemental oxygen, if available. | • Descend at least 2,000 ft (610 m).<br>• Seek medical attention.<br>• **DO NOT** go down alone.<br>• **DO NOT** delay descent.<br>• If immediate descent is not possible:<br>  • Give high-flow supplemental oxygen, if available and you are trained.<br>  • Use a portable hyperbaric chamber, if available and you are trained. | • Descend 4,000 ft (1,219 m).<br>• Seek medical attention.<br>• **DO NOT** go down alone.<br>• **DO NOT** delay descent.<br>• Give high-flow supplemental oxygen, if available and you are trained.<br>• Use a portable hyperbaric chamber, if available and you are trained. |

reduced oxygen causes capillary leakage and swelling of body tissues. Although they are uncommon, both conditions can be fatal in less than 12 hours.

At 18,000 feet (5,486 m), humans reach their ceiling and cannot stay for more than a few weeks. Any person at sea level who is quickly taken to 20,000 feet (6,096 m) will be almost incapacitated in less than half an hour, and death will occur soon thereafter.

## What to Look For

The following symptoms (often mistaken for a cold, flu, or hangover) typically occur during the first 12 hours:

- Headache (most common symptom)
- Loss of appetite
- Nausea
- Insomnia
- Fatigue
- Shortness of breath with exertion

Three-fourths of all people who travel from sea level to above 8,000 feet (2,438 m) have at least one symptom (usually a headache), and the rest have two or more symptoms.

## What to Do

1. Seek medical help if any of the following more serious symptoms appear:
   - Persistent cough
   - Shortness of breath while resting
   - Noisy breathing
   - Loss of balance
   - Confusion
   - Vomiting
2. Have the person rest and let the body acclimatize for a few days.
3. If the person recently ascended to above 6,000 feet (1,829 m) and does not feel better in 1 to 2 days, he or she should see a physician.
4. If it is not possible for the person to see a physician and symptoms continue, the person should descend 2,000 to 3,000 feet (610 to 914 m), rest, and drink plenty of fluids. Aspirin or a similar pain reliever can be taken for a mild headache.
5. If rest and over-the-counter (OTC) medications do not provide relief, consult a physician, who might administer oxygen or prescribe medication.
6. If HACE or HAPE is suspected, early descent is wise, because these conditions are serious. The next best step after descent is to breathe additional oxygen so that the inspired oxygen pressure equals that at sea level. This will relieve the headache and make breathing easier.

## FYI

### Preventing Altitude Illness

You can take several measures to lower your risk of getting altitude sickness. Start slowly and avoid overexerting yourself. If possible, gain altitude slowly to allow your body to adjust. By going easy, you allow your body to acclimatize; that is, adjust to different conditions. Simply put, your body becomes more efficient at using oxygen. Unfortunately, the effects of acclimatization do not last after you return to your normal altitude. You must repeat the process whenever you return to higher elevations.

If you cannot or will not take the time, protective medications are available by prescription. Acetazolamide (Diamox) has been effectively used to prevent AMS for more than 30 years. Acetazolamide also seems to prevent HAPE and HACE, although that is almost impossible to prove because HAPE and HACE are rare.

Side effects of acetazolamide include increased urination and tingling or numbness in the fingers and toes. If you are allergic to sulfa drugs, you may be allergic to acetazolamide. Also, you should wear a sunscreen with a sun protection factor (also called SPF) of at least 15 while taking the drug, since it may increase the risk of sunburn.

Acetazolamide is effective for most lowlanders going to moderate altitudes and perhaps for high-altitude residents returning after a short stay at low altitude. It has been called an artificial acclimatizer. Just how much acetazolamide to take and when to take it are debated. Follow the prescribed dosage; for adults, it is 125 mg twice a day starting as early as 2 days prior to ascent.

Because dehydration can be a factor at high altitudes, drink plenty of fluids such as water and juice. Mountain air is drier than air at lower elevations. You are drinking enough fluid when your urine is clear. Tea, coffee, and alcohol cause more frequent urination and may lead to dehydration. Eat foods that are easy to digest for a few days.

Avoid taking sleeping pills because they tend to cause shallow breathing while you sleep, which can make it difficult for your body to get enough oxygen. Likewise, do not smoke because it increases carbon monoxide levels in the blood, which diminish the body's ability to use oxygen.

## Other Altitude-Related Illnesses

Other altitude-related illnesses include the following:

- *Pharyngitis and bronchitis.* Because of dry air, a sore throat and coughing may develop. Care involves drinking fluids, applying an OTC antibiotic ointment in the nostrils, and sucking on hard candy or throat lozenges.
- *Peripheral edema.* The hands, ankles, and/or face (around the eyes) may swell at high altitude. If possible, raise the affected arms and/or legs. After descending or with acclimatization to higher altitudes, the swelling diminishes. Descend if signs of more serious altitude illness appear.

**Figure 24-7**

Lightning strike.

---

### FYI

**Altitude Increases Sunburn Risk**

Skiers, hikers, and others who enjoy outdoor activities in the mountains have long believed that it takes less time to sunburn in the mountains than at lower levels. Research confirms that the higher the altitude, the quicker a person will develop sunburn. Ultraviolet (UV) light energy readings were taken at solar noon in direct sunlight on cloudless days at Vail, Colorado; Orlando, Florida; and New York, New York. The high-altitude regions in the United States include areas with some of the fastest population growth, and it is vital that people living or visiting these regions recognize the increase in UV exposure at higher altitudes and take precautions to prevent sunburn.

*Source:* Rigel DS, Rigel EG, Rigel AC. Effects of altitude and latitude on ambient UVB radiation. *J Am Acad Dermatol* 1999; 40:114-116.

---

## ▶ Lightning

Lightning is awesome and frightening **Figure 24-7**. The National Oceanic and Atmospheric Administration reports about 10% of lightning strikes to humans result in death. Lightning is one of the leading environmental causes of death in the United States, according to the Centers for Disease Control and Prevention **Figure 24-8**.

In the past, farmers, sailors, and other outdoor workers in isolated areas tended to be the most frequently injured by lightning. Today, a larger proportion of people injured by lightning are hikers, campers, golfers, and others who are outdoors for recreational purposes.

Lightning deaths occur more often during daytime hours when people are active and outdoors. Most occur during the months of June through September, when thunderstorms are most frequent. There are more thunderstorm days in the South than in any other region of the United States. Thunderstorms occur frequently over high mountains. People are better protected in urban areas where high buildings have metal frames and lightning devices.

### How Lightning Injures

Lightning injures in five ways. A direct strike is actually being struck by lightning. Lightning is most likely

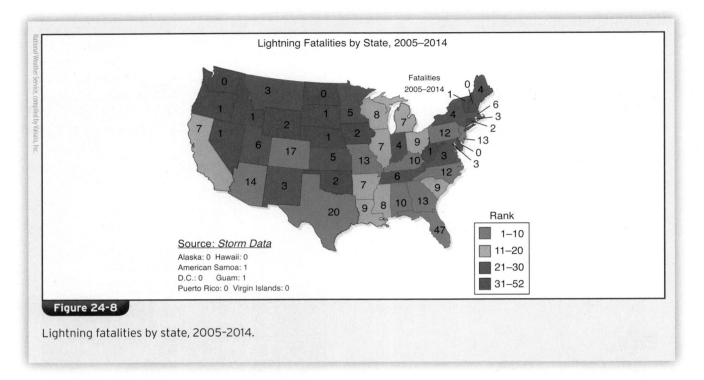

**Figure 24-8**

Lightning fatalities by state, 2005-2014.

## FYI

**Myths About Lightning**

- **Lightning strikes are always fatal.** Actually, studies report that lightning strikes kill only 10% of those struck. Generally, only people who sustain immediate cardiac arrest die.

- **A person who has been struck by lightning retains the charge—is "electrified"—and is dangerous to touch.** This false idea has led to a delay of resuscitation efforts and probably to some unnecessary deaths.

- **Lightning strike injuries allow a long resuscitation effort.** Although rescue breathing (when the person has a pulse) can effectively sustain life for long periods, CPR is usually ineffective after 30 minutes for people in cardiac arrest.

- **Lightning never strikes twice in the same place.** In fact, certain areas are prone to lightning due to height, location, or material. The Willis Tower (Chicago) and the Empire State Building (New York) are hit hundreds of times a year, as are mountaintops and radio and television antennas.

- **A person inside a building is safe from lightning injury.** Electrical current can travel along plumbing fixtures, telephone wires, and other appliances attached to the outside of the house by metal conductors.

to hit a person in the open who has been unable to find shelter. Any conductor of electricity that the person carries, especially if it is metal and carried above the shoulder level (for example, an open umbrella or a bag of golf clubs slung over the shoulder), increases the chances of a direct hit.

A more frequent cause of injury is a splash, which occurs when lightning strikes a tree or a building and splashes onto a person seeking shelter nearby. The electrical current seeks the path of least resistance and may jump to the person because bodies have less resistance than trees or other objects. Frequently, a splash can kill groups of animals as they stand near a fence or seek shelter under trees. Contact injury occurs when a person is holding an object that is directly hit or splashed by lightning.

Ground current is produced when lightning hits the ground or a nearby object. The current spreads like a wave in a pond. Although ground current is less likely to produce fatalities than direct hits or splashes, it often injures multiple people and creates multiple injuries. Large groups have been injured on baseball fields and hiking paths and during military maneuvers.

Finally, people can be injured by the explosive force of the shock wave produced as lightning strikes nearby. People actually can be thrown by this blast effect.

## Differences Between Generated High-Voltage Electricity Injuries and Lightning Injuries

Lightning contact with the body is instantaneous, leading to flashover, where the current flashes over the body and goes through it. With flashover, the person seldom has burns of any magnitude. Lightning injuries disrupt electrical activity in the heart and nervous system. Exposure to household electricity tends to be much more prolonged because the person freezes to the circuit. The electrical energy surges through the tissues with little resistance to flow, causing thermal injury with severe tissue damage that can result in the loss of the damaged extremity. Electric current can also disrupt the body's electrical activity as does lightning.

**Flash-to-Bang: How Close**

Be aware of how close lightning is occurring. The flash-to-bang method is the easiest and most convenient way to estimate how far away lightning is occurring. Thunder always accompanies lightning even though its audible range can be diminished due to background noise in the immediate environment and its distance from you. To use the flash-to-bang method, count the seconds from the time the lightning is sighted to when the clap of the thunder is heard. Divide this number by five to obtain how far away (in miles) the lightning is occurring. For example, if you count 15 seconds between seeing the flash and hearing the bang, 15 divided by 5 equals 3. Therefore the lightning flash is about 3 miles (5 km) away.

| What to Look For | What to Do |
|---|---|
| • No breathing<br>• Seizures, paralysis, and loss of responsiveness (resulting if the central nervous system is damaged)<br>• Minor burns. Most people believe that a person struck by lightning will be severely burned. However, owing to the flashover effect, most people have only the following types of minor burns:<br>　• Punctate burns (small, circular injuries resembling cigarette burns)<br>　• Feathering or ferning burns<br>　• Linear burns<br>　• Burns from ignited clothing and heated metal | 1. If more than one person has been struck by lightning at the same time, go to the quiet and motionless person first, check for breathing and, if absent, begin CPR.<br>2. If the person is unresponsive but breathing, place the person on his or her side.<br>3. Check for and treat injuries (fractures, dislocations, burns).<br>4. Evacuate all people to medical care. |

**FYI**

**30/30 Rule: When to Find Shelter**

The 30/30 rule states that people should seek shelter if the flash-to-bang delay (length of time in seconds between a lightning flash and its subsequent thunder) is 30 seconds or less, and that they remain under cover until 30 minutes after the final clap of thunder.

A 30-second lead time is necessary prior to a storm's arrival because of the possibility of distant strikes. A 30-minute wait after the last thunder clap is heard is necessary because the trailing storm clouds still carry a lingering charge. This charge can—and does—occasionally produce lightning on the back edge of a storm, several minutes after the rain has ended.

Studies have shown most people struck by lightning are struck not at the height of a thunderstorm, but before and after the storm has peaked. **DO NOT** wait for the rain to start before seeking shelter, and do not leave shelter just because the rain has ended. Half of all lightning deaths occur after a storm passes.

## FYI

**Avoid Lightning Injury**

- Be alert about weather conditions and predictions before going outdoors.
- **DO NOT** stand under a natural lightning rod such as a tall, isolated tree in an open area.
- Avoid projecting above the surrounding landscape, as you would do if you were standing on a hilltop, in an open field, on the beach, or fishing from a boat on the open water.
- Get out of and away from open water.
- Get away from tractors and other metal farm equipment.
- Get off and away from motorcycles, scooters, golf carts, and bicycles. Lay down golf clubs.
- Stay away from wire fences, clotheslines, metal pipes, rails, and other metallic paths that could carry lightning to you from some distance away.
- Avoid standing in small, isolated sheds or other small structures in open areas.
- In a forest, seek shelter in a low area under a thick growth of small trees.
- In open areas, go to a low place such as a ravine or valley.
- If you are hopelessly isolated in a level field or prairie and you feel tingling or your hair stand on end—indicating lightning is about to strike—drop to a baseball catcher's crouching position or stance and put your hands over both ears to help avoid an eardrum rupture. **DO NOT** lie flat on the ground. You want as small an area of your body as possible touching the ground to minimize the possibility of your body acting as a conductor.
- If you are indoors during a thunderstorm, avoid open doors and windows, fireplaces, and metal objects such as pipes, sinks, and plug-in electrical appliances. Avoid using the telephone.
- If you are in a motor vehicle (without a cloth top), stay in it. The vehicle will diffuse the current around you to the ground. It is a myth that the rubber tires will provide insulation, but it is true that the metal body affords protection.
- If a group of people is exposed, they should spread out and stay several yards apart. That way, should a strike hit, the smallest number will be seriously injured.

## ▶ Wild Animal Attacks

Despite the fact that few large wild animals (eg, bears, bison, cougars, and alligators) remain in the United States, attacks on humans still occur Figure 24-9 . Wild animal attacks outside the United States are more common. Attacks, especially fatal attacks, are often reported and sensationalized in the media.

**Figure 24-9**

Large animals do not always retreat from humans and may attack rescuers.

The incidence of injuries from wild animal attacks is not known Table 24-2 . Reporting is not mandatory, and many attacks are not recorded. Perhaps one or two deaths occur each year in the United States. Outside the United States, animal attacks by hippopotami, crocodiles, elephants, cape buffalo, lions, and tigers are a much greater cause of injury and death.

Wild animal attacks occur most often in rural or wilderness settings, a long distance from medical care. Preventing wild animal attacks is largely common sense and awareness. An increasing number of parks and wilderness areas are posting warning signs. Recreationalists should be aware of and knowledgeable about the animal habitats through which they travel and take precautions in food handling so as not to attract animals.

Generally, if you encounter a large wild animal, try to remove yourself from the scene quietly and slowly. Running will elicit a predatory response. Never get between an adult animal and its offspring. In most cases, a general rule is to fight back if you are attacked. Vigorous physical resistance, including striking the attacking animal with fists, a weapon, or any other object, has been effective in repelling attacks by cougars, lions, tigers, brown and black bears, and even crocodiles. Exceptions to this recommendation are the grizzly bear and a mother black bear with cubs. In these cases, you should lie down and play dead.

## Table 24-2  Human Deaths from Animal Attacks

| Species | Estimated Deaths Annually | Estimated Attacks Annually | Predominant Area | Comments |
|---|---|---|---|---|
| Humans | 200,000 | --- | Worldwide | Murders only |
| Wolves | 20-50 | 1-5 | Worldwide (mostly Eurasia) | |
| Hyenas | 10-50 | Hundreds | Africa | |
| Domestic dogs | 10-20 | 4.7 million | United States | |
| Other canines | 1-5 | 200-250 | Australia | |
| Tigers | 800 | 800 | India | Frequently maneaters |
| Leopards | 30-100 | 400 | Africa and India | Frequently maneaters |
| Lions | 300-500 | --- | Africa and India | Frequently maneaters |
| Cougars | <1 | <1 | United States | 20 deaths during the last century |
| African buffalo | 20-100 | --- | Africa | |
| Elephants | 600 | --- | Worldwide | |
| Black rhinoceri | 1 | --- | Africa | |
| Hippopotami | 200-300 | --- | Africa | Unpredictable |
| American bison | 3 | 56 | United States | |
| Moose | 3 | 368 injuries | British Columbia, Canada | Auto crashes only |
| Deer | 50 | 1.5 million incidents | United States | Auto crashes only |
| Domestic herbivores | 20-25 | 50,000-100,000 injuries | United States and Australia | |
| Snakes | 100,000 | --- | Worldwide | |
| Crocodiles | 2,000 | --- | Africa | |
| Alligators | 1-2 | --- | United States | |
| Ostrich | 1-2 | --- | Australia | |
| Kangaroos | 1-2 | 100-200 incidents | Australia | Auto incidents only |

## What to Look For

Not all injuries are bites. Severe injuries result from people being thrown in the air, gored by an antler, butted, or trampled on the ground and may include the following:

- Puncture wounds
- Bites
- Lacerations
- Bruises
- Fractures
- Rupture of internal organs
- Evisceration

## What to Do

1. See Chapter 8, *Bleeding*, Chapter 9, *Wounds*, and Chapter 10, *Bandaging Wounds*, for what to do for bleeding and wound care.
2. Depending on the severity of the injury, either evacuate the person to medical care or contact local authorities for evacuation.

## ▶ Wilderness Evacuation

Determining the best way to evacuate a person (helicopter evacuation versus walking the person out versus carrying the person on a litter) must be based on several factors. The following list is adapted from the WMS Practice Guidelines and suggests factors for determining the level of evacuation:

- Severity of the illness or injury
- Rescue and medical skills of the rescuers
- Physical and psychological condition of the rescuers and the ill or injured people
- Availability of equipment and aid for the rescue
- The time it would take to evacuate the person by other means as determined by distance, terrain, weather, and other conditions
- Cost

When requesting outside assistance, you must consider the safety of incoming rescuers, their time commitment, and the cost of the rescue.

As a general rule, you should delay travel plans or start evacuating a person from the wilderness for any of the following reasons:

- The person's condition is not improving.
- The person is experiencing debilitating pain.
- The person is unable to travel at a reasonable pace owing to a medical problem.
- The person is passing blood via the mouth or rectum (not from an obviously minor source).
- The person has signs and symptoms of serious altitude illness.
- Infections are not improving.
- Chest pain is not caused by a rib cage injury.
- Wounds are severe enough to require medical care.
- The person's dysfunctional psychological status is impairing the safety of others.

### When to Evacuate

Use the following guidelines to decide whether a person should be evacuated.

#### Immediate Evacuations
Rapidly evacuate the following injuries, where medical care is needed in 30 to 60 minutes or less:

- Open fractures
- Extremity injuries with deformity
- Extremity injuries in which circulation is absent

- Spinal injuries with no sensation in the fingers or toes or inability of the person to move fingers or toes
- Severe altitude illness (signs of HACE or HAPE)
- Decreased level of consciousness
- Signs of shock
- Severe bleeding

In the wilderness, all bleeding should be controlled. Wounds should be cleaned and irrigated under pressure. The standard rule is not to remove blood-soaked dressings; locate the bleeding vessels and reapply pressure directly over the bleeding vessels. Never attempt to clamp or tie a blood vessel—more damage can result. Do not close a wound with adhesive strips, butterfly bandages, staples, or sutures.

#### Delayed Evacuations
Medical care should be obtained within 6 to 24 hours of injury for the following:

- Limb injuries with deformity, severe pain, or inability to walk
- Severe frostbite
- Open wounds: Evacuate a wounded person so that a physician can suture a wound within 6 hours for hand or foot injuries and within 24 hours for head or trunk injuries. (If necessary, closure can be done by a physician up to about 4 days).
- Hypothermia: It is not necessary to evacuate a person of mild hypothermia if the person has normal mental status and is shivering. Evacuate people who have severe hypothermia (shivering has stopped but the person is still cold, altered mental status). It is impossible to rewarm a person with severe hypothermia in a wilderness or remote location. See Chapter 20, *Cold-Related Emergencies*, for more information.

### Guidelines for Ground Evacuation

If the person is walking out, at least two people should accompany the person. If the person is being carried out, one or two people should be sent to notify authorities that assistance is needed and to give them specifics about the problem.

During a litter evacuation, there should be at least four, and preferably six, litter-bearers at all times. Over rough terrain, eight carriers (six over a smooth trail)

### Hiking: How to Protect One's Health on the Trail

The popularity of backpacking and day hiking has greatly increased, but so have related injuries. A survey of 224 backpackers who hiked the entire 2,100-mile (3,380-km) mountainous Appalachian Trail showed that 82% had injuries (mostly muscle sprains, strains, and stress fractures) and illnesses (mostly diarrhea, skin irritations, foot blisters, and colds). Medical help was needed in 25% of the incidents. Hikers lost an average of 5 days of hiking because of these problems. Because these problems are common, hikers should carry supplies such as water purification equipment, pain medicine, antibiotic ointment, and bandages.

*Source:* Crouse BJ, Josephs D. Health care needs of Appalachian Trail hikers. *J Fam Pract* 1993; 36:521–525.

should carry the litter 100 yards (91 m) and then rest or rotate with eight other carriers. It is very demanding to carry a loaded litter for more than 15 minutes without a break.

### Guidelines for Helicopter Evacuation

Helicopters can reduce the time the person has to wait to receive medical care. Evacuate by helicopter only if the following conditions apply **Figure 24-10**:

- The person's life will be saved or the person will have a significantly better chance for full recovery.
- The pilot believes conditions are safe enough for helicopter evacuation.

- Ground evacuation would be unusually dangerous or excessively prolonged or not enough rescuers are available for ground evacuation.

In general, helicopters are not beneficial if ground transport can get the person to the hospital within 30 to 60 minutes.

## ▶ Signaling for Help

Many emergency conditions require a search for people in distress. Under such circumstances, it is always better if the people being sought know how to make their presence and their location conspicuous.

### Signaling Aircraft

When creating a ground signal that people in an aircraft can see, remember that few straight lines or right angles exist in nature and that things are a lot smaller when viewed from the air. Bigger is almost always better. For ground signals, make a large V for immediate assistance or an X if medical assistance is needed. Make the lines of these signals as large as you can. Construct your signal so that each line is six times as long as it is wide, such as a V with each side 12 feet (4 m) long and 2 feet (1 m) wide. Contrast is another key to ground signals. Examples of materials to use include toilet paper, strips of plastic tarp, strips of tent material, tree branches, logs, and light-colored rocks. In snow and on open ground or sandy shores, signals may be tramped or dug into the surface using shadows to make the signals stand out.

**Figure 24-10**

An EMS helicopter.

*Courtesy of Mark Woolcock*

### CAUTION

**DO NOT** approach a helicopter until one of the aircraft personnel signals it is safe for you to approach.
**DO NOT** approach a helicopter from the rear, where the fast-spinning tail rotor is invisible and dangerous. Many people walk into spinning rotors each year.
**DO NOT** forget to protect against wind chill from the rotor blades in the winter or to protect the eyes against flying dirt and debris.

**DO NOT** approach from the uphill side. The rotor is closer to the ground on the uphill side **Figure 24-11**.
**DO NOT** stand up when approaching a helicopter. Keep as low as possible in a crouched position. Because the blade is flexible, it may dip as low as 4 feet (1 m) off the ground.

**Figure 24-11**

Helicopter safety.

**Figure 24-12**

Signaling.

## Other Signals

A series of three of almost anything indicates "Help." Examples include three shouts, three shots, three blasts from a whistle, or three flashes from a light. Use smoke by day and bright flame by night if other signaling devices are not available. Add engine oil, rags soaked in oil, or pieces of rubber to your fire to make black smoke (best against a light background). Keep plenty of spare fuel on hand. If you are tending a fire as you wait for help, keep fuel handy and throw it on the fire when you hear an aircraft; do not wait, because it takes time for smoke to form and rise. Make sure to start the fire away from combustibles such as grass or trees.

A mirror is an effective means of sending a distress signal. On hazy days, aircraft pilots can see the flash of a mirror before survivors can see the aircraft, so it is wise to flash the mirror in the direction of a plane when you hear it, even when you cannot see it. Mirror flashes have been spotted by rescue aircraft more than 20 miles (32 km) away.

To use a mirror, follow this procedure:

1. Hold the mirror up to the sun with one hand, and stretch your other hand out in front of you. Use your finger or thumb to block your view of your target.
2. Hit your extended finger or thumb with a reflection of the sun from the mirror.
3. Repeatedly flick the spot of light from the mirror across the finger or thumb and the target.
4. Try to hit the aircraft or rescuers with a flash as much as possible. Do not attempt to do series of three flashes—it is too difficult **Figure 24-12**.

### FYI

**Survival Kit: The Bare Essentials**

| Minimal items | Purpose |
|---|---|
| One or two large plastic trash bags or an emergency blanket (space blanket) made of Mylar | Protects against weather (wind, rain, snow). Wear one trash bag by cutting a hole in the bottom of the bag for your head; use the second bag to cover your legs. |
| Whistle (Fox 40 Mini or Windstorm) | Signal for help. |
| Signal mirror | Signal for help. |
| Metal match with striker (magnesium) | Start a fire. |
| Waterproof match case containing windproof and waterproof matches | Start a fire. |
| Waterproof match case or empty film canister containing several cotton balls smeared with petroleum jelly (such as Vaseline) or commercial tinder tabs | Petroleum jelly is flammable. Make tinder using cotton balls smeared with petroleum jelly. When using, open a cotton ball up to catch sparks from metal match. |
| Knife (multitool) and/or wire blade survival saw | Cutting. |
| Food (such as energy bars and MREs [US military surplus meals-ready-to-eat]) | Provides calories and a psychological boost. |

## ▶ Ready for Review

- Be as medically prepared as possible to manage a problem for others and for yourself.
- Prolonged CPR has little use in a wilderness or remote setting. Once started, CPR should be continued for at least 30 minutes.
- In a wilderness situation, reducing some dislocated joints is recommended.
- Always stabilize an unresponsive person.
- People with a femur fracture can have 2 quarts (about 2 L) of blood loss in the thigh and develop massive swelling. These injuries should be splinted.
- Since the early 1970s, the number of deaths caused by avalanches has increased rapidly.
- Altitude illnesses actually are a spectrum of a single problem: hypoxia.
- Determining the best way to evacuate a person must be based on several factors.
- Many emergency conditions require a search for people in distress.

## ▶ Vital Vocabulary

hypoxia A low oxygen content in the blood; lack of oxygen in inspired air.

## ▶ Assessment in Action

You have been enjoying a 5-day backpack trip in the high mountains of Colorado. Being from sea level, you knew the high altitude would take some getting used to, but your group is doing very well. On day 4, you must ascend a 1,000-foot (305-m) pass to get to your final campsite. After an hour of never-ending switchbacks, you arrive at the highest point of the trip—13,500 feet (4,115) above sea level. At this elevation, several members in your group report a severe headache and fatigue. Two members cannot seem to catch their breath.

*Directions:* Circle Yes if you agree with the statement; circle No if you disagree.

Yes    No    **1.** Because you are above 12,000 feet (3,658 m), you suspect they are suffering from HAPE or HACE.

Yes    No    **2.** Plenty of fluids should be given to the people.

Yes    No    **3.** You should stay at this elevation until they feel well enough to hike down the other side of the pass.

Yes    No    **4.** After descent to your final campsite (3,000 feet [914 m] below the pass), if the people's conditions do not improve, you should seek medical care.

## ▶ Check Your Knowledge

*Directions:* Circle Yes if you agree with the statement; circle No if you disagree.

Yes    No    **1.** Injuries in the wilderness rarely happen.

Yes    No    **2.** CPR in the wilderness should be stopped if the person does not respond after 30 minutes.

Yes    No    **3.** Reduction of a dislocation dramatically relieves pain.

Yes    No    **4.** When it comes to spinal stabilization, never improvise!

Yes    No    **5.** After an avalanche, it is easy for people to dig themselves out.

Yes    No    **6.** Speed of ascent can affect altitude illness.

Yes    No    **7.** Headache is a common symptom of altitude illness.

Yes    No    **8.** A person with altitude illness should keep moving.

Yes    No    **9.** Most lightning deaths occur during the night.

Yes    No    **10.** Most people struck by lightning will have only minor burns.

# Rescuing and Moving Injured People

**25**

# Rescue

## ► Water Rescue

*Reach-throw-row-go* identifies the sequence for attempting a water rescue. The first and simplest rescue technique is to reach for the person. Reaching requires a lightweight pole, ladder, long stick, or any object that can be extended to the person. Once you have your "reacher," secure your footing and have a bystander grab your belt or pants for stability. Secure yourself before reaching for the person.

You can throw anything that floats—an empty picnic jug, an empty fuel or paint can, a life jacket, a floating cushion, a piece of wood, or an inflated spare tire—whatever is available Table 25-1. If there is a rope handy, tie it to the object to be thrown so you can pull the person in, or, if you miss, you can retrieve the object and throw it again. The average untrained rescuer has a throwing range of about 50 feet (15 m).

If the person is out of throwing range and there is a rowboat, canoe, motor boat, or boogie board nearby, you can try to row to the person. Maneuvering these craft requires skill learned through practice. Wear a personal flotation device for your own safety. To avoid capsizing, never pull the person in over the side of a boat; instead, pull the person in over the stern (rear end) or tow the person to safety.

**Table 25-1 Effect of Flotation Devices on Survival Times**

| Situation (50°F [10°C] water) | Predicted Survival Time (hours) |
|---|---|
| **No Flotation Device** | |
| Downproofing | 1.5 |
| Treading water | 2.0 |
| **With Flotation Device** | |
| Swimming | 2.0 |
| Holding still | 2.7 |
| HELP (heat escape lessening position) | 4.0 |
| Huddle position | 4.0 |

*Data from:* Collis ML. Survival behaviour in cold water immersion. In: *Proceedings of the Cold Water Symposium.* Toronto: Royal Life-Saving Society of Canada; 1976.

© Jones & Bartlett Learning

If reach, throw, and row are impossible and you are a capable swimmer trained in water lifesaving procedures, you can go to the drowning person by swimming. Entering even calm water makes a swimming rescue difficult and hazardous. All too often, a would-be rescuer drowns as well.

## CAUTION

**DO NOT** swim to and grasp a drowning person unless you are trained in lifesaving.

## FYI

**American Academy of Pediatrics Recommendations for Preventing Childhood Drowning (by Age Group)**

**4 years and younger**
- Never leave children alone in bathtubs, spas, or wading pools or near water-filled buckets, toilets, irrigation ditches, or other standing water.
- Recognize that swimming lessons do not "drown-proof" children.
- Fence the entire pool so that it is separated from the house. Pool covers are not a substitute for fences.
- Learn cardiopulmonary resuscitation (CPR) and keep a telephone and emergency equipment–such as life preservers and a shepherd's crook–poolside.

**5 to 12 years**
- Provide children with swimming lessons that include safety rules.
- Never let the children swim alone or without adult supervision.
- Make sure the children wear approved flotation devices when playing in or near a body of water.
- Teach the children the dangers of jumping or diving into water and of being on thin ice.

**13 to 19 years**
- In addition to relaying the preceding safety tips, counsel about the dangers of substance abuse combined with swimming, diving, or boating.
- Teach adolescents how to perform CPR.

*Source:* American Academy of Pediatrics Committee on Injury, Violence, and Poison Prevention. Prevention of drowning in infants, children, and adolescents. *Pediatrics* 2003;112(2):437-439.

## Drowning

According to the World Health Organization, drowning is the process of experiencing respiratory impairment from submersion/immersion in liquid. This definition, which was adopted by the 2002 World Congress on Drowning, includes all types of liquid except body fluids (eg, vomit, saliva). For drowning to occur, usually at least the person's face (mouth and nose) must be immersed, or covered, in water. During submersion, the entire body, including the face, is under water. Behaviors of a drowning person are found in  .

## FYI

**World Congress on Drowning**

In 2002, experts from all over the world gathered together for the World Congress on Drowning. After considerable debate and dialogue, an internationally accepted definition for drowning was agreed upon. The definition neither describes causes nor classifies the outcome of the drowning process. The congress also concluded that the terms *wet drowning, dry drowning, active drowning, passive drowning, silent drowning,* and *secondary drowning* should no longer be used.

## Table 25-2  Behaviors of a Distressed Swimmer and Drowning Person

| | Distressed Swimmer | Drowning Person–Active | Drowning Person–Passive |
|---|---|---|---|
| Head position | Above water | Tilted back with face looking up | Faceup or facedown in the water; submerged |
| Appearance and, if visible, facial expressions | • Trying to support self by holding or clinging to a lane line or safety line<br>• Expression of concern for personal safety | • Struggling to keep or get the head above the surface of the water<br>• Struggling to reach the surface, if underwater<br>• Expression of panic/ wide-eyed | • Limp or convulsive-like movements<br>• Floating or submerged<br>• Eyes may be closed<br>• If submerged, may look like a shadow |
| Breathing | Is breathing | Struggles to breathe | Not breathing |
| Arm and leg action | • Floating, sculling or treading water<br>• Might wave for help | Arms to sides or in front, alternately moving up and pressing down | None |
| Body position | Horizontal, vertical or diagonal, depending on means of support | Vertical, leaning slightly back | Horizontal or vertical |
| Locomotion | • Little or no forward progress<br>• Less and less able to support self | None | None |
| Sounds | Able to call for help but may not do so | Cannot call out for help | None |
| Location | At the surface | At the surface, underwater or sinking | Floating at the surface, sinking or submerged on the bottom |

## Care for Drowning Person

1. Survey the scene (see Chapter 2, *Action at an Emergency*), then carry out a water rescue **Figure 25-1**.
2. If the person was diving (or it is unknown whether he or she was diving), suspect a possible spinal injury. Support the person on the surface of the water so that he or she is floating faceup with the head and spine in a straight line until properly trained rescuers arrive with a backboard.
3. Check breathing and treat accordingly. Any nonbreathing person who has been submerged in cold water should be resuscitated unless submerged for more than 60 minutes.
4. If no spinal injury is suspected, after the person has been resuscitated, place the person on his or her side to allow fluids to drain from the airway.

## Cold-Water Immersion

Immersion in cold water is a potential hazard for anyone who participates in activities in the oceans, lakes, and streams of all but the tropical regions of the world. The US Coast Guard defines cold water as water with a temperature of less than 70°F (21°C). However, water does not need to be that cold for a person to become hypothermic. A person can become hypothermic in water that is 77°F (25°C). Most North American lakes, rivers, and coasts are colder than that year-round. The risk of immersion hypothermia in North America is nearly universal most of the year. A person immersed in cold water experiences heat loss about 25 times faster than someone exposed to cold air.

**Figure 25-1**

Water rescue. **A.** Reach for the person with a lightweight pole, ladder, long stick, or other object. **B.** Secure your footing before reaching for the person. **C.** Throw anything that floats. **D.** Row to the person if the person is out of throwing range. **E.** Go to the person if reach, throw, and row are impossible and you are trained in water lifesaving procedures.

The US Coast Guard and other rescue organizations recommend that survivors get as much of their bodies out of the water as possible to minimize cooling rate and maximize survival time. A widespread misunderstanding of the concept of wind chill often causes people to conclude that survivors have higher heat losses if they are exposed to wind, especially if they are wet, than if they are immersed in water. During recreational activities at beaches, lakes, and swimming pools, most people have experienced feeling colder after leaving the water than they do while swimming. That reinforces the misunderstanding, which has sometimes led people to abandon a safe position atop a capsized vessel and reenter the water, usually with tragic results.

Cold-water immersion is associated with two potential medical emergencies: drowning and hypothermia. Numerous case histories and statistical evidence document the prominence of cold-water immersion as a cause of drowning and hypothermia. Perhaps the most famous occurrence of cold-water immersion was the sinking of the ocean liner *Titanic* on April 14, 1912. After striking an iceberg, the ship sank in calm seas. Of the 2,201 people on board, only 712 were rescued, all from the ship's lifeboats. The remaining 1,489 people died in the water, despite the arrival of a rescue vehicle within 2 hours. Nearly all of those people were wearing life preservers, yet the cause of death was officially listed as drowning. More likely, the cause of death was immersion hypothermia.

The speed at which a person cools depends on several factors:

- *Body fat.* The more body fat a person has, the slower cooling occurs. More fat increases survival chances.
- *Body type.* Bigger people cool more slowly than smaller people. Children cool faster than adults. Women have more fat but are usually smaller, so they cool at the same rate as men.
- *Physical fitness.* Cardiovascular fitness can help meet the stress of cold-water immersion, but physically fit people usually have less subcutaneous fat for insulation.
- *Water temperature.* The colder the water, the faster a person cools.
- *Clothing.* Clothing can insulate, and some types of fabric, such as wool, are better than others.
- *Alcohol.* People who have been drinking alcohol are more likely to get into dangerous situations. Alcohol impairs judgment and coordination. Research studies have implicated alcohol in 10% to 50% of all drownings. Alcohol dilates the skin's blood vessels, which allows more body heat to escape.
- *Behavior.* Swimming and treading water increase the flow of warm blood from the body's core to the muscles, increasing the cooling rate. Thus, swimmers often die first because they are more likely to try to tread water or swim rather than float. Likewise, so-called drownproofing, a technique of bobbing in the water (like a jellyfish), markedly increases heat loss as water circulates around the head.

A **heat escape lessening position (HELP)** has been devised, in which the person draws the knees up close to the chest, presses the arms to the sides, and remains as quiet as possible **Figure 25-2**. For two or more people, huddling quietly and closely together (huddle position) will decrease heat loss from the groin and the front of the body. Both of these positions require personal flotation devices (life jackets).

Surviving long periods of submersion has been explained by the diving reflex found in mammals. Some say that the diving reflex slows the heart rate, shunts blood to the brain, and closes the airway. Recent research, however, suggests that the diving reflex is present in marine mammals, such as seals, porpoises, whales, and walruses, but not in humans. If the diving reflex is discounted, the most likely explanation for prolonged submersion survival is that cold water produces hypothermia, which reduces the body's demand for oxygen and protects the brain.

## ▶ Ice Rescue

If a person has fallen through the ice near the shore, extend a pole or throw a line with a floatable object attached to it. When the person has hold of the object, pull him or her toward the shore or the edge of the ice.

If the person has fallen through the ice away from the shore and you cannot reach him or her with a pole or a throwing line, lie flat and push a ladder, plank, or

---

**CAUTION**

**DO NOT** go near broken ice without support.

**Figure 25-2**

HELP or huddle. **A.** A person wearing a flotation device can minimize heat loss and increase chances of survival by assuming the heat escape lessening position (HELP) in which the knees are pulled up to the chest and the arms crossed. **B.** Groups of two or more can conserve heat by wrapping their arms around one another and pulling into a tight circle or huddle.

similar object ahead of you **Figure 25-3**. You can also tie a rope to a spare tire and the other end to an anchor point on the shore, lie flat, and push the tire ahead of you. Pull the person ashore or to the edge of the ice.

## ▶ Electrical Emergency Rescue

Electrical injuries can be devastating. Just a mild shock can cause serious internal injuries. A current of 1,000 V or more is considered high voltage, but even the 110 V of household current can be deadly.

When a person receives an electrical shock, electricity enters the body at the point of contact and travels along the path of least resistance (nerves and blood vessels). The current travels rapidly, generating heat and causing destruction.

Most indoor electrocutions are caused by faulty electrical equipment or the careless use of electrical appliances. Before you touch the person, turn off the electricity at the circuit breaker, fuse box, or outside switch box or unplug the appliance if the plug is undamaged.

If the electrocution involves high-voltage power lines, the power must be turned off before anyone approaches the person. If you approach a person and feel a tingling sensation in your legs and lower body, stop. You are on energized ground, and an electric current is entering one foot, passing through your lower body, and leaving through the other foot. You should raise one foot off the ground, turn around, and hop to a safe place. Wait for trained personnel with the proper equipment to cut the wires or disconnect them. If a power line falls over a car, tell the driver and passengers to stay in the car. If a person must get out of the car because of fire or imminent explosion, he or she should jump out so that the ground and car or wires are not touched at the same time.

### CAUTION

**DO NOT** touch an appliance or the person until the current is off.

**DO NOT** try to move downed wires.

**DO NOT** use any object, even dry wood (broomstick, tools, chair, stool), to separate the person from the electrical source.

**Figure 25-3**

Ice rescue: Lie flat to distribute the weight over a larger surface area.

## ▶ Hazardous Materials Incidents

Almost any highway crash scene involves the potential danger of hazardous materials. Clues that indicate the presence of hazardous materials include the following:

- Look for warning signs on the vehicle (eg, "explosive," "flammable," "corrosive"). If you are unable to read the placard or labels, **DO NOT** move closer and risk exposure. If you are able to read the placard with the naked eye, you may be too close and should consider moving farther away. **Figure 25-4** shows a chart illustrating the hazardous materials warning placards, and **Figure 25-5** shows a chart illustrating the warning labels.
- Watch for a leak or spill from a tank, container, truck, or railroad car with or without hazardous material placards or labels.
- A strong, noxious odor can denote a hazardous material.
- A cloud or strange-looking smoke from the escaping substance suggests you should stay away.

Stay well away and upwind from the area. Only people who are specially trained in handling hazardous

materials and who have the proper equipment should be in the area.

## ▶ Motor Vehicle Crashes

In most states, you are legally obligated to stop and give help when you are involved in a motor vehicle crash. If you arrive at a crash shortly after it happens, the law does not require you to stop, although it might be argued that you have a moral responsibility to provide any aid that you can.

1. Stop and park your vehicle well off the highway or road and out of active traffic lanes. Park at least five car lengths from the crash. If the police have taken charge, **DO NOT** stop unless you are asked to do so. If the police or other emergency vehicles have not arrived, call or send someone to call 9-1-1 or the local emergency number as soon as possible. Ways to call include the following:
   - Finding a pay phone or roadside emergency phone
   - Using a cellular phone
   - Using a phone at a nearby house or business

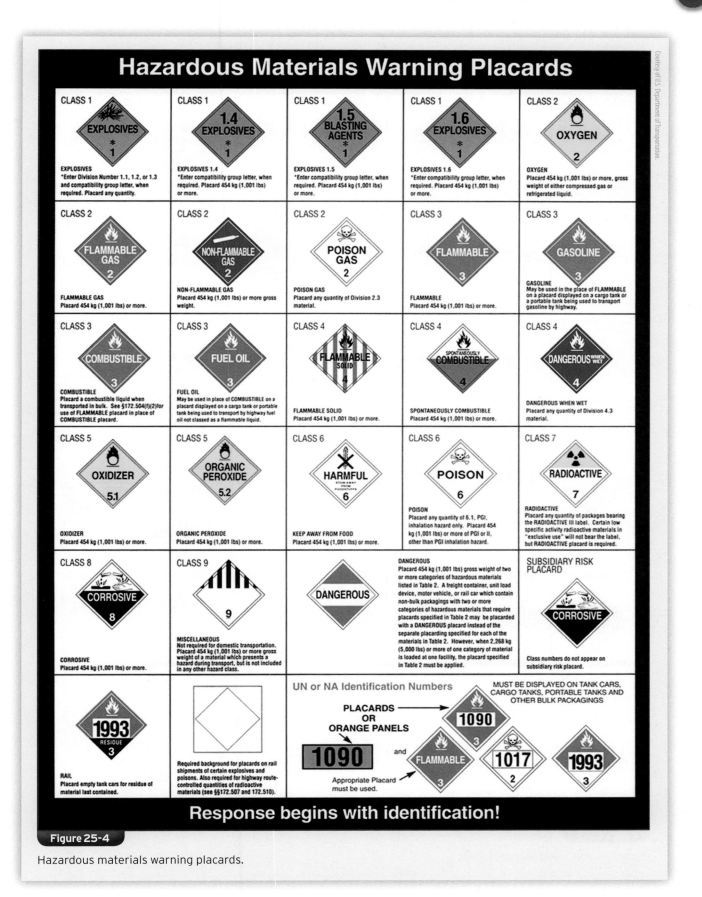

**Figure 25-4**

Hazardous materials warning placards.

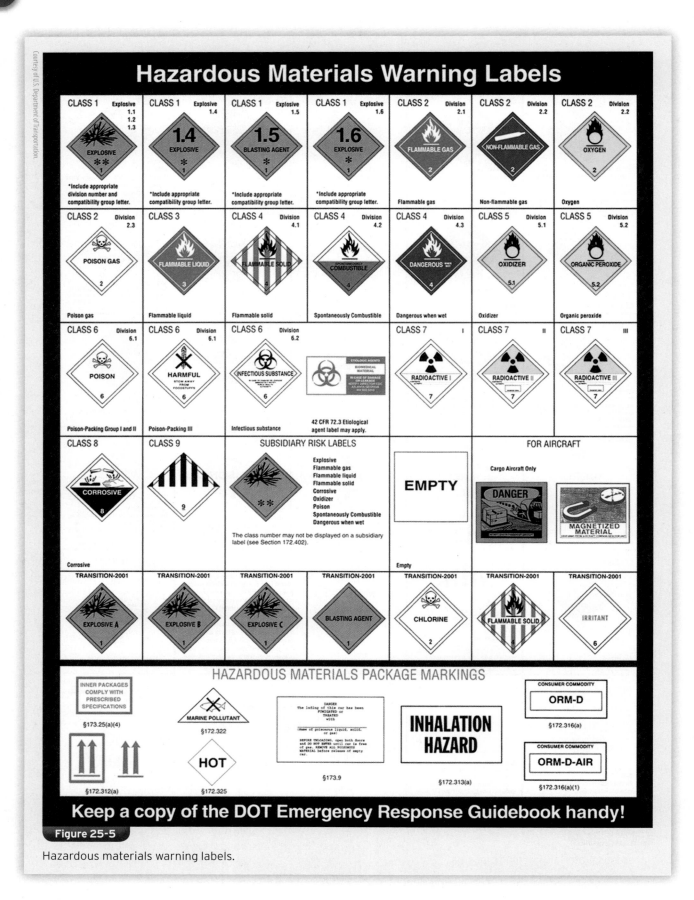

**Figure 25-5**

Hazardous materials warning labels.

2. Turn on your vehicle's emergency hazard flashers.
3. Make sure everyone on the scene is safe.
   - Ask the driver to turn off the ignition or turn it off yourself.
   - Ask bystanders to stand well off the roadway.
   - Place flares or reflectors 250 to 500 feet (76 to 152 m) behind the crash scene to warn oncoming drivers of the crash. **DO NOT** ignite flares around leaking gasoline or diesel fuel.
4. If the driver or passenger is unresponsive or might have spinal injuries, use your hands to stabilize the person's head and neck.
5. Check and keep monitoring the person's breathing. Treat any life-threatening injuries.
6. Whenever possible, wait for EMS personnel to extricate people from vehicles because they have training and the proper equipment. In most cases, keep peoples' conditions stabilized inside the vehicle.
7. Allow EMS to transport people to the hospital.
8. In motor vehicle crashes involving a single vehicle, consider sudden-onset illness (ie, fainting, heart attack, hypoglycemia, etc) as a possible cause.

## CAUTION

**DO NOT** rush to get people out of a car that has been in a crash. Contrary to opinion, most vehicle crashes do not involve fire, and most vehicles stay in an upright position.

**DO NOT** move people or allow people to move unless there is an immediate danger such as fire or oncoming traffic.

**DO NOT** transport people in your car or any other bystander's vehicle.

## ▶ Fires

Should you encounter a fire, you should use the RACE mnemonic to remember what to do:

**R** = *Rescue*. Get all people out of the building and area quickly. Help those in immediate danger get to a safe place.

**A** = *Activate*. Call the emergency telephone number (usually 9-1-1) to report the fire. If the building has an alarm system, pull the nearest fire alarm.

**C** = *Confine*. If it can be done safely, prevent the fire from spreading by closing doors and windows. **DO NOT** lock doors and windows.

**E** = *Extinguish*. If it is safe to do so and you are competent in its use, retrieve and use the nearest fire extinguisher.

You should only fight the fire yourself with a fire extinguisher if the fire is small and if your own escape route is clear. You may be able to put out the fire or at least hold damage to a minimum. Because a fire can spread quickly, efforts to contain it within the first 5 minutes of a blaze can make a substantial difference in the eventual outcome.

To operate a fire extinguisher, use the PASS technique:

**P** = *Pull* the extinguisher's lock pin.

**A** = *Aim* the nozzle at the base of the fire.

**S** = *Squeeze* the handles together.

**S** = *Sweep* from side to side at the base of the flames.

Extinguishers expel their contents quickly; it takes just 8 to 25 seconds for most home models containing dry chemicals to empty.

If clothing catches fire, tear the article off, in a motion away from the face. Keep the person from running, because running fans the flames. Wrap a rug or a woolen blanket around the person's neck to keep the fire from the face or throw a blanket on the person. In some cases, you may be able to smother the flames by throwing the person to the floor and rolling him or her in a rug.

## CAUTION

**DO NOT** let people run if their clothing is on fire.

**DO NOT** become trapped while fighting a fire. Always keep a door behind you so you can exit if the fire gets too big.

## ▶ Threatening Dogs

When you enter any emergency scene, look for signs of a dog and proceed with caution if the animal is not threatening. Ask the owner to control a threatening dog. If you cannot be delayed, consider using a fire extinguisher, water hose, or pepper spray. For a vicious dog, call the police for assistance.

## Farm Animals

Emergencies involving farm animals can be dangerous to rescuers. Horses kick and bite and, if panicked, may trample a person. Cattle may kick, bite, gore, or squeeze people against a pen or barn. Pigs can deliver severe bites.

- Approach a situation involving animals with caution. Whenever possible, obtain help from an experienced animal handler or an Animal Control officer before approaching the scene.
- **DO NOT** frighten or chase an animal. Move slowly and speak quietly to reassure it.
- Be aware of territorial posturing by male livestock, such as bulls, rams, stallions, ganders, or roosters. Avoid making eye contact or facing the animal fully, as this may be interpreted as aggression. If the animal seems to be preparing to charge, back away slowly, as running may provoke it.
- If possible, close gates or fences between you and livestock before assisting injured people.
- **DO NOT** attempt to capture a loose or panicking animal. If food is available, use it to lure the animal away from the injured person. Placing food in a bucket and shaking it may be enough to attract and calm the animal, enabling the rescuer to lead it into an enclosure.

## Confined Spaces

A confined space is any area not intended for human occupancy that may have or develop a dangerous atmosphere. They have limited openings for entrance and exit. There are three types of confined spaces: below ground, ground level, and above ground. Below-ground confined spaces include manholes, below-ground utility vaults and storage tanks, old mines, cisterns, and wells. Ground-level confined spaces include industrial tanks and farm storage silos. Above-ground confined spaces include water towers and legged storage tanks.

An incident in a confined space demands immediate action. If someone enters a confined space and signals for help or becomes unresponsive, follow these steps:

1. Call 9-1-1 for immediate assistance.
2. **DO NOT** rush in to help. If you do, you risk needing rescue as well.

3. When help arrives, try to rescue the person without entering the space.
4. If rescue from the outside cannot be done, only trained and properly equipped (respiratory protection plus safety harnesses or lifelines) rescuers should enter the space and remove the person.
5. Once the person is removed, provide care. Additional training is required for first aid providers who are on-call for helping rescue people in a confined space.

# Triage: Prioritizing Multiple Injured People

Situations requiring first aid usually involve only one person. Rarely will you encounter a large-scale event involving more than one person who needs care. Such events may seem commonplace because, when they do occur, they are frequently reported in the mass media Table 25-3.

When many people are injured, use a process called **triage** (a French word meaning "to sort") to distinguish among:

- Those needing immediate care for one of the "killers"—closed airway and severe bleeding
- Those who can wait for care until after others have been triaged
- Those who are deceased (dead)

The intent of triage is to provide the greatest good for the greatest number of people. Some people have a greater need for emergency care than others. Someone has to go

© Jones & Bartlett Learning

| Table 25-3 Examples of Disasters Involving Two or More People | |
|---|---|
| Natural Disasters | Human-caused Disasters |
| Earthquakes | Highway crashes |
| Tornadoes | Air crashes |
| Hurricanes | Train derailments |
| Floods | Terrorist attacks |
| Lightning strikes | Mass shootings |
| Winter storms | Explosions |
| Heat waves | |

last. Triage is especially effective in situations in which more injured people than first aid providers and rescuers are present, and in situations where time is critical.

© Jones & Bartlett Learning

## Q&A

**What is the origin of the word triage?**
*Triage* is a French word meaning to sort, separate, or select. It refers to the procedure of prioritizing people's care based on the severity of their condition. Several triage methods exist, varying among countries (even within a country) and the type of care provider (eg, paramedic, nurse, first aid provider) involved. The idea originated in World War I with French physicians treating the battlefield wounded at aid stations behind the front lines of battle.

## ▶ Triage Categories

During triage, evaluate and sort every injured person into one of three categories  Table 25-4 .

While EMS personnel may have ribbons, cards, or tags to place on people to identify their category, you will rarely have these items. You can, however, improvise (eg, write on a piece of tape placed on the person's forehead or around the wrist). After triage, take injured people, according to their category, to a medical facility, if available, or to an area designated for medical treatment.

## ▶ Conducting Triage

**Step 1:** Conduct a voice triage by calling out, "If you can walk, come to me." People who can get up and walk rarely have life-threatening injuries. **DO NOT**

force a person to move if he or she complains of pain. People who can walk can be placed in the "delayed" category. Direct them to a designated safe area; have them sit down and stay together. If you need more assistance, you can ask for volunteers from this group to help.

**Step 2:** Start surveying each person who did not get up and walk. Begin with the person closest to where you are standing. Quickly get to each person and sort each by his or her need for care. Tag everyone as "immediate," "delayed," or "dead." **DO NOT** stop to treat anyone during triage except to quickly open the airway and control severe bleeding.

When performing triage  Flowchart 25-1 :

- If a person fails one of the tests (or checks), tag him or her as immediate.
- If a person passes all of the tests (or checks), tag as delayed.
- Everyone should get a tag.

Reassess people regularly for changes in their condition. Only after people with immediate life-threatening conditions receive care should people with less serious conditions be given care. You may have to care for multiple people without adequate help until more highly trained emergency personnel arrive, at which point you may be asked to provide first aid, help move people, or help with ambulance or helicopter transportation.

# Moving People

A person should not be moved until he or she is ready for transportation to a hospital, if required. All necessary first aid should be provided before moving a

| Table 25-4 | Triage Categories |
|---|---|
| Category | Description |
| Immediate | Person has life-threatening injuries (airway closed or severe bleeding) demanding immediate action to save his or her life. |
| Delayed | Person's life is not threatened. He or she may need care, but it can be delayed while other people are triaged. |
| Dead/deceased | Person is not breathing after his or her airway has been opened. There may be no time or people to do CPR when others need immediate help. A volunteer from the walking-wounded group might be able to perform compression-only CPR or, if trained, CPR.<br>An exception to bypassing the dead to treat the moderately or severely injured occurs when a lightning strike involves multiple people; in this event, CPR should be given to those who are motionless and appear to be dead *before* aiding people in other categories. (See Chapter 24, *Wilderness First Aid*, for more information.) |

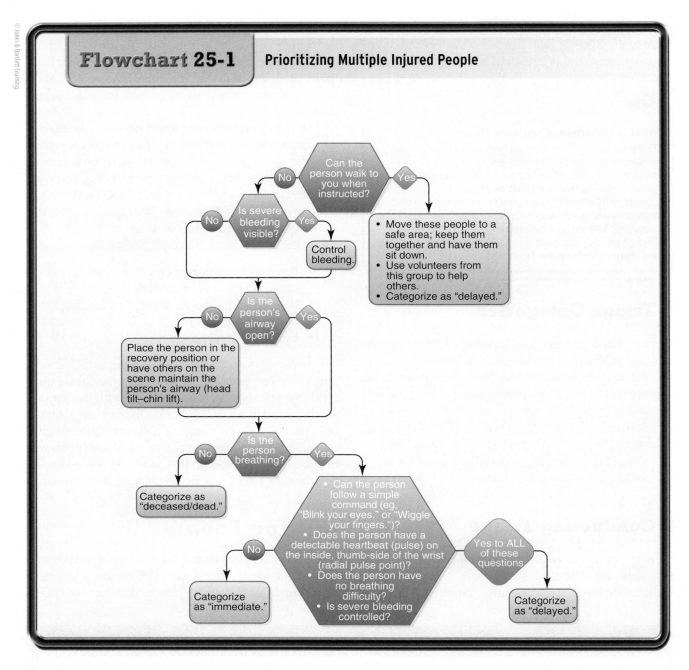

**Flowchart 25-1**   Prioritizing Multiple Injured People

Can the person walk to you when instructed?

No / Yes

Is severe bleeding visible?

No / Yes

Control bleeding.

- Move these people to a safe area; keep them together and have them sit down.
- Use volunteers from this group to help others.
- Categorize as "delayed."

Is the person's airway open?

No / Yes

Place the person in the recovery position or have others on the scene maintain the person's airway (head tilt–chin lift).

Is the person breathing?

No / Yes

Categorize as "deceased/dead."

- Can the person follow a simple command (eg, "Blink your eyes." or "Wiggle your fingers.")?
- Does the person have a detectable heartbeat (pulse) on the inside, thumb-side of the wrist (radial pulse point)?
- Does the person have no breathing difficulty?
- Is severe bleeding controlled?

No

Categorize as "immediate."

Yes to ALL of these questions

Categorize as "delayed."

person. A person should be moved only if there is an immediate danger, such as the following:

- There is a fire or danger of a fire.
- Explosives or other hazardous materials are involved.
- It is impossible to protect the scene from hazards.
- It is impossible to gain access to other people in the situation who need lifesaving care (such as in a motor vehicle crash).

A person with cardiac arrest is usually moved unless he or she is already on the ground or floor because CPR must be performed on a firm, level surface.

## ▶ Emergency Moves

The major danger in moving a person quickly is the possibility of aggravating a spinal injury. In an emergency, every effort should be made to pull the person in the direction of the long axis of the body to provide

**Principles of Lifting**

- Know your capabilities. **DO NOT** try to handle a load that is too heavy or awkward; seek help.
- Use a safe, non-slip grip. Use as much of your palms as possible.
- Keep your back straight. Tighten the muscles of your buttocks and abdomen.
- Bend your knees to use the strong muscles of the thighs and buttocks.
- Keep your arms close to your body and your elbows flexed.
- Position your feet shoulder width apart for balance, one in front of the other.
- When lifting, keep and lift the person close to your body.
- While lifting, **DO NOT** twist your back; pivot with your feet.
- Lift and carry slowly, smoothly, and in unison with the other lifters.
- Before you move a person, explain to him or her what you are doing.

as much protection to the spinal cord as possible. If the person is on the floor or ground, you can move him or her away from the scene by using the various techniques shown in **Figure 25-6** to **Figure 25-19** . Refer to **Flowchart 25-2** for additional information regarding emergency rescue moves.

## ▶ Nonemergency Moves

All injured parts should be stabilized before and during moving. If rapid transportation is not needed, it is helpful to practice on another person about the same size as the injured person.

**Figure 25-7**

Ankle drag. This is the fastest method for a short distance on a smooth surface.

**Figure 25-6**

Shoulder drag. Use for short distances over a rough surface; stabilize the person's head with your forearms.

**Figure 25-8**

Blanket pull. Roll the person onto a blanket, and pull from behind the person's head.

**Figure 25-9**

Human crutch (one person helps the person to walk). If one leg is injured, help the person to walk on the good leg while you support the injured side.

**Figure 25-11**

Firefighter's carry. If the person's injuries permit, you can travel longer distances if you carry the person over your shoulder.

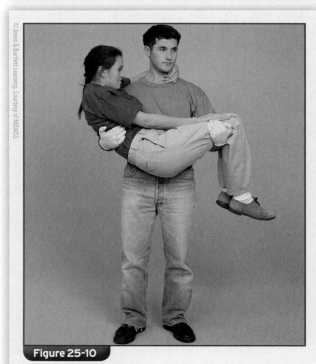

**Figure 25-10**

Cradle carry. Use this method for children and lightweight adults who cannot walk.

**Figure 25-12**

Pack-strap carry. When injuries make the firefighter's carry unsafe, this method is better for longer distances.

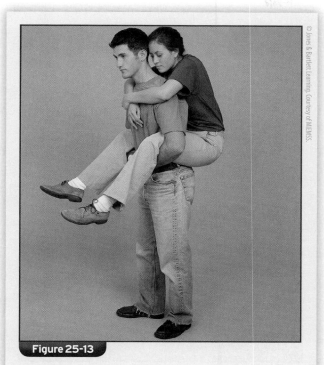

**Figure 25-13**

Piggyback carry. Use this method when the person cannot walk but can use the arms to hang onto the rescuer.

**Figure 25-15**

Two-handed seat carry.

**Figure 25-14**

Two-person assist. This method is similar to the human crutch.

**Figure 25-16**

Four-handed seat carry. This is the easiest two-person carry when no equipment is available and the person cannot walk but can use the arms to hang onto the two rescuers.

**Figure 25-17**

Extremity carry.

**Figure 25-18**

Chair carry. This method is useful for a narrow passage or up or down stairs. Use a sturdy chair that can take the person's weight.

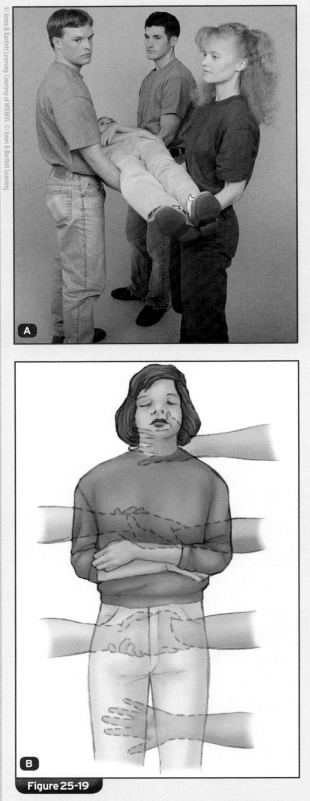

**Figure 25-19**

**A.** Hammock carry. **B.** Three to six people stand on alternate sides of the injured person and link hands beneath the person.

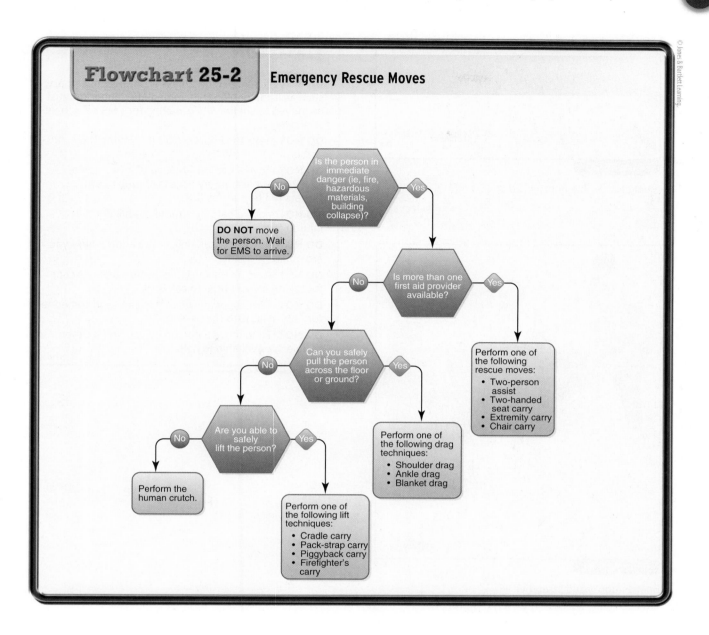

**Flowchart 25-2** | **Emergency Rescue Moves**

Is the person in immediate danger (ie, fire, hazardous materials, building collapse)?
— No → **DO NOT** move the person. Wait for EMS to arrive.
— Yes → Is more than one first aid provider available?
— No → Can you safely pull the person across the floor or ground?
— Yes → Perform one of the following rescue moves:
- Two-person assist
- Two-handed seat carry
- Extremity carry
- Chair carry

Can you safely pull the person across the floor or ground?
— No → Are you able to safely lift the person?
— Yes → Perform one of the following drag techniques:
- Shoulder drag
- Ankle drag
- Blanket drag

Are you able to safely lift the person?
— No → Perform the human crutch.
— Yes → Perform one of the following lift techniques:
- Cradle carry
- Pack-strap carry
- Piggyback carry
- Firefighter's carry

## Stretcher or Litter

The safest way to carry an injured person is on some type of stretcher or litter, which can be improvised. Before using it, test an improvised stretcher by lifting a rescuer about the same size as the injured person.

- *Blanket-and-pole improvised stretcher.* If the blanket is properly wrapped, the person's weight will keep it from unwinding **Figure 25-20** .

- *Blanket with no poles.* The blanket is rolled inward toward the person and grasped for carrying by four or more rescuers.
- *Board-improvised stretcher.* These are sturdier than a blanket-and-pole stretcher but heavier and less comfortable. Tie the person on to prevent him or her from rolling off **Figure 25-21** .
- *Commercial stretchers and litters.* These usually are not available except through EMS.

**Figure 25-20**

Blanket-and-pole improvised stretcher.

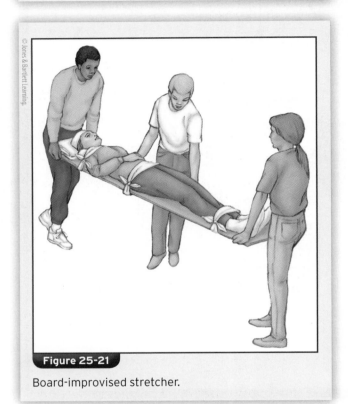

**Figure 25-21**

Board-improvised stretcher.

## CAUTION

**DO NOT** move a person unless absolutely necessary, such as if the person is in immediate danger or must be moved to shelter while waiting for EMS personnel to arrive.

**DO NOT** make the injury worse by moving the person.

**DO NOT** move a person who could have a spinal injury unless absolutely necessary due to other threats to life, such as fire.

**DO NOT** move a person without stabilizing the injured part.

**DO NOT** move a person unless you know where you are going.

**DO NOT** leave an unconscious person alone except for taking a short time to call 9-1-1.

**DO NOT** move a person when you can send someone for help. Wait with the person.

**DO NOT** try to move a person by yourself if other people are available to help.

# prep kit

## ▶ Ready for Review

- *Reach-throw-row-go* identifies the sequence for attempting a water rescue.
- If a person has fallen through the ice near the shore, extend a pole or throw a line with a floatable object attached to it.
- Electrical injuries can be devastating.
- Almost any highway crash scene involves the potential danger of hazardous chemicals.
- In most states, you are legally obligated to stop and give help when you are involved in a motor vehicle crash.
- Should you encounter a fire, you should:
  - Get all people out fast.
  - Call 9-1-1.
- When you enter any emergency scene, look for signs of an animal and proceed with caution if the animal is not threatening.
- Emergencies involving farm animals can be dangerous to rescuers.
- A confined space is any area not intended for human occupancy that may have or develop a dangerous atmosphere.
- The goal of triage is to do the greatest good for the greatest number of people.
- A variety of systems are used to identify care and transportation priorities.
- A person should not be moved until he or she is ready for transportation to a hospital, if required.
- The major danger in moving a person quickly is the possibility of aggravating a spinal injury.
- All injured parts should be stabilized before and during moving.

## ▶ Vital Vocabulary

**drowning** The process of experiencing respiratory impairment from submersion/immersion in liquid.

**heat escape lessening position (HELP)** The recommended position (knees pulled up, arms crossed) for a person who is in cold water and wearing a flotation device; meant to minimize heat loss and increase chances of survival.

**triage** A system used for sorting people to determine the order in which they will receive medical attention.

## ▶ Assessment in Action

You are fishing at the nearby lake. Several swimmers and others in canoes are also enjoying the lake. One swimmer decides to swim to the other side but begins to struggle about 30 feet (9 m) off shore.

*Directions*: Circle Yes if you agree with the statement; circle No if you disagree.

Yes   No   **1.** This type of drowning situation is called distressed nonswimmer.

Yes   No   **2.** You are a very strong swimmer so you should immediately jump in the lake to rescue the person.

Yes   No   **3.** You could try throwing a floating object to the person.

Yes   No   **4.** The best option in this situation would be to use a canoe to rescue the person.

## ▶ Check Your Knowledge

*Directions*: Circle Yes if you agree with the statement; circle No if you disagree.

Yes   No   **1.** You should attempt to move downed power lines away from a person by using a broom or other wooden object.

Yes   No   **2.** Strong, unusual odors or clouds of vapor are possible indications of the presence of hazardous materials.

Yes   No   **3.** To keep from becoming trapped while attempting to extinguish a fire, you should always keep a door behind you for rapid exit.

Yes   No   **4.** In a situation involving several people, those with breathing difficulties need immediate attention.

Yes   No   **5.** A major concern in moving a person quickly is the possibility of aggravating a spinal injury.

Yes   No   **6.** *Row-throw-reach-go* represents the safe order for executing a water rescue.

Yes   No   **7.** In most states, you are legally obligated to stop and give help when you are involved in a motor vehicle crash.

Yes   No   **8.** The first thing to do in case of a fire is to use a fire extinguisher and try to put out the fire.

Yes   No   **9.** When using a fire extinguisher, aim it at the base of the flames.

Yes   No   **10.** When several people are injured, those crying or screaming should receive your attention first.

# Disaster Preparedness

**26**

## Disaster Preparedness

Disasters are a fact of life. Each year thousands of disasters, large and small, natural and caused by humans, strike somewhere in the world. Many people have survived disasters, thanks to good luck and willpower, but that is not enough. Training about disasters needs to be modified from "nice to know" to "must know." Every American will likely experience or witness at least one disaster during his or her lifetime. The tragedy is that each citizen can be better prepared than he or she is now for that disaster. When a disaster strikes, you must be ready to act.

Valuable information about disasters is discussed in this chapter. This information is adapted from US government documents provided by the Federal Emergency Management Agency (FEMA), the US Department of Homeland Security, the National Weather Service, the US Department of Labor, and the US Geological Survey.

## ▶ Natural Disasters

Natural disasters such as earthquakes, floods, hurricanes, and tornados claim many lives each year. Becoming informed about the dangers of natural disasters and the steps you can take to protect yourself and others can help minimize injuries and deaths.

## Earthquake

An earthquake is a sudden, rapid shaking of the earth caused by the breaking and shifting of rock deep beneath the earth's surface. This shaking can cause buildings and bridges to collapse; disrupt gas, electric, and phone service; and sometimes trigger landslides, avalanches, flash floods, fires, and huge, destructive ocean waves known as tsunamis. Earthquakes can occur at any time of the year **Figure 26-1**.

### What To Do During an Earthquake

Follow these safety guidelines if you experience an earthquake:

- If you are indoors, take cover under a sturdy desk, table, or bench or against an inside wall. If the earthquake is severe, crouch next to a large, sturdy object such as a refrigerator or file cabinet. Should the ceiling collapse, a triangle of space next to the object will provide a safe place. Stay away from glass, windows, outside doors, walls, and anything that could fall. If there is no table or desk nearby, cover your face and head with your arms and crouch down; a door frame may offer some protection.
- Stay inside until the shaking has stopped and you are sure exiting is safe. It is dangerous to try to leave a building during an earthquake because objects can fall on you. Beware of aftershocks, and follow the same precautions as for an earthquake.

**Figure 26-1**

Devastation resulting from the California earthquake that crippled San Francisco in 1989.

- If you are in bed, stay there, and protect your head with a pillow, unless you are under a heavy light or fan fixture that could fall. If the earthquake is severe, move to the floor next to, but not under, the bed. This will also provide a safe space if the ceiling collapses.
- If you are in a high-rise building, expect the fire alarms and sprinklers to go off during an earthquake. **DO NOT** use the elevators; use the stairs.
- If you are outdoors, find a clear spot away from buildings, trees, streetlights, and power lines. Drop to the ground and stay there until the shaking stops.
- If you are in a vehicle, pull over and stay there with your seat belt fastened until the shaking has stopped. If the earthquake is severe and you are under a highway overpass, exit your car and lie next to, but not underneath, your vehicle. The falling debris may crush the roof of the car, but beside the car will be a safe place for you to stay until help arrives.
- If you are trapped in debris, do not panic. Move carefully.
  - **DO NOT** use a flame for light because gas leaks.
  - **DO NOT** move about or kick up dust.
  - Cover your mouth with a handkerchief or clothing.
  - Tap on a pipe or wall so rescuers can locate you.
- Learn how to turn off your gas supply where it enters the house. Turn off the gas if you smell gas or have to evacuate.
  - If you smell gas, **DO NOT** use light switches or any other devices that can spark.

## Flood

With the exception of fire, floods are the most common and widespread of all natural disasters. Most communities have experienced some type of flooding after heavy storms or winter snow thaws **Figure 26-2**. Pay attention to flash flood warnings in your area even if skies are clear because runoff can occur from storms miles away. Be especially aware of storms in hills above you. Flash floods occur when heavy rain causes runoff into

**Figure 26-2**

Hurricane Katrina (2005) caused massive floods in New Orleans.

channels and low-lying areas. The flood can be very fast and can occur miles from the rain, often catching people off guard.

## What To Do During a Flood

Follow these safety guidelines if conditions exist that could cause a flood:

- Be aware of the likelihood of flooding in your area. If there is any possibility of a flood or flash flood, move immediately to higher ground. Be aware of streams, drainage channels, canyons, and other areas prone to flooding quickly and suddenly.
- Listen to your local radio or television stations or check social media outlets for information.
- If local authorities issue a flood watch, prepare to evacuate.
- Secure your home, if you have time. Move essential items to upper floors.
- If instructed, turn off utilities at the main switches or valves. Disconnect electrical appliances. **DO NOT** touch electrical equipment if you are wet or standing in water.
- If you are not evacuating, you still need to prepare for the worst. If you do not have access to adequate bottled water, you can fill the bathtub with water in case water becomes contaminated or services are cut off. Before filling the tub, sterilize it with a diluted bleach solution (1 part bleach to 10 parts water).
- **DO NOT** walk through moving water. Six inches (15 cm) of moving water can knock you off your feet. Use a stick or pole to check the firmness of the ground and water depth in front of you.

- **DO NOT** drive into flooded areas. A foot of water can float a vehicle. Two feet (61 cm) of water can carry away most vehicles, including sport utility vehicles and pickups.
- If flood water rises around your car and you cannot drive out, abandon the car and move to higher ground, but only if you can safely do so.

## Heat Wave

In extreme heat and high humidity, cooling of the body by evaporation is slowed and it is difficult for the body to maintain normal temperature **Figure 26-3**. People living in urban areas may be at greater risk from the effects of a prolonged heat wave than those living in rural areas. Asphalt and concrete store heat longer and gradually release heat at night. A devastating heat wave struck Europe in 2003, resulting in thousands of injuries and deaths.

## What To Do During a Heat Wave

Follow these safety guidelines if you experience a heat-wave emergency:

- Stay in the coolest available location. Stay indoors as much as possible. If air-conditioning is not available, stay on the lowest floor out of the sunshine. Circulate the air with a fan, and use cool, wet cloths to help keep your body temperature down.
- Drink plenty of water regularly, even if you do not feel thirsty.
- Avoid drinking alcoholic beverages because they cause further dehydration.
- Never leave children or pets alone in vehicles.
- Dress in loose-fitting clothes. Lightweight, light-colored clothing reflects heat and sunlight and helps maintain normal body temperature.
- Protect your face and head outdoors by wearing a wide-brimmed hat.
- Avoid too much sunshine. Sunburn slows the skin's ability to cool itself.
- Avoid strenuous work during the warmest part of the day (usually at 1000 to 1500 hours).
- Spend at least 2 hours of the day in an air-conditioned place. If your home is not air-conditioned, consider spending the warmest part of the day in public buildings (for example, libraries, movie theaters, and shopping malls).

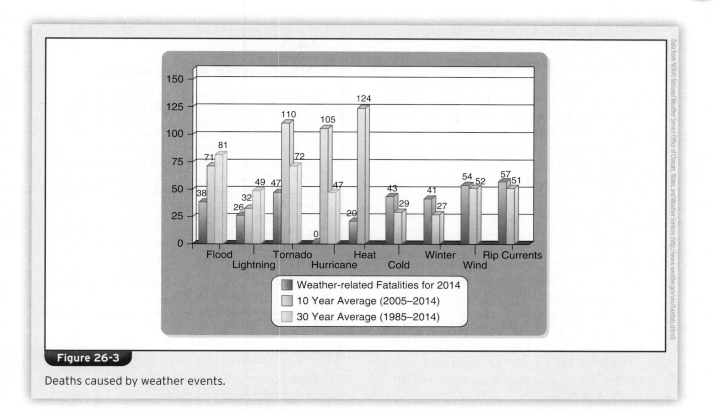

**Figure 26-3**

Deaths caused by weather events.

- Check on family, friends, and neighbors who do not have air-conditioning and who spend much of their time alone. Refer to Chapter 19, *Bites and Stings*, for first aid procedures for heat-related emergencies (for example, heatstroke, heat exhaustion, and heat cramps).

## Hurricane

A **hurricane** is a tropical storm with winds that have reached a constant speed of at least 74 miles per hour (119 kph). As a hurricane nears land, it can bring torrential rains, high winds, and flooding from the ocean, called storm surges. All Atlantic and Gulf of Mexico coastal areas are subject to hurricanes or tropical storms. August and September are the peak months of hurricane activity during the storm season, which lasts from June to November **Figure 26-4**. In the Pacific Ocean, these storms are called typhoons.

### What To Do During a Hurricane

Follow these safety guidelines if you experience the threat of a hurricane:

- Listen to your local radio or television stations or check social media outlets for information. If a hurricane watch is issued, you usually have 24 to 36 hours before the hurricane hits land.

**Figure 26-4**

Hurricanes are among the most costly and dangerous disasters.

- Secure your home. Close any storm shutters. Secure outdoor objects or bring them indoors. Attach boards to window frames or tape windows to prevent or reduce the risk of broken glass. Park cars remaining at home along the side of the house. Make sure that all vehicles have a full tank of gas.

- If you are not evacuating, you need to prepare for the worst. Gather several days' supply of water and food for each household member. If you do not have access to adequate bottled water, fill the bathtub with water in case water becomes contaminated or services are cut off. Before filling the tub, sterilize it with a diluted bleach solution (1 part bleach to 10 parts water).
- If you are evacuating, prepare backpacks to take your disaster supplies with you to the shelter.
- When preparing to evacuate, fuel your vehicle and review evacuation routes. If instructed, turn off utilities at the main valves or switches before departing your residence.
- Evacuate to an inland location early if:
  - Local authorities announce an evacuation and you live in an evacuation zone.
  - You live in a mobile home near the path of the hurricane.
  - You live in a high-rise building near the path of the hurricane.
  - You live on the coast, on a flood plain near a river, or near an inland waterway.
  - You think you are in danger.
- Leave immediately if local authorities order an evacuation. Follow evacuation routes; stay away from coastal areas, riverbanks, and streams; and tell others where you are going.
- If you are not required to evacuate or are unable to evacuate, stay indoors and away from windows and glass doors during the hurricane.
- To protect yourself against the strong wind:
  - Take refuge in a small interior room, closet, or hallway.
  - Close all interior doors; secure and brace exterior doors.
  - In a multiple-story building, go to the first or second floor and stay in interior rooms away from the windows.
  - Lie on the floor under a table or other sturdy object if a hurricane or any associated tornado approaches.
- Phone lines are likely to be busy with emergency traffic. Avoid using the phone except for serious emergencies.

## Q&A

**What part does first aid play in disasters?**

The value of first aid training for laypeople has increased during natural and man-made disasters. When a sudden disaster strikes, survivors often constitute the only source of initial help because medical help takes time to mobilize or is insufficient.

Reports from bombings in New York and London state that first aid by bystanders saved lives. In the Madrid bombings, 67% of the injured people arrived at the hospital in nonambulance vehicles. Transport by bystanders occurs in many mass casualty disasters if ambulance transport is lacking. Officials interviewed after disasters strongly agree that first aid training for laypeople decreases death.

*Source:* Van de Velde S, et al. Effectiveness of nonresuscitative first aid training in laypeople: a systematic review. *Ann Emerg Med* 2009; 54(3):447-457.

## Landslides

Landslides occur in almost every US state when masses of rock, earth, or debris move down a slope. They may be small or large and can move at slow or high speeds. They are usually associated with periods of heavy rainfall or rapid snowmelt.

### What To Do During a Landslide

Follow these safety guidelines if conditions exist that could cause a landslide:

- Stay alert. Many landslides occur when people are sleeping.
- If you are in an area susceptible to landslides, consider evacuating if it is safe to do so.
- Listen for unusual sounds that might indicate moving debris, such as trees cracking, boulders knocking together, or rumbling.
- If you are near a stream or channel, be alert for any sudden increase or decrease in water flow and for a change from clear to muddy water. Such changes may indicate landslide activity upstream, so be prepared to move quickly.
- Be alert when driving. Embankments along roadsides are susceptible to landslides. Watch the road for collapsed pavement, mud, fallen rocks, and other indications of possible debris flow.
- If you remain at home, move to a second level if possible to distance yourself from the direct path of landslide debris.

## Tornado

A tornado is a violent windstorm characterized by a twisting, funnel-shaped cloud. It is spawned by a thunderstorm (or sometimes as a result of a hurricane). Tornado season is generally March through August, although tornadoes can occur at any time of the year. Every state is at some risk from this hazard, but tornados are most frequently reported east of the Rocky Mountains Figure 26-5 .

### What To Do During a Tornado

Follow these safety guidelines if you experience a tornado. If you are at home:

- Go immediately to a windowless interior room, storm cellar, basement, or the lowest level of the building. If there is no basement, go to an inner hallway or a smaller inner room without windows, such as a bathroom or closet.
- Get under a piece of sturdy furniture (such as a heavy table or desk) and hold on to it.

If you are outdoors:

- If possible, get inside a building.
- If shelter is not available or there is no time to get indoors, lie in a ditch or low-lying area or crouch near a strong building.

If you are at work or school:

- Avoid places with wide-span roofs such as auditoriums, cafeterias, large hallways, and shopping malls.
- Go to a predetermined shelter area (signs are usually posted).
- Get under a piece of sturdy furniture (such as a heavy table, desk, or workbench).

If you are in a vehicle:

- **DO NOT** try to outrun a tornado.
- Get out of the vehicle immediately and take shelter in a nearby building. If there is no time to get indoors, get out of the car and lie in a ditch or low-lying area away from the vehicle.

## Tsunami

A **tsunami** (pronounced soo-NAHM-ee) is a series of waves generated by an undersea disturbance (for example, an earthquake). From the area of disturbance, the waves travel outward in all directions, much like the ripples caused by throwing a rock into a pond. Tsunamis reaching heights of more than 100 feet (30 m) have been recorded near coastlines, although most waves are less than 18 feet (5 m) high. Areas of greatest risk are less than 50 feet (15 m) above sea level and within 1 mile (2 km) of the shoreline. Drowning is the most common cause of death due to a tsunami.

### What To Do During a Tsunami

Follow these safety guidelines if conditions exist that could cause a tsunami:

- Listen to your local radio or television stations or check social media outlets for information. If you are advised to evacuate, do so immediately.
- Stay away from the area until local authorities say it is safe to return.
- **DO NOT** go to the shoreline to watch for a tsunami. If you can see the wave, you are too

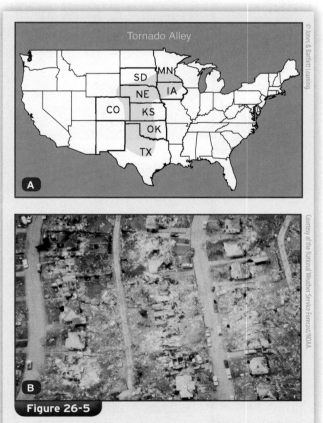

**Figure 26-5**

**A.** Tornados are most frequently reported east of the Rocky Mountains. **B.** The tornado in Wichita Falls, Texas, in 1979 was one of the worst tornadoes in US history.

close to escape it. Because a tsunami is a series of waves, do not assume that one wave means the danger is over.

## Volcano Eruption

A volcano is a mountain that opens downward to a reservoir of molten rock below the earth's surface. When the pressure from gases and molten rock becomes strong enough to cause an explosion, eruptions occur. Gases and rock shoot up through the opening and spill over the mountainsides and/or spew into the air. Most injuries and deaths are due to ash, falling rocks, landslides, and floods, rather than hot flowing lava.

### What To Do During a Volcano Eruption

Follow these safety guidelines if a volcano erupts:

- Follow the evacuation order issued by local authorities. Avoid areas downwind from the volcano.

If caught indoors:

- Close all windows, doors, and chimney and stove dampers.

If caught outdoors:

- Seek shelter indoors.
- Avoid low-lying areas where poisonous gases can collect and flash floods and lava and mudflows can be dangerous.
- Put all machinery inside a garage or barn.

Protect yourself:

- Wear long-sleeved shirts and pants.
- Use goggles to protect your eyes.
- Use a dust mask or hold a damp cloth over your face to keep from breathing in the hot ash or gases.
- Stay out of the area around the erupting volcano. Trying to watch an erupting volcano can be deadly.

## Wildfire

Forest, brush, and grass fires can occur at any time of the year, but mostly during long, dry hot spells. The majority of these fires are caused by human carelessness or ignorance **Figure 26-6**.

## What To Do During a Wildfire

Follow these safety guidelines if a wildfire occurs:

- Listen to your local radio or television stations or check social media outlets for information.
- If advised to evacuate, do so immediately. Choose a route away from the fire hazard. Watch for changes in the speed and direction of fire and smoke. **DO NOT** block firefighting entrance routes.

## Winter Storm

Heavy snowfall and extreme cold can immobilize an entire region. Even areas that usually experience mild winters can be hit with a major snowstorm or extreme cold **Figure 26-7**.

**Figure 26-6**

Wildfires can move quickly, threatening lives and homes.

**Figure 26-7**

Major winter snowstorms can tie up a city.

**FYI**

**Storm Watch Versus Storm Warning**

Government agencies such as the National Weather Service issue alerts when threats arise. A watch, such as a tornado watch, is issued when conditions are ripe for the development of that threat. A warning is issued if the threat is actually occurring or has been detected.

## What To Do During a Winter Storm

Follow these safety guidelines if a winter storm occurs. If indoors:

- Listen to your local radio or television stations, social media outlets, or the National Oceanic and Atmospheric Administration (NOAA) weather radio for weather reports and emergency information.
- Conserve fuel by lowering the thermostat to 65°F (18.3°C) during the day and 55°F (12.8°C) at night. Close off unused rooms.
- Eat regularly and drink ample fluids, but avoid caffeine and alcohol.
- If using kerosene heaters, maintain ventilation, refuel the heater outside, and keep heaters at least 3 feet (1 m) from flammable objects.
- Never use heat sources or generators designed for outside use in a closed space.

If outdoors:

- Dress warmly (ie, several layers of loose fitting clothing, a hat, and a scarf to cover your mouth and protect your lungs).
- Avoid overexertion (eg, shoveling snow or pushing a car), which can bring on a heart attack.
- Be aware of signs of frostbite and hypothermia.
- Keep dry by changing wet clothing, which does not insulate well.

If trapped in a vehicle during a winter storm:

- Pull off the highway. Turn on the vehicle's hazard lights. Hang a distress flag from the window or radio antenna.
- Stay inside the vehicle. Rescuers are more likely to find you. **DO NOT** set out on foot unless you can see a building close by where you know you can take shelter.

- Run the engine and heater about 10 minutes each hour to keep warm. When the engine is running, open a window slightly for ventilation, and clear snow from the exhaust pipe to prevent carbon monoxide poisoning.
- Exercise (eg, clap your hands and move your arms and legs occasionally) to maintain body heat, but avoid overexertion.
- In extreme cold, use floor mats, seat covers, road maps, newspapers, and other available resources for insulation. Huddle with other passengers.
- Take turns sleeping. One person should be awake at all times to look for rescue crews.
- Drink fluids to avoid dehydration.
- Watch for signs of frostbite and hypothermia.
- Be careful not to waste battery power.
- At night, turn on the inside light so work crews or rescuers can see you.
- Once the winter storm passes, you may need to leave the car and proceed on foot.

**FYI**

**Winter Travel Supplies**

When traveling during the winter, carry disaster supplies in the vehicle. The kit should include the following:
- Shovel
- Windshield scraper
- Flashlight
- Extra batteries
- Battery-powered radio
- Water
- Snack food
- Gloves and mittens
- Hat
- Blanket
- Tow chain or rope
- Tire chains
- Bag of road salt and sand
- Fluorescent distress flag
- Jumper or booster cables
- Road maps
- Emergency flares
- Cellular telephone
- Emergency heating candles and container

## ▶ Technological Hazards

### Hazardous Materials Incidents

Chemicals are found everywhere. They can become hazardous during their production, storage, transportation, and disposal. It is not always possible to identify a situation as one involving hazardous materials, but clues such as a leaking cargo trailer, color-coded placards (signs) on abandoned drums, and unusual odors can be good indicators **Figure 26-8**.

### What To Do During a Hazardous Materials Incident

Follow these safety guidelines if a hazardous materials incident occurs:

- If you witness an incident that you believe to be a hazardous materials incident, call 9-1-1 or your local emergency telephone number.
- Stay away from the incident site.
- If caught outside, remember that gases and mists are usually heavier than air. Try to stay upstream, uphill, and upwind. Try to go at least one-half mile from the danger area.
- If in a vehicle, stop and seek shelter in a permanent building if possible. If you must remain in the vehicle, keep the windows and vents closed and shut off the air conditioner and heater.
- If asked to evacuate your home, do so immediately.
- If requested to stay indoors rather than evacuate:

  - Follow all instructions and close all exterior doors, windows, vents, and fireplace dampers.
  - Turn off air conditioners and ventilation systems.
  - Go into an above-ground room with the fewest openings to the outside; close the doors and windows; tape around the sides, bottom, and top of the door; and cover each window and vent in the room with a single piece of plastic sheeting.
  - Listen to local emergency broadcasts.
  - When advised that it is safe to leave your shelter, open all doors and windows and turn on air-conditioning and ventilation systems to flush out any chemicals that infiltrated the building.

**Figure 26-8**

Fumes leaking from a cargo truck could be an indication of a hazardous materials incident.

### Nuclear Power Plants

Nuclear power plants operate in most states and produce about 20% of the nation's power. Nearly 6 million Americans live within 10 miles (16 km) of a nuclear power plant, according to the Natural Resources Defense Council. Although these plants are closely monitored and regulated, unintentional radiation exposures are possible. Local and state governments, federal agencies, and electric utility companies have emergency response plans for nuclear power plant incidents.

### What To Do During a Nuclear Power Plant Emergency

Follow these safety guidelines in a nuclear power plant emergency:

- Stay tuned to local radio and television stations. Local authorities will provide specific information and instructions.
- Evacuate if you are advised to do so.
- If told not to evacuate, remain indoors. Close the doors and windows and turn off the air conditioner, ventilation fans, furnace, and other air intakes. Go to a basement or other underground area if possible. Keep a battery-powered radio with you at all times.
- Do not use the telephone unless absolutely necessary. Lines will be needed for emergency calls.
- If you suspect exposure, take a thorough shower. Change clothes and shoes. Put all exposed clothing in a plastic bag. Seal the bag and place it out of the way.
- Seek medical care for any symptoms, such as nausea, that may be related to radiation exposure.

## Disaster Myths

Myth: Disasters are truly exceptional events.

Reality: They are a normal part of daily life and in many cases are repetitive events.

Myth: Disasters kill people without respect for social class or economic status.

Reality: The poor and marginalized are more at risk of death than are rich people or the middle classes.

Myth: People can survive for many days when trapped under the rubble of a collapsed building.

Reality: The vast majority of people brought out alive from the rubble are saved within 24 or perhaps even 12 hours of impact.

Myth: When disaster strikes, panic is a common reaction.

Reality: Most people behave rationally in a disaster. While panic is not to be ruled out entirely, it is of such limited importance that some leading disaster sociologists regard it as insignificant or unlikely.

Myth: After disaster has struck, survivors tend to be dazed and apathetic.

Reality: Survivors rapidly start reconstruction. Activism is much more common than fatalism (this is the so-called "therapeutic community"). Even in the worst scenarios, only 15% to 30% of people show passive or dazed reactions.

Myth: Looting is a common and serious issue after disasters.

Reality: Looting is rare and limited in scope. It mainly occurs when there are strong preconditions, as when a community is already deeply divided.

Myth: Disease epidemics are an almost inevitable result of the disruption and poor health caused by major disasters.

Reality: Generally, the level of epidemiological surveillance and health care in the disaster area is sufficient to stop any possible disease epidemic from occurring. However, the rate of diagnosis of diseases may increase as a result of improved health care.

Myth: In order to manage a disaster well, it is necessary to accept all forms of aid that are offered.

Reality: It is better to limit acceptance of donations to goods and services that are actually needed in the disaster area.

Myth: Unburied dead bodies constitute a health hazard.

Reality: Not even advanced decomposition causes a significant health hazard. Hasty burial demoralizes survivors and upsets arrangements for death certification, funeral rites, and, where needed, autopsy.

Myth: One should donate used clothes to people affected by disasters.

Reality: This often leads to accumulations of huge quantities of useless garments that people cannot or will not wear.

Myth: Companies, corporations, associations, and governments are always very generous when invited to send aid and relief to disaster areas.

Reality: They may be, but in the past disaster areas have been used as dumping grounds for outdated medicines, obsolete equipment, and unusable goods, all under the cloak of apparent generosity.

Myth: There is usually a shortage of resources when disaster occurs and this prevents them from being managed effectively.

Reality: The shortage, if it occurs, is almost always very temporary. There is more of an issue in deploying resources well and using them efficiently than in acquiring them. Often, there is also an issue of coping with a superabundance of certain types of resources.

*Source:* Alexander DE. Misconception as a barrier to teaching about disasters. *Prehosp Disaster Med* 2007; 22(2):95-103.

## ▶ National Security Emergencies

### Terrorism

__Terrorism__ is the use of force or violence against people or property in violation of the criminal laws of the United States for purposes of intimidation, coercion, or ransom. Acts of terrorism range from threats of terrorism, assassinations, kidnappings, hijackings, bomb scares and bombings, and cyber attacks (computer based) to the use of chemical, biologic, and nuclear weapons Figure 26-9 .

The Homeland Security Advisory System is designed to provide quick, comprehensive information about the potential threat of terrorist attacks or threat levels. Threat conditions can apply nationally, regionally, by industry, or by specific target. You should be aware of the current Homeland Security threat level at all times Table 26-1 .

**Figure 26-9**

The September 11, 2001 terrorist attacks on the World Trade Center in New York City.

## Table 26-1 Homeland Security Advisory System

| Threat Level | Protective Measures You Should Take |
|---|---|
| Severe | • Avoid high-risk areas such as public gatherings.<br>• Listen attentively to news for advisories and instructions.<br>• Contact employers to determine work status. |
| High | Review evacuation and sheltering measures for different types of attacks (chemical, biologic, or radiologic). |
| Elevated | Watch and report any suspicious activity. Contact school(s) to determine their emergency procedures. |
| Guarded | • Review home disaster plan and update supplies.<br>• Meet with your family to discuss what to do, where to go, and how to communicate if an attack occurs |
| Low | Develop a home disaster plan and disaster supply kit. |

## Chemical and Biologic Agents

**Chemical warfare agents** are poisonous vapors, aerosols, liquids, or solids that have toxic effects on people, animals, or plants. They can be released by bombs; sprayed from aircraft, boats, or vehicles; or used in liquid form to create a hazard to people and the environment. Some chemical agents may be odorless and tasteless. They can have an immediate effect (a few seconds to a few minutes) or a delayed effect (several hours to several days). Although potentially lethal, chemical agents are difficult to deliver in lethal concentrations. Outdoors, the agents often dissipate rapidly.

**Biologic agents** are organisms or toxins that can kill or incapacitate people, livestock, and crops. The three basic groups of biologic agents likely to be used as weapons are bacteria, viruses, and toxins.

### What To Do During a Chemical or Biologic Attack

If a chemical or biologic weapon attack occurs near you, authorities will instruct you on the best course of action, which may be to evacuate the area immediately, seek shelter at a designated location, or take immediate shelter where you are and seal the premises. The best way to protect yourself is to take emergency preparedness measures ahead of time and get medical attention as soon as possible, if needed.

Follow these additional safety guidelines if a chemical or biologic attack occurs:

- Listen to your local radio or television stations or check social media outlets for instructions from authorities, such as whether to remain inside or to evacuate.
- If instructed to remain in your home, office building, or other shelter during a chemical or biologic attack:
  - Turn off all ventilation, including furnaces, air conditioners, vents, and fans.
  - Seek shelter in an internal room, preferably one without windows. Seal the room with duct tape and plastic sheeting.
  - Avoid the furnace or utility room.
  - **DO NOT** use any major appliances (for example, the furnace, oven or range, clothes dryer, or washing machine).
- Remain in protected areas where toxic vapors are reduced or eliminated, and take a battery-operated radio with you.
- If caught in an unprotected area, try to get upwind of the contaminated area, try to find shelter inside a building as quickly as possible, and listen to your local radio or television stations or check social media outlets for official instructions.

## Nuclear and Radiologic Weapons

Nuclear explosions can cause deadly effects such as blinding light, intense heat (thermal radiation), initial nuclear radiation, blast fires started by the heat pulse, and secondary fires caused by the destruction. Surface-level explosions also produce radioactive particles called fallout that can be carried by wind for hundreds of miles.

Terrorist use of a radiologic dispersion device—often called a dirty bomb—is considered far more likely than use of a nuclear device. These radiologic weapons are a combination of conventional explosives and radioactive material designed to scatter dangerous and sublethal amounts of radioactive material over a general area. There is no way of knowing how much warning time there would be before an attack by a terrorist using a nuclear or radiologic weapon.

## What To Do During a Nuclear or Radiologic Attack

Follow these safety guidelines if a nuclear or radiologic attack occurs:

- Avoid looking at the flash or fireball; it can blind you.
- If you hear an attack warning:
  - Take cover as quickly as you can, below ground if possible, and stay there until instructed to do otherwise.
  - If caught outside and unable to get inside immediately, take cover behind anything that might offer protection. Lie flat on the ground and cover your head.
  - If the explosion is some distance away, it could take 30 seconds or more for the blast wave to hit. Be aware of a second, returning blast wave.
  - Protect yourself from radioactive fallout by taking shelter, even if you are many miles from the source of the explosion.
  - Keep a battery-powered radio with you, and listen for official information. Follow the instructions given. Local instructions should always take precedence; officials in your area know the local situation best.

**FYI**

**Disaster Preparedness**

The US Department of Homeland Security offers these general guidelines for food and water needs for survival during emergency situations.

**Water**

- One gallon (4 L) of water per person per day, for drinking and sanitation.
- Keep at least a 3-day supply of water per person.
- Children, nursing mothers, and people who are ill may need more water.
- If you live in a warm-weather climate, more water may be necessary.

**Food**

- Store at least a 3-day supply of nonperishable food.
- Select foods that require no refrigeration, preparation, or cooking and little or no water.
- Pack a manual can opener and eating utensils.
- Choose foods your family will eat:
  - Ready-to-eat canned meats, fruits, and vegetables
  - Protein or fruit bars
  - Dry cereal or granola
  - Peanut butter
  - Dried fruit
  - Nuts
  - Crackers
  - Canned juices
  - Nonperishable pasteurized milk
  - High-energy foods
  - Vitamins
  - Food for infants
  - Comfort foods

**First Aid Kit**

- See Appendix A for suggestions for your first aid kit.

# prep kit

## ▶ Ready for Review

- Disasters are a fact of life, and you need to be prepared.
- Natural disasters such as earthquakes, floods, hurricanes, and tornados claim many lives each year.
- Chemicals are found everywhere; they can be hazardous during their production, storage, transportation, and disposal.
- Terrorism is the use of force or violence against people or property in violation of the criminal laws of the United States for purposes of intimidation, coercion, or ransom.
- When disaster strikes, you must be ready to act.

## ▶ Vital Vocabulary

**biologic agents** Organisms or toxins that can kill or incapacitate people, livestock, and crops.

**chemical warfare agents** Poisonous vapors, aerosols, liquids, or solids that have toxic effects.

**hurricane** A tropical storm with winds that have reached a constant speed of at least 74 miles per hour (119 kph). Those in the Pacific Ocean are called typhoons and those in the Indian Ocean are known as cyclones.

**terrorism** Use of force or violence against people or property in violation of criminal laws for purposes of intimidation, coercion, or ransom.

**tsunami** A series of waves generated by an undersea disturbance.

## ▶ Assessment in Action

Seismologists have been predicting a large earthquake for your region of the country within the next 10 years. While at work on the top floor of your three-story office building, the predictions come true. Sudden shaking begins, and you feel the building move. Wall hangings and items on shelves begin to fall to the ground.

*Directions:* Circle Yes if you agree with the statement; circle No if you disagree.

Yes  No  **1.** This is most likely not the "big one," so you can continue your work as normal.

Yes  No  **2.** You should take cover under your desk.

Yes  No  **3.** You should call 9-1-1 to report the emergency.

Yes  No  **4.** You should know all the exit routes from your building.

Yes  No  **5.** If you smell gas, you should not delay your evacuation from the building.

## ▶ Check Your Knowledge

*Directions:* Circle Yes if you agree with the statement; circle No if you disagree.

Yes  No  **1.** Earthquakes most often occur in the winter.

Yes  No  **2.** Never walk through moving water.

Yes  No  **3.** People in urban areas may be at greater risk from the effects of a prolonged heat wave than those in rural areas.

Yes  No  **4.** Hurricane season is from April until August.

Yes  No  **5.** Hide in a room with open windows if you are in the path of a tornado.

Yes  No  **6.** Never go near the shoreline to watch for a tsunami.

Yes  No  **7.** If you are trapped inside your car during a winter storm, run the engine and heater 10 minutes each hour to keep warm.

Yes  No  **8.** If you witness a hazardous materials incident, get up close to find out the name of the hazardous material before calling 9-1-1.

Yes  No  **9.** You should be aware of the Homeland Security threat level at all times.

Yes  No  **10.** All chemical agents have a smell or taste.

# First Aid Supplies

## First Aid Supplies

Many injuries and sudden illnesses can be cared for without medical attention. For these situations and for situations requiring medical attention later, it is a good idea to have useful supplies on hand for emergencies.

Supplies in a first aid kit should be customized to include those items likely to be used on a regular basis. For example, a first aid kit for the home may be different from one at a workplace or one found on a boat.

The list in Table A-1 includes nonprescription (over-the-counter [OTC]) medications. Some drug products lose their potency over time, especially after they have been opened. Therefore, buying a large, family size of a product that you use infrequently may not be economical. Note the expiration date on every medication.

Keep all medicines out of the reach of children. Read and follow all directions for properly using medications. Consider keeping your first aid supplies in either a fishing tackle box or a tool box.

### Table A-1 Sample Items for a First Aid Kit

| **Items for Bleeding Control** | |
|---|---|
| Disposable medical exam gloves (non-latex) | Protects against potentially infected blood, body fluids, or contaminated items |
| Hemostatic wound dressing | Use only when direct pressure fails to control bleeding. |
| Tourniquet | Use only when direct pressure fails to control bleeding. |
| **Items for Wound Care** | |
| Alcohol hand sanitizer (small bottle) | Cleans hands and the area around the wound (not inside wound) |
| Antibiotic ointment (Polysporin, Neosporin, Bacitracinor triple-antibiotic ointment) | Reduces healing time and reduces the risk of skin infections that are associated with shallow wounds and small second-degree burns |
| Surgical tape (Micropore paper tape) (1 in. and 2 in. [3 cm and 5 cm]) | Covers blisters |
| Elastic tape (Elastikon) (2 in. and 4 in. [5 cm and 10 cm]) | Covers wounds and blisters |
| Blister pad (Spenco 2nd Skin) (1 in. and 3 in. [3 cm and 7 cm]) | Covers wounds and blisters |
| Adhesive bandages (1 in. × 3 in. [3 cm × 7 cm] and other various sizes) Figure A-1 | Covers minor wounds |
| Sterile gauze pads (3 in. × 3 in. and 4 in. × 4 in. [7 cm × 7 cm and 10 cm × 10 cm]; individually wrapped) Figure A-2 | Covers wounds |
| Nonstick pads (3 in. × 4 in. [7 cm × 10 cm]) | Covers burns, blisters, and scrapes |
| Self-adhering roller gauze bandage (2 in., 3 in., and 4 in. [5 cm, 7 cm, and 10 cm] wide) Figure A-3 | Holds dressings in place |
| Sterile trauma pad (5 in. × 9 in., 8 in. × 10 in. [13 cm × 23 cm, 20 cm × 25 cm]) Figure A-4 | Covers large wounds |

*(Continues)*

## Table A-1 Sample Items for a First Aid Kit, Continued

| | |
|---|---|
| Triangular bandage (about 40 in. × 40 in. × 56 in. [102 cm × 102 cm × 142 cm]) | When folded (known as a cravat bandage), it can hold dressings and splints in place or it can be applied as a swathe (binder) for an arm sling. |
| Sterile eye pads | Cover both eyes to prevent both eyes from moving, even if only one is injured. |
| **Items for Bone, Joint, and Muscle Care** | |
| Cold pack (instant and disposable) | Use on sprains, dislocations, fractures, and insect stings when ice is not available. |
| Splint (padded and malleable, such as a SAM Splint) | Stabilizes broken bones and dislocations |
| Elastic bandage (3 in. [7 cm] wide) **Figure A-5** | Provides compression to reduce the swelling of joint injuries |
| Plastic bags (sealable) | Holds ice to apply on insect stings and bone, joint, and muscle injuries; contains embedded tick after its removal |
| **Nonprescription (OTC) Medications** *Keep all medications out of the reach of children and use child-resistant containers. For schools and worksites, giving oral medications is often prohibited; check the policies.* | |
| Glucose tablets | Treats hypoglycemia (low blood sugar) |
| Acetaminophen (Tylenol) | Treats pain and fever |
| Ibuprofen (Advil) | Treats pain, fever, and inflammation |
| Aspirin (Motrin) | Treats pain, fever, and inflammation; may be used for suspected heart attack. **DO NOT** give aspirin to children. |
| Antihistamine (Benadryl) *Warning*: First aid kits at workplaces, schools, and public places should not contain products known to cause drowsiness. | Relieves allergy symptoms; treats poison ivy or oak itching and rash; reduces nausea and motion sickness; causes drowsiness and induces sleep |
| Hydrocortisone cream, 1% | Relieves itchiness and skin-related reactions, including rashes associated with insect bites and stings, poison ivy and oak, and other allergic skin rashes. It may be too weak for some conditions. |
| Aloe vera gel (100% gel) **Figure A-6** | Treats sunburn or superficial frostbite |
| Sports drink packets (eg, Gatorade, Powerade) | Treats heat stress, dehydration, and water intoxication when too much water has been consumed and sodium has been depleted from the body |
| Antacids tablets (eg, Tums and Rolaids) | Treats heartburn and acid indigestion (upset stomach) |
| Antidiarrheal tablets (eg, Pepto-Bismol and Imodium A-D) | Treats diarrhea |
| Anticonstipation/laxative tablets (eg, Metamucil) | Treats constipation |
| **Equipment** | |
| Cardiopulmonary resuscitation (CPR) breathing barrier device (with 1-way valve) | Protects against potential infection during CPR |
| Scissors (various types available) **Figure A-7** | Cuts dressings, bandages, and clothing |
| Tweezers (angled tip) | Removes splinters and ticks |
| Safety pins (2 in. [5 cm] long) **Figure A-8** | Creates sling from shirttail or sleeve, secures dressings, and drains blisters |
| Emergency blanket (eg, state highway department trash bags; household polyethylene trash bags; space blanket made of Mylar, although it may tear in wind) | Protects against body heat loss and weather (wind, rain, and snow) |
| *First Aid and CPR Guide* (first aid booklet from Jones & Bartlett Learning) | Provides quick reference during an emergency and for review of first aid procedures |

Figure A-1

Adhesive bandages.

Figure A-2

Gauze pads and nonstick pads.

Figure A-3

Gauze rolls and self-adhering roller bandages.

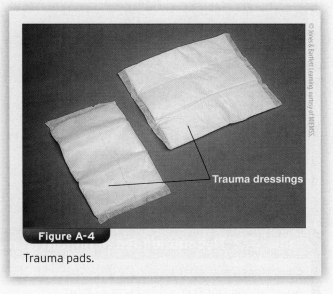

Figure A-4

Trauma pads.

## Workplace First Aid Kit Contents

In the absence of a medical facility in close proximity to a workplace, the Occupational Safety and Health Administration (OSHA) requires that the workplace have adequate supplies readily available and a person or people at the workplace who are adequately trained to render first aid to all injured employees. Neither OSHA's general industry standard 1910.151 nor its construction standard 1926.50 require specific contents be included in the workplace first aid kit.

OSHA refers to the American National Standard (ANSI) z308.1, *Minimum Requirements for Workplace First Aid Kits*, for minimum items to include in a workplace first aid kit. These items, as well as other recommended supplies, are included in Table A-2 .

Figure A-5

Elastic roller bandages.

Figure A-7

EMT shears, bandage scissors, regular scissors, and tweezers.

Figure A-6

Aloe vera gel, instant ice pack, burn dressing, and optional first aid kit items (insect repellent, sunscreen, and lip balm).

Figure A-8

Emergency blanket, cotton-tipped swabs, safety pins, and SAM splint.

## Table A-2 Recommended Minimum Items for a Workplace First Aid Kit

| Equipment | Minimum Quantity |
| --- | --- |
| Adhesive bandage (1 in. × 3 in. [3 cm × 7 cm]) | 16 |
| Adhesive tape (1 in. [3 cm] width) **Figure A-9** | 1 roll |
| Antibiotic ointment | 10 packets |
| Antiseptic towelette/swab **Figure A-10** | 10 packets |
| Aspirin (chewable; 81 mg each) | 2 packets |
| Burn dressing (gel soaked; 4 in. × 4 in. [10 cm × 10 cm]) | 1 packet |

(Continues)

## Table A-2 Recommended Minimum Items for a Workplace First Aid Kit, Continued

| | |
|---|---|
| Burn treatment | 10 packets |
| Cold pack (instant, disposable) | 1 |
| CPR breathing barrier (face mask with 1-way valve) **Figure A-11** | 1 |
| Disposable medical exam gloves (non-latex, large size) **Figure A-12** | 2 pairs |
| Elastic bandage (3 in. or 4 in. [7 cm or 10 cm] width) | 1 |
| Eye covering (0.25 in. [0.64 cm] thick) | 2 pads |
| Eye/skin wash (4-oz [118-mL] bottle) | 1 bottle |
| *First Aid and CPR Guide* (booklet from Jones & Bartlett Learning) | 1 |
| Hand sanitizer (alcohol) | 1 small bottle or 10 packets |
| Roller gauze bandage (3 in. [7 cm] width) | 2 |
| Roller gauze bandage (4 in. [10 cm] width) | 1 |
| Scissors | 1 |
| Splint (malleable, padded such as SAM Splint, 4 in. × 36 in. [10 cm × 91 cm]) | 1 |
| Sterile gauze pad (3 in. × 3 in. [7 cm × 7 cm]) | 4, individually wrapped |
| Sterile trauma pad (5 in. × 9 in. [13 cm × 23 cm]) | 2, individually wrapped |
| Tourniquet | 1 |
| Triangular bandage (40 in. × 40 in. × 56 in. [102 cm × 102 cm × 142 cm]) | 2 |

*Note:* Nonprescription medications can be put in first aid kits if packaged in single dose, tamper-evident packaging and labeled as required by FDA regulations. OTC drug products should not contain ingredients known to cause drowsiness.

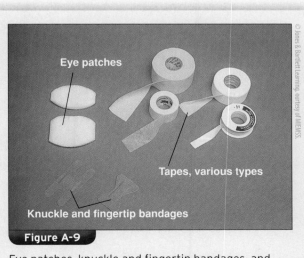

**Eye patches**

**Tapes, various types**

**Knuckle and fingertip bandages**

© Jones & Bartlett Learning, courtesy of MIEMSS.

**Figure A-9**

Eye patches, knuckle and fingertip bandages, and tape.

**Antiseptic towelettes**   **Alcohol prep pads**

© Jones & Bartlett Learning, courtesy of MIEMSS.

**Figure A-10**

Antiseptic towelettes and alcohol prep pads.

Figure A-11

Face mask.

Figure A-12

Exam gloves.

# Medication Information

As a first aid provider, you might be in a situation that requires you to give a person certain medications (or to assist a person in taking his or her own medication). A knowledgeable first aid provider should be familiar with the following medications:

- Over-the-counter pain relievers:
  - Acetaminophen
  - Aspirin
  - Ibuprofen
  - Naproxen
- Physician-prescribed medications:
  - Metered-dose inhaler
  - Nitroglycerin
  - Epinephrine
- Over-the-counter medications carried in a first aid kit or available from the person:
  - Oral glucose

## ▶ Pros and Cons of Popular Pain Relievers

### Acetaminophen

*Brand name:* Tylenol

*Advantages:* Relieves pain and fever, does not irritate stomach

*Disadvantages:* Can damage liver with heavy or prolonged use

### Aspirin

*Brand names:* Bufferin, Anacin, Bayer

*Advantages:* Relieves pain, fever, inflammation; useful for heart attacks and their prevention

*Disadvantages:* Interferes with blood clotting; might trigger stomach bleeding; can cause Reye syndrome in children with viral infections

### Ibuprofen

*Brand names:* Advil, Nuprin, Motrin

*Advantages:* Relieves pain, fever, and inflammation

*Disadvantages:* Interferes with clotting; can cause stomach bleeding, ulcers, irritation; heavy or prolonged use can damage liver and kidneys

### Naproxen

*Brand name:* Aleve

*Advantages:* Relieves pain, fever, and inflammation; one dose lasts 8 to 12 hours

*Disadvantages:* Can cause stomach bleeding, ulcers, irritation; prolonged use can harm kidneys

## ▶ Nitroglycerin

Give a person nitroglycerin (Nitrostat) if the following conditions exist:

- The person is an adult.
- The person has chest pain.
- The person has physician-prescribed sublingual tablets or spray.

**DO NOT** give a person nitroglycerin if any of the following conditions applies:

- The person has a head injury.
- The person is an infant or a child.
- The person has already taken three doses.

### Medication Forms

Tablet (about one-tenth the size of an aspirin), sublingual spray, and patch.

## Dosage

One dose.

## Procedure

Once you have decided to administer nitroglycerin, follow these steps:

1. Check the expiration date of the nitroglycerin.
2. Ask the person about the previous dose taken (time and amount taken).
3. Ask the person to lift his or her tongue. Place the tablet or spray dose under the tongue or have the person do so. Do not touch the tablet; wear gloves because your skin can absorb nitroglycerin, which could affect your blood pressure.
4. Have the person keep his or her mouth closed (if doing so will not interfere with easy breathing) with the tablet under the tongue (without swallowing) until the tablet dissolves and is absorbed.

## Actions

Nitroglycerin takes the following actions:

- Relaxes (dilates) blood vessels
- Reduces the workload of the heart

## Side Effects

Side effects of nitroglycerin include the following:

- Lower blood pressure (person should sit or lie down)
- Headache
- Heart rate changes

## ▶ Epinephrine Auto-injector

Give a person epinephrine (Adrenalin, EpiPen) if both of the following conditions exist:

- The person exhibits signs of a severe allergic reaction (including breathing distress or shock).
- The person has physician-prescribed medication.

## Medication Form

Liquid from automatic needle-and-syringe injection system

## Dosage

- Adult: One adult auto-injector (0.3 mg)
  **Figure B-1**
- Child/infant: One infant/child auto-injector (0.15 mg)

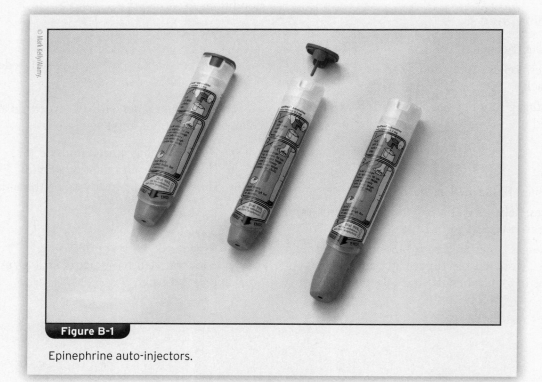

**Figure B-1**

Epinephrine auto-injectors.

## Procedure

Use these steps when administering epinephrine:

1. Obtain the person's physician-prescribed auto-injector.
2. Remove the safety cap.
3. Place the tip of the auto-injector against the person's thigh.
4. Push the injector firmly against the thigh until you hear it click to inject medication.
5. Hold the injector in place for 10 seconds.
6. When a person with anaphylaxis does not respond to the first dose and the arrival of emergency medical services will exceed 5 to 10 minutes, a second dose may be considered.
7. Call 9-1-1.

## Actions

Epinephrine takes the following actions:

- Dilates the bronchioles (small tubes in lungs)
- Constricts blood vessels

## Side Effects

Epinephrine has the following side effects:

- Increased heart rate
- Dizziness
- Headache
- Chest pain
- Nausea
- Vomiting
- Anxiety

## ▶ Metered-Dose Inhaler

Give a person a metered-dose inhaler (Albuterol, Proventil, Ventolin) if the person is experiencing asthma, or difficulty breathing with wheezing.

## Dosage

Adult/child: one to two inhalations

## Procedure

Use these steps when administering a metered-dose inhaler  **Figure B-2** :

1. Shake the inhaler several times, remove the cap, and apply the spacer, if available.
2. Holding the inhaler upright, tell the person to place his or her lips around the inhaler or spacer.
3. For greater benefit, the person can take a breath and then exhale fully. Then, while the person breathes in slowly and deeply, depress the inhaler to release the medication.
4. If using a spacer, press down on the inhaler and then have the person wait 5 seconds before breathing in.
5. Tell the person to hold his or her breath for 10 seconds and to breathe out slowly.
6. A second dose may be given in 30 to 60 seconds.

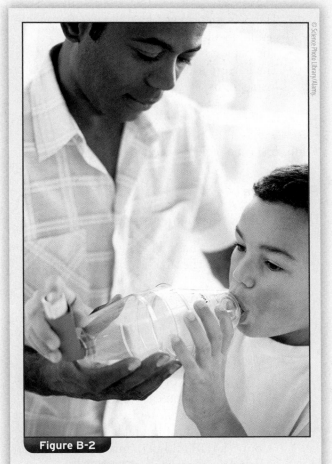

**Figure B-2**

Metered-dose inhaler.

## Actions

A metered-dose inhaler takes the following actions:

- Stimulates the nervous system
- Causes bronchodilation

## Side Effects

A metered-dose inhaler has the following side effects:

- Hypertension
- Increased heart rate
- Anxiety
- Restlessness

**Figure B-3**

Glucose tablets.

## ▶ Oral Glucose

Give a person oral glucose if all of the following conditions exist:

- The person has low blood glucose (hypoglycemia, insulin reaction).
- The person is able to swallow.
- The person is alert and able to follow instructions.

## Dosage

Adult: one tube of gel or three tablets

## Procedure

Use these steps when administering oral glucose:

1. If the person has a blood glucose monitor, allow him or her to check his or her blood glucose.
2. Use the Rule of 15 when:
   - Testing is not possible,
   - Testing shows a low blood glucose level, or
   - Profuse sweating or shaking occurs in a person with diabetes.

   The Rule of 15 works as follows:
   - Have the person eat 15 grams of sugar (ie, 3 to 5 glucose tablets, 3 to 5 teaspoons [15 mL to 25 mL] of table sugar, or 4 ounces [118 mL] of orange juice or regular soft drink [not diet]) **Figure B-3**.

- Wait 15 minutes for the sugar to get into the blood.
- Recheck the blood glucose level. If it is still low or no testing is available, give the person 15 more grams of sugar to consume.

If the person experiences a decline in responsiveness or there is no improvement in the person after 15 minutes, repeat the dose, and if the condition remains the same after another 15 minutes, call 9-1-1.

## Actions

When oral glucose is absorbed by the body, it provides glucose for cell use.

## Side Effects

Oral glucose has the following side effects:

- Nausea
- Vomiting

# Health Care Provider Basic Life Support

Examples of health care providers include physicians, dentists, nurses, paramedics, and athletic trainers. Health care providers work in a variety of settings such as emergency medical services, hospitals, medical and dental clinics, and athletic facilities. These professionals perform basic life support techniques differently than laypeople.

## ▶ One-Rescuer Adult CPR

If you find a collapsed, motionless person, make a quick check for dangerous hazards and other clues as to what happened. Refer to **Skill Sheet C-1** for the appropriate steps and techniques for one-rescuer adult cardiopulmonary resuscitation (CPR).

## ▶ Two-Rescuer Adult CPR

Lifeguards and other health care providers are often taught two-rescuer CPR procedures. Having two or more rescuers present has the following advantages:

- One rescuer can activate the emergency response system and obtain an automated external defibrillator (AED).
- It is less exhausting for the rescuers. One rescuer can give chest compressions while the other performs rescue breathing. Additionally, the rescuers can switch positions after every five sets of CPR or sooner if the rescuer giving chest compressions becomes fatigued.
- There is less interruption between the compressions and breaths.

## Skill Sheet

### C-1    One-Rescuer Adult CPR

*Note:* Whenever possible, use a mouth-to-barrier device to prevent disease transmission.

**1** **Check responsiveness.** Tap the person on the shoulder and shout, "Are you okay?"

If the person responds:

- Ask the person about chief complaints.
- Use the SAMPLE (signs and symptoms, allergies, medications, pertinent past medical history, last oral intake, events leading up to the illness or injury) history questions.
- Check the person for DOTS (deformities, open wounds, tenderness, and swelling) if an injury is suspected.

If the person does not respond, continue to Step 2.

(Continues)

# Skill Sheet Continued

## C-1    One-Rescuer Adult CPR

**2**  **Shout for help.**
- If you are alone, leave the person to activate the emergency response system and get an automated external defibrillator (AED) before starting CPR.
- If another person arrives or is nearby, have him or her activate the emergency response system and get an AED.

*Note:* You can either activate the resuscitation team at this time or after checking for breathing and pulse.

**3**  **Open the person's airway.**
- Take your hand nearest the person's head and place it on his or her forehead; apply pressure to tilt the head back.
- Place two fingers of your other hand under the bony part of the person's jaw (near the chin) and lift. Avoid pressing on soft tissues under the jaw.
- Tilt the head backward.

If you suspect a spinal neck injury, **DO NOT** move the person's head or neck. Use the jaw-thrust method to open the airway. With both hands, one on each side, place your fingers behind the angles of the jaw and lift upward. Your thumbs can be used to pull down the person's lower jaw to allow breathing through the mouth.

If you see liquid or semiliquid in the person's mouth, wear gloves and use a cloth over your fingers to wipe the liquid out of the person's mouth. If you see a solid object, wear gloves and remove the object by using a hooking motion. If you see dentures, leave them in place unless they are loose and cannot be kept in place.

**4**  **Check for breathing.**
- While keeping the airway open, place your ear near the person's mouth and listen and feel for breathing. Observe the person's chest for movement (rise and fall).
- If the person is not breathing or is only gasping, continue to Step 5.
- If the person is breathing normally, continue to monitor his or her breathing until emergency responders arrive.

**5**  **Check for pulse.** (This step can be done simultaneously with Step 4 in less than 10 sec.)
- Maintain the head tilt, with your hand nearest the person's head placed on the person's forehead.
- Locate the larynx (Adam's apple) using two or three fingers of your hand nearest the person's feet.
- Slide your fingers down into the groove of the person's neck on the side nearest you; **DO NOT** use your thumb because you may feel your own pulse.
- Feel for a carotid pulse (take 5 to 10 sec). The carotid artery is used because it lies close to the heart and is easily accessible.
- If the person has a pulse and is breathing, keep the airway open and monitor breathing.
- If the person has a pulse but is not breathing:
  - Provide rescue breaths (1 breath every 5 to 6 sec, or about 10 to 12 breaths per min).

# Skill Sheet Continued

**C-1**   **One-Rescuer Adult CPR**

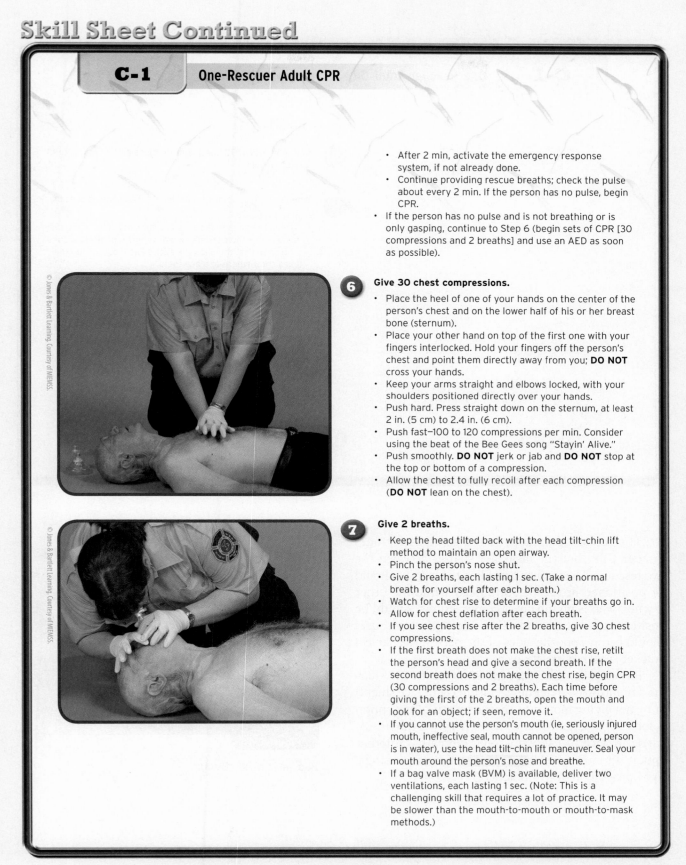

- After 2 min, activate the emergency response system, if not already done.
- Continue providing rescue breaths; check the pulse about every 2 min. If the person has no pulse, begin CPR.
- If the person has no pulse and is not breathing or is only gasping, continue to Step 6 (begin sets of CPR [30 compressions and 2 breaths] and use an AED as soon as possible).

**6**   **Give 30 chest compressions.**

- Place the heel of one of your hands on the center of the person's chest and on the lower half of his or her breast bone (sternum).
- Place your other hand on top of the first one with your fingers interlocked. Hold your fingers off the person's chest and point them directly away from you; **DO NOT** cross your hands.
- Keep your arms straight and elbows locked, with your shoulders positioned directly over your hands.
- Push hard. Press straight down on the sternum, at least 2 in. (5 cm) to 2.4 in. (6 cm).
- Push fast—100 to 120 compressions per min. Consider using the beat of the Bee Gees song "Stayin' Alive."
- Push smoothly. **DO NOT** jerk or jab and **DO NOT** stop at the top or bottom of a compression.
- Allow the chest to fully recoil after each compression (**DO NOT** lean on the chest).

**7**   **Give 2 breaths.**

- Keep the head tilted back with the head tilt–chin lift method to maintain an open airway.
- Pinch the person's nose shut.
- Give 2 breaths, each lasting 1 sec. (Take a normal breath for yourself after each breath.)
- Watch for chest rise to determine if your breaths go in.
- Allow for chest deflation after each breath.
- If you see chest rise after the 2 breaths, give 30 chest compressions.
- If the first breath does not make the chest rise, retilt the person's head and give a second breath. If the second breath does not make the chest rise, begin CPR (30 compressions and 2 breaths). Each time before giving the first of the 2 breaths, open the mouth and look for an object; if seen, remove it.
- If you cannot use the person's mouth (ie, seriously injured mouth, ineffective seal, mouth cannot be opened, person is in water), use the head tilt–chin lift maneuver. Seal your mouth around the person's nose and breathe.
- If a bag valve mask (BVM) is available, deliver two ventilations, each lasting 1 sec. (Note: This is a challenging skill that requires a lot of practice. It may be slower than the mouth-to-mouth or mouth-to-mask methods.)

*(Continues)*

## Skill Sheet Continued

### C-1    One-Rescuer Adult CPR

**8** Continue sets of 30 chest compressions and 2 breaths until an AED arrives.

**9** When an AED becomes available, use it as soon as possible.
- Turn on the AED.
- Attach the pads to the person's bare, dry chest. (You may need to dry the person's skin or remove medical patches or hair so that the pads will stick.) The diagrams on the pads show where to place them.
- Make sure no one is touching the person. Say, "Clear!"
- Allow the AED to analyze the heart rhythm (push the Analyze button, if necessary) and follow the AED's voice prompts.
- If no shock is advised, immediately resume 5 sets of 30 chest compressions and 2 breaths (2 min).
- If shock is advised, do not touch the person. Give 1 shock and immediately resume 5 sets of 30 chest compressions and 2 breaths (2 min).

The AED will prompt you to stop CPR every 2 min to reanalyze the heart rhythm.

**10** When a second rescuer arrives, provide two-person CPR and use the AED.

The sequence of steps is the same as for one-rescuer CPR, but the tasks are shared between the two rescuers. The rescuer providing the breaths should be positioned at the person's head while the other rescuer, who is giving chest compressions, should be positioned at the person's side. Ideally, the rescuers should be on opposite sides of the person to enable a quicker switch of positions.

Protect against disease transmission by not sharing a mouth-to-barrier device (ie, mask or face shield) or by not giving mouth-to-mouth breaths. One option is for each rescuer to have his or her own mouth-to-barrier device to use while giving breaths. Another option is to use a BVM **Figure C-1**; however, using a BVM properly requires practice.

**Figure C-1**

Bag valve mask (BVM).

# FEMA Disaster Supplies Checklists

### Table D-1 First Aid Supplies

| Supplies | Home | Vehicle | Work |
|---|---|---|---|
| Adhesive bandages, various sizes | | | |
| Sterile dressing (5 in. [13 cm] × 9 in. [23 cm]) | | | |
| Conforming roller gauze bandage | | | |
| Triangular bandages | | | |
| Sterile gauze pads (3 in. [8 cm] × 3 in. [8 cm]) | | | |
| Sterile gauze pads (4 in. [10 cm] × 4 in. [10 cm]) | | | |
| Roll of cohesive bandage (3 in. [8 cm]) | | | |
| Germicidal hand wipes or waterless, alcohol-based hand sanitizer | | | |
| Antiseptic wipes | | | |
| Pairs of large, medical grade, nonlatex gloves | | | |
| Tongue depressor blades | | | |
| Adhesive tape (2 in. [5 cm] wide) | | | |
| Antibacterial ointment | | | |
| Cold pack | | | |
| Scissors (small, personal) | | | |
| Tweezers | | | |
| Assorted sizes of safety pins | | | |
| Cotton balls | | | |
| Thermometer | | | |
| Tube of petroleum jelly or other lubricant | | | |
| Sunscreen | | | |
| CPR breathing barrier, such as a face shield | | | |
| First aid manual | | | |

## Table D-2  Nonprescription and Prescription Medicine Kit Supplies

| Supplies | Home | Vehicle | Work |
|---|---|---|---|
| Aspirin and non-aspirin pain reliever | | | |
| Antidiarrhea medication | | | |
| Antacid (for stomach upset) | | | |
| Laxative | | | |
| Vitamins | | | |
| Prescriptions | | | |
| Extra eyeglasses/contact lenses | | | |

## Table D-3  Sanitation and Hygiene Supplies

| Item | |
|---|---|
| Washcloth and towel | |
| Towelettes, soap, hand sanitizer | |
| Toothpaste, toothbrushes | |
| Shampoo, comb, and brush | |
| Deodorants, sunscreen | |
| Razor, shaving cream | |
| Lip balm, insect repellent | |
| Feminine supplies | |
| Heavy-duty plastic garbage bags and ties for personal sanitation uses and toilet paper | |
| Medium-sized plastic bucket with tight lid | |
| Disinfectant and household chlorine bleach | |
| A small shovel for digging a latrine | |
| Toilet paper | |
| Contact lens solution | |
| Mirror | |

## Table D-4  Equipment and Tools

| Tools | | Kitchen Items | |
|---|---|---|---|
| Portable, battery-powered radio or television and extra batteries | | Manual can opener | |
| National Oceanic and Atmospheric Administration (NOAA) Weather Radio, if appropriate for your area | | Mess kits or paper cups, plates, and plastic utensils | |
| Flashlight and extra batteries | | All-purpose knife | |
| Signal flare | | Household liquid bleach to treat drinking water | |
| Matches in a waterproof container (or waterproof matches) | | Sugar, salt, pepper | |
| Shut-off wrench, pliers, shovel, and other tools | | Aluminum foil and plastic wrap | |
| Duct tape and scissors | | Resealable plastic bags | |
| Plastic sheeting | | Small cooking stove and a can of cooking fuel (if food must be cooked) | |
| Whistle | | | |
| Small canister, ABC-type fire extinguisher | | **Comfort Items** | |
| Tube tent | | Games | |
| Compass | | Cards | |
| Work gloves | | Books | |
| Paper, pens, and pencils | | Toys for kids | |
| Needles and thread | | Food | |
| Battery-operated travel alarm clock | | | |

## Table D-5  Food and Water

| Supplies | Home | Vehicle | Work |
|---|---|---|---|
| Water | | | |
| Ready-to-eat meats, fruits, and vegetables | | | |
| Canned or boxed juices, milk, and soup | | | |
| High-energy foods such as peanut butter, jelly, low-sodium crackers, granola bars, and trail mix | | | |
| Vitamins | | | |
| Special foods for infants or persons on special diets | | | |
| Cookies, hard candy | | | |
| Instant coffee | | | |
| Cereals | | | |
| Powdered milk | | | |

## Table D-6 Clothes and Bedding Supplies

| Item | |
|------|--|
| Complete change of clothes | |
| Sturdy shoes or boots | |
| Rain gear | |
| Hat and gloves | |
| Extra socks | |
| Extra underwear | |
| Thermal underwear | |
| Sunglasses | |
| Blankets/sleeping bags and pillows | |

## Table D-7 Documents and Keys

| Item | Location Where Stored |
|------|----------------------|
| Personal identification | |
| Cash and coins | |
| Credit cards | |
| Extra set of house keys and car keys | |
| Copies of the following: | |
|   Birth certificate | |
|   Marriage certificate | |
|   Driver's license | |
|   Social Security card | |
|   Passport | |
|   Will | |
|   Deeds | |
|   Inventory of household goods | |
|   Insurance papers | |
|   Immunization records | |
|   Bank and credit card account numbers | |
|   Stocks and bonds | |
|   Emergency contact list and phone numbers | |
|   Map of the area and phone numbers of places you could go | |

# Answer Key

## ▶ Assessment in Action

### Chapter 1
1. No; 2. Yes; 3. No; 4. No

### Chapter 2
1. Yes; 2. No; 3. Yes; 4. Yes

### Chapter 3
1. No; 2. No; 3. Yes; 4. No

### Chapter 4
1. No; 2. Yes; 3. Yes; 4. Yes

### Chapter 5
1. Yes; 2. No; 3. No; 4. Yes; 5. Yes; 6. Yes

### Chapter 6
1. Yes; 2. Yes; 3. No; 4. Yes; 5. No

### Chapter 7
1. Yes; 2. Yes; 3. No; 4. No

### Chapter 8
1. Yes; 2. Yes; 3. No; 4. Yes

### Chapter 9
1. No; 2. No; 3. Yes; 4. No

### Chapter 10
1. Yes; 2. Yes; 3. Yes; 4. No; 5. Yes

### Chapter 11
1. No; 2. No; 3. Yes; 4. Yes; 5. Yes

### Chapter 12
1. No; 2. Yes; 3. Yes; 4. No

### Chapter 13
1. Yes; 2. Yes; 3. No; 4. Yes; 5. Yes

### Chapter 14
1. Yes; 2. Yes; 3. Yes; 4. No; 5. Yes

### Chapter 15
1. Yes; 2. Yes; 3. No; 4. Yes

### Chapter 16
1. Yes; 2. Yes; 3. No; 4. Yes

### Chapter 17
1. No; 2. Yes; 3. Yes; 4. Yes

### Chapter 18
1. No; 2. No; 3. Yes; 4. Yes

### Chapter 19
1. No; 2. No; 3. No; 4. Yes; 5. Yes

### Chapter 20
1. Yes; 2. Yes; 3. No; 4. Yes; 5. Yes

### Chapter 21
1. No; 2. Yes; 3. Yes; 4. No; 5. Yes; 6. Yes

### Chapter 22
1. No; 2. No; 3. No; 4. Yes; 5. Yes

### Chapter 23
1. Yes; 2. Yes; 3. Yes; 4. Yes; 5. No

### Chapter 24
1. Yes; 2. Yes; 3. No; 4. Yes

### Chapter 25
1. No; 2. No; 3. Yes; 4. Yes

### Chapter 26
1. No; 2. Yes; 3. No; 4. Yes; 5. Yes

## ▶ Check Your Knowledge

### Chapter 1
1. No; 2. Yes; 3. No; 4. No; 5. Yes; 6. No; 7. Yes; 8. Yes; 9. Yes; 10. No

## Chapter 2

1. Yes; 2. No; 3. Yes; 4. Yes; 5. Yes; 6. Yes; 7. Yes; 8. Yes; 9. Yes; 10. No

## Chapter 3

1. No; 2. No; 3. Yes; 4. Yes; 5. No; 6. Yes; 7. No; 8. Yes; 9. Yes; 10. Yes

## Chapter 4

1. Yes; 2. No; 3. Yes; 4. No; 5. Yes; 6. No; 7. Yes

## Chapter 5

1. Yes; 2. Yes; 3. Yes; 4. Yes; 5. No; 6. Yes; 7. Yes; 8. Yes; 9. No; 10. Yes

## Chapter 6

1. Yes; 2. Yes; 3. No; 4. No; 5. No; 6. Yes; 7. No; 8. Yes; 9. Yes; 10. No

## Chapter 7

1. No; 2. Yes; 3. No; 4. No; 5. Yes; 6. Yes; 7. Yes; 8. Yes; 9. Yes; 10. No

## Chapter 8

1. No; 2. No; 3. Yes; 4. No; 5. Yes; 6. No; 7. Yes; 8. Yes; 9. Yes; 10. Yes

## Chapter 9

1. Yes; 2. No; 3. Yes; 4. Yes; 5. Yes; 6. No; 7. Yes; 8. No; 9. No; 10. Yes

## Chapter 10

1. No; 2. Yes; 3. Yes; 4. No; 5. No; 6. Yes; 7. No; 8. No; 9. Yes; 10. Yes

## Chapter 11

1. No; 2. No; 3. Yes; 4. No; 5. Yes; 6. Yes; 7. Yes; 8. No; 9. Yes; 10. No

## Chapter 12

1. No; 2. No; 3. No; 4. Yes; 5. No; 6. Yes; 7. No; 8. Yes; 9. Yes; 10. Yes

## Chapter 13

1. Yes; 2. No; 3. No; 4. No; 5. Yes; 6. Yes; 7. No; 8. Yes; 9. No; 10. Yes

## Chapter 14

1. Yes; 2. Yes; 3. Yes; 4. Yes; 5. No; 6. No; 7. No; 8. Yes; 9. No; 10. Yes

## Chapter 15

1. Yes; 2. No; 3. Yes; 4. No; 5. No; 6. Yes; 7. Yes; 8. No; 9. No; 10. Yes

## Chapter 16

1. Yes; 2. No; 3. Yes; 4. Yes; 5. No; 6. Yes; 7. No; 8. No; 9. Yes; 10. Yes

## Chapter 17

1. Yes; 2. Yes; 3. Yes; 4. Yes; 5. Yes; 6. No; 7. Yes; 8. No; 9. Yes; 10. Yes

## Chapter 18

1. Yes; 2. No; 3. No; 4. No; 5. No; 6. No; 7. Yes; 8. Yes; 9. Yes; 10. Yes

## Chapter 19

1. Yes; 2. No; 3. No; 4. Yes; 5. Yes; 6. Yes; 7. Yes; 8. No; 9. No; 10. Yes

## Chapter 20

1. Yes; 2. No; 3. Yes; 4. Yes; 5. Yes; 6. No; 7. No; 8. Yes; 9. Yes; 10. No

## Chapter 21

1. Yes; 2. Yes; 3. Yes; 4. Yes; 5. Yes; 6. No; 7. Yes; 8. No; 9. Yes; 10. Yes

## Chapter 22

1. Yes; 2. No; 3. No; 4. Yes; 5. No; 6. Yes; 7. Yes; 8. No; 9. Yes; 10. Yes

## Chapter 23

1. Yes; 2. Yes; 3. No; 4. Yes; 5. No; 6. No; 7. Yes; 8. No; 9. Yes; 10. No

## Chapter 24

1. No; 2. Yes; 3. Yes; 4. No; 5. No; 6. Yes; 7. Yes; 8. No; 9. No; 10. Yes

## Chapter 25

1. No; 2. Yes; 3. Yes; 4. Yes; 5. Yes; 6. No; 7. Yes; 8. No; 9. Yes; 10. No

## Chapter 26

1. No; 2. No; 3. Yes; 4. No; 5. No; 6. Yes; 7. Yes; 8. No; 9. Yes; 10. No

# Index